SURGICAL DERMATOLOGY

ADVANCES IN CURRENT PRACTICE

EDITED BY

RANDALL K. ROENIGK, MD
CONSULTANT, DEPARTMENT OF DERMATOLOGY, MAYO
FOUNDATION, ASSOCIATE PROFESSOR OF DERMATOLOGY,
MAYO MEDICAL SCHOOL, ROCHESTER, MINNESOTA, USA

HENRY H. ROENIGK JR, MD
PROFESSOR AND PAST CHAIRMAN, DEPARTMENT OF
DERMATOLOGY, NORTHWESTERN UNIVERSITY MEDICAL
SCHOOL, CHICAGO, ILLINOIS, USA

MARTIN DUNITZ

© 1993 Martin Dunitz

First published in the United Kingdom in 1993 by Martin Dunitz Ltd, 7–9 Pratt Street, London NW1 0AE

All rights reserved. No part of this publication may be reproduced, stored in a retrieval system, or transmitted, in any form or by any means, without prior permission of the publisher.

A CIP catalogue record of this book is available from the British Library

ISBN: 1–85317–061–5

Editorial note: The International System of Units has been used throughout the text.

Material in this text reflects work done outside Mayo Foundation and therefore should not be construed as an endorsement by that institution.

Composition by Scribe Design, Gillingham, Kent
Printed and bound in Spain by Printeksa

CONTENTS

List of contributors **vii**

Preface **xv**

Acknowledgments **xvi**

I CLINICAL CONCEPTS

1. New developments in local anesthesia **3**
   Michael J. Auletta

2. Sedation for dermatologic surgery
   Paul J. Weber, Joseph C. Gretzula, Carlos Sacasa **13**

3. Antibiotic use in dermatologic surgery **31**
   Joseph R. Terracina, Richard F. Wagner Jr

4. HIV and dermatologic surgery **41**
   Gwendolyn A. Crane, Henry H. Roenigk Jr

5. Growth factors and wound healing **47**
   Vincent Falanga

6. The sun, ozone depletion and skin cancer **55**
   Quan H. Nguyen, Ronald L. Moy

7. New indications for cryosurgery in infected patients **61**
   Gloria F. Graham, Douglas Torre

II CUTANEOUS ONCOLOGY

8. Actinic keratoses (solar keratoses) **73**
   Ronald Marks

9. Advances in cryosurgery for cutaneous oncology **85**
   Gloria F. Graham, Douglas Torre

10. Characteristics of giant basal cell carcinoma **93**
    Henry W. Randle, Randall K. Roenigk

11. Basal cell carcinoma recurring following radiotherapy **101**
    Steven P. Smith, Donald J. Grande

12. Metastatic basal cell carcinoma **109**
    Jacob S. Lo, Stephen N. Snow, Frederic E. Mohs

13. Mohs micrographic surgery: European experience **125**
    António Picoto, Francisco Camacho, Neil P.J. Walker, Alejandro Camps-Fresneda

14. Immunohistochemical diagnosis of skin tumors **131**
    Ken Hashimoto, Mitsuru Setoyama, Eugene Hashimoto

15. Surgical margins for nonmelanoma skin cancers **139**
    David G. Brodland

16. The role of embryologic structural development in the spread of cutaneous carcinoma **145**
    J. Michael Wentzell, June K. Robinson

17. Treatment and prevention of basal cell carcinoma with oral isotretinoin **155**
    Gary L. Peck, John J. DiGiovanna, Kenneth H. Kraemer, Joseph A. Tangrea, Earl G. Gross

18	Interferon for skin cancer **165** Hubert T. Greenway	32	Human papillomavirus **307** Mark W. Cobb
19	The risk of developing another skin cancer **177** Michael M. Schreiber	33	The laser plume **319** Neil P.J. Walker
20	Metastasis: basic mechanisms and applications in dermatology **181** David G. Brodland	34	Superficial vascular lasers: yellow light and 532NM **323** Timothy J. Rosio
21	Dermatofibrosarcoma protuberans **191** Edmund R. Hobbs	35	Psychological disabilities of hemangioma **341** J.A. Cotterill
22	Atypical fibrous xanthoma and malignant fibrous histiocytoma **201** Marc D. Brown	36	Photodynamic therapy for skin cancer **347** Scott M. Dinehart, Stephen Flock
23	Sebaceous carcinoma of the eyelid **211** Duane C. Whitaker	37	The Q–switched ruby and Nd–YAG lasers **357** Ronald G. Wheeland
24	Management of neoplasms in the nail **219** Robert Baran, Eckart Haneke	38	Neodymium YAG laser **369** Dudley Hill, Diamondis J. Papadopoulos, Hubert T. Greenway
25	Excisional biopsy and wide excision for malignant melanoma **235** Michael Landthaler	**IV**	**RECONSTRUCTIVE SURGERY**
26	Current management of thin melanoma **241** Sandhya Yadav, Darrell S. Rigel	39	Retinoids, dermabrasion, chemical peel and keloids **375** Kevin S. Pinski, Henry H. Roenigk Jr
27	Mohs micrographic surgery for melanoma **251** Frederic E. Mohs	40	Dermabrasion for scar revision **385** Bruce E. Katz
28	Metastasis and death from thin melanoma **263** Edward T. Creagan	41	Cultured epidermal grafts **395** Youn H. Kim, David T. Woodley
		42	Advances in flaps and grafts in dermatologic surgery **403** Eckart Haneke
III	**LASERS**		
29	Low–fluence CO_2 laser irradiation **271** Jeffrey S. Dover, Mitra Mofid	**V**	**COSMETIC SURGERY**
30	The superpulsed CO_2 laser **279** Richard E. Fitzpatrick, Javier Ruiz–Esparza	43	Sclerotherapy: advances in treatment **425** Mitchel P. Goldman
31	Newer uses for the CO_2 laser **293** Pamela K. Miller, Rokea A. el–Azhary, Randall K. Roenigk	44	Soft tissue augmentation: new techniques and recent controversies **441** Jeffrey L. Melton, C. William Hanke

45 Microlipoinjection **451**
   Kevin S. Pinski, Henry H. Roenigk Jr

46 New trends in liposuction **461**
   William P. Coleman III

47 Facial chemical peel with trichloroacetic acid **469**
   Randall K. Roenigk, David G. Brodland

48 Chemical peel with phenol **479**
   Thomas H. Alt

49 Dermabrasion: rejuvenation and scar revision **509**
   Henry H. Roenigk Jr

50 Minigrafts in hair replacement **517**
   Jean Arouete

51 Newer techniques in hair replacement **527**
   Pierre Bouhanna

Index **555**

LIST OF CONTRIBUTORS

Thomas H. Alt
Medical Director
Alt Cosmetic Surgery Center
4920 Lincoln Drive
Edina
MN 55436
USA

Jean Arouete
Chief Serv. Adjt.
Rothschild Foundation
67 Boulevard Lannes
75116 Paris
France

Michael J. Auletta
Director, Dermatologic Surgery
Robert Wood Johnson Medical School
Division of Dermatology
One Penn Plaza
New Brunswick
NJ 08901
USA

Robert Baran
Chief of the Dermatology Unit
Centre Hospitalier
06407 Cannes
France

Pierre Bouhanna
174 Boulevard Malesherbes
75017 Paris
France

David G. Brodland
Senior Associate Consultant and
Assistant Professor
Department of Dermatology
Mayo Foundation and Mayo
Medical School
200 First Street SW
Rochester
MN 55905
USA

Marc D. Brown
Assistant Professor of Dermatology
Director, Mohs Surgery Unit
Department of Dermatology
University of Rochester
2180 South Clinton Avenue
Rochester
NY 14618
USA

Francisco Camacho
Departamento Dermatologia
Medico – Cirurgica y Venereologia
Faculdad de Medicina
Avda. Dr Fedriani S/N
41009 Sevilla
Spain

Alejandro Camps–Fresneda
Servicio Dermatologia Hospital General
de Cataluna
Balmes 347
Barcelona 21
Spain

LIST OF CONTRIBUTORS

Mark W. Cobb
Department of Dermatology
National Naval Medical Center
Bethesda
MD 20889–5000
USA

William P. Coleman III
Associate Clinical Professor
Department of Dermatology
Tulane University School of Medicine
New Orleans
LA 70118
USA

J.A. Cotterill
Consultant Dermatologist
The General Infirmary at Leeds
Great George Street
Leeds LS1 3EX
UK

Gwendolyn A. Crane
Crane–Carr Dermatologic Professional
Association
1200 Broad Street
Durham
NC 27705
USA

Edward Creagan
American Cancer Society Professor of
Clinical Oncology
Consultant, Department of Oncology
Mayo Foundation
200 First Street SW
Rochester
MN 55905
USA

John J. DiGiovanna
Investigator
Dermatology Branch
Building 10, Room 12N238
NCI, National Institutes of Health
Bethesda
MD 20892
USA

Scott M. Dinehart
Associate Professor
Department of Dermatology
Arkansas Cancer Research Center
4301 West Markham, Slot 580
Little Rock
AR 72205
USA

Jeffrey S. Dover
Assistant Professor of Dermatology
Harvard Medical School
Chief of Dermatology
New England Deaconess Hospital
110 Francis Street
Boston
MA 02215
USA

Rokea el–Azhary
Senior Associate Consultant and
Assistant Professor
Department of Dermatology
Mayo Foundation and Mayo
Medical School
4500 San Pablo Road
Jacksonville
FL 32224
USA

Vincent Falanga
University of Miami School of Medicine
Department of Dermatology
and Cutaneous Surgery
PO Box 016250
Miami
FL 33101
USA

Richard E. Fitzpatrick
Dermatology Associates of San Diego
County, Inc.
477 N. El Camino Real
Suite B–303
Encinitas
CA 92024
USA

LIST OF CONTRIBUTORS

Stephen Flock
*Assistant Professor
Department of Otolaryngology/Head and Neck Surgery
Co–Director, Philllips Classic Laser Research Laboratory
Arkansas Cancer Research Center
4301 West Markham, Slot 580
Little Rock
AR 72205
USA*

Mitchel P. Goldman
*Dermatology Associates of San Diego County, Inc.
850 Prospect Street, Suite 2
La Jolla
CA 92037
USA*

Gloria F. Graham
*Clinical Professor
Department of Dermatology
School of Medicine
University of North Carolina
Chapel Hill
North Carolina
USA*

Donald J. Grande
*Associate Professor and Vice Chairman
Chief, Cutaneous and Mohs Micrographic Surgery
Department of Dermatology
Tufts University School of Medicine
New England Medical Center
750 Washington Street
Boston
MA 02111
USA*

Hubert T. Greenway Jr
*Head, Mohs Surgery and Cutaneous Laser Unit
Division of Dermatology and Cutaneous Surgery
Scripps Clinic and Research Foundation
10666 North Torrey Pines Road
La Jolla
CA 92037
USA*

Joseph C. Gretzula
*1301 North Congress Avenue
Suite 350
Boynton Beach
FL 33426
USA*

Earl G. Gross
*Assistant Professor
Division of Dermatology
University of Connecticut Health Center
263 Farmington Avenue
Farmington
CT 06030
USA*

Eckart Haneke
*Direktor der Hautklinik
Ferdinand Sauerbruch Klinikum
Arrenberger Strasse 20–24
5600 Wuppertal 1
Germany*

C. William Hanke
*Professor of Dermatology, Pathology, Otolaryngology
Indiana University School of Medicine
Regenstrief 524
1050 Walnut
Indianapolis
IN 46202
USA*

LIST OF CONTRIBUTORS

Eugene Hashimoto
*Research Assistant
Department of Dermatology and
Syphilology
Wayne State University School of
Medicine
5E University Health Center
4201 St Antoine
Detroit
MI 48201
USA*

Ken Hashimoto
*Professor and Chairman
Department of Dermatology and
Syphilology
Wayne State University School of Medicine
5E University Health Center
4201 St Antoine
Detroit
MI 48201
USA*

Dudley Hill
*Senior Dermatologist
Royal Adelaide Hospital
50 Hutt Street
Adelaide 5000
Australia*

Edmund R. Hobbs
*Clinical Associate Professor of Medicine
University of Texas Health Science Center at San Antonio
5282 Medical Drive, Suite 518
San Antonio
TX 78229
USA*

Bruce E. Katz
*Assistant Clinical Professor
Department of Dermatology
College of Physicians and Surgeons
Columbia University
14 East 82nd Street
New York
NY 10028
USA*

Youn H. Kim
*Assistant Professor of Dermatology
Department of Dermatology
Stanford University School of Medicine
Edwards Building, Room R–144
Stanford
CA 94305
USA*

Kenneth H. Kraemer
*Research Scientist
Laboratory of Molecular Carcinogenesis
Building 37, Room 3D06
NCI, National Institutes of Health
Bethesda
MD 20892
USA*

Michael Landthaler
*Professor and Chairman
Department of Dermatology
University of Regensburg
Franz–Josef–Strauss–Allee 1
D–8400 Regensburg
Germany*

Jacob S. Lo
*Director, Mohs Surgery Center
Department of Dermatology
Southern California Permanente Medical Group
9985 Sierra Avenue
Fontana
CA 92335
USA*

Ronald Marks
*Professor of Dermatology
Department of Dermatology
University of Wales College of Medicine
Heath Park
Cardiff
CF4 4XN*

LIST OF CONTRIBUTORS

UK

Jeffrey L. Melton
Assistant Professor
Director of Dermatologic and Mohs
Surgery
Section of Dermatology
Loyola University of Chicago
2160 South First Avenue
Maywood
IL 60153
USA

Pamela K. Miller (Phillips)
Pariser Dermatology Specialists, Ltd
601 Medical Tower
Norfolk
VA 23507
USA

Mitra Mofid
Harvard Medical School
Cambridge
MA 02138
USA

Frederic E. Mohs
The Mohs Surgery Clinic
Department of Surgery
The University of Wisconsin Hospital and
Clinics
2880 University Avenue
Madison
WI 53705
USA

Ronald L. Moy
Co-Chief, Division of Dermatology
UCLA Medical Center
200 Medical Plaza, Suite 450
Los Angeles
CA 90024-6957
USA

Quan H. Nguyen
Division of Dermatology
UCLA Medical Center
200 Medical Plaza, Suite 450
Los Angeles
CA 90024-6957
USA

Diamondis J. Papadopoulos
Division of Dermatology and Cutaneous
Surgery
Scripps Clinic and Research Foundation
La Jolla
CA 92037
USA

Gary L. Peck
Professor of Dermatology
Department of Dermatology
University of Maryland School of
Medicine
405 W Redwood Street, 6th Floor
Baltimore
MD 21201
USA

António Picoto
Administracao Regional de Saude de
Lisboa
Centro de Dermatologia
Medico Cirurgica
rua Jose Estevao, 135
1100 Lisboa
Portugal

Kevin S. Pinski
Instructor in Dermatology
Department of Dermatology
Northwestern University Medical School
Chicago
IL 60611
USA

LIST OF CONTRIBUTORS

Henry W. Randle
Consultant and Associate Professor
Department of Dermatology
Mayo Foundation and Mayo
Medical School
4500 San Pablo Road
Jacksonville
FL 32224
USA

Darrell S. Rigel
Clinical Associate Professor
NYU School of Medicine
Ronald O Perelman Department of
Dermatology
562 First Avenue
New York
NY 10016
USA

June K. Robinson
Professor of Dermatology and Surgery
Northwestern University Medical School
Tarry Building 4–767
303 East Chicago Avenue
Chicago
IL 60611–3008
USA

Henry H. Roenigk Jr
Professor of Dermatology
Northwestern University Medical School
Chicago
IL 60611
USA

Randall K. Roenigk
Consultant and Associate Professor
Department of Dermatology
Mayo Foundation and Mayo
Medical School
200 First Street SW
Rochester
MN 55905
USA

Timothy J. Rosio
Epstein Photomedicine Institute at
Marshfield Clinic
Department of Dermatology and
Cutaneous Surgery
1000 North Oak Avenue
Marshfield
WI 54449–5777
USA

Javier Ruiz–Esparza
480 Fourth Avenue
Suite 500
Chula Vista
CA 91910
USA

Carlos Sacasa
2881 East Oakland Park Boulevard
Commonwealth Building, Suite 333
Fort Lauderdale
FL 33306
USA

Michael M. Schreiber
Senior Clinical Lecturer
Dermatology Department
University of Arizona Cancer Center
6369 E Tanque Verde Road
Suite 200
Tucson
AZ 85715
USA

M. Setoyama
Assistant Professor
Department of Dermatology
Kagoshima University
School of Medicine
Kagoshima
Japan

LIST OF CONTRIBUTORS

Steven P. Smith
Assistant Professor
Tufts University School of Medicine
Mohs Micrographic Surgeon
Department of Dermatology
New England Medical Center
750 Washington Street
Boston
MA 02111
USA

Stephen N. Snow
Mohs Surgery Clinic
Department of Surgery
University of Wisconsin Hospital and Clinics
2880 University Avenue
Madison
WI 53705
USA

Joseph A. Tangrea
Deputy Branch Chief
Cancer Prevention Studies Branch, DCPC
Executive Plaza North, Room 211
NCI, National Institutes of Health
Bethesda
MD 20892
USA

Joseph R. Terracina
Division of Dermatologic Surgery and Cutaneous Oncology
Department of Dermatology
The University of Texas Medical Branch
Galveston
TX 77555-0783
USA

Douglas Torre
Clinical Professor
Cornell University Medical College
New York
Staff, Memorial Sloan–Kettering Cancer Center
320 East 65th Street
First Floor
New York
NY 10021
USA

Richard F. Wagner Jr
Division of Dermatologic Surgery and Cutaneous Oncology
Department of Dermatology
The University of Texas Medical Branch
Galveston
TX 77555-0783
USA

Neil P.J. Walker
Senior Lecturer
The St John's Institute of Dermatology
St Thomas's Hospital
London SE1 7EH
UK

Paul J. Weber
2881 E Oakland Park Blvd
Commonwealth Building, Suite 333
Fort Lauderdale
FL 33306

J. Michael Wentzell
Head of Dermatologic Surgery
Billings Clinic
2825 Eighth Avenue North
PO Box 35100
Billings
MT 59107-5100
USA

LIST OF CONTRIBUTORS

Ronald G. Wheeland
Professor and Chairman
Department of Dermatology
University of California – Davis
1700 Alhambra Boulevard, Suite 200
Sacramento
CA 95816
USA

Duane D. Whitaker
Associate Professor
Director of Dermatologic Surgery
Department of Dermatology
University of Iowa Hospitals and Clinics
Iowa City
IA 52242
USA

David T. Woodley
Professor and Chairman
Department of Dermatology
Northwestern University
School of Medicine
303 East Chicago Avenue
Chicago
IL 60611–3008
USA

Sandhya Yadav
NYU School of Medicine
Ronald O Perelman Department of Dermatology
562 First Avenue
New York
NY 10016
USA

PREFACE

Surgical Dermatology: Advances in Current Practice is a cooperative effort between 72 authors to summarize some of the newest ideas in the practice of dermatologic surgery. This text is not intended to be all inclusive or a basic text. Readers looking for basic information may refer to other textbooks including our own (Roenigk R.K., Roenigk H.H., Jr (eds) *Dermatologic Surgery: Principles and Practice*, Marcel Dekker, New York, 1989). *Surgical Dermatology: Advances in Current Practice* presents what we feel are the most important developments in dermatologic surgery in the past few years. It is undeniable that cutaneous oncology has been and will continue to be the major focus of a dermatologist's surgical practice. Much of this book is focused on clinical concepts related to the preoperative evaluation, as well as the appropriate surgical management of specific skin tumors. A logical extension of this practice has been the growth of cutaneous reconstructive surgery performed by dermatologists. In addition, the importance of lasers in our field continues with new instruments being developed that provide the 'magic bullet' for specific cutaneous problems. Finally, there continues to be a strong demand for cosmetic dermatologic surgery, specifically sclerotherapy, soft tissue augmentation, chemical peel and hair replacement with micrografts. Dermabrasion, an older technique, has newer indications such as aging skin and scar revision.

'The best interest of the patient is the only interest to be considered ...' (Dr William J. Mayo, June 15, 1910). It is with this philosophy in mind that dermatologists have ventured into the surgical arena over the past 25 years, with the greatest increase occurring in the 1980s. We expect this trend to continue in the 1990s given the current medical economic climate, especially in the United States. The cost of hospitalization and operating room usage is skyrocketing. We can save tremendous amounts of money and provide quality care by performing procedures with local anesthesia and mild sedation in an office or outpatient setting. We feel this book reflects the 'cutting edge' of dermatologic surgery that is now becoming part of a standard surgical dermatology practice. While written predominantly by dermatologists, we feel that procedures discussed in this book are not limited to the practice of dermatology but should be of interest to otolaryngologic/head and neck surgeons, ophthalmoplastic surgeons, plastic surgeons, and some general surgeons or family practitioners. We hope that any physician who practices in the area of cutaneous medicine and surgery finds the information in *Surgical Dermatology: Advances in Current Practice* useful.

Randall K. Roenigk, MD
Henry H. Roenigk, Jr, MD

ACKNOWLEDGMENTS

We are indebted to our wives, Julie and Kathie, for their love and support. Professionally, we are thankful for our colleagues at Mayo and Northwestern, our contributing authors, our fellows and residents, and the *invaluable* assistance of our paramedical staff and secretaries. Most importantly, we would like to acknowledge our patients for whom we develop our skills and disseminate our experience.

Section I

CLINICAL CONCEPTS

1. NEW DEVELOPMENTS IN LOCAL ANESTHESIA
   Michael J. Auletta

2. SEDATION FOR DERMATOLOGIC SURGERY
   Paul J. Weber, Joseph C. Gretzula, Carlos Sacasa

3. ANTIBIOTIC USE IN DERMATOLOGIC SURGERY
   Joseph R. Terracina, Richard F. Wagner Jr

4. HIV AND DERMATOLOGIC SURGERY
   Gwendolyn A. Crane, Henry H. Roenigk Jr

5. GROWTH FACTORS AND WOUND HEALING
   Vincent Falanga

6. THE SUN, OZONE DEPLETION AND SKIN CANCER
   Quan H. Nguyen, Ronald L. Moy

7. NEW INDICATIONS FOR CRYOSURGERY IN INFECTED PATIENTS
   Gloria F. Graham, Douglas Torre

Chapter 1

NEW DEVELOPMENTS IN LOCAL ANESTHESIA

Michael J. Auletta

The safe and efficient delivery of local anesthesia is a critical part of dermatologic surgery. In the last few years, a number of important advances have been made in addressing some of the problems which have limited the use of local anesthetics in the past. One area of active investigation is the development of a more effective way to provide surface anesthesia. Until recently, topical anesthetic agents, which offered extended periods of anesthesia, were only effective on mucosal surfaces. Use of these agents on intact skin was inefficient due to their slow and erratic penetration, thus necessitating lengthy periods of application before any surface anesthesia was achieved. Over the last few years, new ways of providing anesthesia to the skin surface have been developed, which make the delivery of topical anesthesia more practical.

Another area of investigation has been to find ways of increasing the maximal dosage of lidocaine which can be safely delivered during one sitting. Up to this point, the size and complexity of procedures performed by the dermatologic surgeon were limited by the maximal volume or dosage of lidocaine (7.0 mg/kg)[1] which could be used. This became a critical issue when performing liposuction surgery and lead to the development of tumescent local anesthesia. Tumescent local anesthesia uses large volumes of very dilute anesthetic solutions and allows the surgeon to safely exceed the currently recommended limits on the dosage of lidocaine. This major advance is now being applied to other areas of cutaneous surgery. Consequently, this has expanded the list of procedures which can be performed safely under local anesthesia.

TOPICAL ANESTHETIC AGENTS

Topical anesthetic agents offer obvious theoretical advantages as compared to the infiltration of local anesthesia. These include a lack of discomfort and absence of distortion of tissue, usually with little systemic absorption of the drug. Although topical anesthesia has been relatively easy to achieve through mucosal surfaces, the timely percutaneous absorption of an anesthetic through intact skin in quantities sufficient to provide anesthesia has been difficult to achieve.

The ideal topical anesthetic agent would be one which is safe and inexpensive to use and provides anesthesia of intact skin, on any body surface, down to the level of the dermis within 15 min of application. Such an agent would have many uses in dermatologic surgery, including provision of anesthesia for shave biopsies, electrodesiccation of skin lesions, cauterization of telangiectasias, and laser surgery for superficial disorders. While no single agent to date fulfills all of these criteria, major advances have been made in reaching this goal.

Cryoanesthesia

Cryoanesthesia, or the external application of a cold material to the skin surface, is one of the oldest methods of inducing surface anesthesia. The chief benefit of using this procedure is that the anesthesia is almost immediate.[1] Cryoanesthesia may be induced by either the use of a refrigerant spray or with ice. One advantage of using ice is that it is readily available and inexpensive. Ice, applied directly to the skin surface for approximately 30 s, provides surface anesthesia adequate to allow for the painless insertion of a needle.[2] Another advantage of using ice rather than refrigerant sprays is that it is a material which is familiar to the patient and thus is less likely to induce anxiety.[2] Temporary hardening of the skin is one drawback with the use of cryoanesthesia. This is more likely to occur with refrigerant sprays due to their colder temperatures.[2]

Several other methods have recently been developed to induce cryoanesthesia. The use of an uncapped syringe containing crushed ice is one convenient way of delivering ice to the skin.[2] Another method is to apply a chilled cryogel ice pack to the skin surface.[3] The anesthesia produced by cryoanesthesia is of very short duration (2–5 s), but is sufficient to reduce the discomfort caused by the insertion of a needle.[2]

Adjuvant cryoanesthesia for liposuction surgery

Cryoanesthesia can also be a useful adjuvant towards increasing the patient's comfort during liposuction surgery. Popularized by Fournier, two methods of cryoanesthesia have been employed.[4] In the first method, large ice bags can be applied directly to the operative site. This is often used in combination with tumescent local anesthesia (see page 7). Since the ice bags are often left in place for at least 10–15 min, care must be taken to avoid injury to the skin surface. This can be best accomplished by wrapping the ice bags in a cloth prior to application.

The second, more commonly used method of adjuvant cryoanesthesia for liposuction surgery, is to refrigerate the saline used for tumescent local anesthesia prior to mixing and injecting it into the operative site. The major advantage of using adjuvant cryoanesthesia is that it tends to improve the depth of anesthesia and decreases the chances of bleeding.[4] An occasional patient may develop 'shaking chills' if large volumes of chilled solution are injected.[5]

Lidocaine

Several topical preparations of lidocaine are commercially available.[1] A preparation of 2% lidocaine jelly is very useful in providing anesthesia to mucosal surfaces within 5–10 min of application. However, use of this preparation to provide topical anesthesia on cutaneous surfaces has been limited due to its relatively slow penetration through intact skin. Application for more than 2 h is required to achieve any demonstrable surface anesthesia.[1]

Lidocaine for Mohs micrographic surgery

Although of limited benefit on intact skin, topical preparations of lidocaine can be useful in providing anesthesia to open wounds. This is particularly useful during Mohs micrographic surgery when it is occasionally necessary to maintain anesthesia for a prolonged period. The use of 2% lidocaine jelly on an open wound defect can extend the period of anesthesia of injected 1% lidocaine by at least 48%.[6] An alternative way of achieving this same goal is to saturate a gauze with the same anesthetic solution used for injection. This will provide surface anesthesia to the wound bed. In addition, bleeding will be minimized if epinephrine is also used.[1] It should be remembered that the application of a local anesthetic to an open wound is equivalent to intravenous dosing[6] — care must be taken to ensure that overdosing does not occur. Severe toxic side-effects have been reported following the excessive use of topical lidocaine jelly.[7]

30% Lidocaine in acid mantle cream

Although commercially available preparations of lidocaine for topical use are of limited benefit in providing surface anesthesia on intact skin, the use of 30% lidocaine in acid mantle cream applied under occlusion for 30 min can provide insensitivity to a needle prick on facial skin.[1,8] Equivalent anesthesia on the extremities can be achieved after 1 h under occlusion. The duration of anesthesia is approximately 1–2 h and is dependent on the length of time the cream is on the skin.[9] The use of 30% lidocaine cream has been shown to be effective in providing anesthesia to shave excise nevi and in the use of electrocautery on genital condylomas.[9] This cream has also been helpful in minimizing the discomfort experienced during pulsed dye laser surgery, especially on the face.

The preparation of 30% lidocaine in acid mantle cream is no longer manufactured, but may be compounded since the vehicle, acid mantle cream, is still available (Sandoz Pharmaceutical Corp., Hanover, NJ). The lidocaine base molecule is better absorbed through the skin and should be used for compounding instead of the hydrochloride salt. A major advantage of using this preparation is that it is relatively inexpensive.

EMLA

The Eutectic Mixture of Local Anesthetics (EMLA), is a topical anesthetic combining 2.5% prilocaine with 2.5% lidocaine in an oil-in-water base.[1,10] This eutectic mixture permits better penetration of the skin than would be possible by either agent alone. EMLA is not presently FDA approved but can be ordered from its manufacturer in Europe (Astra Pharmaceutical, Frolunda, Sweden).

EMLA has been found to be effective for a number of minor surgical procedures. On mucosal surfaces, EMLA can induce topical anesthesia within 5–10 min, which is a sufficient amount of time to permit cauterization of condylomas.[11] Anesthesia to a pin prick on intact skin occurs after a 1 h application under occlusion.[12,13] However, more substantial anesthesia of the dermis requires application of the cream for at least 1h 30 min[10,12,14] and will permit the harvesting of a split-thickness skin graft to a depth of 0.5 mm.[10]

EMLA has been noted to have a biphasic effect on cutaneous blood flow to the skin, which can affect the duration of anesthesia. Initially, EMLA may produce blanching of the treated skin, which may be followed by hyperemia if EMLA is left on the skin for an extended period of time.[11] This phenomenon is explained by the effect that differing tissue levels of lidocaine have on arterioles. With short application times of EMLA (approximately 1 h), low tissue levels of lidocaine induce vasoconstriction. As the application time of EMLA is increased (more than 2 h), higher levels of lidocaine produce vasodilation.[15] This vasodilation does seem to have an effect on shortening the duration of anesthesia,[10] since systemic absorption is increased. Thus, the depth and duration of anesthesia with EMLA is related to how long the material is left in contact with the skin — longer application times produce better anesthesia up to a point.[16] The application of EMLA to mucosal surfaces for more than 15 min or to intact skin for more than 3 h results in decreased anesthetic efficacy.[10,11]

EMLA has been reported to be useful for a number of procedures in which surface anesthesia is desirable, including the cautery of skin lesions,[11] treatment of molluscum,[17] epilation,[18] harvesting of skin grafts[10] and pulsed dye laser surgery.[19] The temporary vasoconstriction induced by EMLA does not seem to have an effect on the efficacy of pulsed dye laser treatment for port-wine stains.[19] Contact sensitivity to both prilocaine and lidocaine has been reported.[20]

Iontophoresis

Normally, the epidermis is a formidable barrier to the percutaneous absorption of charged molecules into the skin. However, it is possible to overcome this barrier, at least in part, by the use of iontophoresis. Iontophoresis is the process of using an electric current to introduce small, ionized molecules (such as lidocaine) into tissue.[21] A preparation of the ionized drug (lidocaine) is placed on the skin surface and covered with an electrode of the same charge. Using a small, battery-powered iontophoresis unit (Iomed, Salt Lake City, Utah) (Figure 1.1) a galvanic current is then applied to move the drug into the skin.

The anesthetic which is often used with this iontophoresis unit is 4% lidocaine in a salt-free solution, with or without epinephrine.[22–24] Iontophoresis is usually painless, however, some patients occasionally complain of a tingling or pulling sensation.[22] After 10–15 min of iontophoresis, the treated skin is rendered sufficiently insensitive to perform a shave biopsy,[22] cauterization of telangiectasias[23] or superficial laser surgery[24] without discomfort. The duration of anesthesia can last up to 1 h if epinephrine is also used.[23,24] The anesthesia provided by iontophoresis is inadequate for procedures requiring anesthesia down to the subcutaneous layer.[22]

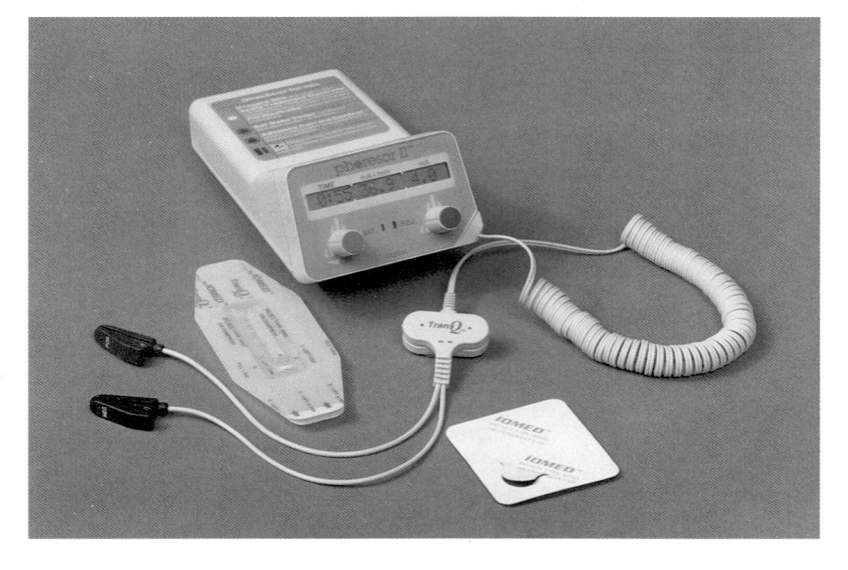

Figure 1.1
Iontophoresis unit used to deliver topical anesthesia (courtesy of Iomed Inc., Salt Lake City, UT).

Iontophoresis of local anesthetics works best on relatively thin-skinned areas, such as the face. Areas with thicker skin, such as the palms or soles, are relatively resistant to this treatment.[22] Other disadvantages of the use of iontophoresis include the relatively high cost of inducing anesthesia,[22] the limited area of anesthesia based on the size of the medication-delivery electrode[24] and a theoretical risk of electrical burns if the electrodes are not placed properly onto the skin.[22] The use of epinephrine in the anesthetic preparation may decrease the effectiveness of the pulsed dye laser in treating port-wine stains.[24]

Use of topical anesthesia

Topical anesthetic agents are particularly useful in areas which are painful to anesthetize, such as the nose, hands, feet and genitalia. They are also useful for younger patients who are poorly tolerant of needle sticks. It should be noted that although they are capable of eliminating the pain from a needle insertion, none of the discussed agents are effective in reducing the discomfort associated with the infiltration of an anesthetic[12] or providing anesthesia to the subcutaneous layer.

Each method of delivering surface anesthesia has its advantages and disadvantages. Choice of a particular method should be dictated by the specific needs of the contemplated procedure. If the situation calls for immediate surface anesthesia, such as preventing pain from a needle stick, the use of cryoanesthesia would be most effective. If surface anesthesia for an extended period of time is needed within a limit of 15 min, iontophoresis should be considered. Anesthetic creams represent a much less expensive way of achieving the same goal, but need to be applied for at least 30 min prior to the procedure.

A helpful hint when using topical anesthetic creams is to remember that drug penetration is enhanced by covering the applied cream with an occlusive dressing. A clear plastic polyurethane or polyethylene film covering is often used. Degreasing the skin prior to the application of these agents may also help penetration.

TUMESCENT LOCAL ANESTHESIA

Dermatologic surgery in the past has principally been cutaneous surgery which may be performed under local anesthesia. Previously, both the size and complexity of procedures performed by dermatologic surgeons were restricted due to limitations on the recommended dosage of lidocaine. This became a particularly important issue when dermatologists became interested in performing liposuction surgery and lead indirectly to a major advance in the delivery of local anesthesia.

When the procedure was first introduced over 15 years ago, suction-assisted lipectomy was performed under general anesthesia. However, performing liposuction under general anesthesia without the aid of a local anesthetic, termed the 'dry technique', was associated with significant incidences of morbidity and in rare cases, mortality, due in part to bleeding complications.[25] Interest on the part of dermatologic surgeons in performing this technique led to the desire to perform it more safely, using local anesthetics. Initially, a modification of the Illouz wet technique[26] was developed in which standard concentrations of lidocaine (0.5–1.0%) with epinephrine (1:100 000) were injected into the surgical site to achieve anesthesia. However, when using this technique, the upper limit of lidocaine dosage still applies,[1] thus limiting the volume of tissue that can be effectively anesthetized at one sitting. Since the anesthesia provided by the wet technique was limited, the adjuvant use of preoperative sedatives and/or analgesics was often necessary.

A major advance in providing anesthesia for liposuction surgery was achieved by Klein, who found that large volumes of very dilute (0.05–0.1%) lidocaine (Table 1.1) could be injected safely and were adequate to provide anesthesia for liposuction surgery.[27,28] Use of this dilute lidocaine solution, termed the 'tumescent technique' of anesthesia,[27] allows one to increase the dosage of lidocaine to 35–50 mg/kg[5,27,29] without developing toxic blood levels of lidocaine.[30] Large areas of skin could now be safely anesthetized using local anesthetics. Four reasons have been proposed to explain this:[1]

1. During the liposuction procedure, a small portion of the anesthetic solution is aspirated.
2. Since adipose tissue is relatively avascular, the rate of absorption into the circulation is decreased.
3. The lipophilic portion of the lidocaine molecule permits absorption into the fat. This also delays release into the circulation. Peak plasma concentrations of lidocaine occur between 10 and 15 h after injection.[5]
4. The use of a lower concentration of lidocaine reduces the concentration gradient of the anesthetic into the circulation. Since this also abates the diffusion of the anesthetic, new methods had to be developed to deliver tumescent local anesthesia.

Methods of delivery

When using lower concentrations of local anesthetics, such as with tumescent local anesthesia, it is important to evenly distribute the anesthetic solution over the surgical site. Several methods of delivery have been developed to administer tumescent local anesthesia. Since large volumes of anesthetic solution are administered (Table 1.2), the use of different types of refilling syringes connected to the intravenous bag

Table 1.1
Formula for Tumescent Local Anesthesia[a]

50 ml 1% plain lidocaine
1 ml 1:1000 epinephrine
12.5 ml sodium bicarbonate (1 mEq/ml)
1 liter 0.9% sodium chloride intravenous bag

[a]Formula produces a solution which contains 0.05% lidocaine, epinephrine 1:1 000 000, 12.5 mEq/ml sodium bicarbonate and 0.84% sodium chloride.[28] If 0.1% lidocaine mixture is desired, use an additional 50 ml of lidocaine.

Table 1.2
Regional Tumescent Local Anesthesia Requirements

Area	Approximate volumes (ml)
Chin	75–150
Knees	500–1000
Male breasts	750–1500
Flank	750–2000
Lateral thighs	1000–2000
Abdomen	1000–2000

containing the anesthetic solution (Table 1.1) has been employed. Both McGhan Medical (Santa Barbara, CA) and Byron Medical (Tucson, AZ) (Figure 1.2) manufacture spring loaded disposable re-filling syringes which facilitate the administration of the tumescent local anesthesia.

Attachment with a 25-gauge, 3-inch needle offers an easy way to inject the solution throughout the subcutaneous layer utilizing multiple injection sites.[1] The use of a needle larger than 20 gauge is usually not tolerated well without prior analgesia. Discomfort during the administration of the tumescent local anesthetic can be minimized by slowly injecting the solution. However, an occasional patient may still require preoperative sedatives and/or analgesics.[5]

An alternative approach to delivering tumescent local anesthesia is through the use of the Klein needle (Jeff Klein Surgical Inc., San Clements, CA), which is a blunt-tipped 30 cm long, 4 mm diameter, steel

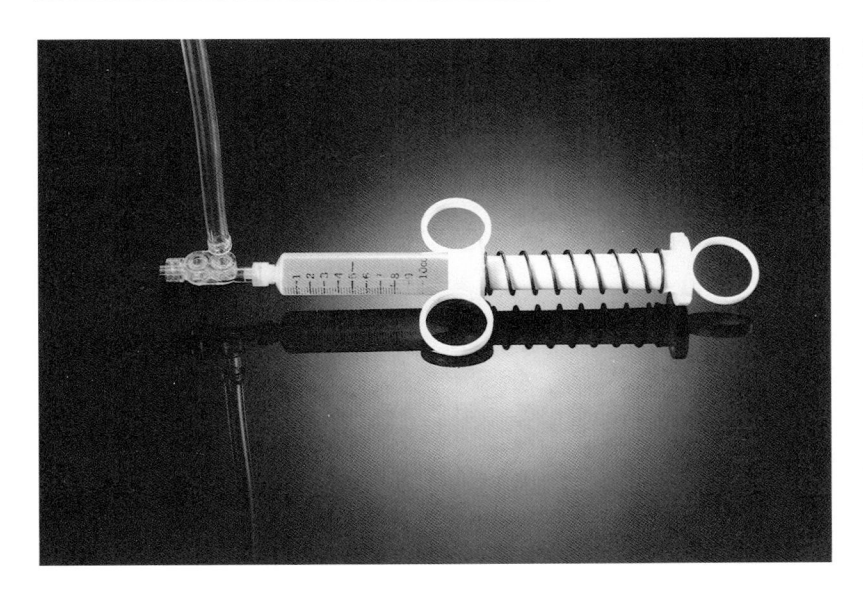

Figure 1.2
Re-filling spring-loaded syringe used to deliver tumescent local anesthesia (courtesy of Byron Medical, Tucson, AZ).

catheter which allows one to anesthetize the entire operative site through the same stab incision used for liposuction.[28,29] If preoperative intravenous analgesia is not being employed, this needle is usually used after prior injection with a small gauge needle, since the Klein needle will produce considerable discomfort in non-anesthetized skin. It is advisable in this situation to test the completeness of anesthesia prior to liposuction surgery.[28,29]

The tumescent local anesthetic is usually prepared in an intravenous bag (Table 1.1). Normally, the concentration of lidocaine is either 0.05 or 0.1%. The higher concentration is usually employed if larger cannulas (greater than 4 mm in diameter) are to be used.[28] After thorough injection of the surgical site with the tumescent local anesthetic, anesthesia is usually complete in 15–20 min.[5] The duration of anesthesia using the tumescent technique is approximately 8–10 h.[5] However, partial anesthesia lasts up to 18 h, thus minimizing the need for post-operative analgesics.[29] When using this technique, 50 ml/kg of aspirate can be safely removed with minimal blood loss, without the need for sedatives or analgesics,[5] especially if smaller (less than 4 mm in diameter) cannulas are used. The tumescent anesthetic solution makes up approximately 15–30% of the final volume of the aspirate during liposuction surgery.[31]

Advantages of tumescent local anesthesia

The advantages of using tumescent local anesthesia for liposuction include: a more cooperative patient, since the patient is alert during the procedure; minimal blood loss if epinephrine is incorporated in the tumescent mixture;[5] and more effective liposuction since the tissue has increased firmness[26,28] and depth.[29] The need for intravenous fluid replacement is obviated by fluid absorption using the subcutaneous route from the tumescent local anesthetic solution.[5,28,29] This greatly simplifies the approach to fluid management as compared to the dry technique.

Post-operative bruising and swelling are minimal, therefore, compression bandages do not need to be applied for as long a period of time as they do with the dry technique.[5,28] This results in a more rapid recovery following liposuction surgery with less discomfort when compared to treatment under general anesthesia.[28] There is also an extremely low incidence of infection using this technique as compared to the dry technique.[5]

Other uses of tumescent local anesthesia

The ability to safely anesthetize large areas of skin with tumescent local anesthesia should be helpful for a number of other uses of the suction-assisted lipectomy method, which include undermining and defatting of large skin flaps for reconstruction,[32] removal of lipomas,[33] treatment of axillary hyperhidrosis[25,34] and gynecomastia.[35] In addition, tumescent local anesthesia has also been used to provide anesthesia for hair transplantation, scalp reduction and dermabrasion.[36] There is little doubt that this new method of anesthesia will find many other uses in dermatologic surgery.

REFERENCES

1. Auletta MJ, Grekin RC, *Local anesthesia for dermatologic surgery* (Churchill Livingstone: New York 1991).
2. Holmes HS, Options for painless local anesthesia, *Postgrad Med* (1991) **89**(3):71–2.
3. Swinehart JM, The ice–saline–Xylocaine technique, *J Dermatol Surg Oncol* (1992) **18**:28–30.
4. Fournier PF, Reduction syringe liposculpturing, *Dermatol Clin* (1990) **8**(3):539–51.
5. Lillis PJ, The tumescent technique for liposuction surgery, *Dermatol Clin* (1990) **8**:439–50.
6. Robins P, Ashinoff R, Prolongation of anesthesia in Mohs micrographic surgery with 2% lidocaine jelly, *J Dermatol Surg Oncol* (1991) **17**:649–52.
7. Lie RL, Vermeer BJ, Edelbroek PM, Severe lidocaine intoxication by cutaneous absorption, *J Am Acad Dermatol* (1990) **23**(5):1026–8.
8. Lubens HM, Sanker JF, Anesthetic skin patch, *Ann Allergy* (1964) **22**:37–41.
9. Lubens HM, Ausdenmoore RW, Shafer AD et al, Anesthetic patch for painful procedures such as minor operations, *Am J Dis Child* (1974) **128**:192–4.
10. Ohlsen L, Englesson S, Evers H, An anaesthetic lidocaine/prilocaine cream (EMLA) for epicutaneous application tested for cutting split skin grafts, *Scand J Plast Reconstr Surg* (1985) **19**:201–9.
11. Ljunghall K, Lillieborg S, Local anaesthesia with a lidocaine/prilocaine cream (EMLA) for cautery of condylomata acuminata on the vulval mucosa: the effect of timing of application of the cream, *Acta Derm Venereol (Stockh)* (1989) **69**:362–5.
12. Jones SK, Handfield-Jones S, Kennedy CT, Does EMLA reduce the discomfort associated with local-anaesthetic infiltration?, *Clin Exp Dermatol* (1990) **15**:177–9.
13. Gunawardene RD, Local application of EMLA and glyceryl trinitrate ointment before venipuncture, *Anaesthesia* (1990) **45**:52–4.
14. Arendt-Nielsen L, Berring P, Laser induced pain for evaluation of local anesthesia: a comparison of topical application (EMLA) and local injection (lidocaine), *Anesth Analg* (1988) **67**:115–23.
15. Johns RA, DiFazio CA, Longnecker DE, Lidocaine constricts or dilates rat

arterioles in a dose-dependent manner, *Anesthesiology* (1985) **62**:141–4.
16. McCafferty DF, Woolfson AD, Boston V, In vivo assessment of percutaneous local anaesthetic preparations, *Br J Anaesth* (1989) **62**:17–21.
17. de Waard-van der Spek FB, Oranje AP, Lillieborg S et al, Treatment of molluscum contagiosum using a lidocaine/prilocaine cream (EMLA) for analgesia, *J Am Acad Dermatol* (1990) **23**:685–8.
18. Hjorth N, Harring M, Hahn A, Epilation of upper lip hirsutism with a eutectic mixture of lidocaine and prilocaine used as a topical anesthetic, *J Am Acad Dermatol* (1991) **25**:809–11.
19. Ashinoff R, Geronemus RC, Effect of the topical anesthetic EMLA on the efficacy of pulsed dye laser treatment of port-wine stains, *J Dermatol Surg Oncol* (1990) **16**:1008–11.
20. Curley RK, Macfarlane AW, King CM, Contact sensitivity to the amide anesthetics lidocaine, prilocaine and mepivacaine, *Arch Dermatol* (1986) **122**:924–6.
21. Sloan JB, Soltani K, Iontophoresis in dermatology: a review, *J Am Acad Dermatol* (1986) **15**:671–84.
22. Maloney JM, Local anesthesia obtained via iontophoresis as an aid to shave biopsy, *Arch Dermatol* (1992) **128**:331–2.
23. Bezzant JL, Stephen RL, Petelenz TJ et al, Painless cauterization of spider veins with the use of iontophoretic local anesthesia, *J Am Acad Dermatol* (1988) **19**:869–75.
24. Kennard CD, Whitaker DC, Iontophoresis of lidocaine for anesthesia during pulse dye laser treatment of port-wine stains, *J Dermatol Surg Oncol* (1992) **18**:287–94.
25. Coleman WP, The history of dermatologic liposuction, *Dermatol Clin* (1990) **8**(3):381–3.
26. Illouz YG, Body contouring by lipolysis: a 5-year experience with over 3,000 cases, *Plast Reconstr Surg* (1983) **72**:591–7.
27. Klein JA, The tumescent technique for liposuction surgery, *Am J Cosmet Surg* (1987) **4**:263–7.
28. Klein JA, The tumescent technique: anesthesia and modified liposuction technique, *Dermatol Clinics* (1990) **8**:425–37.
29. Klein JA, Tumescent technique for regional anesthesia permits lidocaine doses of 35 mg/kg for liposuction: peak plasma lidocaine levels are diminished and delayed 12 hours, *J Dermatol Surg Oncol* (1990) **16**:248–63.
30. Lillis PJ, Liposuction surgery under local anesthesia: limited blood loss and minimal absorption, *J Dermatol Surg Oncol* (1988) **14**:1145–8.
31. Bridenstein J, Letter to the editor, *J Dermatol Surg Oncol* (1989) **15**:775–6.
32. Field LM, Spinowitz AL, Flap elevation and mobilization by blunt liposuction cannula dissection in reconstructive surgery, *Dermatol Clin* (1990) **8**:493–9.
33. Pinski KS, Roenigk HH, Liposuction of lipomas, *Dermatol Clin* (1990) **8**:483–92.
34. Lillis PJ, Coleman WP, Liposuction for treatment of axillary hyperhidrosis, *Dermatol Clin* (1990) **8**:479–82.
35. Dolsky RL, Gynecomastia: treatment by liposuction subcutaneous mastectomy, *Dermatol Clin* (1990) **8**:469–78.
36. Coleman WP, Klein JA, Use of the tumescent technique for scalp surgery, dermabrasion and soft tissue reconstruction, *J Dermatol Surg Oncol* (1992) **18**:130–5.

Chapter 2

SEDATION FOR DERMATOLOGIC SURGERY

Paul J. Weber
Joseph C. Gretzula
Carlos Sacasa

Dermatologic surgery has recently grown tremendously in both the scope and complexity of its procedures. During surgery, the choice of sedation for adequate patient comfort is crucial. The most frequently used agents and coagents, their pharmacology, drug interactions, benefits and problems, as well as the equipment involved in sedating and monitoring dermatologic surgery patients, will be discussed.

DEFINITIONS

Before discussing dermatologic surgical sedation, some definitions are in order:

1. General anesthesia: a recent California legislative statute defines general anesthesia as 'a controlled state of depressed consciousness or unconsciousness, accompanied by partial or complete loss of protective reflexes ...'.[1] However, a simpler and equally appropriate definition is, 'a state of unconsciousness ... with absence of pain over the entire body and a ... degree of muscular relaxation'.[2]
2. Analgesia: absence of sensibility to pain; designating particularly the relief of pain without loss of consciousness.[2]
3. Conscious: capable of an appropriate response to command with protective reflexes intact, including the ability to maintain an airway.[3]
4. Sedation: the pharmacologic induction of an elevated anxiety threshold without loss of consciousness.[3]

    'Conscious' sedation is a state of sedation in which the conscious patient is rendered free of fear, apprehension and anxiety through the use of pharmacologic agents.[2]

Since sedation in the above definition implies consciousness, it appears that the term 'conscious sedation' is redundant. It is probably more appropriate to use the terms 'sedation' or 'pharmacosedation'.[3] In general, use of sedation in the field of dermatology is reserved for surgical purposes. Therefore, the term 'surgical sedation' is used in this chapter.

SURGICAL SEDATIVES

Guedel's four generally accepted stages of general anesthesia are: I, analgesia; II, delirium; III, surgical anesthesia: IV, medullary depression. Stage I ends with loss of consciousness.[4] Physicians wishing to perform surgical sedation would like their patients to remain in Guedel's stage I. Characteristic of stage I anesthesia are normal respiratory and ocular movements, as well as intact protective reflexes. Amnesia may or may not result from stage I anesthesia.[3]

Some of the objectives and benefits of surgical sedation include the following: tranquil patient mood, maintenance of patient cooperation and protective reflexes, increased pain threshold, minor deviation in vital signs, and, potentially, some degree of amnesia. Amnesia, if it occurs, takes place during the surgical induction period. Amnesia is desirable since the most anxiety-producing and painful portions of cutaneous surgical procedures may be performed during the induction process.[3]

Surgical sedation is useful if extensive local anesthesia is employed.[3] Patients may dislike extensive local anesthesia because they choose to be unaware of the operation, fear numerous injections, worry that the anesthesia will 'wear off' prematurely, or fear a 'reaction'.[5] Psychogenic reactions to local anesthesia include fainting, hostility and agitation. The latter two consequences often occur with accompanying sweating, blood pressure, heart rate and respiratory changes.[6] It is possible that psychogenic reactions to local anesthesia may be allayed by using surgical sedation and good preoperative indoctrination.

Surgical sedation allows the intraoperative continuance of verbal rapport between patient and physician. Such verbal rapport contributes to the success of the sedation. In addition, good verbal rapport reduces the overall dosage of both narcotics and sedative drugs necessary during surgical procedures.[7] For verbal rapport to be effective it must be established well in advance of the surgery and continued throughout the procedure. During the procedure it may be best that communication occurs unilaterally, from doctor to patient, since excessive patient talking during surgical sedation may increase the blood pressure by 10%.[7]

Many authorities prefer the intravenous route of sedative administration to the intramuscular route since it is more difficult to anticipate the clinical results of the latter. Many intravenous sedatives discussed here are rapid-acting. Their onset of action is primarily limited by the arm to brain circulation time, about 26 s. Intramuscular administration of most sedative drugs requires approximately 15 min before onset of clinical action, and 30 min to peak effect. This delay causes difficulty in titration that may result in overdosage or underdosage, necessitating additional injections of either antagonistic drugs or additional sedative agents. In addition, drugs given by the intramuscular route may result in a prolonged duration of clinical action eventuating in a recovery time that may exceed 4 h. The intravenous recovery period may be shorter.[3]

Relative contraindications to intravenous sedation include: age (older than 65 or less than 6); significant hepatic disease; pregnancy; hyperthyroidism; hypothyroidism; adrenal insufficiency; monoamine oxidase (MAO) inhibitor or tricyclic antidepressant use; extreme obesity; psychiatric disorders; lack of easily accessible veins; or a history of adverse reactions to the intravenous sedatives proposed for use.[3]

Traditionally, the primary drugs used for surgical sedation fall into the following categories: sedative-hypnotics; narcotics; and inhalation anesthetics. Some agents may be effectively used singly or combinations of agents may be used over time. Combinations of minute doses of several drugs may be safer, and less depressing to the cardiovascular and respiratory systems, than a single large dose of an individual drug. Myriads of drug combinations are possible. Favorite intravenous 'cocktail' mixtures have been described.[7] The benefits or problems arising with surgical sedation are not totally the result of drug pharmacology but are closely related to the skill of the administering personnel.

Sedative hypnotics

The classification of sedative-hypnotic agents includes the benzodiazepines, barbiturates and ethanol. These pharmacologic agents are often used orally to produce drowsiness or to promote sleep.[4]

Sedation, semiconsciousness and unconsciousness (general anesthesia) are part of a central nervous system (CNS) depression spectrum. Most hypnotic drugs, in high doses, are capable of inducing all three parts of this CNS depression spectrum. Fortunately the benzodiazepines are incapable of inducing general anesthesia. True general anesthesia does not occur with benzodiazepines because awareness usually persists and relaxation is insufficient for surgery. To render true surgical anesthesia, benzodiazepines must be given concomitantly with other CNS depressants.[4]

The barbiturate class of sedative hypnotics will not be discussed at length since the barbiturates, as a group, produce more profound behavioral, cardiovascular and psychological effects than the benzodiazepines and since most barbiturates possess steep dose–response curves, making them relatively unsafe. Furthermore, barbiturates do not affect the pain threshold without altering the level of consciousness. Barbiturates may even render patients hypersensitive to stimulation. Adverse responses to pain may also occur, especially when barbiturates are used as the sole agent. Outside of opioids the barbiturates are the most likely drug group to produce respiratory depression.[3] Therefore, the discussion will be limited to the benzodiazepine class of sedative hypnotics used in surgical sedation. Special emphasis will be placed on the agents diazepam, midazolam and flumazenil, the first benzodiazepine antagonist, recently introduced in the USA.

Benzodiazepines

Benzodiazepines, unlike the barbiturates, are not general neuronal depressants. Their most prominent effects are on the CNS and include sedation, hypersuggestibility, decreased anxiety, muscle relaxation and anticonvulsant activity. The currently accepted mechanism of CNS action for benzodiazepines is potentiation of gamma-aminobutyric acid neuronal inhibition.[4]

Benzodiazepines are popular because their amnesia effect creates a feeling of general anesthesia for the patient.[4] Benzodiazepines appear to attenuate the emotional response to pain more than the actual pain sensation.[3]

Other noteworthy benzodiazepine effects include coronary vasodilatation and neuromuscular blockade. The cardiovascular effects of benzodiazepines are minor except in severe intoxication. Given alone, the benzodiazepines are only moderately depressive of the circulatory and respiratory systems. Diazepam may, in preanesthetic doses, decrease the hypoxic, not the hypercapnic, respiratory drive, resulting in acidosis. Also, benzodiazepines decrease blood pressure and increase heart rate.[4]

Side-effects of benzodiazepines include light-headedness, lassitude, increased reaction time, motor incoordination, ataxia, mental and psychomotor function impairment, disorganized thought, dysarthria, amnesia, dry mouth, and, paradoxically, hallucinations, euphoria, restlessness and hypomanic behavior. Serious complications of benzodiazepine use include coma, but coma is uncommon in the absence of another CNS depressant.[4] The benzodiazepines and the sedative antihistaminics have been reported to cause an increased pharmacologic effect of coumarin anticoagulants and may theoretically cause bleeding in these patients.[6] Serious interaction may occur between benzodiazepines and ethanol.[4] Contraindications to benzodiazepines include narrow- and open-angle glaucoma.[3] Otherwise, benzodiazepines are relatively safe.[4]

When intravenous sedation with multiple agents is conducted, the sedative-hypnotic agent should be administered prior to a narcotic agent since the sedative hypnotic is the primary sedating agent.[3]

Diazepam Diazepam, the prototypical benzodiazepine, has a long history of use in surgical sedation. Diazepam is also an excellent muscle relaxant and is even successful in the treatment of tetanus.[4] Diazepam exerts this effect via central nervous postsynaptic inhibition. Conversely, monosynaptic reflexes are relatively unaffected. Diazepam has been popular in multiple-drug sedating regimens and intravenous 'cocktails'. Caution must be exercised, however, in mixing diazepam in the same syringe with other agents since it is lipid soluble. As with the other sedative hypnotics, when diazepam is administered with an opioid, the dose of the opioid should be reduced by at least one-third.[3]

The maximal amnesiac effect of diazepam occurs 10 min after intravenous administration. Therefore, the more painful portions of the surgery, for example local anesthesia, should be planned to occur during the amnesiac phase. These amnesiac properties may be enhanced by concomitant scopolamine administration. Unfortunately, diazepam has occasionally been associated with an additional episode of amnesia, 24 h postoperatively, in patients who received over 30 mg during surgical sedation.[3]

The usual sedating dose of intravenous diazepam is between 5 and 15 mg. Although diazepam's plasma half-life is 30 h, its effective intravenous surgical sedation life is 45 min. Peak intravenous effects usually occur between 2 and 15 min postinjection. Also, intravenous diazepam may be redistributed into the gall bladder and intestines, as well as the fat. After surgery, when the patient is able to eat, this redistribution may cause a rebound or second peak diazepam effect 1 h postprandially.[3]

The effects of diazepam may last three times longer than normal because of the metabolites nordiazepam and oxazepam.[4] These metabolites are excreted renally. Therefore, caution is advised in patients with renal failure.[3] Caution is also recommended in diazepam administration to the elderly and those with hepatic dysfunction.[8] In the elderly, the half-life of diazepam may be extended by four times compared to that of the young adult; hepatic disease may have the same effect.[4] It is also felt that a decreased protein binding of diazepam in the elderly provides increased amounts of free unbound drug to the CNS.[3] Intravenous aminophylline (1–2 mg/kg) may be used to reverse CNS depression from diazepam. Benzodiazepine metabolism may be inhibited by disulfiram, cimetidine, isoniazid and oral contraceptives. Heavy cigarette smoking may decrease the effectiveness of the benzodiazepine, so smokers may require greater diazepam doses for sedation.[4] Smokers may also be at greater risk for emphysema, chronic obstructive pulmonary disease, and other respiratory disorders which may lead to increased respiratory problems with diazepam.

The most frequently reported adverse reaction for intravenous diazepam is thrombophlebitis primarily due to the 40% propylene glycol vehicle. The 40% propylene glycol is also probably responsible for the burning sensation on intravenous injection. Slowing the rate of delivery reduces these phenomena.[3] Other possible adverse reactions include hives, laryngospasm, hiccups, headaches, dysarthria, ataxia, spasticity, bradycardia, hypotension, cardiovascular collapse, incontinence, urinary retention, as well as oversedation, dry mouth, recurrent amnesia and the paradoxical reactions of excitement, anxiety, hallucinations, muscle spasticity and rage.[3]

The paradoxical reactions are manifestations of emergence delirium. Emergence delirium usually takes place during recovery from diazepam or scopolamine sedation. In this situation the patient may speak unintelligibly and become hyperactive. Physostigmine is the best antidote for emergence delirium in the surgical-sedation setting.[3]

Midazolam Midazolam is a short-acting benzodiazepine. It is solubilized in an acidic buffered aqueous solution. Therefore, irritating vehicles and solvents like propylene glycol are unnecessary. Some studies concur that intravenous midazolam causes less burning and thrombophlebitis than diazepam;[3] yet other studies indicate the opposite relationship or no difference.[9,10]

Midazolam is clinically three to four times as potent per milligram as diazepam, yet the clinical effects of midazolam do not directly correlate with blood levels. In surgical sedation, it may be used alone intravenously before short procedures or in combination with a narcotic or nitrous oxide in longer procedures. Midazolam may also be used intramuscularly for preoperative sedation and anterograde amnesia. When given intramuscularly, midazolam yields anterograde amnesia in 70% of recipients. Intramuscular midazolam doses of 0.07–0.08 mg/kg (5 mg in the average adult) do not depress the carbon dioxide ventilatory response.[11]

Midazolam's alleged advantages over diazepam include a more rapid onset of sedation, less pain during injection, more profound enterograde amnesia, fewer postoperative complications and more rapid recovery.[12,13] However, during dental sedation studies using intravenous midazolam, respiratory side-effects such as hiccups, brief apnea following induction, and airway obstruction during maintenance were markedly greater for midazolam than diazepam.[14] Other reports have revealed that diazepam and midazolam induce relatively equivalent respiratory depression.[15] Midazolam's short duration of action after a single dose is due to its lipid solubility and rapid distribution from the central to the peripheral compartments as well as hepatic clearance.[16] The usual intramuscular premedicating doses do not depress respiration reflexes, while the higher induction doses do. Recent reports of apnea, respiratory depression, cardiac arrest, hypoxic encephalopathy and death have prompted the maker (Roche) to send warning literature to physicians in November 1987. This warning literature stressed the need for resuscitative equipment, drugs and trained personnel when using midazolam as an intravenous sedative as is necessary in all surgical sedation. The report emphasized that the intramuscular route of administration of midazolam may possibly provide clinical efficacy while controlling the more serious side-effects.[11]

The suggested initial intravenous dose of midazolam should be between 1 and 2.5 mg. Most importantly, midazolam should not be administered as a bolus.[9] A total dose between 2.5 and 7.5 mg is usually sufficient for sedation. A rate of administration of 2.5 mg/min is considered safe.

Sedation after intravenous injection occurs in 3–5 min. Clinical recovery from either midazolam or diazepam usually appears to be complete within 1 h following administration.[3] Intramuscular sedative effects begin 15 min and peak 30–60 min after intramuscular injection.

The most frequent complaint following midazolam administration is dizziness.[15] Other adverse reactions include hives, laryngospasm, nausea, vomiting, arrythmias, retrograde amnesia, emergence delirium, tonic–clonic movements, muscle tremor, paresthesias, visual disturbances, pinpoint pupils and vertigo.[11] Midazolam in large doses decreases cerebral bloodflow and intracranial pressure.[17]

The elderly population is more susceptible to midazolam overdosage and therefore extreme caution is required in this age group.[13] Because the midazolam is significantly impaired by alcoholic cirrhosis, caution is advised when administering midazolam to patients with this condition.[19] Care should also be exercised in the face of chronic obstructive pulmonary disease[11] because these patients are especially sensitive to the respiratory depressive effects of midazolam.

Flumazenil Flumazenil is the first and only benzodiazepine antagonist which can restore patients to consciousness in less than 1 min, maintaining analgesia and removing sedation. Flumazenil is an imidazobenzodiazepine derivative. It antagonizes the action of benzodiazepines on the CNS, inhibiting their action on the gamma-aminobutyric acid receptors. Resedation can occur and, therefore, patients should be monitored closely.[20] A dose of just 0.2 mg repeated once or twice will usually preserve analgesia and remove sedation.

The use of flumazenil can produce seizures, most frequently seen in benzodiazepine-dependent patients or those on tricyclic antidepressants. Flumazenil should not be administered to patients who take benzodiazepines to control seizure disorders. Other adverse reactions include nausea, vomiting, anxiety and confusion as the patient awakens. There are also reports of sweating, blurred vision, pain at the injection site and headache.[20]

Opioid agents

The term opioid designates the group of drugs with properties somewhat similar to those of opium or morphine.[4] The opioids interact with the mu, kappa, delta or sigma receptors of the endorphins, enkephalins and dynorphins, which are the endogenous opioid peptides.[21] The term narcotic, derived from the Greek word for sleep, was originally used synonymously with opioids, but because it is now applied to other medications as well, its original meaning has been lost and it is now obsolete.[4] Therefore, the term opioid is preferred.

Presently, there is no perfect opioid classification. Goodman and Gilman divide opioids into three groups: morphine-like opioid agonists; opioid antagonists; and mixed-action opioids.[4] Naloxone, an opioid antagonist, will be discussed briefly later because it should be readily available whenever opioids are used.

New compounds with differing properties appear with every modification of morphine or thebaine molecules. None, however, has been clinically proven to be superior to morphine in pain relief.[4] Morphine remains the standard of pain relief to which other opioid compounds are compared. Today, morphine is rarely used for outpatient surgical sedation because of its relatively prolonged duration of action.[3] A brief discussion of morphine and morphine-like opioids will aid in the understanding of opioid properties in general. Following this discussion, three phenylpiperidine-based opioids, which are among the most popular in surgical sedation, will be discussed.

Morphine-like drugs

Morphine-like drugs produce analgesia, drowsiness, mood alterations, and mental clouding. More specifically, these effects may include euphoria, apathy, mentation difficulties, lethargy and decreased visual acuity. Patients also claim a comfortable feeling, heaviness in the extremities, bodily warmth, facial itching (especially nasal) and dry mouth.[4]

Opioids have varying analgesic effects, depending on the type of pain being treated. At low doses, continuous dull pain is better relieved than sharp intermittent pain. Most notably, opioid-induced analgesia occurs without loss of consciousness.

Also, opioid-induced analgesia may be relatively selective in that sensory modalities, excluding pain, are not obtunded. During opioid analgesia, patients commonly claim that the pain may be present but not uncomfortable. Although the ability to perceive pain may be unaltered, the pain threshold is raised because the patient's affective responses to pain are mitigated. For example, anxiety, fear and panic tend to enhance one's expectations of pain.[4] Lessening these expectations lessens the pain.

The respiratory, cardiovascular and gastrointestinal systems are among those affected by opioids. Morphine-like opioids directly affect the brain stem to produce respiratory depression. In fact, respiratory arrest is the cause of almost all morphine-induced deaths. Maximal respiratory depression caused by intravenous morphine usually occurs within 7 min. The 7 min may be extended to 30 or 90 min, respectively, when using the intramuscular and subcutaneous routes.[4]

Morphine-like opioids may also stimulate the medullary chemoreceptor trigger zone in the brain stem, causing nausea and vomiting. Other gastrointestinal effects include decreased gastric acid and biliary and pancreatic secretions, and decreased intestinal propulsive contractions.[4]

The cardiovascular effects of therapeutic doses of morphine-like opioids in the supine patient are almost always minimal.[4] Nonetheless, significant hypotension, hypertension and arrythmias have been associated with almost all opioids.[21] Morphine produces peripheral arteriolar and venous dilatation that may aggravate hypovolemic shock. Concomitantly administered phenothiazines may increase this risk of hypovolemic shock. The vasodilatation is, in part, mediated by opioid-induced histamine release. This vasodilatation is effectively reversed by naloxone and much less effectively by (H1) antihistamines. The warm, flushed feeling in the face, neck and upper thorax felt by patients receiving therapeutic doses of morphine is in part secondary to this vasodilatation.[4] Opioid-induced pruritus may also be due to vasodilatation from histamine release.

Opioids can increase muscle tone, causing severe rigidity, especially of the thoracic and abdominal muscles. Fortunately, this opioid-induced rigidity usually occurs in unconscious patients during general anesthesia; however, it is occasionally encountered in conscious patients. Concomitant use of nitrous oxide gas and opioids increases the occurrence of this phenomenon.[21]

Opioid dosage adjustments are necessary in the elderly since blood levels of medication are higher due to decreased blood volume.[22] Because of their respiratory depressive capabilities, morphine and related opioids must be used cautiously in patients with decreased respiratory capability. Emphysema, chronic obstructive pulmonary disease, kyphoscoliosis and severe obesity must be considered in this regard.[4]

Rapid intravenous injection of opioids should be avoided since it increases the incidence of adverse reactions such as severe respiratory depression, apnea, hypotension, peripheral circulatory collapse, thoracic muscle rigidity and cardiac arrest.[11]

Meperidine

Meperidine is a synthetic piperidine derivative exhibiting analgesic and spasmolytic properties.[7] It was originally synthesized in the 1930s as an anticholinergic, and its vagolytic actions may cause a dry mouth.[3] Low-dose meperidine provides pain relief without sleepiness. Larger doses are sedating and may potentiate the hypnotic effects of surgical hypnotics.[7] Meperidine is also popular in surgical sedation combination therapy because it provides additional analgesia and some euphoria.[3] Unfortunately, meperidine has its disadvantages.

One of meperidine's biggest drawbacks in surgical sedation use is its greater frequency of nausea and vomiting compared with fentanyl.[7] The nausea and vomiting are due to sensitivity of the labyrinthine apparatus to meperidine. Another problem with meperidine is that toxic doses may cause CNS excitation manifested by tremors and seizures.[4] As with other opioids, meperidine may release histamine. Meperidine is notable for its occasional striking localized histamine release, causing 'tracking' weals in the skin over the injected vein. This phenomenon may also be manifested by diffuse or blotchy erythema and is usually self-limited and short-lived, lasting only 5 min.[3] At equivalent doses, meperidine produces respiratory depression similar to that produced by morphine, a depression that may last as long as 4 h.[4] Other effects of meperidine include an increased pulse rate, decreased respiration, increased cerebrospinal fluid pressure and syncopal reactions. Meperidine has been reported to have a disadvantageous hypotensive effect.[7] Intravenous meperidine frequently produces an increased heart rate that may be alarming, but this is uncommon with intramuscular administration.[4] Meperidine should not be used in patients with myocardial disease, patients taking digitalis, or those with atrial arrythmias.[7]

Meperidine is principally metabolized in the liver to normeperidine, meperidinic acid and normeperidinic acid. Normeperidine may induce seizures.[21]

Total doses between 38 and 50 mg of meperidine are sufficient for sedation. Intravenous meperidine should not be administered in concentrations exceeding 10 mg/ml or a total dose exceeding 50 mg.[3] Unfortunately, intramuscular administration of meperidine will result in erratic absorption.[4] Although meperidine itself is excreted by the kidney, metabolite elimination is via renal and hepatic mechanisms.[21] Therefore, overdosage may occur with either renal or hepatic disease.[22] Oral contraceptives have been shown to impair meperidine metabolism.[6]

Meperidine given with MOA inhibitors can result in adverse interactions, including: delirium, hyperpyrexia, convulsions or severe respiratory depression. Meperidine, given with chlorpromazine and tricyclic antidepressants, results in respiratory depression.[3,4] Unpredictable fatal reactions have occurred following administration of meperidine to patients who have received MOA inhibitors within 14 days.[11] It is of interest that amphetamines enhance meperidine's analgesic effects.

The most frequently observed adverse reactions to meperidine include dizziness, nausea, vomiting and sweating. Other adverse effects are headaches, hallucinations, visual disturbances, arrythmias, urinary retention, localized injection phlebitis, constipation and biliary spasm.[11]

In summary, caution should be exercised in the administration of meperidine to pregnant women and to patients with asthma and other respiratory conditions, supraventricular tachycardias, seizure tendencies, impaired hepatic or renal function, hypothyroidism and urinary retention.[11]

Fentanyl

Fentanyl is a synthetic piperidine-based opioid. It is a frequently used opioid because of its short (30–60 min, i.v.) duration of action and infrequent production of nausea and vomiting. A 0.1-mg dose (i.v. or i.m.) of fentanyl is equivalent to 10 mg morphine or 75 mg meperidine.[7] Fentanyl accumulates in the skeletal muscle and fat and is slowly released into the blood.[11] Fentanyl, however, has an extremely rapid onset of action if given intravenously because of its lipid solubility, and therefore has faster CNS penetration than morphine. Fentanyl differs from other opioids in that complete anesthesia can be produced without altering cardiovascular function.

Whereas morphine and other morphine-like opioids should not be used in patients with very compromised cardiac function, fentanyl is well suited. In fact, during anesthetic induction studies with fentanyl, blood pressure, cardiac rate, cardiac output and pulmonary vascular parameters remained unaltered.[21] Fentanyl produces less vasodilatation and histamine release than morphine.[23] Rarely, fentanyl has been reported to produce bradycardia-induced hypotension that is responsive to atropine.[21,24]

Fentanyl may cause significant respiratory depression.[25] Large doses of fentanyl may even produce apnea. Although the action of intravenous fentanyl is almost immediate, the maximal respiratory effects may take several minutes.[11] Reduction in respiratory rate rarely occurs over 30 min after administration. However, the respiratory depressant effects of fentanyl may outlast the analgesic effects.[3] Fentanyl may also cause rigidity of the muscles of respiration. This rigidity may require treatment with neuromuscular blocking agents.[11] Although any opioid may cause chest rigidity, fentanyl usually causes this problem, especially when it is given in combination with nitrous oxide.[3] The combination of fentanyl and nitrous oxide therapy has recently become popular. However, the combination of nitrous oxide and most narcotics produces cardiovascular depression.[21] Unfortunately, the combination of diazepam and fentanyl has also been reported to produce similar cardiovascular effects.[26,27]

Fentanyl dosing should be tailored to each patient. A total dose of up to 2 µg/kg is considered low, suitable for minor surgical analgesia. 'Moderate'-dose fentanyl (2–20 µg/kg), in addition to increased analgesia and patient relaxation, could necessitate artificial ventilation because of respiratory depression.[11]

The usual sedating total dose of fentanyl is between 0.05 and 0.06 mg.[3] However, it has been reported that a history of smoking plus alcohol and caffeine use may increase fentanyl requirements for general anesthesia.[21]

Fentanyl primarily undergoes hepatic metabolism (90%), so dosage adjustments are appropriate for hepatic disease.[21] Care is also advised in giving fentanyl to renally compromised patients. Caution should be exercised, as well, in the face of cardiac bradyarrhythmias, impaired respiration, pregnancy and patients using CNS depressant drugs (for example barbiturates, narcotics and general anesthetics).[11]

Additional adverse reactions to fentanyl include euphoria, bradycardia, laryngospasm, bronchoconstriction, hypotension and visual disturbances.[11]

Sufentanyl

Sufentanyl is another synthetic piperidine-based opioid whose analgesic effect is 5 to 10 times more potent than that of fentanyl. Its high lipid solubility and lower elimination half-time allow a very rapid penetration into the blood–brain barrier. Side-effects are similar to those of fentanyl.[28]

Small doses of 10–20 µg are more than enough to maintain sedation and a pain-free state. Monitoring of the respiratory rate is imperative. Lower dosing is recommended in elderly and debilitated patients.[29]

Naloxone

Naloxone is an opioid antagonist and a synthetic congener of oxymorphone.[7] Naloxone is the only pure opioid antagonist available in the USA.[3] It does not produce respiratory depression, psychomimetic effects or pupillary constriction. Naloxone is primarily used to reverse postoperative respiratory depression.[21] It should only be employed for clinically significant respiratory or cardiovascular depression.[11] Naloxone should not be used for patients who appear sluggish after surgical sedation in which opioids have been used because naloxone also reverses the opioid's analgesic effects.[3,7] Naloxone may also be used to reverse postoperative rigidity and to resuscitate patients in opioid-induced shock.[21]

Naloxone has significant cardiovascular effects, including hypertension, pulmonary edema, cardiac arrythmias and arrests.[21] Adverse effects of naloxone include nausea, vomiting, sweating, tachycardia, increased blood pressure and tremulousness.[3]

Naloxone's main use should be to reverse opioid toxicity or severe side-effects. The classic triad of coma, pinpoint pupils and decreased respiration strongly suggests opioid overdosage. Tonic–clonic seizures may be seen when meperidine is the opioid. These seizures are also ameliorated by naloxone. Pulmonary edema may also occur. The treatment of opioid poisoning primarily involves the establishment of an open airway, ventilation and repetitive small doses of naloxone, 0.4 mg, every 2–3 min. The diagnosis of opioid poisoning is in question if naloxone, 4–10 mg, has been given without effect.[4] Even if naloxone reverses the opioid-induced respiratory depression, the respiratory effect may return in 30 min, depending on the opioid half-life. Therefore, no patient should be discharged within an hour of naloxone administration.[3]

INHALATION SEDATIVES

The following two sedatives enter the patient via the gaseous phase. They may have a wider safety margin than the previously described sedative hypnotics and opioid agents.

Methoxyflurane

Methoxyflurane (MOF) is an inhalational anesthetic and analgesic. It is a volatile liquid at room temperature with a boiling point of 105°C and is nonflammable within its recommended concentrations for use. Methoxyflurane is one of the most soluble inhalation anesthetics, possessing a blood–gas coefficient of 13.0 as opposed to 2.4 for halothane or 0.5 for nitrous oxide.[3] Methoxyflurane is readily metabolized in the human body, only 20% of inhaled MOF being recovered in the exhaled air. Urinary exretion of organic fluorine, fluoride and oxalic acid accounts for 30% of the inhaled MOF uptake.[11]

Methoxyflurane has been reported to be useful in dermatologic surgery when given by hand-held inhaler.[30] Obstetricians have used it successfully in combination with nitrous oxide–oxygen sedation during delivery.[11] Dentists also report good experiences with MOF for surgical sedation.[31] Methoxyflurane has fallen out of favor with anesthesiologists because of its significant nephrotoxicity. The apparently dose-related renal manifestations range from reversible alterations to occasional failure.[11] The suspected, but unproven, nephrotoxic mechanism is fluoride ion release.[31-34] In addition, MOF may cause a mild metabolic acidosis. According to the manufacturer, no reported clinical or subclinical nephrotoxicity has been associated with a 15-ml volume of MOF in the hand-held inhaler (personal communication from Abbott Laboratories, Chicago, IL).

Methoxyflurane is, indeed, best suited in dermatologic surgery when delivered by hand-held inhaler.[30] The authors have achieved good results with 3–5-ml volumes of MOF placed within the device. Similar conservative dental usage has also been described.[31] The maximum recommended volume of MOF to be given in the inhaler is 15 ml. Because it may be difficult to control the level of MOF intake over short periods of time with this volume and device, it is recommended that MOF not be used as a light anesthetic for more than 4 h.[11]

Patients with renal disease or altered renal function should not receive MOF. Fatal renal toxicity has resulted from the concomitant use of MOF and tetracycline. This occurrence has prompted the manufacturer to recommend against MOF usage in patients on any nephrotoxic drug. It may be prudent as well to avoid using MOF in the obese patient because of unpredictable metabolism.[35] Caution should also be exercised in giving MOF to persons with diabetes, or in combination with narcotics and barbiturates. The administration of general anesthetics to patients receiving antidepressant and antihypertensive drugs may result in hypotension.[3]

Other adverse reactions to MOF include hepatic dysfunction, jaundice, hepatic necrosis, cardiac arrest, malignant hyperpyrexia (dantrolene is a treatment), prolonged postoperative somnolence, respiratory depression, laryngospasm, nausea, vomiting and hypotension.[11] Like other inhalational anesthetics, MOF may decrease the isocapnic hypoxemic ventilatory response.[34]

Nitrous oxide–oxygen sedation

Nitrous oxide is an inert, sweet-tasting and -smelling, colorless gas.[7] It is the only inorganic gas practical for clinical anesthesia. Nitrous oxide is also a powerful analgesic with little or no toxicity during ordinary clinical use.[4] Commercially available nitrous oxide is approximately 99.5% pure. Nitrous oxide supports combustion as actively as oxygen, but is not flammable or explosive.[3]

A 20% nitrous oxide/80% oxygen mixture is equivalent to 15 mg morphine.[3] Nitrous oxide is also an excellent supplemental agent in anesthesia and surgical sedation. In fact it is the most common supplement used by anesthesiologists with intravenous opioids.[21]

In the lungs and body nitrous oxide replaces nitrogen.[7] It is not metabolized nor is it absorbed permanently by the body. It is relatively insoluble in the blood.[3] It is eliminated almost entirely by the lungs.[7] It exerts its sedating effects by depressing the cortex, thalamus, hypothalamus, reticular activating system and limbic system.[3]

Advantages of nitrous oxide–oxygen sedation include safety nonallergenicity, no need for preoperative fasting or medicine, rapid onset of action, adjustable depth of sedation, rapid recovery, complete recovery and low cost.[3] The onset, peak and reversal times are 2–3, 3–5 and 10 min, respectively.[3,7] Patients are conscious and can obey instructions, and are also in a hypersuggestible state.[3] Reflexes are well maintained, especially the cough reflex, while sensations, including sight, hearing, taste and smell, are decreased. Nitrous oxide appears to have another beneficial effect: it has been reported to raise the toxicity threshold to intravenous lidocaine.[36]

Although nitrous oxide is a safe agent, it may not benefit every patient due to its lowered potency when mixed with 20% oxygen. In fact, nitrous oxide is the least potent of the anesthetic gases. Unfortunately, even in expert hands, at least 5% of the general population are not candidates for nitrous oxide analgesia and will require other means of sedation. In addition, pain is not consistently controlled with nitrous oxide, and, therefore, concomitant use of local anesthetics is often necessary.[3]

Nitrous oxide should be used in combination with at least 30% oxygen at all times during surgical sedation procedures. Some authors feel that the optimal nitrous oxide concentration for analgesia, while still maintaining patient cooperation, is approximately 35%.[3] However, it may be best not to administer more than 30% nitrous oxide because it may produce irrational behavior, possibly bordering on unconsciousness.[7] Inasmuch as nitrous oxide for dermatologic surgical purposes must be administered in concert with oxygen, the term nitrous oxide–oxygen sedation will be applied to describe the process.

Nitrous oxide is absorbed rapidly from the lungs to the blood and from the blood to the brain. Because the lag time between administration and clinical effect is 3–5 min, patients should be maintained at the same concentration of nitrous oxide for 3–5 min prior to any concentration increase.[3]

Nitrous oxide replaces the nitrogen in the blood and the closed air-filled spaces 35 times more rapidly than the nitrogen it is replacing can leave. This rapid and imbalanced diffusion may cause intestinal distention, middle ear expansion and pneumothorax.[3]

Nitrous oxide's extremely rapid exit from the bloodstream into the alveoli significantly dilutes the alveolar oxygen. This may bring about diffusion hypoxia.[3] It may also occur because alveolar carbon dioxide is lowered, resulting in decreased respiratory drive. The resulting hypoventilation produces hypoxia and occasionally concomitant nausea or vomiting.[7] The incidence of nausea is related to the depth and duration of nitrous oxide analgesia. Nausea is also related to the number of nitrous oxide concentration changes. Therefore, the frequency of changes should be kept as low as possible. Diffusion hypoxia and nausea may be prevented by administering 100% oxygen during the final 5 min of the procedure.[3]

Other adverse reactions to nitrous oxide include dizziness, headache, loss of control, excessive talking, shivering from vasodilatation, noncompliance and vivid dreams.[3] Patients receiving as little as 25% nitrous oxide have experienced blood pressure, pulse and respiration alterations secondary to hypoxia or hypercarbia.[7] Although commonly used with intravenous opioids, this combination may produce significant cardiovascular depression.[22] Signs of oversedation include mouth breathing, sleepiness, dreaming, incoherent speech, irrational or sluggish responses, poor coordination, inappropriate laughing, crying, noncompliance and complaints of discomfort. Fortunately, treatment may be as simple as decreasing the nitrous oxide concentration by 5–10%.[3]

Another drawback to nitrous oxide use includes potential for abuse; 7% of dentists admit recreational use of nitrous oxide. A disabling, primarily sensory, peripheral neuropathy has been associated with professional use and abuse.[3,37] However, long-term exposure to high concentrations of nitrous oxide appears necessary for development of this neuropathy. The chronic exposure levels, to which the surgeon and assistants must be exposed, can be decreased by use of scavenging nasal hoods, vacuums, air sweep fans and well-ventilated operating rooms. Another serious drawback of nitrous oxide is induction of sexual fantasies.[38] There are no absolute contraindications to nitrous oxide as long as it is given with at least 20% oxygen. However, nitrous oxide should not be given to patients with impaired nasal breathing, including those with upper respiratory infections. Relative contraindications include pregnancy, claustrophobia, upper respiratory infections, chronic mouth breathing, middle ear disease, chronic obstructive pulmonary disease (emphysema and chronic bronchitis), other severe pulmonary diseases (for example tuberculosis), and compulsivity and other personality disorders.[3] Of all the agents discussed in this chapter, nitrous oxide provides the greatest margin of safety.

SEDATING ANTIHISTAMINES

Hydroxyzine may be a beneficial addition to surgical sedation. It is the prototypical sedating antihistamine. Intravenously, it potentiates the other CNS depressant sedatives. In addition, hydroxyzine possesses antiemetic, antigaging, antinausea, bronchodilatory, antisalivary and mental dissociatory properties. As opposed to diazepam, hydroxyzine in high doses has some intrinsic analgesic potential and is nonirritating to the cerebral cortex. Also, hydroxyzine has minimal blood pressure and pulse effects.[7] Unfortunately, hydroxyzine is irritating to the veins, with a high rate of phlebothrombosis which is unacceptable to some authorities.[3]

Propofol

Propofol (2,3-diisopropylphenol) has been available in the USA since late 1989. The compound is virtually insoluble in water and highly soluble in fat. The high lipid solubility requires it to be mixed in an emulsion of soybean oil, glycerol and lecithin. Propofol has a unique pharmacokinetic profile in that its clearance is 10 times as fast as the metabolic clearance of thiopental. High lipid solubility contributes to a rapid onset (less than 60 s) of unconsciousness following intravenous administration. Compared to barbiturates, there is less postoperative sedation (that is hangover effect).[16]

The FDA has recently approved propofol for maintenance of sedation. However, the doses required are far less than those needed for maintenance of anesthesia. When used for maintenance of sedation, propofol requires an infusion pump. Most patients require an infusion of 25–70 μg/kg per min. Additive effects are observed when opioids are used concomitantly or when it is used in elderly or debilitated patients. Therefore, the infusion dose must be decreased according to those risk factors.[39]

Anaphylactic reactions have been reported, most probably attributed to lecithin. Cardiovascular effects include a decrease in mean arterial blood pressure producing arterial and venous vasodilatation. Its mild negative inotropic and chronotropic effects necessitate caution with its use. Propofol causes apnea in hypnotic doses and its respiratory depressant effect is enhanced by concurrent administration of opioids. Central nervous system effects are similar to those of barbiturates: decreased cerebral bloodflow, intracranial pressure and cerebral metabolism. Other side-effects include pain on injection (especially when injected into a small vein), involuntary skeletal muscle movements, coughing and hiccups.[16]

Suggestions, Standards, Precautions and Monitoring

Every office performing sedation should have a trained staff and 'state of the art' emergency equipment appropriate for all reported complications of the agents employed. Prior to surgery, a good medical and drug history must be obtained. Particular attention should be paid to potential drug interactions and side-effects, and appropriate adjustments must be made.

There is no substitute for excellent intraoperative clinical monitoring of patient alertness, wound bleeding, depth and ease of respirations, neuromuscular control and skin color. The physician should periodically communicate with the patient to check mental and physical status. Inappropriate communication by the patient may indicate oversedation or a compromised airway. This situation necessitates stopping the procedure and evaluating the patient's status.[3] The depth of sedation relies on clinical recognition and judgment as well. Amnesia may be clinically determined by noting the presence of either nystagmus or exotropia (divergence of the eyeballs). Although careful clinical observation may be a surgical sedation prerequisite, it may fall short in some instances. Altered coordination and muscle twitches are early indications of hypoxemia but are difficult to ascertain during surgery. Blood pressure changes and cyanosis may, unfortunately, be late indicators of hypoxemia. The pulse rate is a more accurate index of hypoxemia than even hyperapnea, since tachycardia is inversely proportional to the arterial oxygen saturation.[7]

Some anesthesiology texts and authorities recommend an intravenous catheter for surgical procedures lasting longer than 15 min if the patient has been fasting.[22] We believe that the nature of the procedure and possible complications should determine the necessity for an intravenous infusion or heparin lock. For example, liposuction may merit an intravenous infusion, yet a small to medium scalp reduction may not. There are disadvantages to intravenous infusions, including bacteremia.[40] An intravenous line being used to deliver sedatives may have the dual role of an emergency drug route. However, some authorities believe that of all peripheral veins, only the antecubital veins should be used for cardiopulmonary resuscitation drug administration.[41] Although the previously mentioned arm-to-brain or arm-to-heart circulation time was under 15 s, during circulatory compromise (that is arrest) a significant delay may result.[40,42,43] Thus, it is recommended to raise the extremity and infuse rapidly a 50-ml bolus of fluid after medicating from peripheral intravenous sites.[40]

The incidence of cardiac arrythmias varies with the diligence with which they are sought. Many who practice surgical sedation routinely use the electrocardiogram. In most clinical situations, only one electrocardiogram lead is sampled (usually lead II because of its better P-wave demonstration). However, recent evidence indicates that lead V best indicates cardiac ischemia.[6] It may therefore be best to monitor both leads II and V. Unfortunately, electrocardiogram monitors may not display abnormalities until the patient has been hypoxic or apneic for a considerable time. Irreversible brain damage may occur prior to electrocardiographic alteration.

Hypoxia is probably the most serious peril encountered in sedation techniques and is a major contributor to anesthetic morbidity and mortality. Therefore, a method for early detection of hypoxia has long been sought to help insure safe anesthesia and sedation. In the past, one had to rely on clinical signs subject to human error in an attempt to diagnose low arterial oxygen saturation. Due to the subjectivity of these clinical signs, the pulse oximeter has come to the forefront in the detection of low arterial oxygen saturation. The pulse oximeter is widely used in many clinical situations and is now considered the standard of care.[44]

The pulse oximeter detects the oxygen saturation of hemoglobin by combining the techniques of spectrophotometry and plethysmography. The oximeter provides continuous measurements of blood oxygen saturation by identifying pulsatile changes of laser light absorbance in arterial blood components.[44]

The use of noninvasive blood pressure monitoring devices (Dynamap) provides a physiological hemostatic outlook and is now considered a standard of care in many hospital- and office-based practices. The most common technique of blood pressure measurement involves variations of the Riva–Rocci method. The appropriate cuff size is imperative to identify the correct systolic, mean and diastolic blood pressure.

In summary, monitoring is suggested for all patients receiving surgical sedation. Suggested monitoring devices include:

1. Electrocardiogram (with a reliable P-wave display).
2. Noninvasive blood pressure monitoring device.
3. Pulse oximeter.
4. Intraoperative sedation chart (recommended).

Baseline vital signs, including respiratory rate, should be charted at least every 15 min throughout the procedure.[3]

Patients should never be discharged from the office alone following intravenous sedation during surgery. The procedure should be rescheduled if the patient cannot be accompanied by a relative or close friend. A taxi may not be a good alternative.[3]

In conclusion, we have stressed many of the negative and some of the positive aspects of sedation used before or during surgery. Prior to administering any of these drugs, the physician must be familiar with the possible side-effects and their treatment. The problems with surgical sedation often arise not from the drugs or techniques themselves but rather from how the drugs are administered.

REFERENCES

1. Legislation and litigation (no author), *J Am Dent Assoc* (1987) **114**:273.
2. *Dorland's Illustrated Medical Dictionary*, 26th edn (WB Saunders: Philadelphia 1981).
3. Malamed SA, *Sedation, a guide to patient management* (CV Mosby Co.: St Louis 1985).
4. Gilman AG, Goodman LS, Gilman A (eds), *The pharmacological basis of therapeutics*, 7th edn (Macmillan Publishing: New York 1985).
5. Dripps RD, Eckenhoff JE, Vandam LD, *Introduction to anesthesia. The principles of safe practice*, 5th edn (WB Saunders: Philadelphia 1977).
6. Orkin FK, Cooperman LH (eds), *Complications in anesthesiology* (JB Lippincott: Philadelphia 1983).
7. Shane SM, Rogers MC, *Conscious sedation for ambulatory surgery* (University Press: Baltimore 1983).
8. Klotz U, Avant GR, Hoyumpa A et al, The effects of age and liver disease on the disposition and elimination of diazepam in adult man, *J Clin Invest* (1987) **55**:347–59.
9. Margary JJ, Rosenbaum NL, Partridge M et al, Local complications following intravenous benzodiazepines in the dorsum of the hand. A comparison between midazolam and Diazemuls in sedation for dentistry, *Anaesthesia* (1986) **41**:205–7.
10. Clark RN, Rodrigo MR, A comparative study of intravenous diazepam and midazolam for oral surgery, *J Oral Maxillofac Surg* (1986) **44**:860–3.
11. *Physician's Desk Reference* (Medical Economics Inc.: Oradell, NJ 1986).
12. Al-Khudhairi D, Whitwam JG, McCloy RF, Midazolam and diazepam for gastroscopy, *Anaesthesia* (1982) **37**:1002–6.
13. Aun C, Flynn PJ, Richards J, Major E, A comparison of midazolam for intravenous sedation in dentistry, *Anaesthesia* (1984) **39**:589–93.
14. Forster A, Gardaz JP, Suter PM, Gemperle M, Respiratory depression by midazolam and diazepam, *Anesthesiology* (1980) **53**:494–7.
15. Connor JT, Katz RL, Pafano RR, Graham CW, RO 21-3981 for intravenous surgical premedication and induction of anesthesia, *Anesth Analg* (1978) **57**:1.
16. Stoelting RK, *Pharmacology and physiology in anesthetic practice* (JB Lippincott: Philadelphia 1987).
17. Nugent M, Artru AA, Michenfelder JD, Cerebral metabolic, vascular and protective effects of midazolam maleate. Comparison to diazepam, *Anesthesiology* (1982) **56**:172–6.
18. Bell GD, Spickett GP, Reeve PA et al, Intravenous midazolam for upper gastrointestinal endoscopy: a study of 800 consecutive cases relating dose to

age and sex of patient, *Br J Clin Pharmacol* (1987) **23**:241–3.

19. MacGilchrist AJ, Rirnie GG, Cook A, Scobie G, Murray T, Watkinson G, Brodie MJ, Pharmacokinetics and pharmacodynamics of intravenous midazolam in patients with severe alcoholic cirrhosis, *Gut* (1986) **27**:190–5.

20. Mazicon. Product monograph, Hoffman-LaRoche, 1992.

21. Miller RD (ed.), *Anesthesiology*, 2nd edn (Churchill Livingston: New York 1986).

22. Szeto HH, Inturrisi CE, Houde R et al, Accumulation of normeperidine, an active metabolite of meperidine, in patients with renal failure or cancer, *Ann Intern Med* (1977) **86**:738–41.

23. Roscow CE, Philbin DM, Keegan CR et al, Hemodynamics and histamine release during induction with sufentanil or fentanyl, *Anesthesiology* (1984) **60**:489–91.

24. Hill AB, Nahrwold ML, de Rosayro M et al, Prevention of rigidity during fentanyl-oxygen induction of anesthesia, *Anesthesiology* (1981) **55**:452–4.

25. Stanley TH, Webster LR, Anesthetic requirements and cardiovascular effects of fentanyl-oxygen and fentanyl-diazepam-oxygen anesthesia in man, *Anesth Analg* (1978) **57**:411–16.

26. Baily PL, Wilbrink J, Zwanikken P et al, Anesthetic induction with fentanyl, *Anesth Analg* (1985) **64**:48–53.

27. Tomichec RC, Roscow CE, Schneider RC et al, Cardiovascular effects of diazepam-fentanyl anesthesia in patients with coronary artery disease, *Anesth Analg* (1983) **61**:217–18.

28. Bowill JG, Sebel PS et al, The pharmacokinetics of Sufentanyl in surgical patients, *Anesthesiology* (1984) **61**:502–6.

29. Matteo RS, Ornstein E et al, Pharmacokinetics of Sugentanyl in the elderly, *Anesth Analg* (1986) **65**:594.

30. Lewis LA, Methoxyflurane for office surgery, *J Dermatol Surg Oncol* (1984) **10**:85–6.

31. Edmunds DH, Rosen M, Inhalation sedation for conservative dentistry. A comparison between nitrous oxide and methoxyflurane, *Br Dent J* (1975) **139**:398–40.

32. Carter R, Heerdt M, Acchiardo S, Fluoride kinetics after enflurane anesthesia in healthy and anephric patients and in patients with poor renal function, *Clin Pharmacol Ther* (1976) **20**:565–70.

33. Weiss V, de Carlini Ch, Methoxyflurane and serum fluoride concentrations during anaesthesia and postoperative renal function, *Anaesthetist* (1975) **24**:60–6.

34. Knill RL, Clement JL, Variable effects of anaesthetics on the ventilatory response to hypoxaemia in man, *Can Anaesth Soc J* (1982) **29**:93–9.

35. Samuelson PN, Merin RG, Taves DR et al, Toxicity following methoxyflurane anaesthesia. IV. The role of obesity and the effect of low dose anaesthesia on fluoride metabolism and renal function, *Can Anaesth Soc J* (1976) **23**:465–79.

36. Prince DA, Robson JG, Concentrations of lignocaine in the blood after intravenous, intramuscular, epidural, and endotracheal administration, *Anaesthesia* (1961) **16**:461–78.

37. Layzer RB, Fishman RA, Schafer JA, Neuropathy following abuse of nitrous oxide, *Neurology* (1978) **28**:504–6.

38. Jastak JT, Malamed SF, Nitrous oxide and sexual phenomena, *J Am Dent Assoc* (1980) **101**:38–40.

39. Shaffer SL, Stanski DR, Intravenous Anesthesia; 1991 Annual Refresher Course. American Society of Anesthesiologists, Oct. 26–30, 1991, San Francisco.

40. Albarran-Sotelo R, Atkins JM, Bloom RS et al, *Textbook of advanced cardiac life support* (American Heart Association: Dallas 1987).

41. Standards and guidelines for cardiopulmonary resuscitation (CPR) and emergency cardiac care (ECC), *JAMA* (1986) **255**:2905–89.

42. Kuhn GJ, White BC, Swetnan RE et al, Peripheral vs central circulation times during CPR: a pilot study, *Ann Emerg Med* (1981) **10**:417–19.

43. Hedges JR, Barsan WB, Doan LA et al, Central versus peripheral intravenous routes in cardiopulmonary resuscitation, *Am J Emerg Med* (1984) **2**:385–90.

44. Tinker JH, Dull DL, Caplan RA et al, The role of monitoring devices in prevention of anesthetic mishap: a closed claims analysis, *Anesthesiology* (1989) **71**:541–6.

Chapter 3

ANTIBIOTIC USE IN DERMATOLOGIC SURGERY

Joseph R. Terracina
Richard F. Wagner Jr

The expanding knowledge of microbiology, along with the development of new and more potent antibiotics, has made dermatologic surgery more complex. Many guidelines for antibiotic use have omitted cutaneous surgery. Thus, many indications for antibiotic use in dermatologic surgery are extrapolations from animal studies or from closely related surgical fields. The purpose of this chapter is to summarize current information about the use of antibiotics in dermatologic surgery, to give specific guidelines about their use, and to present new information about emerging trends in antibiotic utilization. This chapter will consider what we think are the three most fundamental challenges for the dermatologic surgeon. First we will deal with issues relating to the risk of endocarditis and apply this information to dermatologic surgery. Next, we will discuss preoperative antibiotic management. Finally, new antimicrobials which may have relevant use in dermatologic surgery will be reviewed.

ENDOCARDITIS PROPHYLAXIS

The current trend in antimicrobial prophylaxis against pathogens which cause endocarditis has been to pinpoint therapy in order to simplify it and to better prevent these occurrences. Clear-cut guidelines concerning antibiotic use in cutaneous surgery are lacking, leaving the physician to decide the proper circumstance for implementation. Since bacterial endocarditis carries a substantial morbidity and mortality, it may seem as though the choice to use antibiotic prophylaxis is an elemental one. However, only 10–15% of all cases of bacterial endocarditis can be linked to previous dental, medical and surgical procedures. Compounding this problem is the fact that controlled clinical trials to define the pathogenesis of endocarditis are limited by ethical considerations. The potential risk–benefit ratio should be a prime consideration.

There is no doubt that certain pre-existing cardiac conditions increase the risk for developing bacterial endocarditis. The American Heart Association (AHA) has defined cardiac conditions which increase patient risk (Table 3.1).[1] Several conditions such as congenital or acquired valvular dysfunction, prosthetic valves, or previous history of endocarditis are well-defined risks. Whether mitral valve prolapse (MVP) should be included has inspired much controversy. The concern over this seemingly simple problem is based on two

Table 3.1
Cardiac conditions and endocarditis risk.

I. Cardiac conditions not associated with an increased risk of endocarditis.

   Secundum atrial septal defects
   History of coronary artery bypass procedures
   Nonpathogenic murmurs
   History of rheumatic fever or Kawasaki's disease without residual valve dysfunction
   Pacemakers or defibrillators
   Isolated mitral valve prolapse
   Following surgical repair of any septal defect (beyond 6 months)

II. Cardiac conditions associated with an increased risk of endocarditis

   Congenital cardiac anomalies
   Any acquired valvular dysfunction, including prosthetic valve replacement
   History of previous episode of endocarditis
   Congenital or acquired hypertrophic cardiomyopathy
   Valvular regurgitation associated with mitral valve prolapse

overriding considerations. The first problem arises in delineating the true incidence of MVP. Although the exact prevalence is unknown, several studies estimate it to be between 4 and 6% of the population.[2-4] The next difficulty is defining the risk of endocarditis associated with MVP. It has been speculated that the number of endocarditis patients with pre-existing MVP has been grossly underestimated. In one study, 18 of 87 patients admitted with endocarditis were found to have concurrent MVP and regurgitation. However, of the 18 patients with endocarditis and mitral regurgitation, only eight had MVP previously observed.[5] The true correlation between MVP and the risk of endocarditis may be underestimated due to the lack of good documentation prior to patient presentation with infection.

The most recent investigations concerning this dilemma have been aimed at assessing the risk in patients with MVP who have concurrent mitral regurgitation. Data from the Framingham study suggested that only 9% of persons with MVP in the community had concurrent systolic murmurs.[4] Considering this fact, other studies have sought to examine the subset of patients with concurrent systolic murmurs to discern if this was the group at increased risk. In an Australian study, investigators found that the incidence of MVP was 20% in patients with endocarditis as opposed to only 4% in the control population. After further subdividing these groups into those with and without evidence of mitral regurgitation, it was found that 9 of 11 cases of endocarditis and MVP also had concurrent regurgitation murmurs. On final analysis there was no significant increased risk in the subset of patients with isolated MVP.[6] Another study found that male gender and the presence of a systolic murmur, particularly in persons over the age of 45 years, characterized patients with MVP at increased risk for infective endocarditis.[7] Although much controversy still exists over this question, the AHA has recently concluded that isolated MVP does not increase the risk for endocarditis compared with the general population.[1]

Many of the recommendations for endocarditis prophylaxis are based upon dental or surgical procedures which are more likely to initiate the bacteremia that results in endocarditis. No cutaneous surgical procedures are included in this group of high-risk procedures. However, some recent studies have shown that, despite small numbers of occurrences, transient bacteremia ensued after cutaneous surgery was performed on clean, uncontaminated surfaces.[8,9] Other cutaneous surgical procedures which have been associated with significant bacteremia are incision and drainage of soft tissue abscesses. In one small but convincing study 10 patients had pre- and post-procedure blood cultures drawn to document the incidence of bacteremia. Blood cultures were found to be positive in 6 of 10 patients after incision and drainage, revealing organisms similar to those cultured from the wound surface.

In contrast, none of the blood cultures taken prior to the procedure were positive.[10]

Considering these studies, it seems as though the prudent course would be to implement antibiotic prophylaxis for those patients deemed at high risk for endocarditis when any breach of the integument is planned. Individuals with hereditary hemorrhagic telangiectasia (Rendu–Osler–Weber disease) denote a particular subset of patients which should be included in this high-risk group. A recent report suggests that this group is at risk for visceral and central nervous system (CNS) infections with rates reported to be between 5 and 20%.[11]

The next question arises about what organisms should be targeted in the endeavor to pinpoint therapy, maintain a simplified regimen, and facilitate a high rate of compliance. Of all the resident cutaneous flora, *Staphylococcus epidermidis* is one of the most common in normal nondiseased skin[12] and has been found to be the most frequent pathogen causing prosthetic valve endocarditis.[13] It is also well established that *Staphylococcus aureus* is found in high densities on diseased skin and is also a common cause of endocarditis. Important work has been performed in elucidating the role that receptors may play in defining the pathogenicity of an organism for causing endocarditis. In one study, both types of staphylococci previously mentioned adhered readily to aortic valve leaflets in vitro,[14] thereby fulfilling the requirements to be an effective pathogen in endocarditis. Since *Propionibacterium acnes*, *Streptococcus viridans* and other Gram-negative organisms cause endocarditis infrequently, Wagner et al[15] have generally recommended that when prophylaxis is indicated it should be aimed at *Staphylococcus*. This group outlined recommendations that consisted of a two-dose regimen of oral antibiotics. The schedule utilizes dicloxacillin at a dose of 2 g at least 2 h after surgery followed by 1 g 6 h later. An alternative to this regimen in penicillin-allergic patients is the use of 1 g erythromycin at least 1 h before surgery followed by 0.5 g 6 h post-procedure.

Perhaps the most important consideration is physician education regarding appropriate application of endocarditis prophylaxis guidelines. Several studies have recognized three main areas where errors commonly occur. The first step is the identification of a particular patient at risk for endocarditis. Studies reveal that the physician recognizes patients at risk only 50–70% of the time. Individuals with the best understanding of patients at risk included internists, cardiologists and cardiovascular surgeons.[16] The next difficulty arises in selecting the correct regimen for endocarditis prophylaxis, especially for those allergic to penicillin and its derivatives. Dentists consistently out-performed physicians in selecting the AHA-recommended antibiotics by a rate of 58 to 36%.[16] The final difficulty arises when physicians fail to advise and educate high-risk patients about their need for future antibiotic prophylaxis. In one review of patients visiting an outpatient cardiology clinic, more than half the charts (68/134) contained no record of such counsel.[17]

In summary, guidelines based on well-controlled studies to aid the dermatologic surgeon in deciding about endocarditis prophylaxis do not exist. Most recommendations are based on animal studies or extrapolations from other similar medical specialties. We present general guidelines to the dermatologic surgeon based upon our review of the current literature (Table 3.2). Our recommendations about identifying high-risk individuals for endocarditis prophylaxis are consistent with those of the AHA. We include patients with MVP and concurrent mitral regurgitation murmurs. When endocarditis prophylaxis is ordered for most cutaneous surgery, it

Table 3.2
Antibiotic prophylaxis for adult dermatologic surgery[a]

	Primary regimen	Alternative regimen	Timing
Endocarditis	Dicloxacillin[b] 2.0-g loading dose followed by 1.0 g 6 h post-procedure	Erythromycin 1.0-g loading dose followed by 500 mg 6 h post-procedure	Give loading dose least 1 h prior to initiation of procedure
Wound infection prophylaxis	Cephalexin[c] 2.0-g loading dose followed by 500 mg every 6 h post-procedure	Erythromycin 1.0-g loading dose followed by 500 mg every 6 h post-procedure	Give loading dose at at least 1 h prior to initiation of procedure followed by 6-h dosing for 24–48 h

[a] These recommendations may require modification with regard to a specific patient based on the location of surgery and available microbiological studies. Pediatric doses should be based on weight.
[b,c] The authors do not use these antibiotics when there is an allergy to penicillin.

should usually include coverage against Gram-positive organisms, mainly the staphylococci, and should be initiated prior to and given after the procedure. Endocarditis prophylaxis is more complex when cutaneous surgery is planned on moist interiginous regions, mucous membranes or clinically infected tissue and the patient is at high risk for bacterial endocarditis. Under these unusual circumstances we seek specialist consultations for guidance. The incision of an infected loculation should be included on the list of surgical procedures that may place patients at risk for endocarditis.

ANTIBIOTICS TO PREVENT WOUND INFECTION

A critical aspect of surgical management is the prevention of postoperative wound infections. Like endocarditis prophylaxis for cutaneous surgery, this topic is controversial. In addition, bacterial resistance as well as the evolution of innovative broad-spectrum antibiotics has made clinical decisions more complex. One hundred years ago Cabot stated that 'every surgical operation is an experiment in bacteriology'.[18] Efforts beginning with Joseph Lister's use of carbolic acid in 1867 focused on attempting to decrease the incidence of infections. It would be easy to assume that over history the incidence of postoperative wound infections has improved greatly. The reality is that in 1899 Kocher reported a postoperative infection rate of 2.9%.[19] Recent estimates of nosocomial wound infections have placed the figure between 3 and 5%[20] with an estimated annual cost that exceeds one billion dollars.[21] It is with this in mind that we will consider those conditions which challenge the dermatologic surgeon, and attempt to delineate circumstances and guidelines for antibiotic use (Table 3.2).

As is the case with endocarditis prophylaxis, preoperative and postoperative antibiotics are often misused. Some of the most frequent examples of improper use include: (1) excessive length of treatment; (2) incorrect dosing and route of administration; and (3) using antibiotics without a proper indication.[22] It is commonplace to prescribe postoperative antibiotics automatically, without an awareness of the proper timing and duration of therapy which should be followed. In addition, incorrect patient selection is an area which may lead to errors. It has been shown that there are certain subsets of patients who may benefit from antibiotic prophylaxis. These may include: (1) circumstances in which patient history or the innate nature of the procedure may signify a greater than normal incidence of wound infection; (2) those procedures in which infection could be a catastrophic event, especially those involving prostheses; (3) surgical procedures on anatomical sites where increased bacterial colonization is predicted or infection is present; and (4) situations where there is decreased host resistance.[23] Most of these circumstances are well-established situations in which preoperative antibiotics have been shown to be of value. We routinely use antibiotic prophylaxis in immunocompromised patients.

Bacterial contamination of surgical wounds arises from exogenous or endogenous sources. Exogenous sources include contact with the operative team or with the environment via a flaw in aseptic surgical technique. Endogenous contamination occurs from the patient's skin, and respiratory, gastrointestinal and genitourinary tracts, and is the most important source in all types of wound infections except for clean, elective procedures. Surgical incisions can be classified into one of four categories based on the suspected inoculum of contaminants. Clean, uncontaminated incisions carry an infection rate of less than 5% and are performed under elective, ideal operating room conditions. Procedures involving a minor break in surgical technique or where entry into a hollow organ occurs are categorized as clean, contaminated wounds and carry an estimated wound infection rate of 10%. Contaminated wounds have an infection rate of 20% and include open, fresh, traumatic wounds or occur when there have been major errors in sterile technique. The last group includes wounds containing devitalized tissue or foreign bodies which are categorized as dirty wounds. This group has a 30–40% rate of postoperative infection.[24] Most dermatologic surgery is in the category of clean, uncontaminated wounds where the risk of infection is quite low. In one very large study which examined the infection rate from a total of 47 054 clean, uncontaminated wounds, a rate as low as 1.5% was observed.[25]

There are additional factors which may increase the risk of wound infection. It has been shown that the presence of silk or braided sutures in wounds reduces the number of staphylococci needed to induce infection by 10 000-fold.[26] In addition, preparing the operative site by shaving the area has been shown to increase significantly the postoperative infection rate. Seropian and Reynolds[27] studied 406 clean wounds and found infection rates of 5.6% for wounds prepared by shaving with a razor, 0.6% when no shaving was performed, and 0.6% when a depilatory was used. The increased incidence of postoperative infections from shaving has been attributed to minute abrasions produced from the action of the razor on the surface of the skin. Increasing patient age (especially those over 65 years of age) and increasing duration of procedure also increase the risk of postoperative infections, with the rate of infection roughly doubling for each hour of surgery. Factors which have not been shown to reduce wound infection rates include the use of adhesive plastic drapes instead of conventional cotton drapes, using iodophors instead of chlorhexidine scrubs, and utilizing a 10-min surgical scrub instead of a 5-min preparation.[26]

The timing of preoperative antibiotics is as important in preventing wound infection as is selecting the correct antibiotic. Since dermatologic surgery deals mainly with clean, uncontaminated wounds, the risk of pathogen inoculation into the surgical wound during the procedure is minimized. However, since surgery of clinically normal skin can result in transient bacteremia, it is also likely that wound contamination with the same microorganisms occurs.[9] If the cutaneous surface is eroded, as is often the case in dermatologic malignancies, the incidence of transient bacteremia has been noted to be as high as 8.4%.[8] A recent study attempted to determine if curettage of skin lesions would result in transient bacteremia.[28] None of the 22 treated lesions were associated with positive blood cultures.[28] In our experience, eroded skin tumors treated by electrodesiccation and curettage rarely become infected when left to heal by second intention. Thus we seldom use oral antibiotics in an attempt to prevent wound infection in this setting. Similarly, Mohs micrographic surgery wounds left to heal by second intention usually do not require systemic antibiotics.

Elaborate studies to determine optimal timing for antibiotic administration have been performed. One study looked at experimentally inflicted wounds contaminated with staphylococcal organisms at several time intervals both before and after antibiotic administration.[29] Infection rates and speed of healing were equivalent in both the untreated contaminated wound group and those in which the antibiotics were begun after the injuring process. However, in those groups where antibiotics were begun 3 h prior to wound contamination, infection rates and speed of healing were equivalent to those of wounds not contaminated with bacteria. Another study that suggested initiation of antibiotics 48 h prior to and continuing for 48 h after the procedure reported a significantly reduced infection rate.[30] It has been shown in multiple trials that similar results are obtained when dosing is initiated 2 h prior to and continued for as little as 12 h following the procedure.[31–35]

The choice of preoperative antibiotics has been another area of controversy. Since little has been written in the past about this issue with regard to dermatologic surgery, closely related areas must be examined for insights. There are two basic requirements that have to be met in order for an antibiotic to be effective for prophylaxis. First, it must display adequate blood levels along with exhibiting good tissue penetration. Second, the spectrum of activity should be commensurate with the most likely contaminating bacterial flora. Erythromycin is one of the most commonly used antibiotics in dermatology and is a reasonable choice if the oral route is preferred or if the patient is allergic to penicillin. Problems with this selection are its poor tissue penetration after parenteral administration,[36] its erratic oral absorption, and its tendency to elicit poor patient compliance. Perhaps better alternatives for this task are the first-generation cephalosporins, which exhibit excellent Gram-positive coverage, a low incidence of adverse reactions, and stability against beta-lactamase-producing bacteria.[37] Several first-generation cephalosporins are resistant to acid hydrolysis and therefore can be administered orally. These antibiotics have similar spectra of activity and include cephalexin, cephadrine and cefadroxil. The main difference between these antibiotics is the availability of generic forms and cost. In our practice we generally use oral loading doses of cephalexin (2 g) or erythromycin (1 g) followed by 500 mg orally every 6 h for two to four doses.

Universal use of perioperative antibiotics is probably not justified, considering the limited benefit gained in low-risk individuals. Although postoperative infections continue to be an occasional problem in low-risk patients, the additional cost plus the unfavorable risk–benefit ratio argue against preoperative antibiotic use in all situations. However, high-risk patients can benefit from preoperative antibiotic use. To decrease the risk of postoperative wound infections in most clinical encounters, the selected antibiotics should have good Gram-positive coverage, should be initiated at least 2 h prior to the procedure in question, and need be continued no longer than 12–24 h post-procedure. As in endocarditis prophylaxis, dermatologic surgery involving moist intertriginous regions, mucous membranes or clinically infected tissue may require different antibiotics than those usually selected.

NEW ANTIMICROBIALS IN DERMATOLOGIC SURGERY

The purpose of this section is briefly to summarize new antimicrobials which are likely to play an important role in future dermatologic surgery (Table 3.3). We emphasize advances in therapy and their potential use in soft tissue infections, while referring the reader to a general overview of commonly used dermatologic antimicrobials.[38] Recently developed broad-spectrum antimicrobials have simplified the task of treating resistant pathogenic bacteria occasionally encountered in dermatologic surgery. Prominent Gram-positive pathogens in dermatologic surgery have been met with antimicrobials which are extremely effective. Antimicrobials which have been the mainstay of therapy for many years include semisynthetic penicillins, first-generation cephalosporins, tetracyclines and macrolide antibiotics. However, the emergence of resistant organisms in wound infections and the increasing prevalence of Gram-negative organisms have lowered the effectiveness of many of these well-established regimens. It is with this problem in mind that we will review some other approaches to antimicrobial therapy.

The quinoline antibiotics have been available for many years, with nalidixic acid, the prototype within this group, used primarily for its effectiveness in urinary tract infections. A novel fluorinated carboxyquinolone, ciprofloxacin, has been very useful to dermatologic surgeons. The main value has been due to its action on Gram-negative organisms, particularly *Pseudomonas aeruginosa* and other pseudomonal strains. Its mechanism of action is primarily by disruption of DNA synthesis through inhibiting the ATP-dependent DNA-supercoiling reaction catalyzed by DNA gyrase.[39] The quinolones are well tolerated and serum concentrations following oral absorption are excellent. Ciprofloxacin exhibits distribution to most body compartments, with high levels in pulmonary, bronchial and osseous tissues. However, soft tissue levels during therapy have been found to be decreased in comparison to the above locations, thereby decreasing efficacy.[40] Despite this fact, ciprofloxacin has been shown in numerous studies to be equivalent or superior to various regimens of oral, intramuscular or intravenous preparations in the management of Gram-negative infections.[41-43] In one study comparing the efficacy of oral ciprofloxacin with intravenous administration of cefotaxime, various soft tissue infections, including cellulitis, abscesses, ulcers and wound infections, were treated with equivalent regimens. Bacteriologic cure rates were 90% versus 82% in the ciprofloxacin- and cefotaxime-treated

Table 3.3
New antimicrobials

	Generic	Trade Name	Dosage
Fluoroquinolones	Ciprofloxacin	Cipro	500–750 mg twice daily
	Ofloxacin	Floxin	200–400 mg twice daily
Azalides	Azithromycin	Zithromax	250 mg once daily
	Clarithromycin	Biaxin	250–500 mg twice daily

groups respectively. In addition, ciprofloxacin was found to be effective in 90% of the infections caused by *Staphylococcus aureas* and 100% of those caused by *Pseudomonas aeruginosa*.[41] One major difficulty with this antibiotic has been the emergence of bacterial resistance. Several studies have documented that *Pseudomonas* organisms exhibit a decrease in susceptibility as indicated by a four-fold rise in the minimal inhibitory concentration (MIC) during the course of therapy.[44] Despite this fact, most organisms continue to show susceptibility even in the face of this rise in the MIC and clinical cure rates have been consistent. Another fluorinated carboxyquinolone, norfloxacin, is effective in the treatment of auricular perichondritis, which is frequently complicated by *Pseudomonas* infections.[45] Ofloxacin, a recently approved carboxyquinolone, may rival ciprofloxacin in efficacy and perhaps create therapeutic alternatives should resistance become a problem.[46]

Another potentially important class of antibiotics for dermatologic surgery are the azalides. The prototype, azithromycin, is chemically related to erythromycin, has similar Gram-positive activity, and has a significantly greater spectrum of activity against anaerobes and Gram-negative organisms such as *Escherichia coli*, *Hemophilus influenzae* and *Klebsiella pneumoniae*.[47] Azithromycin achieves relatively high tissue concentrations despite low serum levels[48,49] and has excellent activity against cutaneous pathogens such as *Staphylococcus aureas* and *Streptococcus pyogenes*. Its long half-life (2–4 days) allows once-daily dosing and requires a shorter duration of therapy.[50] A large double-blind study comparing azithromycin once daily for 5 days with cephalexin twice daily for 10 days in treating various soft tissue infections showed overall bacteriologic cure rates of 98.5% and 98.3% respectively.[51] Clinical response and side-effect profiles were similar despite the marked difference in the duration of therapy.

References

1. Dajani AS, Bisno AS, Chung KJ et al, Prevention of bacterial endocarditis. Recommendations by the American Heart Association, *JAMA* (1990) **264**:2919–22.
2. Hickey AJ, Wolfers J, Wilcker DEL, Mitral valve prolapse. Prevalence in an Australian population, *Med J Aust* (1981) **1**:31–3.
3. Procacci PM, Savran SV, Schreiter SL et al, Prevalence of clinical mitral-valve prolapse in 1169 young women, *N Engl J Med* (1976) **294**:1086–8.
4. Savage DD, Garrison RJ, Derereux RB et al, Mitral valve prolapse in the general population. Epidemiologic features: the Framingham study, *Am Heart J* (1983) **106**:571–5.
5. Corrigall D, Bolen J, Hancock EW et al, Mitral valve prolapse and infective endocarditis, *Am J Med* (1977) **63**:215–22.
6. Hickey AJ, MacMahon SW, Wilcken DEL, Mitral valve prolapse and bacterial endocarditis: when is antibiotic prophylaxis necessary? *Am Heart J* (1985) **109**:431–4.
7. MacMahon SW, Roberts JK, Kramer-Fox R et al, Mitral valve prolapse and infective endocarditis, *Am Heart J* (1987) **113**:1291–8.
8. Sabetta JB, Zitelli JA, The incidence of bacteremia during skin surgery, *Arch Dermatol* (1987) **123**:213–15.
9. Halpern AC, Leyden JJ, Dzubow LM et al, The incidence of bacteremia in skin surgery of the head and neck, *J Am Acad Dermatol* (1988) **19**:112–16.
10. Fine BC, Sheckman PR, Bartlett JC, Incision and drainage of soft-tissue

abcesses and bacteremia, *Ann Int Med* (1985) **103**:645.

11. Swanson DL, Dahl MV, Embolic abcesses in hereditary hemorrhagic telangiectasia, *J Am Acad Dermatol* (1991) **24**:580–3.

12. Reichert V, Saint-Leger D, Schaefer H, Skin surface chemistry and microbial infection, *Semin Dermatol* (1982) **1**:91–100.

13. Karchmer AW, Treatment of prosthetic valve endocarditis. In: Sande MA, Kaye D, Root RK, eds, *Endocarditis* (Churchill Livingston Inc.: New York 1984) 165–6.

14. Gould K, Ramirez-Ronda CH, Holmes RK et al, Adherence of bacteria to heart valves in vitro, *J Clin Invest* (1975) **56**:1365–70.

15. Wagner RF, Grande DJ, Feingold DS, Antibiotic prophylaxis against bacterial endocarditis in patients undergoing dermatologic surgery. *Arch Dermatol* (1986) **122**:799–801.

16. Nelson CL, Van Blaricum CS, Physician and dentist compliance with American Heart Association Guidelines for prevention of bacterial endocarditis, *J Am Dent Assoc* (1989) **118**:169–73.

17. Pitcher DW, Papouchado M, Channer KS et al, Endocarditis prophylaxis: do patients remember advice and know what to do? *Br Med J* (1986) **293**:1539–40.

18. Cabot AT, Discussion. In: Gerster AG, ed., Aseptic and antiseptic details in operative surgery, *Tr Cong Am Phys Surg* (1891) **2**:51.

19. Kocher T, On some conditions of healing by first intention with special reference to disinfection of hands, *Trans Am Surg* (1899) **17**:116–30.

20. Polk HC, Simpson CJ, Simmons BP et al, Guidelines for prevention of surgical wound infection, *Arch Surg* (1983) **118**:1213–17.

21. Bennett JV, Human infections: economic implications and prevention, *Ann Intern Med* (1978) **89**:761–3.

22. Jogerst GJ, Dipe SE, Antibiotics use among medical specialties in a community hospital. *JAMA* (1981) **245**:842–6.

23. Lewis RT, Antibiotic prophylaxis in surgery, *Can J Surg* (1981) **24**:451–566.

24. DiPiro JT, Record KE, Schanzenback KS et al, Antimicrobial prophylaxis in surgery: Part 1, *Am J Hosp Pharm* (1981) **38**:320–34.

25. Cruse PJE, Foord R, The epidemiology of wound infection. A 10 year prospective study of 62,939 wounds, *Surg Clin North Am* (1980) **60**:27–40.

26. Elek SD, Conen PE, The virulence of staphylococcus pyogenes for man: a study of the problems of infection, *Br J Exp Pathol* (1957) **38**:573–83.

27. Seropian R, Reynolds BM, Wound infections after preventive antibiotic therapy. Timing, duration, and economics, *Am J Surg* (1971) **121**:251.

28. Maurice PDL, Parker S, Acadia BS et al, Minor skin surgery. Are prophylactic antibiotics ever needed for curettage? *Acta Derma Venereol (Stockholm)* (1991) **71**:267–8.

29. Burke JF, The effective period of preventive antibiotic action in experimental incisions and dermal lesions, *Surgery* (1961) **50**:161–8.

30. Bencini PL, Galimberti M, Signorini M et al, Antibiotic prophylaxis of wound infections in skin surgery, *Arch Dermatol* (1991) **127**:1857–60.

31. Polk HC, Lopez-Mayor JF, Postoperative wound infection: a prospective study of determinant factors and prevention, *Surgery* (1969) **66**:97–103.

32. Hirschmann JV, Irui TS, Antimicrobial prophylaxis: a critique of recent trials, *Rev Infect Dis* (1980) **2**:1–23.

33. Kaiser AB, Antimicrobial prophylaxis in surgery, *N Engl J Med* (1986) **315**:1129–2238.

34. Wenzel WP, Preoperative antibiotic prophylaxis, *N Engl J Med* (1992) **326**:336–9.

35. Classen DC, Evans RS, Pestotnik SL et al, The timing of prophylactic administration of antibiotics and the risk of surgical wound infection, *N Engl J Med* (1992) **326**:281–6.

36. Sande MA, Mandell GL, Antimicrobial agents. In: Gilman AG, Goodman LS, Gilman A, eds, *The pharmacologic basic of therapeutics* (Macmillan: New York 1980) 1222–48.

37. Neu HC, The new beta-lactamase-stable cephalosporin, *Ann Intern Med* (1982) **94**:408–18.

38. Feingold DS, Wagner RF, Antibacterial therapy, *J Am Acad Dermatol* (1986) **14**:535–48.

39. Fass RJ, The quinolones, *Ann Intern Med* (1985) **102**:400–2.

40. Neu HC, Clinical use of the quinolones, *Lancet* (1987) **ii**:1319–22.

41. Ramirez-Ronda CH, Saavedra S, River-Vazquez CR, Comparative, double-blind study of oral ciprofloxacin and intravenous cefotaxime in skin and skin structure infections, *Am J Med* (1987) **82**(supplement 4A):220–3.

42. Gentry LO, Ramirez-Ponda CH, Rodriquez-Noriega E et al, Oral ciprofloxacin vs parenteral cefotaxime in the treatment of difficult skin and skin structure infections, *Arch Intern Med* (1989) **149**:2579–83.

43. Self PL, Zeluff BA, Sollo D et al, Use of ciprofloxacin in the treatment of serious skin and skin structure infections, *Am J Med* (1987) **82**(supplement 4A):239–41.

44. Scully BE, Parry MF, Neu HC et al, Oral ciprofloxacin therapy of infections due to *Pseudomonas aeruguinosa*, *Lancet* (1986) **i**:819–922.

45. Thomas JM, Swanson NA, Treatment of perichondritis with a quinolone derivative norfloxacin, *J Dermatol Surg Oncol* (1988) **14**:447–9.

46. Monk JP, Campoli-Richards DM, Ofloxacin: a review of its antibacterial activity, pharmacokinetic properties and therapeutic use, *Drugs* (1987) **33**:346–91.

47. Retsema J, Girard A, Schelky W et al, Spectrum and mode of action of azithromycin (CP-62, 993), a new 15 membered-ring macrolide with improved potency against gram-negative organisms. *Antimicrob Agents Chemother* (1987) **31**:1939–47.

48. Girard AE, Girard D, English AR et al, Pharmacokinetics and in vivo studies with azithromycin (CP-62, 993), a new macrolide with an extended half-life and excellent tissue distribution, *Antimicrob Agent Chemother* (1987) **31**:1948–54.

49. Foulds G, Shephard RM, Johnson RB, The pharmacokinetics of azithromycin in human serum and tissues, *J Antimicrob Chemother* (1990) **25**(supplement A):73–82.

50. Cooper MA, Nye K, Andrews JM et al, The pharmacokinetics and inflammatory fluid penetration of orally administered azithromycin, *J Antimicrob Chemother* (1990) **26**:533–8.

51. Mallory SB, Azithromycin compared with cephalexin in the treatment of skin and skin structure infections, *Am J Med* (1991) **91**(supplement 3A):36–9.

Chapter 4

HIV AND DERMATOLOGIC SURGERY

Gwendolyn A. Crane
Henry H. Roenigk Jr

Medicine continues to be an ever-changing field with the acquisition of knowledge being the driving force. Just 60 years ago, some felt that adequate hygiene and sanitation would cure any ailment.[1] If it were only this simple. During the past decade, the acquired immunodeficiency syndrome (AIDS) has emerged as a dominant concern of the medical profession and society in general. AIDS is a complex illness. It is difficult to keep pace with current events and policy changes in this rapidly evolving field of medicine. A substantial amount of knowledge has been gained about the human immunodeficiency virus (HIV) since it was first reported in 1981.[2] Along with this acquisition of knowledge, a number of questions have been raised regarding moral, ethical and medico-legal issues. Answers to many of these questions have been provided, yet many remain unanswered and generate new questions and controversy. Who should be tested for the HIV virus? Should testing be mandatory? Should HIV-positive health care workers disclose their status to their employers or patients? Should an HIV-positive health care worker perform invasive procedures? As dermatologists, we need to be aware of all aspects of the HIV epidemic. There are a number of skin diseases associated with AIDS which can frequently be the first manifestation of AIDS. Knowledge of policies regarding testing, informed consent and disclosure is important. These policies vary from state to state in the USA. Dermatology is also a surgical specialty and thus being informed about current recommendations on infection control and prevention is equally important.

Transmission of the HIV virus can occur through exposure to blood, semen, vaginal secretions or breast milk.[2] The risk of transmission can be and has been decreased through the use of condoms for sexual intercourse, routine HIV screening for blood and tissue products, avoidance of contaminated needles, and education. Despite this education, the incidence of infection is increasing with a shift in transmission routes.[3] It is no longer a disease only of high-risk groups but has become a disease of the general population. Heterosexual transmission and intravenous drug abuse have become more frequent modes of transmission.[3] Education is no longer being targeted only toward high-risk groups but also toward the general public. The World Health Organization estimates there will be more than three million AIDS-related deaths among women and childen in the

1990s.[4] AIDS is surpassing other leading causes of death. In 1988, it was the third leading cause of death among men 25–44 years of age and the eighth leading cause of death in American women in the same age group.[4]

Occupational transmission is an area of concern for the public and for health care professionals. Occupational risk following a percutaneous injury has been estimated to be 0.3%.[5] There are 65 estimated cases of HIV infection through occupational exposure.[2] It is difficult to determine the risk of transmission from the health care worker to the patient as there is only the one report of transmission from a health care worker to his patients.[5] In this case a dentist transmitted the virus to 5 of his patients (of 850 tested). There have been 'look-back' cases where patients, upon whom invasive procedures were performed by HIV-positive health care workers, were tested. To date, none of the patients have tested HIV positive[5] (with the exception of an intravenous drug abuser thought to be positive prior to surgery).[5,6] The CDC estimates that the probability of transmitting HIV from an infected surgeon to a patient is 1 in 41 667 to 1 in 416 667.[7] The CDC postulates that between 3 and 28 patients may have been infected between 1981 and 1990 from exposure to an HIV-positive health care worker.[7]

The case of transmission from the dentist to his patients in 1990 has disturbed public, medical and legal groups. A compilation of national public opinion surveys from 1988 to 1991 regarding AIDS, drug abuse and sexual orientation revealed the following.[8] The majority (80%) of the public support mandatory testing for high-risk groups such as homosexuals, intravenous drug users, prisoners, health providers, patients and those applying for US residency. Approximately 50% favor testing of the general population. Nine of ten individuals support disclosure of the HIV status of the health care worker and patient. Forty-nine percent of those polled believe an HIV-positive health care worker should not practice and almost two-thirds would not continue to see an HIV-positive individual for medical care.

The concern of physicians as stated by Gostin is 'that they are required by law and ethics to treat AIDS patients, but if they are infected with HIV, they may be left without adequate rights, compensation or compassionate care.'[9] The legal requirement to treat AIDS patients stems from the Federal Rehabilitation Act 1973 and the Americans with Disabilities Act 1990. The Federal Rehabilitation Act 1973 considers individuals with AIDS and AIDS-related complex, asymptomatic seroconverters and those engaging in high-risk behavior as handicapped and protects them from discrimination.[10] Programs receiving federal aid are subject to this Act.[10] In 1990, the Americans with Disabilities Act was passed, expanding protection against discrimination to private areas such as employment, education, transportation and public accommodations and services.[3,10]

The Council on Ethical and Judicial Affairs of the AMA feels a physician has an ethical duty to treat an HIV-positive patient if the patient's medical condition is within that physician's area of competence.[11] If a physician is unable to provide the necessary services to the patient, then adequate referral should be made. Rizzo et al[12] report the results of a 1988 telephone survey of 3506 physicians. Seventy-five percent agree there is an ethical obligation to treat an HIV-positive patient if capable. Sixty-four to sixty-eight percent of general surgeons and surgical specialists feel they have an obligation to treat HIV-positive patients. Seventy-four percent of senior internal medicine and family medicine residents in a 1989 study indicated that they planned to continue to provide primary care to patients with AIDS.[13]

Although the Americans with Disabilities Act 1990 prohibits discrimination against the handicapped in certain areas, a degree of discrimination toward AIDS patients does exist and is likely to continue. Lack of knowledge about the disease and the associated stigma contribute to the discrimination. Health care providers deal not only with treating HIV-positive patients, but also with the possibility of contracting the HIV virus in the process. The American Medical Association, the American Academy of Orthopedic Surgeons, and the American College of Obstetrics and Gynecology feel that certain procedures are associated with a high risk of transmission of the HIV virus from the HIV-positive surgeon to the patient and that the HIV-positive surgeon should not perform those procedures.[14]

Recommendations by the CDC concerning HIV-positive health care providers are: (1) those involved in providing health care should follow guidelines for universal precautions; (2) invasive procedures that are not exposure-prone should not be restricted from the practice of the HIV-positive health care worker as long as universal precautions are taken; (3) exposure-prone procedures should be identified by the organization or institution where the procedures are performed; (4) those health care workers performing exposure-prone procedures should know their HIV status; and (5) HIV-positive health care workers should not perform exposure-prone procedures until they seek counsel from a review panel for advice regarding circumstances under which these procedures should be performed. These circumstances would include patient knowledge of the health care worker's HIV status and informed consent stating this.[5] Features of exposure-prone procedures include 'digital palpation of a needle tip in a body cavity or the simultaneous presence of the health care worker's fingers and a needle or other sharp instrument or object in a poorly visualized or highly confined anatomic site'.[5] The CDC has defined invasive procedures as 'surgical entry into tissues, cavities, or organs or repair of major traumatic injuries associated with any of the following: (1) an operating or delivery room, emergency department, or outpatient setting, including both physicians' and dentists' offices; (2) cardiac catheterization and angiographic procedures; (3) vaginal or caesarean delivery or other invasive obstetric procedure during which bleeding may occur; or (4) the manipulation, cutting or removal of any oral or perioral tissues, including tooth structure, during which bleeding occurs or the potential for bleeding exists'.[5] There is still a great deal of controversy surrounding the CDC guidelines and recommendations. In addition, a new federal law requires states to enact the CDC recommendations or equivalent guidelines by October 1992 in order to receive Public Health Service funds.[15] Texas is the only state which has adopted these guidelines as of December 1991.[15]

How does the medical community feel about mandatory testing? The CDC and the AMA are both opposed.[5,16] The American College of Emergency Physicians, the American Dental Association and the American Nurses' Association are also opposed to mandatory testing.[16] The American Medical Association and American Dental Association both support voluntary disclosure.[16] Orentlicher[14] states that mandatory testing would be needed if the goal is to eliminate any risk of transmission. However, elimination of all risk is an 'illusory goal' as HIV infection can occur at any time and even daily testing will not eliminate all risk.[14]

Legislative bills introduced with regard to disclosure of HIV status and mandatory testing have been numerous. There are currently seven US states with laws for HIV-positive health care providers. These states are California, Florida, Hawaii, Illinois, Louisiana, Maryland and Texas (AIDS Policy Center, Intergovernmental

Table 4.1
Recommended protective equipment for certain dermatologic procedures

	Eye protection	Face shields	Gown	Gloves	Surgical mask	Smoke evacuator
Laser[18,19]	✓		✓	✓	✓	✓
Dermabrasion[19,20]	✓	✓	✓	✓	✓	
Hair transplant[19,21]	✓			✓	✓	

Health Policy Project, The George Washington University, unpublished data). Nineteen states have introduced legislation in the past year (AIDS Policy Center, Intergovernmental Health Policy Project, The George Washington University, unpublished data). Five states have put forth proposals for mandatory testing of health care workers. Twelve states have bills which would require patients to be notified of an HIV-positive health care worker's status. Four states have proposals which prohibit infected health care workers from performing exposure-prone procedures without the patient's knowledge or the health department's approval. Four states propose that HIV-positive health care workers report their status to the department of health or licensing board. Seven states have proposals to impose criminal penalties for HIV-positive health care workers who fail to disclose their HIV status to patients.

This legislative action and concern over transmission of the HIV virus in the workplace has also led to new regulations for infection control. The FDA has established new quality control standards for gloves.[17] The CDC has published new recommendations for preventing transmission of the HIV virus to patients through exposure-prone procedures.[5] The Occupational Safety and Health Administration (OSHA) presented its final rule on 6 December 1991.[2] This ruling became effective on 6 March 1992. The OSHA rule makes employers responsible for their employees' education regarding the transmission of the HIV and hepatitis B virus and sets forth guidelines for infection control and prevention in the workplace.

Table 4.1 lists recommendations for protective attire for dermatologic procedures with a tendency for bloody spatter and/or the aerosolization of particulate matter. Special surgical masks may be preferred for laser or dermabrasion cases.

For any dermatologic procedure involving exposure to blood and certain body fluids, universal precautions should be applied.[22] The protective clothing will vary with the type of surgery being performed. Gloves are advised for any surgical case or examination in which there may be exposure to blood or potentially infectious material.[22,23] Double gloving has become routine in many practices.[24] Masks, gowns and protective eyewear are suggested for situations where spatter and aerosolization of blood is possible.[18,19]

A system or plan for the handling of sharps should be developed by each surgical team. Unnecessary or contaminated sharps should be removed from the surgical field and disposed of in an appropriate manner. Instruments should be used in all aspects of tissue handling with minimal use of fingers in the manipulation of the needle holder.[24,25]

The issues regarding AIDS will no doubt continue to be complex. However, one should be familiar with federal and state legislation regarding disclosure of HIV status, informed consent and confidentiality as well as regulations for the health care provider. Efforts directed toward educating the public should be continued as well as instruction for all health care workers in preventive measures for infection control.

REFERENCES

1. Percival CG, *The royal road* (Tyrrell's Hygienic Institute: New York 1930).
2. Occupational Safety and Health Administration, Occupational exposure to bloodborne pathogens, *Federal Register* (1991) **56**(235):64004–182.
3. Bowleg L, Past, present and future state responses in the first decade of the AIDS epidemic, *Intergovernmental AIDS Reports* (1991) **4**:1–4.
4. Centers for Disease Control, The HIV challenge continues, *CDC HIV/AIDS Prevention Newsletter* (February 1991) 1–5.
5. Centers for Disease Control, Recommendations for preventing transmission of human immunodeficiency virus and hepatitis B virus to patients during exposure-prone invasive procedures, *MMWR* (1991) **40**:1–9.
6. Mishu B, Schaffner W, Horan JM et al, A surgeon with AIDS: lack of evidence of transmission to patients, *JAMA* (1990) **264**:467–70.
7. Rayhawk P, Health care workers with HIV: balancing the rights of patients and health professionals, *Intergovernmental AIDS Reports* (1991) **4**:1–6.
8. Blendon RJ, Donelan K, Knox RA, Public opinion and AIDS: lessons for the second decade, *JAMA* (1992) **267**:981–6.
9. Gostin LO, The surgeon and the HIV-infected patient, *JAMA* (1990) **264**:1408.
10. Gostin LO, The AIDS litigation project: a national review of court and human rights commission decisions, part II: discrimination, *JAMA* (1990) **263**:2086–93.
11. Council on Ethical and Judicial Affairs, Ethical issues involved in the growing AIDS crisis, *JAMA* (1988) **259**:1360–1.
12. Rizzo JA, Marder WD, Wilke RJ, Physician contact with and attitudes toward HIV-seropositive patients: results from a national survey, *Med Care* (1990) **28**:251–60.
13. Hayward RA, Shapiro MF, A national study of AIDS and residency training: experiences, concerns, and consequences, *Ann Intern Med* (1991) **114**:23–32.
14. Orentlicher D, HIV-infected surgeons: Behringer v Medical Center, *JAMA* (1991) **266**:1134–7.
15. Rayhawk P, Health care workers with HIV: the policy confusion continues, *Intergovernmental AIDS Reports* (1991) **4**:4,9.
16. Frandzel S, Organizations defend their positions at CDC conference on HIV-infected health care workers, *AIDS Patient Care* (1991) **15**:129–32.
17. Makulowich GS, FDA establishes new quality standards for gloves, *AIDS Patient Care* (1991) **5**:143–5.
18. Sawchuk WS, Weber PJ, Lowy DR et al, Infectious papillomavirus in the vapor of warts treated with carbon dioxide laser or electrocoagulation: detection and protection, *J Am Acad Dermatol* (1989) **21**:41–9.
19. Sawchuk WS, Infectious potential of aerosolized particles, *Arch Dermatol* (1989) **125**:1689–92.
20. Burks JW, *Dermabrasion and chemical peeling* (Charles C Thomas: Springfield 1979).
21. Unger WP, Nordstrom REA, *Hair transplantation* (Marcel Dekker: New York 1988).

22. Centers for Disease Control, Update: universal precautions for prevention of transmission of human immunodeficiency virus, hepatitis B virus, and other bloodborne pathogens in healthcare settings, *MMWR* (1988) **37**:377–82, 387–8.
23. Freeman WE, Chalker DK, Smith JG, Use of gloves among dermatologists, *J Am Acad Dermatol* (1987) **17**:320–3.
24. Burget GC, Orane AM, Teplica D, HIV-infected surgeons, *JAMA* (1992) **267**:803.
25. Raahave D, Bremmelgaard A, New operative technique to reduce surgeons' risk of HIV infection, *J Hosp Infect* (1991) **18**(supplement A):177–83.

Chapter 5

GROWTH FACTORS AND WOUND HEALING

Vincent Falanga

The rate at which knowledge of the biology of growth factors has accumulated in the last decade has been dramatic. At the moment, the role of these potent peptides in medicine is not completely clear, but an exciting picture is beginning to emerge. Due to the dramatic effects these proteins have on cell proliferation, cell chemotaxis, and the formation of extracellular matrix molecules, a role in wound healing and in the treatment of chronic wounds appears certain. It is likely that surgeons in the not-too-distant future will make use of growth factors perioperatively and during the healing process to improve granulation tissue, enhance tensile strength, and promote re-epithelialization. Ways to antagonize and block the action of these peptides will offer novel approaches to decrease scarring and to prevent keloids. This chapter is written for the dermatologic surgeon. It will emphasize the practical aspects of growth factors, and is meant to summarize and clarify the complex nomenclature and confusing terminology that characterizes this important field.

Growth factors: nomenclature

For those who are unfamiliar with growth factors, the names of these peptides alone is sufficient to cause confusion and inhibit the assimilation of knowledge that has emerged regarding their role in wound repair. Growth factors are proteins, and are also frequently referred to as peptides or polypeptides. However, the major source of confusion is probably the fact that 'growth factor' is a term applied to a variety of growth-promoting substances. This is because these agents were discovered by members of different scientific disciplines. For example, a new growth-promoting substance has generally been called cytokine by cell biologists, interleukin by immunologists, and colony-stimulating factor by hematologists. Ultimately, these are all growth factors, and this term seems to prevail. Thus, the various interleukins (IL-1, IL-2 etc.) are all really growth factors. Interleukins are generally thought of as essential peptides for lymphoid cells, but it should be recognized that they can also act on nonlymphoid cells, such as fibroblasts and keratinocytes. A good example of this is IL-1. Table 5.1 is a partial summary of major polypeptides and their overall effects.[1]

Table 5.1 shows an added difficulty that surfaces with regard to nomenclature. The name of a growth factor generally says little about its most important or prominent effects. A few examples will serve to illustrate this. Epidermal growth factor (EGF) has important effects on nonepidermal cells; fibroblast growth factor (FGF) has endothelial cells and not fibroblasts as its most obvious target; transforming growth factors do not 'transform' cells, or cause other signs of malignancy; platelet-derived growth factor (PDGF) is indeed stored in platelets, but is secreted also by other cells. All of this apparent confusion over names is the result of the fact that the names of growth factors are derived from the initial observation that led to their discovery; the initial context of this discovery is often not representative of the final assessment of biological activity.

Even Table 5.1 and the list of prominent effects of these peptides can be misleading. A number of variables can alter these general guidelines. For example, TGF-beta inhibits endothelial cell and keratinocyte proliferation in vitro but not in vivo. A proliferative effect of TGF-beta on fibroblasts is only observed after prolonged exposure in vitro and after stimulation of PDGF synthesis. The biological activity of acidic FGF is augmented up to 100-fold by the addition of heparin. This multifunctional activity of growth factors has emerged as one of the most important concepts in this field.[2] It offers hope that, depending on the conditions or the presence of other peptides, growth factors can have a variety of roles in the modulation of wound repair.

Mechanism of action of growth factors

A detailed analysis of this subject is outside the scope of this discussion. However, a few basic principles will be outlined because here too the nomenclature can be confusing. Growth factors have their biological effects on cells through highly specific receptors present on the surface of cells. Multiple receptors can exist for each growth factor, and they can bind the peptide with different strengths (affinity). This offers yet another mechanism by which the response of cells and tissues to growth factors can be regulated. Through such receptors, growth factors can exert their effect on distant cells (exocrine mode), neighboring cells (paracrine mode), and on the cell of origin (autocrine mode).

Table 5.1
Some representative growth factors and biological effects

Name	Overall effects
EGF	The first growth factor to be discovered and characterized. It promotes re-epithelialization and angiogenesis. It increases collagenase activity
PDGF	Strong mitogen and chemoattractant for mesenchymal cells, particularly fibroblasts and smooth muscle cells. It enhances extracellular matrix deposition
FGF	A family of peptides that bind heparin and which are normally secreted by cells unless they are injured. They are extremely potent angiogenic agents, and also increase epithelialization
TGF-beta	Initially isolated from tumor cells. They are a very potent stimulus for the deposition of extracellular matrix, including collagen, proteoglycans and fibronectin. TGF-betas have immunosuppressive properties
TNF-alpha	Also called cachectin. A distinct monocyte-derived factor first characterized as protein cytotoxic to tumor cells. It activates neutrophils, and is mitogenic for fibroblasts. It has a number of catabolic activities, including bone and cartilage resorption
IL-1	It is released by activated monocytes and macrophages, and is increased with infection. It is a pyrogen, and is chemotactic for keratinocytes, neutrophils, monocytes and lymphocytes. It increases collagen synthesis

EGF, epidermal growth factor; PDGF, platelet-derived growth factor; FGF, fibroblast growth factor; TGF-beta, transforming growth factor beta; TNF-alpha, tumor necrosis factor alpha; IL-1, interleukin-1

The events following the binding of a growth factor to a receptor are not well understood and are the subject of intense investigation. The signaling mechanisms involved from the initial binding to the cell's surface to a biological response involve protein kinases (which add phosphate groups to other molecules, causing either their activation or inactivation), and various intermediates, such as G-proteins and phospholipase-C-induced products.[1,3]

The molecules involved in the signaling pathways, from the peptides themselves to the receptors and various intermediates, can all fall victim to the mimicry of homologous molecules supplied by oncogenic viruses. The general name of oncogenes is given to these proteins, and they can be of either cellular (c-onc) or viral (v-onc) origin. Proto-oncogenes are oncogene homologues present in normal cells. Because oncogenes can act and substitute in an unregulated fashion for all of the molecules involved in the action of growth factors, they can lead to cellular transformation and cancer.[1] At the moment, it is unclear what relevance this has to the use of growth factors in wounds, and whether this poses a threat of malignant transformation. It appears that this risk is quite remote, although it has caused numerous precautions to be taken during clinical trials. Thus far, no apparent malignant transformation has been reported with their use.

THE PRESENCE OF GROWTH FACTORS IN WOUNDS

Growth factors are likely to be intimately involved in the healing process.[4] We will review some of the events occurring during wound repair from the standpoint of which growth factors are actively engaged in this process. With injury, a host of peptides are released in the wound from platelets, which are rich sources of PDGF and TGF-beta. Platelet-derived growth factor is a potent mitogen for fibroblasts and is chemotactic for a variety of cell types, including fibroblasts, smooth muscle cells and macrophages. TGF-beta is also an extremely potent chemotactic agent for neutrophils and macrophages. It is widely believed that the initial surge of peptides from platelets is essential for proper wound repair.[5] Shortly after wounding, a clot forms at the site. In the formation of a fibrin plug, several peptides are liberated, including fibrinopeptides A and B, which have been shown to be chemotactic for fibroblasts and mononuclear cells. Therefore, the first few minutes and hours of wound repair are characterized by the formation of a provisional matrix, made up of fibrin and other extracellular proteins, and by the release of peptides that amplify the healing response. Neutrophils enter the wound within a few hours after wounding. It is often stated that these cells have as their main role wound debridement through the release of proteolytic enzymes. However, neutrophils themselves are rich sources of growth factors, particularly PDGF-like peptides, which contribute further to fibroblast stimulation and accumulation of extracellular matrix materials and to the recruitment of other cells.[4]

Macrophages are essential cells in the wound-healing process. They enter the wound site after the first 48–72 h[4] and secrete a number of growth factors, including TGF-beta, TNF-alpha and PDGF-like peptides. These peptides continue the ongoing stimulation of extracellular matrix formation and endothelial cell growth. The role of lymphocytes during wound healing is unclear. They are recruited into the wound through specific receptor–ligand interactions with endothelial cells, a process that is modulated by TGF-beta, TNF-alpha, IL-1 and gamma-interferon.[7] Lymphocytes may actually help downregulate and play a role in the remodeling phase of wound repair.[8] Throughout the cascade of events and the release of growth factors during healing, a central phenomenon is that of re-epithelialization. It appears that keratinocyte migration rather than mitosis is a more important component of this wound closure. A number of growth factors probably play a role in epidermal migration, including EGF, TGF-alpha and FGF. Wound fluid is in fact known to contain chemotactic activity for keratinocytes,[9] as well as other mitogens.

The topics we will address in the following sections are whether the growth factors we have just discussed with respect to the process of wound repair can be used in pharmacologic doses to upregulate or downregulate wound repair, and the kinds of wounds that may be amenable to this approach.

Acute and chronic wounds

The terms 'acute' and 'chronic' are obviously relative and cannot be precisely defined. In general, acute wounds are those that do not have an underlying healing defect and which are expected to heal easily without substantial treatment. Examples of acute wounds are simple cuts or injuries, excisions and split-thickness or even full-thickness defects in normal individuals. Chronic wounds are those expressed in tissues or individuals with an underlying healing defect. Examples of these wounds include venous ulcers, arterial ulcers and pressure-induced wounds in patients unable to move or sense their position properly, such as in individuals with diabetes or those confined to a bed or a wheelchair. An important consideration is that acute wounds behave as chronic wounds given an abnormal host. For example, a simple excision may not heal properly and within the expected period of time in a patient on high doses of systemic corticosteroids. Similarly, an injury to the leg of a patient with arterial insufficiency may become a therapeutic problem and be labeled as a chronic wound.

It has been the general expectation that growth factors will be important therapeutic agents in the treatment of chronic wounds. Substantial consideration has been given to the fact that chronic wounds may either lack growth factors or have a disturbed balance of these peptides. For example, wound fluid taken from acute wounds is highly stimulatory to cells in vitro,[10] while fluid taken from chronic wounds may lack this mitogenic activity.[11] Thus, acute wounds may have been partially overlooked thus far as a potential target for growth factors. In fact, dermatologic surgeons often deal with acute wounds that could benefit from an augmentation of the healing process, such as those left after Mohs micrographic surgery. Even after simple excision, the use of growth factors may perhaps result in decreased scarring by allowing faster and better healing. As we shall see later, better scarring may also result from antagonizing the effects of growth factors.

Nevertheless, it is easy to see why chronic wounds have attracted the most attention as a target for growth factors. Due to an ever-increasing elderly population in the USA and the rest of the Western world, the care of chronic wounds and its socio-economic impact have become important considerations. Faster ways to heal wounds would dramatically reduce costs and, given the information provided thus far on growth factors, it is not unreasonable to think that these peptides may be the answer to nonhealing wounds. Moreover, it is hoped that potent agents like growth factors would make up for the general lack of knowledge of the pathogenesis of chronic wounds, as well as our inability to change the underlying defect in these wounds.

Animal studies

As with any other drug, animal testing has been an important component of growth factor research in preparation for their use in human wounds. This approach has been valuable for obtaining safety information and for demonstrating the effectiveness of growth factors in acute wounds. The repair process in experimental animal wounds has been shown to be stimulated by the addition of EGF, PDGF, FGF and TGF-beta, among others.[1] In most animal studies the end-point has been the formation of granulation tissue and tensile strength.[12] However, particularly with EGF, re-epithelialization has also been shown to be augmented.[1] Thus, the evidence is clear that growth factors can accelerate wound repair in animal experimental wounds.

As we stated earlier, the hope has been that growth factors would make a difference in human chronic wounds. However, the problem is that no animal models exist that accurately reflect the pathology encountered in human chronic wounds. Some attempts have been made to re-create the human situation in animals. For example, wound animal models of immunosuppression or diabetes suggest a benefit from the topical application of growth factors. These studies have also suggested that a single growth factor may not be sufficient, and that a combination may have an additive effect. Thus, it was shown that a combination of EGF, PDGF and TGF-beta was superior to each of the growth factors alone in the repair of wounds in animals tested with Adriamycin.[13] However, the addition of FGF and PDGF was not better than either of the growth factors alone in accelerating healing in diabetic mice.[14]

TGF-BETA AND SCARRING

A great deal of interest has been generated recently by the possibility that scarring may be decreased by blocking the action of TGF-beta. There are at least three isoforms of TGF-beta in humans, but TGF-beta 1 and 2 are the best studied.[15] Originally isolated from sarcoma cells, TGF-beta 1 was eventually found to be secreted by most normal cells, and to be stored in platelets in large quantities. Thus, it is inevitable that TGF-beta 1 is present in the initial phases of wound repair. Further investigations have established TGF-beta as an important stimulus for extracellular matrix formation, including collagen, proteoglycans and fibronectin. There is a strong association of TGF-beta with fibrotic states, including scleroderma, cirrhosis and pulmonary fibrosis.[15] Recently, it was found in experimental animal wounds that the injection of antibodies to TGF-beta shortly after wounding markedly decreased subsequent scarring as compared to control animals.[16] This observation suggests that a similar approach may some day be possible in humans to decrease scarring, contractions and the formation of keloids. While the use of antibodies to TGF-beta may not be entirely safe, other safer approaches may be the use of decorin, a proteoglycan that binds TGF-beta, or a soluble form of TGF-beta receptor. These observations also serve to emphasize that augmentation of wound repair will not be the only role of growth factors, and that opposite effects may be achieved depending on how we use them.

HUMAN WOUNDS AND GROWTH FACTORS

The results we have described in the previous sections would suggest that successful use of growth factors in human wounds is well established, and that no doubt can exist as to the usefulness of these agents in human wounds. The reality is different, and we will try to analyze the reasons for this discrepancy.

Several growth factor trials have been done in humans.[17] However, very little of this has been published. The first indication that a growth factor may enhance healing in humans actually came from studies of acute wounds. It was shown that topically applied EGF enhanced re-epithelialization of split-thickness donor sites.[18] The results were encouraging but not dramatic. A double-blind, randomized trial in venous ulcers showed that the wounds treated with topical EGF healed faster than those in the placebo group.[19] However, while the trend favoring EGF was clear, the results were not statistically significant. Topical EGF was also shown to increase the healing of chronic wounds in an uncontrolled trial of chronic wounds.[20] Perhaps the most encouraging result to date is a study demonstrating a statistically significant improvement in venous ulcers treated with topical growth hormone.[21] Even more recent is a study indicating that topical PDGF enhances the healing of pressure sores.[22] In all of these studies the results favoring the growth factor have either been not significant or marginally so. Certainly, the results have not met the expectations derived from in vitro and animal data.

As we mentioned earlier, perhaps the approach with human wounds, particularly chronic wounds, should be a combination of growth factors. There are several obstacles to the implementation of this approach. First, the use of combinations may render more difficult the approval from regulatory agencies. Second, companies may be reluctant to test their product with a growth factor from another company. Third, combinations are expected to be more expensive and more difficult to market. A group led by Knighton et al has circumvented many of these difficulties by marketing a platelet releasate that is prepared from the patient's own platelets and which, in principle, contains a number of growth factors.[23] The results appear to be encouraging, but are still not spectacular, and the financial aspects are controversial.

A fair question is whether growth factors have fulfilled their promise as therapeutic agents for wounds, and whether we will ever see their widespread use. We believe that, ultimately, growth factors will indeed represent a substantial addition to other surgical techniques. We can think of several reasons why the results obtained in clinical trials thus far are not of the degree that was expected. First, the dose used in humans was derived from animal data, and may have been far too low for a chronic wound. Second, the delivery of the peptide remains a problem, particularly in chronic wounds, which are characterized by a microenvironment that is perhaps not suitable for growth factors. Third, the fate of the peptide after its delivery into the wound is virtually unknown, and it is unclear whether it actually stays within the wound.

Conclusions

For dermatologic surgeons, growth factors are likely to be important in ways that are different from other surgical fields. For example, the augmentation of tensile strength by growth factors will have less impact on dermatologic surgery. What will be important is faster re-epithelialization and better cosmetic appearance. Thus, at least potentially, growth factors could become an integral component of the care of Mohs micrographic surgery wounds, which are often very large and expensive to repair. Whether growth factor application will bring substantial benefits to other procedures, such as dermabrasion or hair transplantation, is difficult to predict at this time. One application that is still theoretical at this point is the use of growth factors to decrease wrinkling and aging. Based on what we know of these peptides, this is not an unreasonable expectation. As mentioned earlier, blocking the action of growth factors and thus reducing scarring will probably have an important role in dermatologic surgery.

Acknowledgment

Supported by National Institutes of Health Grant AR39658.

References

1. Rothe M, Falanga V, Growth factors: their biology and promise in dermatologic diseases and tissue repair, *Arch Dermatol* (1989) **125**:1390–8.

2. Sporn MB, Roberts AB, Peptide growth factors are multifunctional, *Nature* (1988) **332**:217–19.

3. Alberts B, Bray D, Lewis J et al, *Molecular biology of the cell*, 2nd edn (Garland Publishing: New York 1989) 681–726.

4. Clark RAF, Cutaneous tissue repair: basic biologic considerations. I, *J Am Acad Dermatol* (1985) **13**:701–25.

5. Knighton DR, Hunt TK, Thakral KK et al, Role of platelets and fibrin in the healing sequence, *Ann Surg* (1982) **196**:379–87.

6. Senior RM, Skogen WF, Griffin GL et al, Effects of fibrinogen derivatives upon the inflammatory response, *J Clin Invest* (1986) **77**:1014–19.

7. Cai J-P, Falanga V, Chin Y-H, Transforming growth factor-beta 1 regulates the adhesive interactions between mononuclear cells and microvascular endothelium, *J Invest Dermatol* (1991) **97**:169–74.

8. Cai JP, Harris B, Falanga V et al, Recruitment of mononuclear cells by endothelial cell binding into wounded skin is a selective, time-dependent process with defined molecular interactions, *J Invest Dermatol* (1990) **95**:415–21.

9. Martinet N, Harne L, Grotendorst GR, Characterization of epidermal chemoattractants, *J Invest Dermatol* (1988) **90**:122–6.

10. Katz MH, Alvarez A, Kirsner R et al, Human wound fluid from acute wounds stimulates fibroblast and endothelial cell growth, *J Am Acad Dermatol* (1991) **25**:1054–8.

11. Bucalo B, Eaglstein WH, Falanga V, The effect of chronic wound fluid on cell proliferation in vitro, *J Invest Dermatol* (1989) **92**:408.

12. Mustoe TA, Pierce GF, Thomason A et al, Accelerated healing of incisional wounds in rats induced by transforming growth factor-beta, *Science* (1987) **237**:1333–6.

13. Lawrence WT, Norton JA, Sporn MB et al, The reversal of an adriamycin induced healing impairment with chemoattractants and growth factors, *Ann Surg* (1986) **203**:142–7.

14. Greenhalgh DG, Sprugel KH, Murray MJ et al, PDGF and FGF stimulate wound healing in the genetically diabetic mouse, *Am J Pathol* (1990) **136**:1235–46.

15. Massague J, The transforming growth factor-beta family, *Annu Rev Cell Biol* (1990) **6**:597–641.

16. Shah M, Foreman DM, Ferguson MWJ, Control of scarring in adult wounds by neutralising antibody to transforming growth factor-beta, *Lancet* (1992) **339**:213–14.

17. Ratafia M, Clinical trials on growth factors for wound healing, *Wounds* (1991) **3**:79–82.

18. Brown GL, Nanney LB, Griffin J et al, Enhancement of wound healing by topical treatment with epidermal growth factor, *N Engl J Med* (1989) **321**:76–9.

19. Falanga V, Growth factors: status and expectations. In: Leaper DJ, ed., *International Symposium on Wound Repair* (Medicom Europe BV: The Netherlands 1991) 87–93.

20. Brown GL, Curtsinger L, Jurkiewicz MJ et al, Stimulation of healing of chronic wounds by epidermal growth factor, *Plast Reconstr Surg* (1991) **88**:189–94.

21. Rasmussen LH, Karlsmark T, Avnstorp C et al, Topical growth hormone treatment of chronic leg ulcers. In: Leaper DJ, ed., *International Symposium on Wound Repair* (Medicom Europe BV: The Netherlands 1991) 257–9.

22. Robson MC, Phillips LG, Thomason A et al, Platelet-derived growth factor BB for the treatment of chronic pressure ulcers, *Lancet* (1992) **339**:23–5.

23. Knighton DR, Ciresi K, Fiegel VA et al, Stimulation of repair in chronic, non-healing, cutaneous ulcers using platelet-derived wound healing formula, *Surg Gynecol Obstet* (1990) **170**:56–60.

Chapter 6

THE SUN, OZONE DEPLETION AND SKIN CANCER

Quan H. Nguyen
Ronald L. Moy

THE OZONE CRISIS

Most of the harmful ultraviolet (UV) radiation from the sun is absorbed by the thin layer of ozone surrounding the earth's atmosphere. This ozone layer is formed by the conversion of some of the oxygen present in the atmosphere by UV radiation. It is divided into the upper stratosphere (10–50 km above sea level) and the lower troposphere (the first 10 km above sea level). The sun emits large amounts of UVC (200–290 nm), UVB (290–320 nm) and UVA (320–400 nm) radiation; however, only UVA and a small amount of UVB actually penetrate the ozone and reach the surface of the earth. The most biologically effective and carcinogenic radiation in the sunlight spectrum is from the UVB region and its penetration is dependent on changes in the atmospheric ozone concentration.[1]

In 1985, Farman et al[2] reported a dramatic decrease of the ozone column over Halley Bay station in Antarctica in the late winter and early spring from the period of 1957 to 1973. The so-called 'Antarctic hole' was later confirmed by the Nimbus-7 satellite measurement and appeared to span the entire continent, and continued to grow larger.[3] This depletion in the stratospheric ozone, as much as 40% during the spring, may cause a great amount of the damaging UV radiation to reach the earth's surface. The International Ozone Trends Panel formed later by NASA concluded that the Antarctic ozone concentration has decreased at an average of approximately 2–3% over the past 20 years.[4] Newer startling evidence from NASA early in 1992 revealed that the ozone hole is not just limited to Antarctica. A new hole in the earth's protective shield could soon open north of the 50° latitude which covers Russia, Scandinavia, Germany, Britain, Canada and northern parts of the USA.

The effects of man-made chlorofluorocarbons (CFCs) are thought to be primarily responsible for this ozone depletion. Chlorofluorocarbons are nonflammable, nontoxic, relatively inert and highly stable compounds, which makes them very valuable commercially. They were initially developed in the 1930s and are used extensively in paints, deodorants, hairsprays, fire extinguishers, insulation, refrigeration, and air conditioners. In the early 1970s, billions of pounds of these compounds were being produced per year and studies have shown that most of these have ended up in the earth's atmosphere without being degraded. The same inert property that makes these compounds popular for technological use also helps them to remain in the atmosphere for up to 100 years. In 1974, Molina and Rowland[5] reported that these CFCs, mainly in the upper stratosphere sink, would be photolyzed by UV radiation to release chlorine atoms. These atoms would then combine with the surrounding ozone to create chlorine oxide and diatomic oxygen, causing a catalytic destruction of the ozone layer and decreasing its ability to absorb UVB radiation.[8] Subsequently, in 1978 the USA banned the use of CFCs in aerosol sprays. However, the nonaerosol uses have since become increasingly popular in developing countries, where CFCs are used as cleansers in the electronic and computer industries.

Other important factors known to be responsible for the reduction of stratospheric ozone are the halons, or bromochlorofluorocarbons, which are also used in major industries. It is believed that these bromine-containing compounds can destroy the stratospheric ozone at a faster rate than CFCs, and that they can cause an extra 4% reduction in the ozone column density in addition to that caused by CFCs. Recent studies also showed that additional ozone depletion can result from the reaction of the ozone with nitric oxide generated by solar protons associated with solar flares.[7]

Ultraviolet radiation and skin cancer

While it is known that increased UVB radiation exposure can cause increased skin cancer risks, evidence for increased UVB flux from stratospheric ozone depletion had not been well documented. Surface measurement of biologically effective solar radiation in the USA from 1974 to 1985 by Scotto et al[8] failed to detect any increase in UVB at ground levels. Climatic, meteorological and environmental factors such as cloudiness and surface reflectivity due to snow cover have been suggested to attenuate the UVB radiation reaching the earth. However, recent studies have indicated a slight increase of about 1% of UVB per year in the Alpine regions from 1981 to 1989.[9] Variations in the earth's atmospheric conditions as described above are now thought to have masked the slight increase in UVB radiation. This trend agrees with the reported 3% ozone reduction in the Northern Hemisphere from 1969 to 1986 by Lindley[10] and a more updated estimate of 4–5% ozone depletion in the past decade by the National Aeronautics and Space Administration in 1991. Earlier predictions had also estimated that up to 2% increase in UVB amount can result from each 1% decrease in stratospheric ozone.[4]

The most effective biological wavelength for producing erythema on Caucasian skin is 297 nm in the UVB spectrum. A small increase in UVB radiation from ozone depletion thus can certainly be detrimental to human health. The most obvious effect would be increased incidences of basal cell and squamous cell carcinomas. Other possible effects include the development of cutaneous melanoma, ocular changes leading to cataracts, and immunologic disturbances.

Most cutaneous basal cell and squamous cell carcinomas occur on the sun-exposed areas of the body. The incidence of these cancers also increases with increasing age and sun exposure. This evidence suggests that sunlight is a significant factor in the development of cutaneous carcinoma. It is estimated that over 600 000 cases of nonmelanoma skin cancers occur each year in the USA. This incidence is continuing to rise with increased exposure to UVB radiation, changes in clothing styles, and increased longevity. This rise in skin cancer incidence cannot be solely due to ozone depletion because ozone measurements have only been recently reported while skin cancers are usually induced over several decades.[11] Nevertheless, if significant stratospheric ozone depletion continues to occur then the incidence of skin cancers will exceed what has already been reported in the past decade. Many studies have estimated an increase of non-melanoma skin cancer of 2–3% for each percentage decrease in ozone.[12,13] Moan et al[14] has calculated that each ozone depletion of 1% will result in an increase in the incidence of basal cell carcinomas of 2.1% and of squamous cell carcinomas of 1.7%. The 1991 International Symposium on the Environmental Threat to the Skin estimated that a 10% reduction in total column ozone by the year 2050 will produce an extra 12 million cases of skin cancer and 200 000 skin cancer deaths in the USA alone.

There is some evidence now suggesting that at least some cutaneous melanomas are related to UVB radiation exposure. In the USA the incidence of melanoma appears to depend on latitude and increases with proximity to the equator. Patients with xeroderma pigmentosum have a higher tendency to develop cutaneous melanoma because they lack the ability to repair DNA damaged by UVB radiation.[15] In addition, studies on animal models have suggested that UVB radiation can induce growth of melanomas.[16] However, there is still no direct relationship between sunlight exposure and melanoma incidence since many melanomas do not occur on sun-exposed body sites.

New findings in photoimmunology have suggested that UVB radiation exposure can cause disturbances in the immune system, leading to increased skin cancer risks. Studies on experimental animals have shown that after exposure to UVB radiation, Langerhans cells are decreased in number and are no longer capable of presenting antigen to helper T-lymphocytes.[17] Also, when a contact allergen is applied to UV-irradiated skin, it fails to induce contact allergy.[18] It was later found that exposure to UVB radiation can result in the generation of T-suppressor lymphocytes that prevent the function of an immune surveillance system responsible for detecting and eradicating UV-induced tumors or transformed cells.[19]

Conclusion

Because of growing scientific evidence and increasing public concerns over the biological hazards of the ozone depletion, a Montreal Protocol on Protection of the Ozone Layer was signed by over 50 industrial nations in September 1987 and took effect in January 1989. Under this agreement, production of the five major CFCs (CFC-11, CFC-12, CFC-113, CFC-114 and CFC-115) and halons 1211 and 1301 would be reduced by 35% and consumption cut by 50% each year. Some of these CFCs are commonly used in refrigerants by dermatologists who perform dermabrasion. Elimination of the refrigerants could affect the future method of skin freezing. This original Montreal Protocol was criticized by many for not going far enough since it has been shown by the US Environmental Protection Agency that an 85% reduction of CFCs would be needed just to stabilize levels in the atmosphere.[20] A second Montreal Protocol was subsequently drawn up in June 1990, planning to phase out production and consumption of CFCs and halons by the year 2000.

The development of alternative compounds is a key factor in the plan to phase out CFCs and halons. Two popular substitute compounds are now being developed: the hydrochlorofluorocarbons (HCFCs), which contain lower levels of the destructive chlorine atoms than CFCs, and the hydrofluorocarbons (HFCs), which contain no chlorine at all. It has been estimated by Dupont, a major manufacturer of CFCs that up to 40% of the demand will be met by these CFC substitutes and another 32% will be met by the nonfluorocarbon products by the end of the century. However, the commercialization and full implementation of these substitute compounds are still years away and developing countries, which are dependent on CFCs, will certainly need assistance in making the economic transition.

The continuing problem of ozone depletion and how we handle it now will certainly affect future generations. As dermatologists we should be educating our patients on wearing protective garments and staying out of the sun. On the international level, we need to work for more cooperation and research to help protect our global atmosphere and human lives from the sun's damaging radiation.

References

1. Amron DM, Moy RL, Stratospheric ozone depletion and its relationship to skin cancer, *J Dermatol Surg Oncol* (1991) **17**:370–2.
2. Farman JC, Gardiner BG, Shanklin JD, Large losses of total ozone in Antarctica reveal seasonal ClOx/NOx interaction, *Nature* (1985) **315**:207–10.
3. Stolarski RS, Krueger AJ, Schoeberl MR et al, Nimbus-7 satellite measurement of the springtime Antarctic ozone decrease, *Nature* (1986) **322**:808–12.
4. Watson RT, Prather MJ, Kurylo MJ, Present state of knowledge of the upper atmosphere in 1988: an assessment report (Reference Publication 1208, NASA: Greenbelt, MD 1988).
5. Molina MJ, Rowland FS, Stratospheric sink for chlorofluoromethanes–chlorine atomic-catalyzed destruction of ozone, *Nature* (1974) **249**:810–12.
6. Prather MJ, McElroy MB, Wofsy SC, Reductions in ozone at high concentrations of stratospheric halogens, *Nature* (1984) **312**:227–31.
7. Stephenson JA, Scourfield WJ, Importance of energetic solar protons in ozone depletion, *Nature* (1991) **352**:137–9.
8. Scotto J, Cotton G, Urbach F et al, Biologically effective ultraviolet radiation: surface measurement in the United States, 1974–1985, *Science* (1988) **239**:762–4.
9. Blumthaler M, Ambach W, Indication of increasing solar ultraviolet-B radiation flux in Alpine regions. *Science* (1990) **248**:206–8.
10. Lindley D, CFCs cause part of global ozone decline. *Nature* (1988) **323**:293.
11. Kripke ML, Impact of ozone depletion on skin cancers, *J Dermatol Surg Oncol* (1988) **14**:853–7.
12. Kelfkens G, DeGruijl FR, VanderLeun JC, Ozone depletion and increase in annual carcinogenic ultraviolet dose, *Photochem Photobiol* (1990) **52**:819–23.
13. Henriksen T, Dahlback A, Larson S et al, Ultraviolet radiation and skin cancer: effect of an ozone layer depletion, *Photochem Photobiol* (1990) **51**:579–82.
14. Moan J, Dahlback A, Henriksen T et al, Biological amplification factor for sunlight-induced nonmelanoma skin cancer at high latitudes, *Cancer Res* (1989) **49**:5207–12.
15. Kraemer KH, Lee MM, Scotto J, DNA repair protects against cutaneous and internal neoplasia: evidence from xeroderma pigmentosum, *Carcinogenesis* (1984) **5**:511–4.
16. Ross PM, Carter DM, Actinic DNA damage and pathogenesis of cutaneous malignant melanoma, *J Invest Dermatol* (1989) **92**:293–6S.

17. Fisher MS, Kripke ML, Suppressor T lymphocytes control the development of primary skin cancers in ultraviolet-irradiated mice, *Science* (1982) **216**:1133–34.

18. Elmets CA, Bergstresser PR, Tigelar RE et al, Analysis of the mechanism of unresponsiveness produced by haptens painted on skin exposed to low dose ultraviolet radiation, *J Exp Med* (1983) **158**:781–94.

19. Morison WL, Effects of ultraviolet radiation on the immune system in humans, *Photochem Photobiol* (1989) **50**:515–24.

20. Koehler J, Hajost SA, The Montreal protocol: a dynamic agreement for protecting the ozone layer, *Ambio* (1990) **19**:82–6.

Chapter 7

NEW INDICATIONS FOR CRYOSURGERY IN INFECTED PATIENTS

Gloria F. Graham
Douglas Torre

There are a number of new innovations in the use of cryosurgery. This chapter will explore some of these with the aim of especially looking at how cryosurgery may be used in an era where AIDS has had a profound impact on the way we manage patients and protect ourselves. There are several specific uses for cryosurgery in treating patients with infectious disorders such as chromoblastomycosis, leishmaniasis, molluscum contagiosum, verruca vulgaris and condyloma acuminata, and these will be explored as well.

Cryosurgery is a relatively risk-free, bloodless therapy which may be used in a variety of conditions and tumors in high-risk patients. For physicians who are dealing with a large population of patients with AIDS and hepatitis, cryosurgery is now becoming a safe alternative to other procedures where more exposure would be anticipated.

AVOIDING CROSS-CONTAMINATION IN CRYOSURGICAL TREATMENT

Use of strict precautions against transfer of the HIV virus from an infected patient to the physician, other health care workers, as well as to another patient has gained worldwide acceptance.[1,2] Although cryosurgery has an advantage over scalpel excision, curettage or electrosurgery in that in most instances the equipment does not touch bleeding surfaces, there is still a danger of cross-contamination. If liquid nitrogen spray is used to treat a lesion which has been biopsied or is ulcerated, contaminated blood can be spattered or rebound on the tip of the spray unit. This holds true even for intact lesions which have been anesthetized by injection. Frequently a drop of blood oozes out of the puncture site. Cryoprobes obviously can even more easily be contaminated. Contamination can also occur from body fluid when moist mucous membranes are treated. The HIV virus gets the most publicity with blood contaminants, but the hepatitis B and C viruses are much more likely to cause infection.

Therefore it is important to use noncontaminated cryosurgical devices for each patient. Cryoprobes and spray tips can be sterilized by autoclave or a dry heat sterilizer. This routinely takes several hours. However, all metal cryoprobes and spray tips can be rapidly sterilized in small ovens at high heat. One that may be used is a toaster oven which heats the equipment to 250°C in less than 5 min (Toaster, Sanyo). An oven thermometer is affixed behind the glass door so the temperature can be confirmed. If the equipment is to be used immediately after sterilization it can be cooled in cold water or by a squirt of liquid nitrogen before handling. The oven is poorly insulated so that the top and sides become quite warm.

DISPOSABLE DEVICES

Disposable devices are helpful in avoiding HIV cross-contamination.[3] Disposable cotton-tipped swabs (such as Q-tips) have been used for many years. However, if the swab is applied to the lesion and redipped in the liquid nitrogen container before reapplication to another lesion on the patient, the container can be contaminated. If a Styrofoam cup is used as the container, it can be discarded with the swab after each patient. Dolezal reported on a special device, the Frigiderm Asepticator (Delasco, Council Bluffs, Iowa), which contains a small stainless steel vessel which can be heat sterilized.[4] However, if the cryosurgeon has a spray apparatus with a luerlock fitting, hollow-shaft swabs with cotton on each end can be used. If the swab is cut in half, a No. 14 hypodermic needle (Figure 7.1) will fit into the hollow shaft and then onto the spray unit so liquid nitrogen can be squirted intermittently into the shaft, saturating the cotton swab at the end. If No. 14 needles are not available, disposable No. 16, 17 or 18 needles may be inserted through the cotton at one end, and the other end used to treat the lesions.[3]

Hypodermic needles can be used as spray tips. All-metal reusable No. 15, 16, 17 and 18 needles with sharp tips removed with a small tube cutter can be heat sterilized between patients. If disposable plastic and metal needles are to be used, it is not necessary to remove the sharp tip (Figure

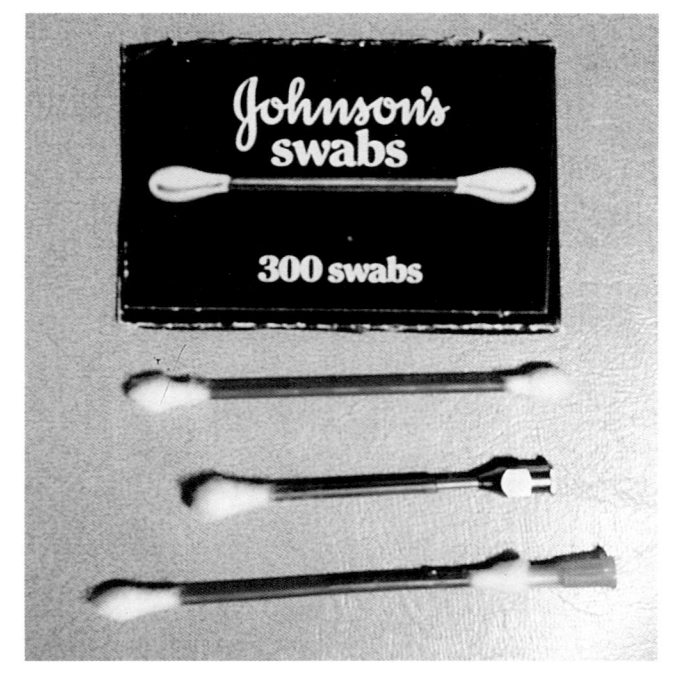

Figure 7.1
Hollow stem swabs for use with spray apparatus.

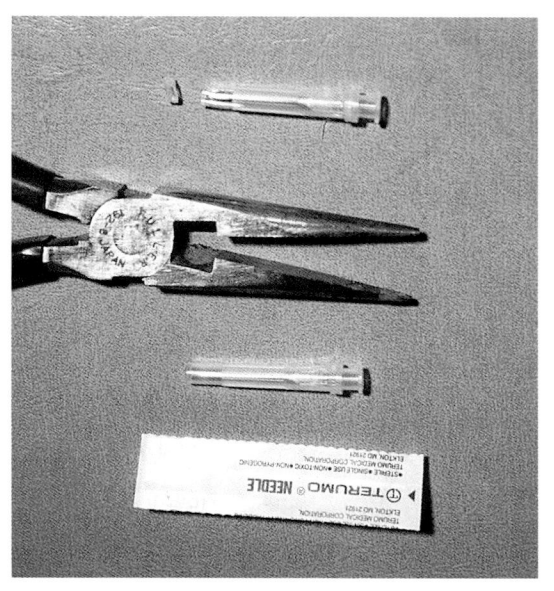

Figure 7.2
Sixteen gauge disposable needles with scabbards in place for liquid nitrogen spray. End of scabbard may be clipped off with cutting pliers.

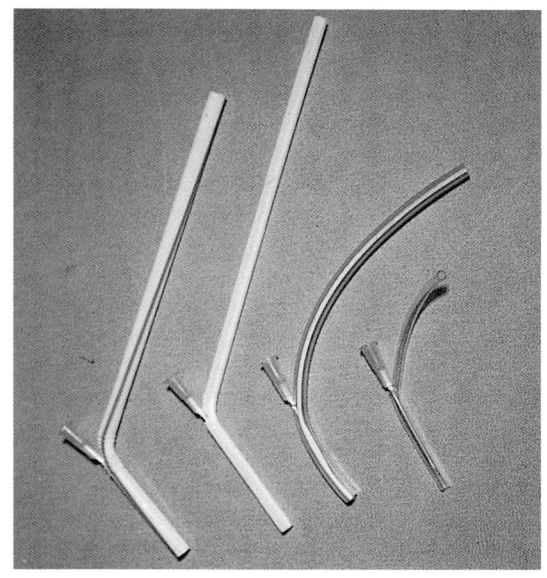

Figure 7.3
Tubing with needle for surface-limiting liquid nitrogen spray.

7.2). The needle is left in its scabbard and the tip of the scabbard clipped off with cutting pliers or a similar instrument. This takes much less time than removing the sharp tip and does not distort the lumen of the needle.

LIMITING DEVICES

A useful device for limiting application of cold is the disposable plastic otoscope cone, which comes with various size openings. An alternative to using otoscope cones is to use disposable segments of plastic tubing with different diameters. By slanting a hypodermic needle through the wall and positioning the needle tip near the tubing opening, we can treat various-diameter areas (Figure 7.3). These surface-limiting devices can be used with pressure as an alternative to cryoprobes. For bleeding or oozing surfaces, Blenderm tape (3M, St Pauls, MN) can be applied over the contact area of the tubing, converting it to a true cryoprobe. Some of these devices have been particularly useful in treating skin lesions frequently seen in AIDS patients such as Kaposi's sarcoma, molluscum contagiosum, and various types of warts, including condylomata acuminata.[3]

TREATMENT OF KAPOSI'S SARCOMA IN AIDS

The goals in treating lesions of Kaposi's sarcoma in AIDS patients are to safely and effectively reduce morbidity and improve cosmetic appearance (Figure 7.4). Cryosurgery works best for small thin lesions in cosmetically sensitive areas (face,

SURGICAL DERMATOLOGY

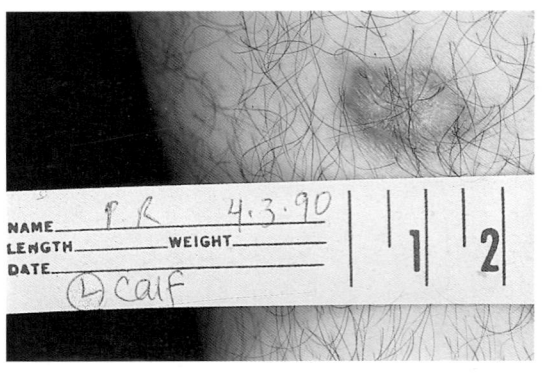

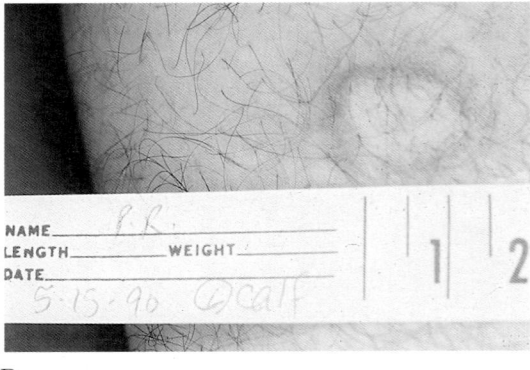

Figure 7.4
(A) Kaposi's sarcoma before cryosurgery. (B) Kaposi's sarcoma 6 weeks after cryosurgery.

ears, hands, forearms) and the earlier these lesions can be treated, the better. Using short applications of liquid nitrogen spray (open spray or limited on surface by disposable otoscope cone or by spraying into a hollow Q-tip or disposable tubing) excellent results can be obtained. A freeze time of 15–30 s with a thaw time of less than 30 s is usually satisfactory for lesions less than 1 cm in diameter. When using restricted spray with otoscope cones, spraying until the lateral spread of freeze extends 2–3 mm peripheral to the cone can be used for depth dose estimation. If one treatment is not sufficient, a repeat at 3–4 weeks is in order. These small lesions, if treated by radiography, end up flat, but with a brown stain that is not well accepted cosmetically.

Large, deep lesions can be treated for palliation but long freezes with a thaw time of 2 min or more may lead to permanent depigmentation and poor cosmetic result. For these lesions radiographic treatment may be superior. Cryosurgery can also be employed concurrently with other treatments.

Tappero et al[5] treated 20 subjects with liquid nitrogen using double freeze–thaw cycles with thaw time ranging from 11 to 60 s per cycle. Treatment was repeated at 2–3-week intervals if indicated and the average number of treatments per lesion was three. There was an 80% complete response with a 50% cosmetic response. Odom[6] also used two freeze–thaw cycles of 30–45 s. Stickler and Friedman-Kien[7] and Serfling and Hood[8] have also used cryosurgery for Kaposi's sarcoma lesions.

MOLLUSCUM CONTAGIOSUM

Molluscum contagiosum, which occurs frequently in AIDS patients,[9] can also be treated by cryosurgery. For individual lesions, spraying liquid nitrogen into an otoscope cone with a small opening is advised. The spray is continued until a white frozen zone about 1 mm in radius appears surrounding the cone. For areas which are studded with numerous mollusca close together, the area can be treated by a brief spray of liquid nitrogen evenly covering the area. It is suggested that the areas involved with mollusca be washed twice daily with an antimicrobial skin cleanser.

CHROMOBLASTOMYCOSIS

Chromoblastomycosis, a chronic fungal infection of the skin and subcutaneous tissues, may be caused by several different fungi, including *Fonsecaea pedrosoi*, *Cladosporium carrionii* and *Phialophora verrucosa*. The lesions are usually on exposed areas and are quite unresponsive to treatment. The most effective chemotherapeutic agents have been 5-fluorocytosine (5-FC) orally or 5-FC plus amphotericin B intravenously.[10]

Ramirez,[11] in 1973, first used cryosurgery to treat chromoblastomycosis. Several other authors, including Lubritz and Spence,[12] Nobre et al[13] and Sittart and Valente[14] reported on its effectiveness. Pimentel et al[15] reported in 1989 on their success in treating 11 cases of chromoblastomycosis with liquid nitrogen over a period of 8 years. The freeze times varied from 30 s up to 3 min and larger lesions were treated with multiple freezing cycles. In the treatment of multiple lesions, a few centimeters of normal skin were left in between to avoid confluence and formation of large ulcers.

After-care includes analgesics, $KMnO_4$ 1:40 000 solution soaks twice daily and occlusive bandages for control of bleeding. Healing is in 3–6 weeks, usually with a flat, smooth, shiny scar. One extensive area on the buttock healed after 10 cryosurgical sessions with no relapse after 53 months. Relapses are treated in the same manner as the primary lesions.[15]

While cryosurgery has proved to be a safe treatment, there are several complications, including exposure of joints in two cases, and scar formation in 11 cases. Eight (72.7%) of 11 patients were cured while three (27.3%) showed some clinical improvement, but with persistent active lesions. Localized lesions (100%) responded better than generalized ones (50%).[15]

Not only did the treatment prove effective, but it was also less costly than 5-FC. Hospitalization was often avoided with cryosurgery and the patients could, in many cases, continue their normal activities at home.[15] Gamboa and Belfort at the 10th Annual Meeting of the American College of Cryosurgery on Marguerita Island, Venezuela, presented three cases of chromoblastomycosis present for 21–35 years. These were controlled with cryosurgery for up to 4 years.

CUTANEOUS LEISHMANIASIS

Cutaneous leishmaniasis due to *L. major* or *L. tropica* is endemic in the Middle East, especially Saudi Arabia. While the disease heals spontaneously and with immunity, treatment is indicated to reduce the reservoir of infections. Morsy et al[16] compared treatment with sodium stibogluconate (Pentostam) in 57 patients and cryosurgery in 38 patients.

The systemic pentavalent antimonial drug is recommended if lesions are inflamed or ulcerated, have lymphatic involvement, are in areas where scarring might prove disfiguring, or involve cartilage. Of 95 patients 38 were treated by cryosurgery using a 1-cm probe. Freeze time was 60–90 s with a 1–2-mm margin of normal skin frozen around the lesion. A double freeze–thaw cycle was used in some. Multiple lesions, usually on the extremities or face, were not uncommon, especially in those patients from nonendemic areas.[16]

Robles reported at the International Course on Cryosurgery, 1992, in Mexico City that leishmaniasis in Guatemala responded to freezing the lesions with liquid nitrogen and monitoring with thermocouple needles to −40°C or −60°C. One hundred patients were treated, with a total of 137 lesions. One hundred and ten lesions (80.3%) were controlled (Figure 7.5).

VERRUCAE

Lembo et al[17] treated 432 consecutive patients with common, filiform, flat, keratotic palmar, plantar and periungual warts by liquid nitrogen spray. One

SURGICAL DERMATOLOGY

A

B

C

D

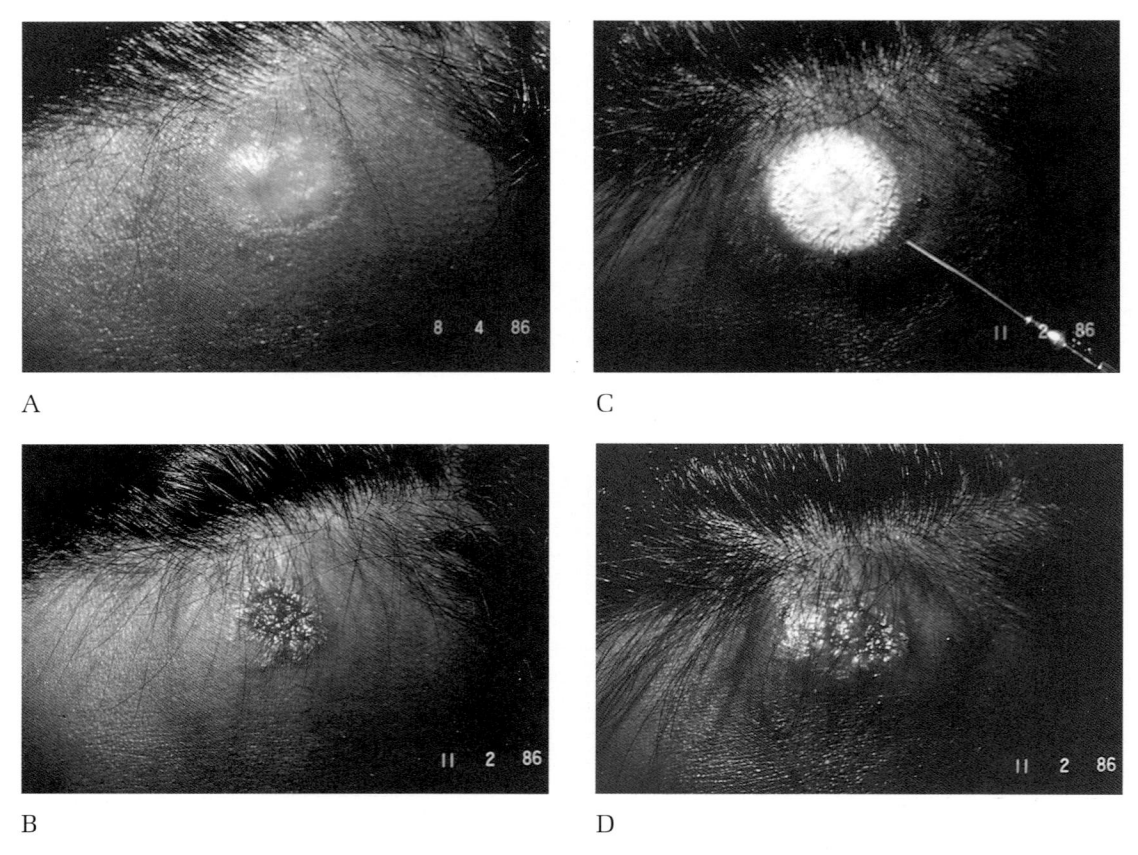

Figure 7.5
Leishmaniasis treated by cryosurgery using liquid nitrogen to freeze lesion on −40 °C. (A) Hypopigmented scar resulting from cryosurgery of lesion of leishmaniasis (August, 1986). (B) Recurrent lesion of leishmaniasis is treated a second time in November, 1986. (C) Site treated by liquid nitrogen spray to −40 °C. (D) Marked edema immediately after cryosurgery. The area cleared after the second freeze. (Courtesy of Dr Eduardo Robles.)

freeze–thaw cycle per visit was used every 2 weeks for flat warts and a double freeze–thaw cycle for other warts. Tangential spray was used for elevated lesions. Pain following treatment of the periungual warts was the primary side-effect.

Clearing occurred in 89.1% of patients with verruca vulgaris on the back of the hand and in 100% of those with warts elsewhere on the face in from one to six treatments. Filiform warts showed a high cure rate of 97.7% after one or two treatments; for verrucae plana, 62.5% of patients were cleared on the face and 75% elsewhere after three to eight sessions (Figure 7.6). Periungual warts were only cleared in 55.5%, palmar in 57.9% and plantar in 52.3% after 5–12 treatments. The authors concluded that while cryosurgery was the treatment of choice for common and filiform

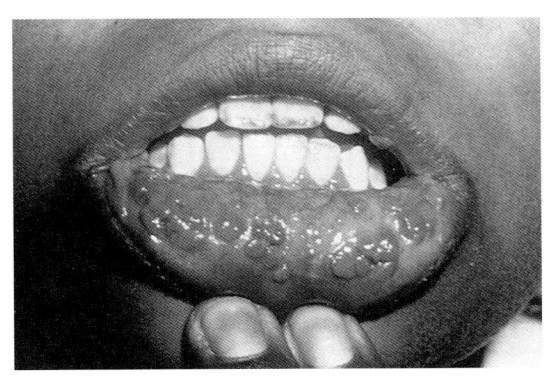

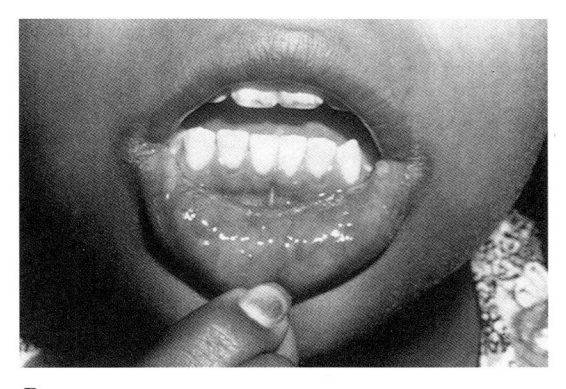

CONDYLOMATA ACUMINATA

While new therapies such as alpha-interferon,[21,22] podophyllotoxin[23] and laser[24] are helping significantly in the treatment of condylomata acuminata, a controlled study by Damstra and Van Vloten[25] of 64 patients using cryotherapy showed 83% of lesions resolving within 4 weeks and 96% after 6 weeks. While they used the Cry-Ac (Brymill Corporation, Vernon, CT), which has stainless steel tips, they found the tips too large and they developed a spray-tip device with a luerlock fitting. Disposable intravenous needles were used instead of the original spray tips. This form of fine-needle cryotherapy using an intermittent-spray technique achieved small regions of cryonecrosis and excellent results.

They compared condylline, podophyllin, electrocautery and cryotherapy using the standard tip and the fine-needle tip. The percentage cleared at 6 weeks was 87% with condylline, 63% with podophyllin, 45.9% with standard cryotherapy and 96% with fine-needle cryotherapy.

SUMMARY

The use of cryotherapy in the era of AIDS and for treatment of infectious conditions is increasing. This technique may help to decrease the chance of infection spreading to physicians and their employees and may also clear some infections that in the past have been difficult to eradicate.

REFERENCES

1. CDC Update: universal precautions for prevention of transmission of human immunodeficiency virus, hepatitis B virus, and other blood borne pathogens in health care settings, *MMWR* (1988) **37**:377–88.

2. Murphy SA, HIV and safety: universal precautions, *Clin Dermatol* (1991) **9**:31–8.

A

B

Figure 7.6
(A) A form of oral verrucae seen in Columbia, South America. (B) Postcryosurgery using liquid nitrogen spray. (Courtesy of Dr Carlos H. Gonzalez.)

warts, topical pharmacologic treatment should be considered first for other warts.[17]

The addition of bleomycin therapy for recalcitrant warts has been quite helpful for some patients.[18] Pretreating warts with pads or films containing salicylic and/or lactic acid speeds recovery and is a first line of therapy for many patients.[19] Carbon dioxide laser therapy shows great promise as well.[20]

3. Boulier J, Myskowshi P, Torre D, Disposable attachments in cryosurgery: a useful adjunct in the treatment of HIV-associated neoplasms, *J Dermatol Surg Oncol* (1991) **17**: 277–8.

4. Dolezal JF, A device to prevent cross contamination when directly applying liquid nitrogen, *J Dermatol Surg Oncol* (1991) **17**:827–8.

5. Tappero JW, Berger TG, Kaplan LW et al, Cryotherapy for Kaposi's sarcoma (KS) associated with acquired immune deficiency syndrome (AIDS): a phase II treatment, *J Acquired Immune Deficiency Syndromes* (1991) **4**:839–46.

6. Odom, RB, The management of AIDS-associated Kaposi's sarcoma, *Cosmet Dermatol* (1991) **10**:199.

7. Stickler MC, Freidman-Kien AE, Kaposi's sarcoma, *Clin Dermatol* (1991) **9**:39–47.

8. Serfling U, Hood AF, Local therapies for cutaneous Kaposi's sarcoma in patients with acquired immunodeficiency syndrome, *Arch Dermatol* (1991) **127**:1479–81.

9. Cockerell CJ, Cutaneous manifestations of HIV infection other than Kaposi's sarcoma: clinical and histologic aspects, *J Am Acad Dermatol* (1990) **22**:1260–9.

10. Bopp C, New method for the treatment of chromoblastomycosis. In: *Proceedings of the International Conference on the Mycoses*, Brasilia, 1977 (PAHO, Scientific Publications: Washington, DC: 1978) 33–4.

11. Ramirez MM, Treatment of chromomycosis with liquid nitrogen, *Int J Dermatol* (1973) **2**:250–4.

12. Lubritz RR, Spence JE, Chromoblastomycosis: cure by cryosurgery, *Int J Dermatol* (1978) **17**:830–2.

13. Nobre G, Oliveira AS, Verde F et al, Chromomycosis: report of a case and management by cryosurgery, topical chemotherapy and conventional surgery, *J Dermatol Surg Oncol* (1982) **5**:36–8.

14. Sittart JAS, Valente NYS, Tratamento da cromomicose pelo nitrogenio liquido, *Med Cutan Ibero Lat Am* (1986) **14**:227–32.

15. Pimentel ERA, Castro LGM, Cuce LC et al, Treatment of chromomycosis by cryosurgery with liquid nitrogen: a report on eleven cases, *J Dermatol Surg Oncol* (1989) **15**:1.

16. Morsy TA, Rahman EGA, Ahmed MM, Treatment of cutaneous leishmaniasis with pentostam or cryosurgery, *J Egyptian Soc Parasitol* (1989) **19**:533–43.

17. Lembo G, De Natale F, Rolando A et al, Cryotherapy of warts: evaluation by morphology and localization, *Ann Inter Dermatol Clin Spec* (1991) **45**:3.

18. Shumer SM, O'Keefe EJ, Bleomycin in the treatment of recalcitrant warts, *J Am Acad Dermatol* (1983) **9**:91–6.

19. Mottaz JH, McKeever PJ, Zelickson AS et al, Transdermal delivery of salicylic acid in the treatment of viral papillomas, *Int J Dermatol* (1988) **27**:596–600.

20. Street ML, Roenigk RK, Recalcitrant periungal verrucae: the role of CO_2 laser vaporization, *J Am Acad Dermatol* (1990) **23**:115–20.

21. Gall SA, Hughes CE, Trofatter K, Interferon for the therapy of condylomata acuminata, a new operative technique, *J Soc Med* (1978) **7**:180–5.

22. Eron LD, Judson F, Tucker S et al, Interferon therapy for condylomata acuminata, *N Engl J Med* (1986) **315**:1059–64.

23. Greenberg MD, Rutledge LH et al, A double-blind, randomized trial of 0.05% Podofilox and placebo for the

treatment of genital warts in women, *Obstet Gynecol* (1991) **75**:737–9.

24. Frirhurst MV, Roenigk RK, Brodland DG, Carbon dioxide laser surgery for skin disease, *Mayo Clin Proc* (1992) **67**:49–58.

25. Damstra RJ, Van Vloten WA, Cryotherapy in the treatment of condylomata acuminata: a controlled study of 64 patients, *J Dermatol Surg Oncol* (1991) **17**:273–6.

Section II

CUTANEOUS ONCOLOGY

8. ACTINIC KERATOSES (SOLAR KERATOSES)
   Ronald Marks

9. ADVANCES IN CRYOSURGERY FOR CUTANEOUS ONCOLOGY
   Gloria F. Graham, Douglas Torre

10. CHARACTERISTICS OF GIANT BASAL CELL CARCINOMA
    Henry W. Randle, Randall K. Roenigk

11. BASAL CELL CARCINOMA RECURRING FOLLOWING RADIOTHERAPY
    Steven P. Smith, Donald J. Grande

12. METASTATIC BASAL CELL CARCINOMA
    Jacob S. Lo, Stephen N. Snow, Frederic E. Mohs

13. MOHS MICROGRAPHIC SURGERY: EUROPEAN EXPERIENCE
    António Picoto, Francisco Camacho, Neil P.J. Walker, Alejandro Camps-Fresneda

14. IMMUNOHISTOCHEMICAL DIAGNOSIS OF SKIN TUMORS
    Ken Hashimoto, Mitsuru Setoyama, Eugene Hashimoto

15. SURGICAL MARGINS FOR NONMELANOMA SKIN CANCERS
    David G. Brodland

16. THE ROLE OF EMBRYOLOGIC STRUCTURAL DEVELOPMENT IN THE SPREAD OF CUTANEOUS CARCINOMA
    J. Michael Wentzell, June K. Robinson

17. TREATMENT AND PREVENTION OF BASAL CELL CARCINOMA WITH ORAL ISOTRETINOIN
    Gary L. Peck, John J. DiGiovanna, Kenneth H. Kraemer, Joseph A. Tangrea, Earl G. Gross

18. INTERFERON FOR SKIN CANCER
    Hubert T. Greenway

19. THE RISK OF DEVELOPING ANOTHER SKIN CANCER
    Michael M. Schreiber

20. METASTASIS: BASIC MECHANISMS AND APPLICATIONS IN DERMATOLOGY
    David G. Brodland

21. DERMATOFIBROSARCOMA PROTUBERANS
    Edmund R. Hobbs

22. ATYPICAL FIBROUS XANTHOMA AND MALIGNANT FIBROUS HISTIOCYTOMA
    Marc D. Brown

23. SEBACEOUS CARCINOMA OF THE EYELID
    Duane C. Whitaker

24. MANAGEMENT OF NEOPLASMS IN THE NAIL
    Robert Baran, Eckart Haneke

25. EXCISIONAL BIOPSY AND WIDE EXCISION FOR MALIGNANT MELANOMA
    Michael Landthaler

26. CURRENT MANAGEMENT OF THIN MELANOMA
    Sandhya Yadav, Darrell S. Rigel

27. MOHS MICROGRAPHIC SURGERY FOR MELANOMA
    Frederic E. Mohs

28. METASTASIS AND DEATH FROM THIN MELANOMA
    Edward T. Creagan

Chapter 8

ACTINIC KERATOSES (SOLAR KERATOSES)

Ronald Marks

INTRODUCTION

Actinic keratoses (AK) are generally categorized as 'premalignant lesions' of epidermis, although their exact relationship to squamous cell carcinoma (SCC) is not as straightforward as the term seems to imply (see pp. 79–80). They may be defined as localized areas of epidermal dysplasia caused by persistent exposure to solar radiation which are clinically evident as pink or gray scaling or warty patches, plaques or nodules. The biological importance of these common lesions is twofold. First, their presence indicates that a significant amount of solar injury has been sustained and that the skin on which they arise may develop a frankly neoplastic lesion. Second, because AKs are common and accessible, they are an excellent model for the study of neoplasia in general and photocarcinogenesis in particular.

Their general clinical importance is growing because of the aging population in most developed countries and of a marked change in social behavior resulting in ever-increasing opportunities for solar exposure. These trends suggest that at least for the foreseeable future these and similar disorders will occupy an ever-increasing proportion of dermatologic practice. Specifically, to the individual patient they are an annoyance: they are itchy and occasionally tender and painful, as well as cosmetically unpleasant.

EPIDEMIOLOGY

Actinic keratoses occur in all lightly pigmented peoples who live in warm sunny climates. The lighter the skin, hair and eye color, the more frequent and prolific are the lesions of AK. They are particularly prevalent in hot subtropical zones which have been colonized by fair-complexioned Europeans. The problem has been particularly well characterized in Australia where in recent years several surveys have been completed. One population survey in Mayborough found a prevalence rate in the adult population of 56.9% for the presence of at least one AK.[1] These lesions are also extremely common in the pale-skinned communities in the southern United States, South Africa and southern Europe.

Those most at risk are the red- or ginger-haired individuals or those with numerous freckles, who are often Irish, Scottish or Welsh descent. However, the susceptibility does not seem to be confined to the very-light-complexioned individuals of Celtic

SURGICAL DERMATOLOGY

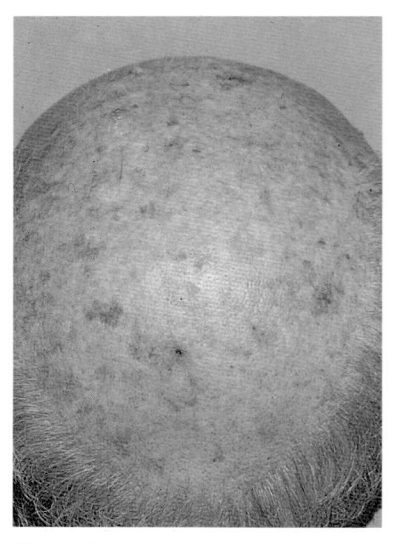

Figure 8.1
Scalp of man aged 65 with many pigmented patches and small scaling pink solar keratoses.

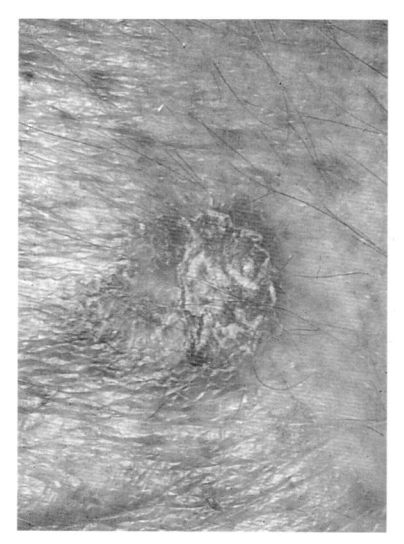

Figure 8.2
Scaling pink solar keratosis on back of hand.

ancestry, as some of the somewhat darker Celtic types are also prone to AKs. It has been suggested that this group of individuals have a minor fault in DNA repair, less than but similar to xeroderma pigmentosum.[2] In a recent survey in South Glamorgan in Wales some 24% (approximately 17% after validation) of the population over the age of 60 were found to have these lesions.[3]

CLINICAL FEATURES

Actinic keratoses may occur anywhere on exposed areas of skin but are seen particularly frequently on the forehead, the nose, the tops of the ears and the upper cheeks on the face. As may be expected, the dorsa of the hands, the extensor aspects of the forearms and the V of the neck are other areas that often have numerous AKs. They are also common on the bald areas of the scalp in men (Figure 8.1) and on the lower legs in women.

The usual clinical appearance is that of a small pink or gray scaling or warty patch or plaque up to 1 cm in diameter (Figure 8.2) but there is considerable variation.

Cutaneous horn

Solar keratosis is one of the common causes of a horny projection developing from a nodule of plaque (Figure 8.3). It was found to account for 23.2% of cutaneous horns by Yu et al.[4] Cutaneous horns were caused by benign epidermal lesions in 63.1% and by SCC in 15.7% in this study. Sometimes these horny lesions become very large, up to 2 cm in length being not especially uncommon.

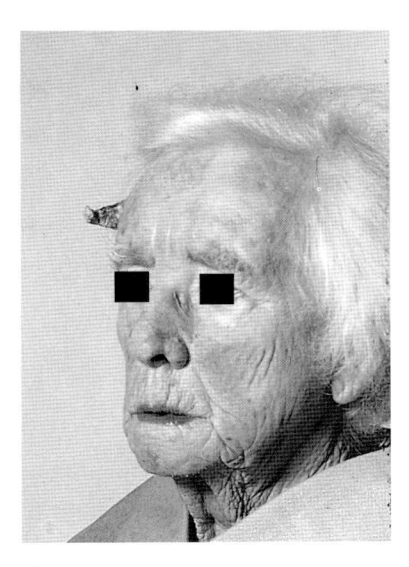

Figure 8.3
Cutaneous horn on side of forehead in elderly woman.

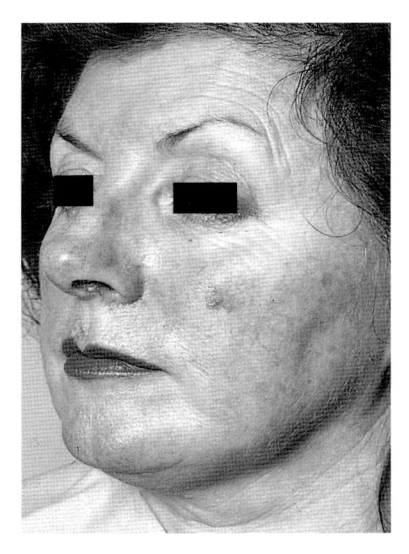

Figure 8.4
Biopsy-proven Lupus erythematosus-like keratosis on cheek of middle-aged woman.

Lupus erythematosus-like keratosis (lupoid AK)

It is quite often very difficult to tell whether a red scaling patch on the cheek or elsewhere on the face is a lesion of lupus erythematosus or an AK (Figure 8.4). In most cases a biopsy will clearly distinguish the two disorders but this is not always so. Severe photodamage and the presence of more easily identified AKs will aid the diagnosis of AK.

Pigmented actinic keratosis (spreading pigmented AK)

Some AKs are pigmented, flat and slightly scaly. Because of this it is difficult to determine, clinically or histologically, whether these lesions are AKs, flat seborrheic keratoses, senile lentigines or even lentigo maligna.[5,6] The lesions are said by James et al[7] to differ from ordinary AKs by their relatively large size (more than 1 cm in diameter) and by their tendency to spread centrifugally. The only difference histologically is the presence of pigment which has been confirmed ultrastructurally by Dinehart and Sanchez.[8]

Mucosal lesions

Dysplastic premalignant epithelial lesions due to chronic solar exposure occur on both the lips and the conjunctiva. Not unexpectedly, dermatologists tend to be consulted about the former but not about the latter. On the lips the disorder is known as solar cheilitis and is much more common on the lower lip. The affected area is less well marginated than on the skin and is characterized as a whitish,

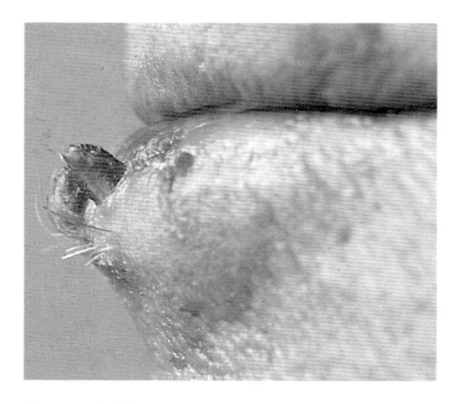

Figure 8.5
Severe solar cheilitis with horny projections suggesting that frank neoplastic change may have taken place.

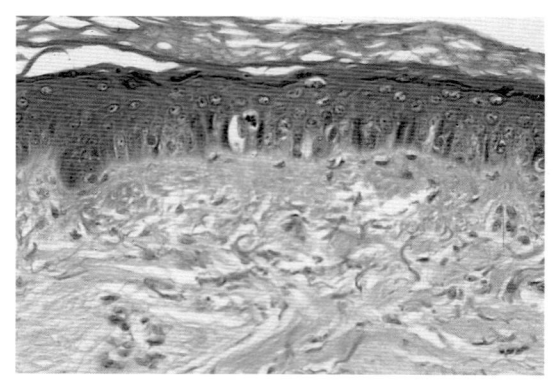

Figure 8.6
Sun-damaged skin showing minor degree of epidermal dysplasia with irregularity of cell size and shape and loss of cell polarity.

thickened, scaling and fissured patch (Figure 8.5).

Pathology and Pathophysiology

In severely photodamaged skin the epidermis shows minor degrees of abnormality in the absence of clinical lesions. There is focal irregularity in cell size, shape and polarity, along with nuclear irregularity and variability in staining (Figure 8.6). These alterations, which are referred to collectively as dysplasia, require a trained eye for detection. They are accompanied by an increase in the rate of epidermal cell replication as judged by the tritiated thymidine autoradiographic labeling indices.[9]

This clinically undetected focal alteration in the structure and behavior of epidermal cells is frequently present in severely photodamaged skin and is regarded as the first morphologically detectable step towards malignancy.

Actinic keratoses represent the next step. The cellular changes seen in AKs are similar to those already mentioned but more extensive. In addition, the cellular and nuclear heterogeneity is more marked and accompanied by a thickened and parakeratotic stratum corneum (Figure 8.7). Furthermore, AKs possess several quite typical features that are not present in minor degrees of dysplasia.

1. Alterations to the epidermal profile occur with irregular thickening and small bud-like downgrowths. Sometimes, however, instead of overall thickening there is flattening of the dermoepidermal junction and thinning of the epidermis (atrophic keratosis').
2. When a sweat duct drains to the surface via the affected epidermis its constituent cells are quite clearly normal and different from the surrounding dysplastic epidermis. This gives a funnel-like appearance within the lesion—the so-called 'Freundenthal funnel' (Figure 8.8).

ACTINIC KERATOSES (SOLAR KERATOSES)

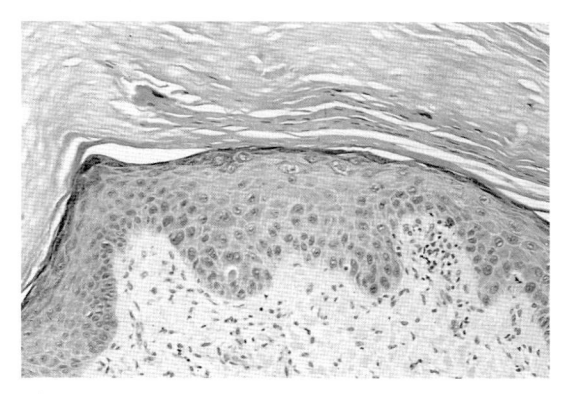

Figure 8.7
Solar keratosis showing nuclear irregularity and some parakeratosis.

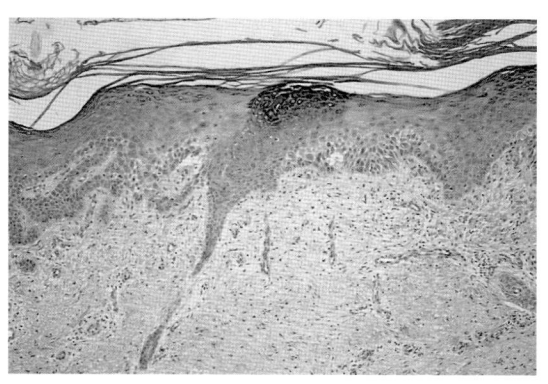

Figure 8.8
'Freundenthal funnel': note the abnormal appearance of the cells around the intraepidermal portion of the sweat duct.

3. Sheets of abnormal cells from the AK lesion may follow the margins of hair follicles at the edge of the AK and track downwards.
4. The abnormal cells of the keratosis are quite plainly delineated from the more normal tissue on either side, and the margin of the lesion is usually oblique rather than vertical, giving a wedge-shaped profile to the lesions (Figure 8.9).
5. Premature individual cell keratinization may occur within the body of the lesion (malignant dyskeratosis) in some thicker AK lesions and these cells are recognized as eosinophilic homogeneous bodies.

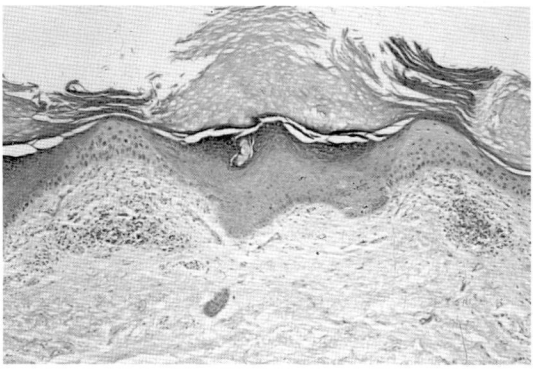

Figure 8.9
Solar keratosis. The abnormal cells are separated from the more normal cell population by an oblique border, making wedge-shaped areas of abnormality.

HISTOLOGIC VARIANTS

Lichenoid keratosis

Most AKs attract a degree of inflammatory cell infiltrate composed primarily of T lymphocytes. In some cases the infiltrate is dense and 'lichenoid' in that it hugs the dermoepidermal junction (Figure 8.10). Indeed, the similarity to lichen planus does not stop there, as basal liquefactive degenerative change occurs and cytoid bodies are

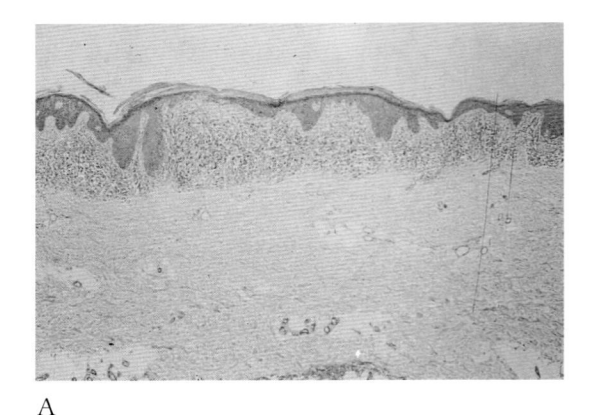

Figure 8.10
(A) Lichenoid solar keratosis showing inflammatory cells in a bank-like distribution beneath the epidermis.

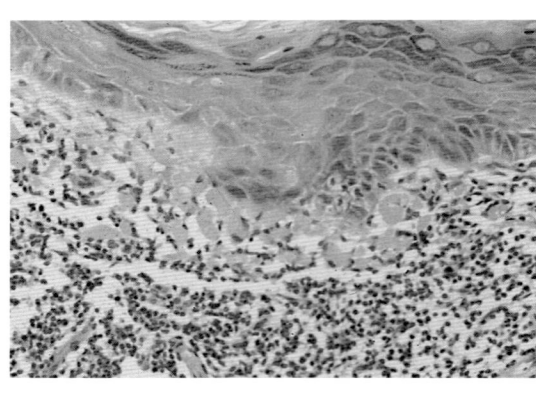

(B) Lichenoid keratosis. Notice the heavy infiltrate of lymphocytes and many cytoid bodies at the epidermal junction.

sometimes found. These 'lichenoid keratoses' are less uncommon than may be thought. In 212 lesions examined retrospectively, 6.1% exhibited the characteristic changes of lichenoid keratosis while the phenomenon occurred in 3 of 28 lesions (10.7%) studied prospectively.[10] The issue is discussed below (p. 80).

Bowenoid keratosis

In this lesion there is more marked dysplasia than in the ordinary AK and the abnormal cells occupy most of the thickness of the epidermis, so that the area looks somewhat like Bowen's disease histologically. In fact, the distinctions between this lesion and an ordinary solar keratosis on the one hand and between the Bowenoid keratosis and frank Bowen's disease on the other are those of degree and not kind. They may represent different points of development on the spectrum of 'premalignancy'. Clinically, the lesions do not differ from histologically less dysplastic lesions.

Darier-like keratosis

In some AKs the abnormally appearing cells become separated from the rest of the epidermis, making a cleft between the two sorts of epidermis. Because the cleft and the presence of dyskeratotic cells give a superficial resemblence to Darier's disease, these lesions are known as Darier-like keratoses, or sometimes 'carcinoma segregans.'[11] They are also known as acantholytic solar keratoses,[12] since in addition to the clefting described, individual cells may separate one from the other, giving a pemphigus-like acantholytic picture (Figure 8.11). The cleft is sometimes associated with a zone of vacuolation of epidermal cells or spongiosis.

The changes of Darier-like keratosis are by no means rare. We encountered them in 27% of 52 lesions examined prospec-

ACTINIC KERATOSES (SOLAR KERATOSES)

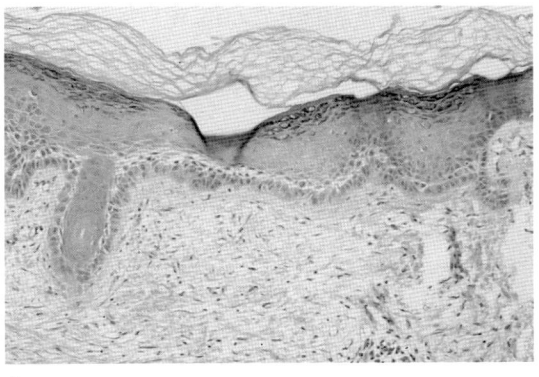

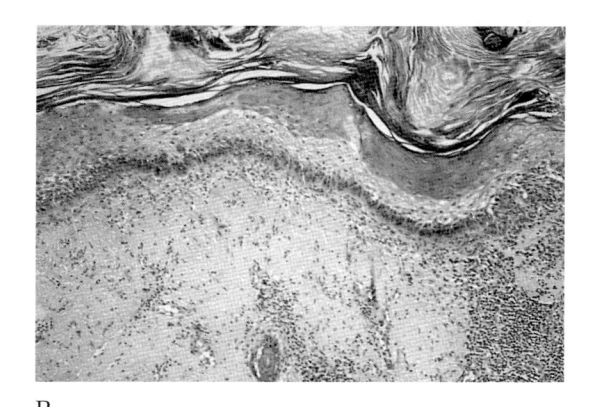

Figure 8.11
(A) Darier-like keratosis. There is a sheet of abnormal epidermal cells tracking at the base of the epidermis but separated from it. (B) Solar keratosis. There is an odd layered appearance to this histologic section of a solar keratosis, with a sheet of abnormal basaloid cells separating from more normal appearing epidermis. This is one appearance in Darier-like keratoses.

tively.[13] In our study the changes were found more commonly on the face and the lesions tended to be larger and histologically thicker and more dysplastic.

CAUSES OF KERATOSES OTHER THAN SOLAR EXPOSURE

There are several other agents and physical modalities that may cause premalignant lesions of the epidermis. These are in every way similar to AKs, but are much less common and occur at different sites. Keratoses occur in areas of erythema ab igne and indeed it is well established that chronic heat injury acts as a stimulus to carcinogenesis.[14] Keratoses may also occur anywhere on the skin surface, but seem curiously prone to develop on the palms and soles in chronic arsenical toxication. This was at one time not uncommon when arsenic was given in medication as a 'tonic'. Areas of radiation atrophy may develop premalignant epidermal lesions and these may well have a greater propensity to transform to SCC.

Erythroplasia of Queyrat is also a premalignant lesion that presents as an odd velvety plaque affecting the glans penis and has been related to HPV infection. Other mucosal sites on which development of premalignant epithelial lesions may occur include the vulvovaginal mucosa and the buccal mucosa; however, a full discussion of these lesions is outside the remit of this chapter (see Chapter 32).

NATURAL HISTORY AND IMMUNOLOGICAL ASPECTS

It is now quite clear that AKs do not transform into SCC as often as was once believed. Careful follow-up studies of patients with AKs in Australia by Robin Marks and his colleagues,[15] as well as our own work,[3] suggest that less than 0.1% transform into frankly malignant lesions and that a small proportion of lesions (perhaps 1–2% per annum) spontaneously remit. The mechanism of their spontaneous remission is unclear, but it seems likely that immunological mechanisms are involved. It would be reasonable to interpret the lichenoid keratosis described above as an attempt at immunological rejection. Certainly the presence of many T-helper cells and killer T-cells,[16] together with vacuolar degenerative change and cytoid body formation, is suggestive of immune attack.

Presumably, immunological mechanisms are provoked by a change in the antigenic status of the dysplastic epidermal cells. Neoantigens have not been found in AKs, but there appears to be a partial deletion of the normal complement of antigens on the cell surface, the extent of which parallels the degree of dysplasia. This is certainly the case for the pemphigus antigen,[17] blood-group substance A,[18] class I MHC antigens[19] and the EGF receptor.[20] Perhaps the loss of these antigens in some way allows access to cellular sites and substances not usually in contact with the immune system and thus not recognized as 'self'. If this were the case, an immunological attack on the cells that contain them might well ensue.

It is also the case that immunosuppressed individuals are prone to nonmelanoma skin cancer and premalignant lesions. This is certainly so with renal-transplant patients, as several studies have shown.[21] Our own studies found that the overall prevalence of nonmelanoma skin cancer and AKs was 25% in 85 renal-transplant patients but that in those who had transplants more than 80 months previously the prevalence was 38%.[22]

Transplant patients are also prone to viral warts, and it is sometimes quite difficult to distinguish these lesions from AKs clinically or histologically. In fact *in situ* hybridization studies have identified the viral genome in lesions that appear to be AKs in these patients[23] and it seems likely that viral oncogenesis has occurred.

Because of the apparent pronounced inflammatory response that some AKs generate and the profusion of lesions in immunosuppressed patients, it could be supposed that the usual low rate of transformation in subjects with normal immune systems might be due to their being held in check by immunological mechanisms. In order to test this hypothesis we transplanted AKs into nude mice where the absence of delayed hypersensitivity should allow them to progress uninhibited by immune influences. In fact, although the lesions 'survived', they did not progress as was predicted[24] so that further studies are required to determine the exact role of the cell-mediated hypersensitivity in the biology of AKs and SCC.

TREATMENT

As AKs rarely progress into more aggressive lesions and sometimes resolve spontaneously, it is reasonable to treat patients only when there are special considerations. These are: (1) when there are large numbers of lesions constituting a cosmetic or mechanical disability, (2) when individual lesions cause symptoms such as pain, tenderness and/or irritation, or (3) when there is doubt as to the diagnosis of any particular lesion. In this context it has to be said that accuracy in clinical diagnosis of nonpigmented small skin tumors is no better than for pigmented lesions (that is, 60–70%).[25]

When treatment is required, curettage with electrocautery of the base, light cryotherapy with liquid nitrogen, chemexfoliation with trichloroacetic acid or excision are the most frequently used measures.

Chemotherapy

Chemotherapy with topical 5% fluorouracil ointment (Efudix, Roche), used daily for 10–21 days to a few lesions at any one time, has proved very successful for many patients, causing resolution in 60–70% of patients after the first treatment. This treatment can cause local irritation and sometimes marked photosensitivity. Weekly treatment with 5% fluorouracil solution to all affected areas cleared 98% of the lesions in 10 patients.[26] This weekly 'pulse dosing' for 9-week treatment periods seems a sensible approach when there are large numbers of lesions.

Both oral and topical retinoids have been used. Oral retinoids are certainly effective while given but are only rarely indicated because of the significant side-effects with which they are associated. Moriarty et al[27] used etretinate (1 mg/kg per day) in a double-blind study in patients with multiple actinic keratoses and recorded a dramatic reduction in numbers of AKs in treated subjects. Our own studies with an arotinoid (Ro13–6298),[28] etretinate[29,30] and acitretin all confirm that oral retinoids cause regression of AKs. The most recent results are with acitretin and are seen in Table 8.1, from which it is also evident that the lesions recur when the treatment stops. Studies with isotretinoin in xeroderma pigmentosum[31] suggest that this drug would have similar effects. Oral retinoids are clearly only indicated in the most severely affected patients.

Table 8.1
Results of 3 months' oral treatment with acitretin (Ro 10–1670) and 9 months' follow up, in patients with solar keratoses (n=12)

Months	0	1	2	3	6	9	12
No. of keratoses (mean)	16.5	12.7	10.8	7.7	11.5	14.8	16.1
(±SD)	±13.4	±8.3	±7.5	±7.5	±5.8	±9.0	±8.7

Topical retinoids also have a useful therapeutic effect, although they may need to be given for long periods or in combination with another treatment modality such as topical 5-fluorouracil. Topical tretinoin 0.05% cream has been used in a large multicentre trial and shown to be effective (Table 8.2).[32]

Another topical retinoid, Ro14–9706 (the arotenoid methyl sulfone), was compared with topical 0.05% tretinoin over a 16-week trial period. The arotinoid methyl sulfone appeared better tolerated and slightly more effective than tretinoin (approximately 38% reduction, compared to approximately 30% reduction for the tretinoin-treated areas).[33]

Table 8.2
Results of an open multicenter study of the treatment of solar keratoses with 0.05% tretinoin cream. (Adapted from ref. 32.)

	6 months (n = 93)		9 months (n = 88)		12 months (n = 25)		15 months (n = 24)	
	Pre	Post	Pre	Post	Pre	Post	Pre	Post
Mean lesion count	11.2	8.9	11.2	7.9	14.4	8.84	14.0	7.4
Decrease	2.23		3.3		5.56		6.6	
P	<0.001		≤0.001		<0.003		<0.001	
Mean lesion size (mm)	84.1	62.2	84.7	55.4	131.7	72.8	124.1	61.4
Decrease	21.9		29.3		58.9		62.7	
P	<0.001		≤0.001		<0.014		<0.009	

Recent studies with topical isotretinoin indicates that this drug is also effective for the treatment of keratoses.

A novel antineoplastic agent, masoprocol (meso-nordihydroguariaretic acid—a dicatechol compound) which is also a potent 5-di-lipoxygenase inhibitor, has been used at a 10% concentration twice daily for the topical treatment of AKs on the head and neck. In one trial in which 113 patients used the 10% masoprocol there was a mean decrease of 15–5.4 AKs after treatment for 14–28 days.[34] This novel compound appears to hold promise for the treatment of multiple lesions and may be less irritating than 5-fluorouracil.

When very large lesions are present there is one further modality that can be used and which has been successful—intralesional interferon α2β.[35] However, because of the necessity of injection three times per week over a 3-week period, this treatment is not suitable for many patients.

Conclusion

Actinic keratoses are fascinating premalignant epidermal lesions which represent the tip of the dysplastic iceberg, as the exposed skin on which they arise is usually also severely sun-damaged despite the absence of focal clinical lesions. Because very few progress, they do not represent a sinister threat, but do indicate that a significant degree of sun damage has been sustained, and that more serious neoplastic lesions may arise nearby. In addition, their frequency and accessibility give an important opportunity for investigation of neoplastic progression in particular and photocarcinogenesis in general.

References

1. Marks R, Ponsford MW, Selwood TS et al, Non-melanotic skin cancer and solar keratoses in Victoria—clinical studies II, *Med J Aust* (1983) **ii**: 619–22.
2. Abo-Darub JM, MacKie R, Pitts JD, DNA repair in cells from patients with actinic keratosis, *J Invest Dermatol* (1983) **80**: 241–4.
3. Harvey I, Rankel SJ, Shalom D et al, Non melanoma skin cancer: questions concerning its distribution and natural history, *BMJ* (1989) **299**: 1118–20.
4. Yu RCH, Pryce DW, MacFarlane AW et al, A histopathological study of cutaneous horns, *Br J Dermatol* (1991) **124**: 449–52.
5. Rafal ES, Griffiths EM, Ditre CM et al, Topical tretinoin (retinoic acid) treatment for liver spots associated with photodamage, *New Eng J Med* (1992) **326**: 368–74.
6. Lever LR, Marks R, Pigmented facial macules: a sign of photoaging? In: Marks R, Plewig G, eds, *The environmental threat to the skin* (Martin Dunitz: London 1992) 91–6.
7. James MP, Wells GC, Whimster IW, Spreading pigmented actinic keratosis, *Br J Dermatol* (1977) **98**: 373–9.
8. Dinehart SM, Sanchez RL, Spreading pigmented actinic keratosis, *Arch Dermatol* (1988) **124**: 680–3.
9. Pearse AD, Marks R, Actinic keratoses and the epidermis on which they arise, *Br J Dermatol* (1977) **96**: 45–50.
10. Tan CY, Marks R, Lichenoid solar keratoses: prevalence and immunological findings, *J Invest Dermatol* (1982) **79**: 365–7.
11. Jablonsk S, Chorzelski T, Dyskeratoma and epithelioma (carcinoma): dyskeratoticum segregans, *Dermatologica* (1961) **123**: 24–37.
12. Carapeto FJ, Garcìa-Pérez A, Acantholytic keratosis, *Dermatologica* (1974) **148**: 233–9.
13. Lever L, Marks R, The significance of the Darier-like solar keratosis and acantholytic change in preneoplastic

lesions of the epidermis, *Br J Dermatol* (1989) **120**: 383–9.

14 Shahrad P, Marks R, The wages of warmth: changes in erythema ab igne, *B J Dermatol* (1977) **97**: 179–86.

15 Marks R, Rennie G, Selwood TS, Malignant transformation of solar keratoses to squamous cell carcinoma, *Lancet* (1988) **i**: 795–7.

16 Habets JMW, Tank B, van Joost Th, Characterisation of the mononuclear infiltrate in Bowen's disease (squamous cell carcinoma in situ). Evidence for a T-cell mediated antitumour immune response, *Virchows Archiv A Pathol Anat* (1989) **415**: 125–30.

17 De Morgans JM, Winkelmann RK, Jordon RE, Immunofluorescence of epithelial skin tumours I. Patterns of intercellular substance, *Cancer* (1970) **25**: 1399–1403.

18 Marks R, Pearse AD, Holt PJA et al, Evidence for changes in antigeneity in premalignant lesions of the epidermis, *Les Colloques de l'INSERM* (1978) **80**: 247–54.

19 Turbitt ML, Mackie RM, Loss of β2 microglobulin from the cell surface of cutaneous malignant and premalignant lesions, *Br J Dermatol* (1981) **104**: 507–13.

20 Nazmi MN, Dykes PJ, Marks R, Epderminal growth factor receptors in human epidermal tumours, *Br J Dermatol* (1990) **123**: 153–61.

21 Boyle J, Briggs JD, MacKie RM et al, Cancer, warts and sunshine in renal transplant patients, *Lancet* (1984) **i**: 702–5.

22 Shuttleworth D, Marks R, Griffin PJA et al, Dysplastic epidermal change in immunosuppressed patients with renal transplants, *Q J Med* (1987) **64 (243)**: 609–16.

23 Benton EC, McLaren K, Barr BB et al, Human papilloma virus infection and its relationship to skin cancer in a group of renal allograft recipients, *Curr Probl Dermatol* (1989) **18**: 168–77.

24 Thomas SE, Pearse AD, Marks R, Transplantation of human malignant and premalignant lesions of epidermis to nude mice. *Eur J Cancer Clin Oncol* (1985) **21(9)**: 1093–8.

25 Perednia DA, Gaines JA, Rossum AC, Variability in physician assessment of lesions in cutaneous images and its implications for skin screening and computer-assisted diagnosis, *Arch Dermatol* (1992) **128**: 357–64.

26 Pearlman DL, Weekly pulse dosing: effective and comfortable topical 5-fluorouracil treatment of multiple facial actinic keratoses, *J Am Acad Dermatol* (1991) **25**: 665–7.

27 Moriarty M, Dunn J, Darragh A et al, Etretinate in the treatment of actinic keratosis. A double blind, cross-over study, *Lancet* (1982) **i**: 364–5.

28 Kingston T, Gaskell S, Marks R, The effects of a novel potent oral retinoid (Ro13–6298) in the treatment of multiple solar keratoses and squamous cell epithelioma, *Eur J Cancer Clin Oncol* (1983) **19(9)**: 1201–5.

29 Hughes BR, Marks R, Pearse AD et al, Clinical response and tissue effects of etretinate treatment of patients with solar keratoses and basal cell carcinoma, *J Am Acad Dermatol* (1988) **18**: 522–9.

30 Shuttleworth D, Renal transplantation, immunity, skin cancer and retinoids. In: Marks, R ed. *Retinoids in cutaneous malignancy* (Blackwell Scientific Publications; Oxford 1991) 118–32.

31 Kraemer KH, DiGiovanna JJ, Moshell AB et al, Prevention of skin cancer in xeroderma pigmentosum with the use of oral isotretinoin, *New Eng J Med* (1988) **318**: 1633–7.

32 Kligman AM, Thorne EG, Topical therapy of actinic keratoses with tretinoin. In: Marks R, ed. *Retinoids in cutaneous malignancy* (Blackwell Scientific Publications: Oxford 1991) 66–73.

33 Misiewicz J, Sendagorta E, Golebiowsha A et al. Topical treatment of multiple actinic keratoses of the face with arotinoid methyl sulfone (Ro 14–9706) cream versus tretinoid cream: a double-blind, comparative study, *J Am Acad Dermatol* (1991) **24**: 448–51.

34 Olsen EA, Abernethy MK, Kulp-Shorten C et al, A double-blind vehicle-controlled study evaluating masoprocol cream in the treatment of actinic keratoses on the head and neck, *J Am Acad Dermatol* (1991) **24**: 738–43.

35 Shuttleworth D, Marks R, A comparison of the effects of intralesional interferon α–2b and topical 5% 5-fluorouracil cream in the treatment of solar keratoses and Bowen's disease, *J Dermatol Treat* (1989) **1**: 65–8.

Chapter 9

ADVANCES IN CRYOSURGERY FOR CUTANEOUS ONCOLOGY

Gloria F. Graham
Douglas Torre

There have been several advances in the use of cryosurgery for treatment of skin tumors. Techniques for treatment of keloids will be discussed.[1,2] Work from Germany on the use of cryosurgery as a new, standardized wound-healing model to test the efficacy of a cream containing hyaluronic acid will be presented.[3] Another look at face peeling of sun-damaged skin by using liquid nitrogen spray is promising.[4]

Breitbart[5,6,7] has evaluated freezing for melanomas after measuring the depth of lesions with ultrasound. Weshahy[8] has developed a type of intralesional cryosurgery using needles, and Castro Ron has used intralesional probes. Torre[9] is working with helium as a cryogen and Graham and Graham have evaluated selected cutaneous tumors before and after cryosurgery.[10] The many uses of cryosurgery make this one of the most widely utilized techniques in dermatology as well as in other specialties, such as the treatment of liver metastasis with cryosurgery.

Keloids

Aranzana et al[1] presented material on the combined treatment of shave excision and cryosurgery for keloids at the XIIth International Congress of Dermatologic Surgery (ISDS) in Munich. The treatment was repeated every other month for 2 months and combined with intralesional injections of triamcinolone (40 mg/ml). The final cosmetic result was excellent. Graham[2] has described a similar technique in a patient with extensive keloids on the neck. He was treated initially under general anesthesia.

Robles reported at the International Course of Cryosurgery on 7 May 1992 that freezing keloids to −40°C or −60°C resulted in necrosis of the keloid, separation of the entire keloid as an escar resulting in satisfactory cosmetic results. No surgery was done prior to freezing and no intralesional steroids were used (Figure 9.1).

Wound healing after cryosurgery

Hoffman[3] at the XIIth International Congress of Dermatologic Surgery in Munich in October 1991 reported on the use of hyaluronic acid verum cream (Jossalind (Jossa-arznei, Germany)) in wound healing after cryosurgery of basal cell carcinoma in a randomized, placebo-controlled double-blind study. The

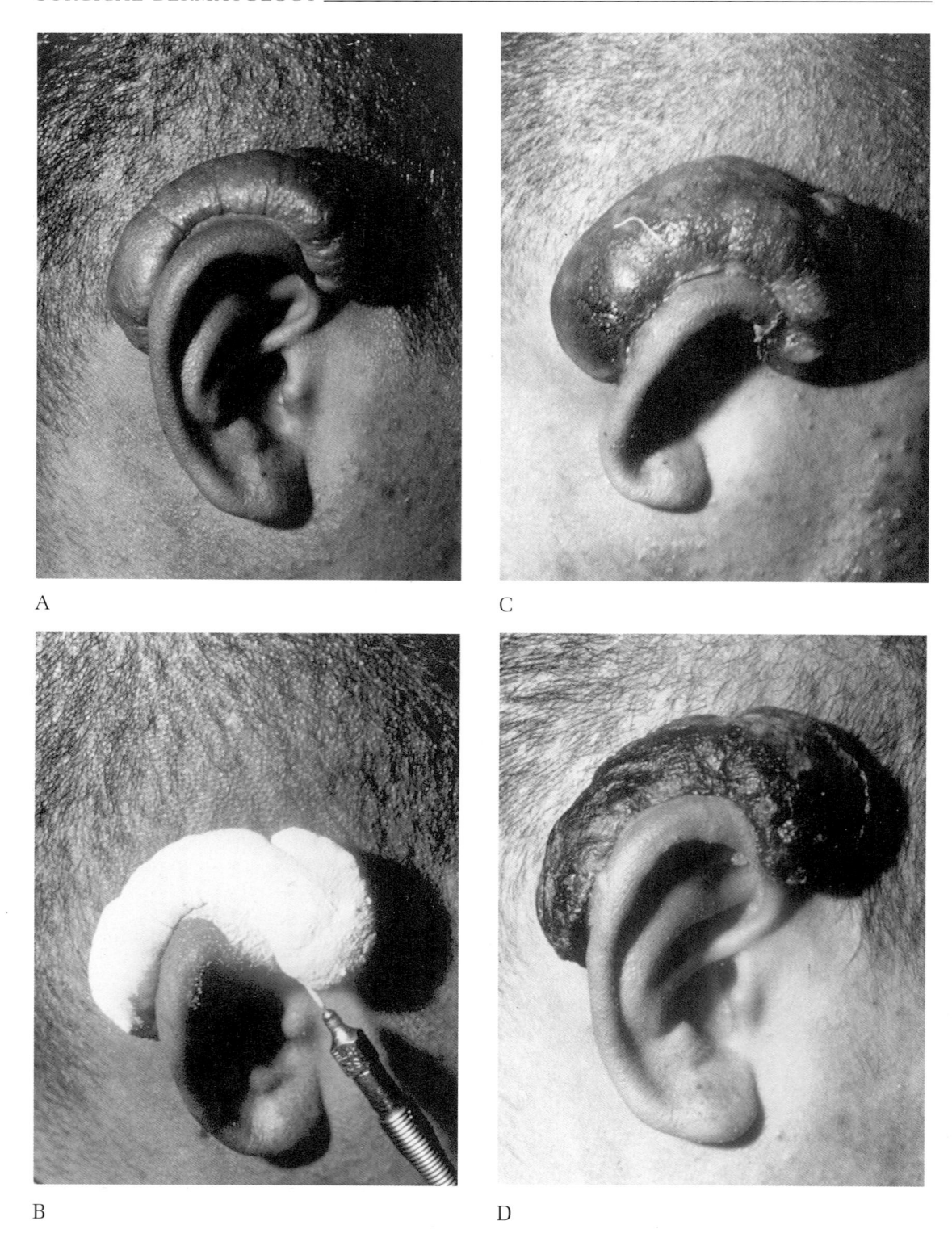

SURGICAL DERMATOLOGY

A

B

C

D

ADVANCES IN CRYOSURGERY FOR CUTANEOUS ONCOLOGY

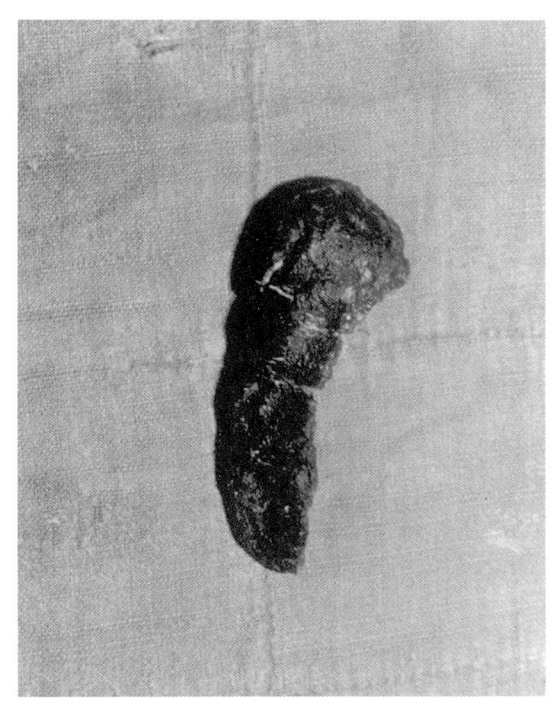

Figure 9.1
(A) Keloid of ear prior to treatment. (B) Keloid of ear during freezing to −40 °C. (C) Exudative reaction week following freezing. (D) Necrotic escar several weeks after freezing. (E) Escar after separation. (F) Ear well healed and free of keloid postcryosurgery. (Courtesy of Dr Eduardo Robles.)

E

F

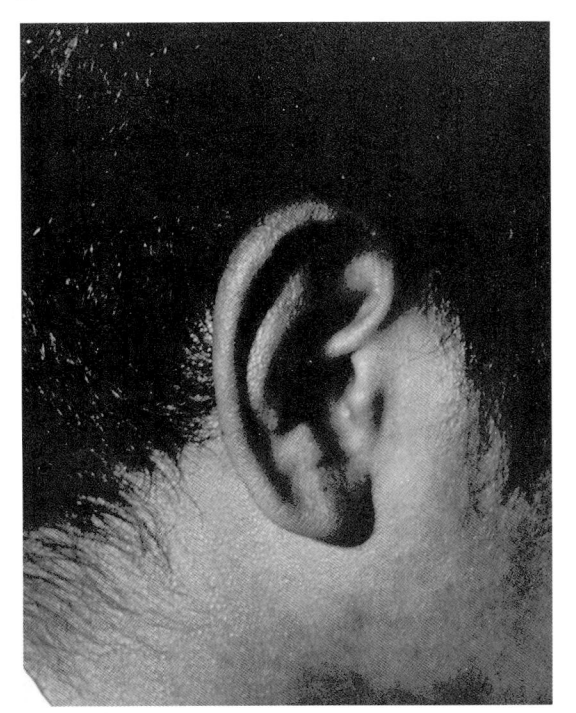

cryosurgical wound serves as a good wound-healing model since the defect is standardized by the use of a probe and the placement of a thermometer needle under the tumor to measure the temperature gradient. Jossalind cream was applied three times a day postoperatively for 3 weeks. Ultrasound using a 20-MHz B-scanner was used for evaluating the results. Healing was documented with ultrasound images and polaroid photographs. The median healing time with verum was 17.5 days and with the placebo 21 days. This work may be the first step in providing for more rapid wound healing following cryosurgery as well as other surgical procedures.

FULL-FACE CRYO PEELING

Chiarello[4] has described a technique for full-face liquid nitrogen cryo spraying of actinically damaged skin which not only destroys actinic keratoses and pigmented lesions but also leaves the skin healthier, pinker and smoother. This technique has previously been described for treating acne scars, and involves en bloc freezing of sheets of skin as is also done prior to dermabrasions. Permanent hypo-hyperpigmentation has been rare.

The face is divided into six sections and the liquid nitrogen is sprayed in a paint brush pattern covering each individual segment. Freeze time may be 30 s or even longer depending on the depth needed for eradication.

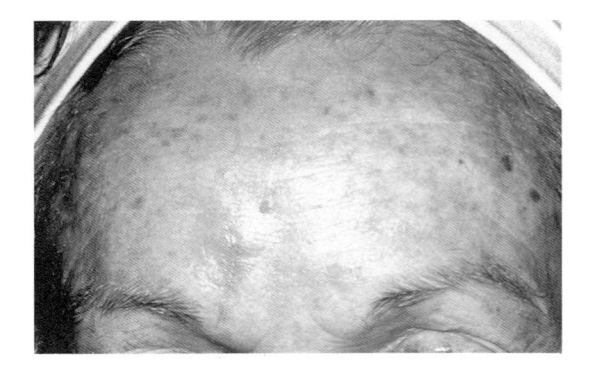

A

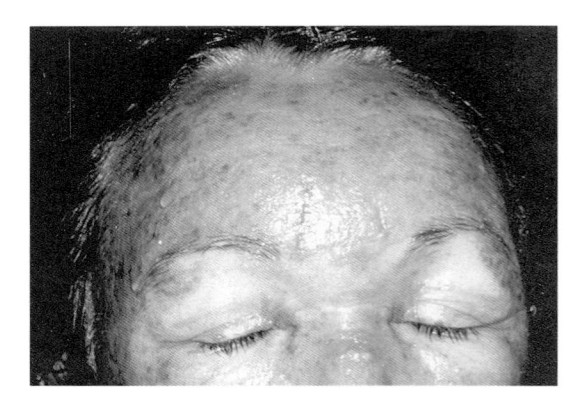

B

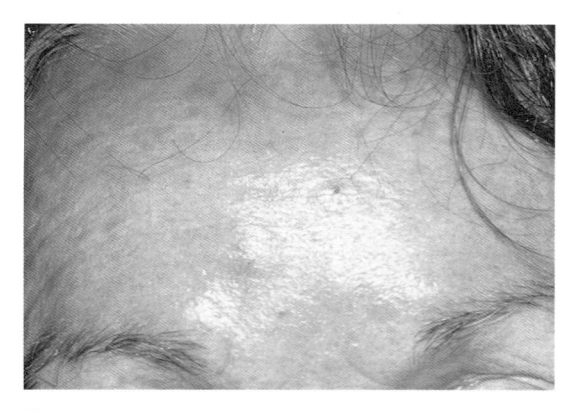

C

Figure 9.2
(A) Actinic damage and seborrheic keratoses prefreezing. (B) One day postfreezing. (C) A nice cosmetic result with clearing of actinic and seborrheic keratoses 3 weeks postcryo peel. (Courtesy of Dr Stephen Chiarello.)

The results of this form of face peeling are gratifying. Healing is complete, usually in 10 days. Swelling and blistering have subsided by the fifth day. The end result is smoother skin free of actinic keratoses and other blemishes. Even fine wrinkles are smoother. Since all the exposed skin is treated, the nidus for further actinic keratoses is removed.

Pictures can be used to show the patient how they will look during the swelling, blistering and oozing stage. Hyper-hypopigmentation is transient. The patient's treated skin is lightened homogeneously (Figure 9.2). The brown, leathery skin becomes pinker, smoother-textured skin and, in contrast to the results of spot freezing, is even-colored rather than splotchy.

Sun protection is essential for at least 10 days postoperatively and then a No. 30 sunscreen and broad-brimmed hat are essential. The skin is kept moist with white petrolatum or antibiotic ointment and the crusts are washed with lipid-free cleansing lotion and antiseptic soaps. Hydroxyzine and low-potency topical steroid may be used to prevent pruritus. Tretinoin is started 2–4 weeks after cryopeeling.

A problem is the pain of freezing, which is short-lived. Analgesia during the procedure is accomplished with 30–60 mg Toradol (Syntex, Palo Alto, CA) (ketorolac), a nonsteroidal anti-inflammatory agent which is given 30–45 min before the procedure. Toradol, a non-narcotic, has few side-effects, the most common being sedation.[4]

CUTANEOUS MALIGNANT MELANOMA (CMM)

In the Department of Dermatology of the University of Hamburg, Germany, between 1977 and 1983, 67 patients with malignant melanoma were treated by cryosurgery.[5,6] This technique for melanoma was based on several facts and assumptions:

'1. The cold-induced destruction of melanoma cells occurs at temperatures of −4°C to −7°C, while connective tissue destruction is observed at temperatures below −20°C.
2. Electron microscopic investigations of the cryolesions have shown that cell membranes, intracellular organelles and the nucleus are destroyed.[7]
3. There are indications that humoral as well as cell-mediated immune responses are induced by cryotherapy. The destroyed tumor remains in situ, giving rise to the possibility of prolonged exposure (about 72 h) of tumor antigens to the host's immune system.' The tissue thus destroyed may be capable of immune stimulation by the release of auto-antigens into the bloodstream because of cell membrane destruction or alteration of membrane molecular surface structure so that the immune system mistakes them for foreign antigens. If a large lesion is treated, more antigenic material is released.[5]

Cryosurgery for melanoma has been used for primary malignant melanoma and palliative cryosurgery for metastases. For successful cryotherapy of CMM, the following conditions are necessary:

'1. High-velocity cooling at 100°C/min (necessary for homogeneous nucleation).
2. A temperature of −21°C must be reached in the precautionary safety zone beneath the tumor.
3. Low thawing velocity at 10°C/min
4. Repeated freeze–thaw cycles (at least two).[5]'

The preferred cooling agent is liquid nitrogen and the preferred method is the spray, which in studies in living pig skin was capable of inducing deeper necrosis than the contact method. The depth of tumor invasion is determined by ultrasound. A moulage covering is used as a protection for tissue around the tumor. The biopsy is obtained while the tissue is frozen. During removal of the tissue, no tearing of the tissue occurs. The tissue is placed in formalin *while* frozen. The control of the ice ball extension is measured by temperature and impedance methods.

At the time of the publication in 1990,[5] no recurrence of CMM had been observed. From 1977 to 1983, 67 patients were treated for primary CMM. In 1987, when no tumor progression was apparent in the 67 patients, a prospective, randomized, controlled clinical study, comparing conventional surgery with cryosurgery, was begun. Only patients with an intermediate-risk melanoma in clinical stage I are admitted. Total T cells, T-helper cells, T-suppressor cells, Il2+ cells, HLA-DR+ cells, total B cells and natural killer cells are monitored using monoclonal antibodies.

Sixteen patients have been included in the study, eight with conventional surgery and eight with cryosurgery. The difference in immunologic parameters has been striking with a significant increase ($P > 0.001$) in the cryosurgery groups. This includes total T cells, T-helper cells, T-suppressor cells and HLA-DR+ cells. There were no differences in Il2+ cells, total B cells or natural killer cells. More patients and longer follow-up are needed in this important trial before we can draw conclusions concerning the use of cryosurgery as a primary therapy for malignant melanoma.

THE USE OF ULTRASOUND IN DERMATOLOGY

Breitbart[5,6,7] has evaluated the use of ultrasound in measuring the in vitro depth of skin tumors with a high degree of accuracy for 10 years using equipment developed by Sonometrics in New York: the ophthalmo scan connected to a 20-MHz transducer made by Panametrics. This is a combined A-mode and B-scan unit.

Before using this method, Breitbart and co-workers validated the technique in a study comparing 100 measurements of skin thickness with other methods, including histology. They then used ultrasound for 4 years as part of a diagnostic procedure for all types of skin tumors.[7] They compared the results of ultrasound measurements of malignant melanoma invasion depth in 202 cases with histopathology. Melanomas are thicker in sonometry than in pathological fixed specimens, probably due to shrinkage artifact in paraffin-embedded sections. They established a regression coefficient to estimate the sonometric tumor thickness with invasion depth using Breslow thickness.[7] Melanomas were not difficult to examine on ultrasound and showed a homogeneous internal echo with no inner echoes. Other tumors showed very different echo patterns.

They now feel that because of reliable results using ultrasound to measure depth of invasion of malignant melanoma, this should be done routinely. For cryosurgeons, ultrasound can give reliable information on the extent of the tumor and its invasion depth prior to treatment.

After visiting the University of Hamburg and reviewing the work of Dr Breitbart and his colleagues, Graham acquired (on loan) the use of the Dermascan-C from Denmark. This is a high-resolution scanner which views layers and structures in the skin as thin as 0.05 mm in three dimensions. It offers A, B, C and M modes of operation. This unit was used to evaluate tumors in a general dermatology practice where cryosurgery was used often in the treatment of skin cancers. While lentigo maligna is treated by cryosurgery, malignant melanoma has not been treated in this manner in our practice.

Benign lesions evaluated were hydrocystoma, actinic keratosis, seborrheic keratosis, dermatofibroma, disseminated superficial actinic porokeratosis and vascular hamartoma. Malignant lesions were basal and squamous cell carcinoma. Attempts were made to differentiate benign tumors from malignant and scar tissue from tumor. Histological verification of clinical diagnosis was carried out on most lesions with the exception of vascular and some benign lesions that were clinically obvious. In some tumors, positioning of the thermocouple needle was possible using ultrasound and after shave excision of tumors, evaluation of the remaining tumor using Cleocin-T/Gel (UpJohn, Kalamazoo, MI) as a coupling medium was useful. The most important contribution that ultrasound makes to the cryosurgeon is to determine the size, shape and depth of a lesion prior to therapy.

NEW EQUIPMENT

Castro-Ron, at the International Course of Cryosurgery, May, 1992, in Mexico City, presented his use of a flat probe for intralesional treatment of deep hemangiomas with minimal damage to overlying epidermis. An incision is made lateral to the lesion, and the probe is inserted below the epidermis, but above the angioma. As the upper surface is insulated, the epidermis is not destroyed as the angioma is being frozen.

Weshahy[8] at a recent ISDS meeting showed angulated or hook-shaped hollow needles which could be placed intradermally for cryosurgery. Treatment of hidradenitis suppurativa would be one indication for such a technique.

Torre[9] has been experimenting with helium gas cooled by liquid nitrogen for cryosurgery. This system offers many advantages, some of which are:

1. The temperature can be easily varied by mixing cooled and warm gas in various proportions.

2. Very thin flexible probes for intralesional use are possible.
3. Balloon probes for intralesional or intracavitary use are possible.
4. Accurate quantitative heat exchange with tissue easily determined.[9]

Graham and Graham[10] studied biopsies of solar keratoses, basal cell carcinomas and melanocytic nevi before and after cryosurgery. Most biopsies were obtained 2 months following freezing. Common lesions of solar keratosis were eradicated with 10 s of liquid nitrogen spray (LNSP) whereas hypertrophic types and bowenoid and clonal solar keratoses required 20–30 s of freezing before they were destroyed.

Junctional nevi were removed by 10–15 s of freezing but compound and intradermal nevi required 25–30 s. With the results obtained by Breitbart[5] in treating melanocytic lesions and in possibly generating an immune response following freezing, careful study of selected cases with many nevi may lead to more efficient and effective methods of therapy for many forms of pigmented lesions.

OTHER TUMORS

Castro-Ron at the International Course on Cryosurgery, May, 1992, in Mexico City, presented extensive cases of verrucous epidermal nevi treated effectively by cryosurgery. He has also treated numerous cases of lymphangioma circumscripta successfully. Ojeda et al[11] reported on five cases treated with excellent results and low recurrence rates.

SUMMARY

While there are new methods being developed for treatment of cutaneous tumors, cryosurgery continues to be an economical, effective, efficient modality yielding good cosmetic results. Cryosurgery may stimulate an immune response in certain pigmental lesions, including malignant melanoma. The clearing of multiple facial lesions with a cryopeel and eradication of large areas of verrucous epidermal nevi and lymphangioma circumscripta are other examples of the versatility of cryosurgery.

Many dermatologists use cryosurgery for benign and premalignant lesions. An increasing number of dermatologists treat malignant lesions by this method, so cryosurgery is becoming one of the more widely used techniques for eradicating skin tumors worldwide.

REFERENCES

1. Aranzana A, Conje-Min JS, Camacho F, Combined treatment of cryosurgery and surgery in keloids (001464), *Zbl Haut* (1991) **159**:354.
2. Graham G, Cryosurgery for acne. In: Zacarian SA, ed., *Cryosurgery for skin cancer and cutaneous disorders* (CV Mosby: St Louis 1985).
3. Hoffman K, Cryosurgery as a new, standardized wound healing model: a placebo controlled randomized double-blind study with hyaluronic acid (001463), *Zbl Haut* (1991) **159**:353.
4. Chiarello SE, Full face cryo peeling, *J Dermatol Surg Oncol* (1992) **18**:329–32.
5. Breitbart EW, Cryosurgery in the treatment of cutaneous malignant melanoma, *Clin Dermatol, Adv Cryosurg* (1990) **8**:96–100.
6. Breitbart EW, Cryosurgical considerations for melanoma. In: Zacarian A, ed., *Cryosurgery for skin cancer and cutaneous disorders* (CV Mosby: St Louis 1985) 215–37.
7. Breitbart EW, Rehpenning W, Bohnsack S, Hautdickenmessung: Vergleich der Hautfalten-, der Ultraschallmebtechnik und der

8. Weshahy AH, Intralesional cryosurgery — 'Weshahy's technique;' an effective method for treating deep and dynamic skin lesions (001465) and a combination between intralesional cryosurgery (Weshahy's technique) and surface cryosurgery (probe technique) in treatment of large plantar warts (001466), *Zbl Haut* (1991) **159**:354.

9. Torre D, Cryosurgical instrumentation and depth dose monitoring, *Clin Dermatol* (1990) **8**:48–60.

10. Graham GF, Graham JH, Histopathologic evaluation of selected cutaneous tumors before and after cryosurgery, *J Am Soc Dermatopathol* (1991) **18**:371 (abst).

11. Ojeda A, Sanchez Conejo-Min J, Perez Bernal A et al, Lymphangioma circumscription: evaluation of cryosurgical therapy, *Actas Dermo Sif* (1991) **10**:683–5.

(Reference 7 continued:)
Histometrie mit der direkten MeBmethode. Poster 50, X. Jahrestagung der ADF Münster/Westf, 1982.

Chapter 10

CHARACTERISTICS OF GIANT BASAL CELL CARCINOMA

Henry W. Randle
Randall K. Roenigk

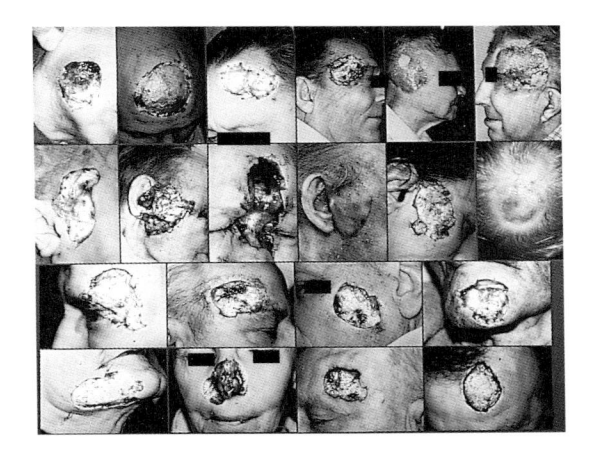

INTRODUCTION

Giant basal cell carcinoma (BCC) is a clinical expression for a large-sized BCC. There is no general consensus on what constitutes large or 'giant'. Sizes range from greater than 2 cm[1] to greater than 3 cm[2] to greater than 10–12 cm.[3] The size limit established by the American Joint Committee on Cancer,[4] in which the largest category is 5 cm or greater in diameter, will be used in this chapter to designate giant BCCs. These BCCs have been reported under a variety of synonyms: giant basaloma;[5] horrifying;[6] giant exophytic;[3] basaloma terebrans,[5] ulcus terebrans[7] and forme bourgeonnate et vegetante.[8]

Fewer than 1% of all BCCs reach this size, although in one series of cases treated by Mohs micrographic surgery, the percentage of BCCs 5 cm or greater in diameter was 8.8.[9] The majority of reported cases of giant BCCs have been case reports, often from the surgical literature related to reconstruction. This chapter reviews many of these case reports, including two larger series, and discusses the parameters associated with the development of giant BCCs, the potential complications, and the treatment of these large cancers.

ASSOCIATIONS

Basal cell carcinomas develop most commonly on the head and neck of older, fair-skinned individuals, more commonly in males with a significant history of sun exposure.[10,11] Most of these cancers result in minimal morbidity. However, a few BCCs become large and are capable of significant local destruction and disfigurement. Why do these few cancers reach such a giant size?

It has been stated that giant BCCs often are a consequence of deterioration or neglect by a patient.[5] Clearly, if a patient refuses to have a BCC treated, it will continue to grow to a large size and potentially metastasize.[12] However, many patients with giant BCCs do not neglect their cancers; they see physicians regularly, and receive treatment, often several times. In fact, the majority of giant BCCs represent recurrences.[13] The following sections will review the host, tumor and environmental factors that have been reported to be associated with the development of giant BCCs.

Duration of tumor, age of patient

While it seems intuitive that giant BCCs should be present for several years and seen in older individuals, it has been suggested that aggressive cancers occur in young adults and behave differently and grow more rapidly.[14] These are the exceptions. Most giant BCCs have been present for many years. In a large series most of the giant BCCs were present for at least several years and none were seen in patients under the age of 44 years.[13] The average age was 72 years. In general, size appears to be related to duration of tumor growth rather than a rapid rate of growth.

Neglect

One of the historical explanations for BCCs growing to a giant size was that the patient neglected seeking treatment. Neglect may be the result of cognitive impairment, such as Alzheimer's, mental disease, cancerophobia, being 'too busy' to seek treatment, or other reasons as listed below.

A 58-year-old male teacher did not seek medical treatment for a BCC on the back for over 30 years because of religious reasons, allowing the tumor to follow its natural course and grow to 25 cm in diameter and metastasize to the axillary lymph node.[12] In another report, a physician had elected not to treat a BCC because of a patient's advanced age and leukemia. It grew to 12 × 9 cm before it was successfully excised by Mohs micrographic surgery.[15]

Neglect was unrelated to lack of access to medical care in one series.[13] Overall, neglect seems to be one of several factors contributing to the development of giant BCCs.

Recurrence

Many giant BCCs have not been neglected but represent recurrent lesions.[13] Some have been treated several times. Why do these cancers recur and reach a giant size despite surgical care? Recurrent disease may reflect a new primary but more likely represents initial inadequate treatment.[16,17]

Five-year recurrence rates for most treatment modalities of primary BCC lesions are less than 10%.[16] However, five-year recurrence rates for treatment of recurrent lesions (previously treated) are much higher and range from 5.6% for Mohs micrographic surgery to 40% for electrodesiccation and curettage.[17] Clearly, the type of treatment selected for recurrent tumors is of considerable importance in preventing another recurrence and ultimately in limiting the development of giant BCCs.

Histological subtype

Thackray, in 1951,[18] was the first to correlate the histology of BCCs with their clinical behavior. In 1977, Sloane[19] stressed the value of histological subtyping of BCCs to predict recurrence after surgical excision. He indicated the importance of reporting the subtype of BCCs in the pathologist's report.

Certain histological patterns (morpheaform, micronodular and metatypical) have been associated with an aggressive course. These frequently have a sclerosing stroma with infiltrating islands of tumor,[20,21,22] a tendency for local spread by perineural, perivascular and periadnexal subclinical extension,[23] and a tendency to recur following treatment.[1,22,24,25] Nodular BCCs may also have an area of sclerosis and be at risk for recurrence.[26] An average of 7.2 mm of subclinical tumor extension was found in morpheaform BCCs as compared with 2.1 mm of extension in well-circumscribed nodular lesions.[23] In addition, morpheaform BCCs have biological features that distinguish them from the nodular subtypes and may play a role in their aggressiveness, such as the ability to synthesize type IV collagenase,[27] distinct nuclear morphometric features,[28] and a high number of nucleolar organization regions.[29] Because of these features, these subtypes are not amenable to treatment with 'blind techniques' such as electrodesiccation and curettage, cryosurgery or radiotherapy. Thus, there is an implied relationship between histological appearance and behavior which has both diagnostic and prognostic value.[14] A much higher percentage of aggressive histological subtypes was found in giant BCCs as compared to smaller tumors.[13]

Often there are mixed histological subtypes in the same tumor. It may be that in some instances one of the components may have been eradicated, leaving the other component to give rise to a recurrence.[22]

The effects of radiation exposure

A considerable number of patients with giant BCCs have had previous radiation exposure.[6,13] They either were treated with radiation or had environmental exposure to radioactive material. Ionizing radiation can produce malignant degeneration in the skin. It is a matter of conjecture whether, in isolated cases, radiation energy can transform a low-grade cutaneous carcinoma into a biologically more aggressive cancer.[30] It has recently been demonstrated that BCCs which recur after radiation therapy are often larger cancers than those treated initially by other means.[31] Several factors have been postulated to account for the larger size of the BCCs following radiation. Intrinsic to the tumor: (1) histological change; and (2) increase in biological aggressiveness not reflected by tumor histology. Extrinsic to the tumor: (1) decrease in local host defenses; (2) entrapment of tumor cells in scar tissue; (3) sequestration of residual tumor cells within a relatively larger area of scar tissue of radiation dermatitis; (4) the effect of scar tissue formation in preventing upward migration of residual malignant cells, forcing them in horizontal and deep directions; and (5) deep invasion due to radiation damage to bone and/or cartilage that may adversely alter their protective ability.[31]

The effects of wound grafting

Some authors report that in an appreciable number of cases, tumor dissemination was related to incomplete excision of large invasive tumors followed by immediate wound closure, particularly by grafting,[32,33] and that recurrences under grafts are difficult to detect and treat.[9] It has been suggested that the scar that holds the graft in place is impenetrable and prevents residual tumor from reaching the skin surface. The tumor expands in the direction of least resistance under the plane of the scar before it resurfaces in an adjacent area. This would not only contribute to the development of a giant BCC but would also enhance the risk for metastasis. These authors deemed it advisable to defer wound grafting of large defects whenever possible for at least 6 months after excision to monitor for residual neoplasm before reconstructive surgery is begun. Seven of 50 giant BCCs in a large series were covered by a graft compared with only one in a comparable number of smaller tumors.[13]

Genetics

Individuals with the autosomal dominantly inherited basal cell nevus syndrome have been reported to develop extensive uncontrolled BCC of the face resulting in death from direct cerebral invasion via the orbit, facial nerve palsy, bilateral eye enucleation, and severe facial mutilation in young adults.[34]

Immunity

Depressed systemic immunity has been associated with large tumors.[35] The incidence of BCCs increases with age. Depression of cell-mediated immunity is most pronounced after the age of 50 years.[36] Whether age-related declining cellular immunity plays a role in the development of giant BCCs is unclear.

Immunosuppressed patients who have undergone renal transplantation have a markedly increased incidence of squamous cell carcinoma compared with normal subjects but only a modest elevation in BCC occurrence,[37,38] so this may have only a minor role in the development of giant BCCs. Weimar et al were the first to report giant BCCs in patients with chronic lymphocytic leukemia and lymphoma.[15] A recent report of a patient with a giant (and metastatic) BCC in AIDS-related complex may indicate another group of immunosuppressed individuals at risk for giant BCCs.[39] Decreased local immunity as measured by the sparse infiltrate surrounding BCC tumor islands may contribute to the development of giant BCCs[40] in some cases.

Tumor location

Special privileged sites have been implicated in the development of giant BCCs. Single case reports of giant mutilating BCCs have been reported on the face.[41,42] The occurrence of large aggressive BCCs has been reported to be unique to the scalp. These have been said to occur principally in young adults,[43] attributed to previous treatment of tinea capitis by radiotherapy,[44] inadequate treatment,[45,46,47] and neglect.[48] Several of these papers were written by reconstructive surgeons and dealt primarily with the reconstruction of defects of cosmetically and functionally important sites. The risk factors for these special sites were the same as those reported for other locations, that is neglect, aggressive histology, prior treatment with radiation, and concealment by graft.

A few giant exophytic, vegetative, sessile BCC plaques up to 20 cm in diameter have occurred on the back.[3,12,49–53] The majority of these tumors represented patient neglect and the patient sought treatment only after family members complained of the odor of the tumor. Large series of giant BCCs reveal that most occur on the head and neck, like smaller BCCs.[6,13]

COMPLICATIONS OF GIANT BCCS

The size of the tumor is very important in predicting a successful outcome after treatment. The greater the diameter of the lesion, the greater the likelihood of recurrence. For BCCs treated with Mohs micrographic surgery by one surgeon, recurrences ranged from 1.4% for lesions less than 1 cm in diameter up to 7.8% for lesions more than 5 cm in diameter.[54] Giant BCCs may lead to disfigurement and be life-threatening because of the tendency to erosion, hemorrhage and meningeal complications if the skull is penetrated.[44]

Metastatic BCCs are rare but giant BCCs are often implicated in metastasis. Rizovsky et al.[55] discussed 'the hazard of metastasis in the case of very old and very *large* BCCs'. 'The primary lesion in metastatic BCC typically begins as a neglected, *large*, ulcerated, locally-invasive, and destructive neoplasm that recurs despite repeated surgery or radiotherapy'.[56] Blewitt[57] concluded that large size of the primary lesion is the most outstanding feature of metastatic disease and that metastatic potential is related to depth of invasion.

TREATMENT

We have learned to recognize BCCs based on different histological subtypes and patient characteristics that place them at risk for recurrence or the subsequent development of a giant BCC (Table 10.1).

Table 10.1
Giant BCC characteristics

1. Host — tumor of long duration
   Neglect
   Recurred after treatment
     Radiation
     Concealed by graft
   Genetically predisposed (basal cell nevus syndrome)
2. Tumor — 'aggressive' histological subtype
3. Environment — ionizing radiation exposure

Treatment by electrodesiccation and curettage, simple excision, radiotherapy or cryotherapy is adequate for the majority of BCCs, but those with an aggressive histological subtype, that have recurred after previous treatment, or that occur in patients with a history of exposure to ionizing radiation, should be approached in a different manner. They should be treated by Mohs micrographic surgery. Patients once treated for a skin cancer are at risk for recurrence. Therefore, follow-up evaluation is important in limiting the occurrence of giant BCCs.

Once giant BCCs occur, they may require a multidisciplinary approach, initially using total microscopic margin control, to achieve superior local excision. Other surgical subspecialists in reconstructive surgery, neurosurgery, ophthalmic surgery, head and neck surgery and medical oncology should be involved when appropriate to remove tissue in deeper structures and help with reconstruction.

REFERENCES

1. Roenigk RK, Ratz JL, Bailin PL et al, Trends in the presentation and treatment of basal cell carcinomas, *J Dermatol Surg Oncol* (1986) **12**:860–5.

2. Mohs FE, *Chemosurgery, microscopically controlled surgery for skin cancer* (Charles C. Thomas: Springfield 1978).

3. Curry MC, Montgomery H, Winkelmann RK, Giant basal cell carcinoma, *Arch Dermatol* (1977) **113**:316–19.

4. American Joint Committee on Cancer, *Manual for staging of cancer*, 3rd edn. (JB Lippincott: Philadelphia 1988).

5. Braun-Falco O, Plewig G, Wolff H et al, *Dermatology* (Springer-Verlag: Berlin 1991).

6. Jackson R, Adams RH, Horrifying basal cell carcinoma: a study of 33 cases and a comparison with 435 non-horror cases and a report on four metastatic cases, *J Surg Oncol* (1973) **5**:431–63.

7. Weidner F, Stolte M, Multizentrisches Metatypisches Kopfhautbasaliom (Typ Ulcus terebrans) mit Perforationen der Schädelkalotte, *Der Hautarzt* (1974) **25**:68–72.

8. Degos R, *Dermatologie* (Flammarion: Paris 1953) 848.

9. Robins P, Chemosurgery: my 15 years of experience, *J Dermatol Surg Oncol* (1981) **7**:779–89.

10. Broders AC, Basal-cell epithelioma, *JAMA* (1919) **72**:856–60.
11. Chuang T, Popescu A, Daniel Su WP et al, Basal cell carcinoma: a population-based incidence study in Rochester, Minnesota, *J Am Acad Dermatol* (1990) **22**:413–17.
12. Wendt JR, Houck JP, A giant basal cell carcinoma with lymph node metastases: case report and review of the literature, *Contemp Surg* (1988) **32**:33–8.
13. Randle HW, Roenigk RK, Brodland DG, Giant basal cell carcinoma: who is at risk? (Submitted for publication.)
14. Leffell DJ, Headington JT, Wong DS et al, Aggressive-growth basal cell carcinoma in young adults, *Arch Dermatol* (1991) **127**:1663–7.
15. Weimar VM, Ceilley RI, Goeken JA, Aggressive biologic behavior of basal- and squamous-cell cancers in patients with chronic lymphocytic leukemia or chronic lymphocytic lymphoma, *J Dermatol Surg Oncol* (1979) **5**:609–14.
16. Rowe DE, Carroll RJ, Day CL Jr, Long-term recurrence rates in previously untreated (primary) basal cell carcinoma: implications for patient follow-up, *J Dermatol Surg Oncol* (1989) **15**:315–28.
17. Rowe DE, Carroll RJ, Day CL Jr, Moh's surgery is the treatment of choice for recurrent (previously treated) basal cell carcinoma, *J Dermatol Surg Oncol* (1989) **15**:424–31.
18. Thackray AC, Histological classification of rodent ulcers and its bearing on their prognosis, *Br J Cancer* (1951) **5**:213–24.
19. Sloane JP, The value of typing basal cell carcinomas in predicting recurrence after surgical excision, *Br J Dermatol* (1977) **96**:127–32.
20. Jacobs GH, Rippey JJ, Altini M et al, Prediction of aggressive behavior in basal cell carcinoma, *Cancer* (1982) **49**:533–7.
21. Hashimoto K, Mehregan A, *Tumors of the epidermis* (Butterworths: Boston 1990) 128–9.
22. Lang PG Jr, Maize JC, Histologic evolution of recurrent basal cell carcinoma and treatment implications, *J Am Acad Dermatol* (1986) **14**:186–96.
23. Salasche SJ, Amonette RA, Morpheaform basal-cell epitheliomas, a study of subclinical extensions in a series of 51 cases, *J Dermatol Surg Oncol* (1981) **7**:387–94.
24. Levine HL, Bailin PL, Basal-cell carcinoma of the head and neck: identification of the high risk patient, *Laryngoscope* (1980) **90**:955–61.
25. Howell JB, Caro M, Morphea-like epithelioma, *Arch Dermatol* (1957) **75**:517–24.
26. Freeman RG, Duncan WC, Recurrent skin cancer, *Arch Dermatol* (1973) **107**:395–9.
27. Barsky SH, Grossman DA, Bhuta S, Desmoplastic basal cell carcinomas possess unique basement membrane-degrading properties, *J Invest Dermatol* (1987) **88**:324–9.
28. deRosa G, Vetrani A, Zeppa P et al, Comparative morphometric analysis of aggressive and ordinary basal cell carcinoma of the skin, *Cancer* (1990) **65**:544–9.
29. deRosa G, Staibano S, Barra E et al, Nucleolar organizer regions in aggressive and nonaggressive basal cell carcinoma of the skin, *Cancer* (1992) **69**:123–6.
30. Conway H, Hugo NE, Metastatic basal cell carcinoma, *Am J Surg* (1965) **110**:620–4.
31. Smith SP, Foley EH, Grande DJ, Use of Moh's micrographic surgery to establish quantitative proof of

heightened tumor spread in basal cell carcinoma recurrent following radiotherapy, *J Dermatol Surg Oncol* (1990) **16**:1012–16.

32. Mikhail GR, Nims LP, Kelly AP Jr et al, Metastatic basal cell carcinoma, *Arch Dermatol* (1977) **113**:1261–9.

33. Mikhail GR, Boulos RS, Knighton RS et al, Cranial invasion by basal cell carcinoma, *J Dermatol Surg Oncol* (1986) **12**:459–64.

34. Southwick GJ, Schwartz RA, The basal cell nevus syndrome, *Cancer* (1979) **44**:2294–305.

35. Dellon AL, Potvin C, Chretien PB et al, The immunobiology of skin cancer, *Plastic Reconstruc Surg* (1975) **55**:341–54.

36. Lattes R, Kessler RW, Metastasizing basal-cell epithelioma of the skin: report of two cases, *Cancer* (1951) **4**:866–77.

37. Miller SJ, Biology of basal cell carcinoma, Part I, *J Am Acad Dermatol* (1991) **24**:1–13.

38. Miller SJ, Biology of basal cell carcinoma, Part II, *J Am Acad Dermatol* (1991) **24**:161–75.

39. Sitz KV, Keppen M, Johnson DF, Metastatic basal cell carcinoma in acquired immunodeficiency syndrome-related complex, *JAMA* (1987) **257**:340–3.

40. Myskowski PL, Safai B, The immunology of basal cell carcinoma, *Int J Dermatol* (1988) **27**:601–7.

41. Dvoretzky I, Fisher BK, Haker O, Mutilating basal cell epithelioma, *Arch Dermatol* (1978) **114**:239–40.

42. Bianchini R, Wolter M, Fatal outcome in a metatypical giant, 'horrifying' basal cell carcinoma, *J Dermatol Surg Oncol* (1987) **13**:556–7.

43. Binstock JH, Stegman SJ, Tromovitch TA, Large aggressive basal-cell carcinomas of the scalp, *J Dermatol Surg Oncol* (1981) **7**:565–9.

44. Gormley DE, Hirsch P, Aggressive basal cell carcinoma of the scalp, *Arch Dermatol* (1978) **114**:782–3.

45. Gaisford JC, Hanna DC, Susen AF, Major resection of scalp and skull for cancer with immediate complete reconstruction — fourteen cases, *Plastic Reconstr Surg* (1958) **21**:335–44.

46. Bakamjian VY, Morain WD, Phelan JT, Massive basal cell carcinoma of the scalp: successful management by cooperation of chemosurgeon and reconstructive surgeon, *Ann Plastic Surg* (1978) **1**:421–8.

47. Peters CR, Dinner MI, Dolsky RL et al, The combined multidisciplinary approach to invasive basal cell tumors of the scalp, *Ann Plastic Surg* (1980) **4**:199–204.

48. Jones NF, Hardesty RA, Swartz WM et al, Extensive and complex defects of the scalp, middle third of the face, and palate: the role of microsurgical reconstruction, *Plastic Reconstr Surg* (1988) **82**:937–50.

49. Love GL, Sarma DP, Giant polyploid basal cell carcinoma, *J Surg Oncol* (1985) **28**:230.

50. O'Brien CJ, Harvey KM, Harris JP et al, Shoulder girdle resection for giant basal cell carcinoma, *Br J Plastic Surg* (1984) **37**:556.

51. Beck H, Andersen JA, Bickler NE et al, Giant basal cell carcinoma with metastasis and secondary amyloidosis: report of case, *Acta Dermatol Venereol (Stockholm)* (1983) **63**:564.

52. Canterbury TD, Wheeler WE, Madan E, Giant basal cell carcinoma of the back, *West Virginia Med J* (1990) **86**:291–2.

53. Kleinberg C, Penetrante RB, Miltrom H

et al, Metastatic basal cell carcinoma of the skin, *J Am Acad Dermatol* (1982) **7**:655–9.

54. Rigel DS, Robins P, Friedman RJ, Predicting recurrence of basal-cell carcinomas treated by microscopically controlled excision, *J Dermatol Surg Oncol* (1981) **7**:807–10.

55. Rizovsky R, Bourlond A, Mairesse M et al, Epithelioma basocellulaire etendu de la nuque, *Arch Belges Dermatol* (1974) **30**:263–8.

56. Lo JS, Snow SN, Reizner GT et al, Metastatic basal cell carcinoma: report of twleve cases with a review of the literature, *J Am Acad Dermatol* (1991) **24**:715–19.

57. Blewitt R, Why does basal cell carcinoma metastatize so early? *Int J Dermatol* (1980) **19**:44–6.

Chapter 11

BASAL CELL CARCINOMA RECURRING FOLLOWING RADIOTHERAPY

Steven P. Smith
Donald J. Grande

Historical Background

Basal cell carcinoma (BCC) is a relatively slow-growing neoplasm with an extraordinarily small metastatic potential. The large majority of primary tumors are eradicated with any of several well-established treatment modalities. However, BCCs which recur are a therapeutically challenging entity, with higher recurrence rates than primary BCCs, regardless of subsequent treatment modality.

Among recurrent BCCs, those following treatment with radiotherapy have proven to be particularly difficult to eradicate (Table 11.1). Three series investigated BCCs recurring after radiotherapy and subsequently treated with standard surgical excision. Cobbett's[1] series of 96 postradiation BCCs had a recurrence rate of 16.7%. Hayes[2] showed a 24.3% recurrence rate for his series of recurrent BCCs, of which 191 of 220 (87%) were initially treated with radiotherapy. Rank and Wakefield[3] noted a 14.7% recurrence rate for 197 tumors, all but one of which had been irradiated as initial treatment.

Recurrence rates have been even higher for series where radiotherapy has been employed as a treatment for BCC recurring after previous radiotherapy. Churchill-Davidson and Johnson[4] treated 26 BCCs recurring after radiotherapy with a second course of radiation and found that 69.2% persisted or recurred. Hansen and Jensen[5] reported a 48.3% recurrence rate for a

Table 11.1
Recurrence rates following treatment of basal cell carcinomas recurring after radiotherapy

Series	Postradiotherapy BCCs	Recurrence rate (%)
Surgical excision		
Rank and Wakefield[3]	196	14.7
Hayes[2]	191	24.3
Cobbett[1]	96	16.7
Additional radiotherapy		
Churchill-Davidson and Johnson[4]	26	69.2
Hansen and Jensen[5]	197	48.3

BCC, basal cell carcinoma.

larger series of 197 patients with similarly treated BCCs.

These high recurrence rates suggest a particularly aggressive and invasive behavior among BCCs recurring after radiotherapy. Further evidence of such behavior is found in the literature, in the form of reports of incurable and metastasizing tumors. Hirshowitz and Mahler[6] described four incurable BCCs of the midface, all of which were initially treated with radiotherapy. Of 33 'horrifying' BCCs reviewed by Jackson and Adams,[7] 16 had been treated initially with radiotherapy. In Pierce et al,[8] all 33 of the BCCs in a series of incurable 'horror' tumors had received radiotherapy and in 26 of the cases it was the initial treatment modality. The majority of the reported cases of metastasizing BCCs in the world literature were initially treated by irradiation.[6]

Mohs micrographic surgery (MMS) is generally accepted as the treatment of choice for recurrent BCC. A recent review of the literature[9] showed recurrence rates for MMS of previously treated BCCs to be substantially less than those for other treatment modalities (standard surgical excision, electrodesiccation and curettage, cryotherapy, radiotherapy). However, prior to our work[10,11] there had been no study evaluating MMS as a therapy for recurrent BCCs after previous treatment with radiotherapy.

Current data

We examined 27 BCCs recurring following radiotherapy alone or in addition to other therapeutic modalities and treated with MMS at the Tufts-New England Medical Center from 1983 to 1989. All cases were reviewed and analyzed in terms of age, sex, location (forehead, periauricular, periorbital, cheek, nose, trunk), clinically apparent preoperative tumor area and final postoperative defect area. The mean age at the time of surgery was 66.8 years.

Fourteen of the tumors occurred in men and 13 in women. Of the tumors, 70.4% were located in the mid-third of the face. The average preoperative tumor size was 2.1 cm. Over the same period, 791 BCCs recurring after one or more nonradiotherapy treatment modalities (standard surgical excision, electrodesiccation and curettage, cryotherapy, radiotherapy, 5-fluorouracil) were excised by MMS at our institution. Twenty-seven of these cases were matched by computer to the postradiation tumors for age, sex, location and clinically apparent preoperative tumor area, and formed a control group.

The Mohs technique itself was then employed as a tool in an attempt to quantitate the seemingly aggressive, invasive behavior of BCC recurring after radiotherapy. Both above-mentioned groups of tumors were evaluated by three parameters. The number of Mohs excision stages necessary to achieve a tumor-free plane for each lesion was tabulated, and the mean value was calculated for each group. Secondly, the percentage area increase (PAI), a figure expressing the final postoperative defect area as a percentage of the clinically apparent preoperative tumor area, was determined for all tumors. The mean PAI was then calculated for each group. Finally, all tumors were analyzed in terms of invasion of deep subcutaneous tissue (perichondrium, periosteum, cartilage, bone) by review of MMS operative reports. The percentage of tumors in each group displaying such invasion was then calculated.

Overall, we noted a clear-cut difference between the two tumor groups. First, the mean number of Mohs excision stages required to achieve a tumor-free plane was larger for the postradiation group, 2.11 ± 1.09 versus 1.74 ± 0.59. The larger mean number of Mohs excision stages for the postradiation group, although not statistically significant ($P = 0.13$, student's two-tailed T test), suggests deeper and/or wider tumor extension. This parameter is probably the weakest of the three, however, as the dimensions of a Mohs stage (layer) are variable, depending on several factors, including the surgeon and the anatomical site involved. Nevertheless, previous studies have shown a heightened recurrence rate for both BCCs and squamous cell carcinomas (SCCs) excised with a large number (four or more) of Mohs stages.[12]

The discrepancy between the mean PAIs for both groups was statistically significant. In fact, the mean PAI for the postradiation group was more than twice that of the nonradiation group, 859 ± 1016 versus 372 ± 504 (P <0.05, student's two-tailed T test). The Mohs technique excises tumor completely, yet with only microscopically small margins. Accordingly, the final postoperative defect dimensions very closely approximate to the true horizontal tumor extension. This makes the PAI a valuable tool for quantitative comparison of horizontal growth among tumors with contiguous growth patterns. In this study, the two groups were so closely matched in terms of clinically apparent preoperative tumor area (mean values of 4.96 cm^2 versus 4.92 cm^2) that the difference in mean PAIs provided solid quantitative evidence of heightened horizontal extension for postradiation BCCs. It especially reflects the number of postradiation lesions exhibiting large PAIs (15 PAIs of greater than 400 and five greater than 1400, versus seven and one, respectively, for the nonradiation BCCs).

Lastly, 59% of the postradiation tumors displayed invasion of deep subcutaneous tissue, as opposed to only 22% of the nonradiation tumors. This difference was the most statistically significant of the three parameters ($P < 0.01$, two-tailed chi-square test). It clearly quantitates both increased vertical extension of postradiation tumors and their heightened level of invasive behavior.

HYPOTHESES AND EXPLANATIONS

Our quantitative results strongly support the previously discussed clinical impression that BCC recurring following radiotherapy demonstrates a particularly aggressive, invasive behavior. There has been a good deal of conjecture and debate in the literature as to why previously irradiated tumors act in such a manner. The possible etiologies may be grouped into two major categories: the effects of radiotherapy on the tumor itself and the effects on neighboring host tissue.

Irradiation may cause the tumor to change histologically and/or biologically. Among their previously mentioned series of 197 tumors, Rank and Wakefield[3] found a number of cases where classical basal cell tumors became mixed cell lesions or typical SCCs subsequent to treatment. In a study of 100 recurrent BCCs, Menn et al[13] discovered a tendency for the architecture to change from solid nests of tumor cells within a mucinous stroma in primary lesions to infiltrating elements encased in a dense connective tissue stroma among recurrent cancers. In comparing the pretreatment and posttreatment histology of a series of 53 recurrent BCCs and SCCs, Freeman and Duncan[14] noted a significant increase in the number of sclerosing and invasive tumors among the posttreatment carcinomas. Radiotherapy could also alter the biological nature of BCCs without causing histological change. Jackson and Adams[7] found their series of 'horrifying' BCCs to be histologically identical to ordinary BCCs and postulated such a change in innate tumor biology as one possible explanation for the aggressive clinical behavior of these tumors. Hirshowitz and Mahler[6] also questioned possible 'biological changes in the tumor cell leading to greater invasiveness' as one explanation for their series of incurable postradiation BCCs.

Radiotherapy may also elicit change from tissue surrounding the BCC. Both Hirshowitz and Mahler[6] and Jackson and Adams[7] have suggested that irradiation may decrease local host defenses, allowing heightened tumor spread. Several authors have advanced the hypothesis that scar formation with entrapment of residual tumor can make recurrent BCCs very difficult to eradicate.[1,8,13,15–17] Radiotherapy might result in the fibrotic scar tissue of radiation dermatitis, which could encompass a far greater area than the scarring that follows surgical excision, electrodesiccation and curettage, or cryotherapy. Sequestration of residual tumor cells within such a relatively large zone would correlate well with the significantly heightened horizontal extension for postradiation BCCs seen in our series. Mora and Robins[16] proposed that scar tissue may act as an overlying barrier to the spread of residual tumor, forcing it in horizontal and deep directions. In the region of the midface, where the majority of the recurrent BCCs in our series are found, this could lead to the tracking of tumor along periosteum and perichondrium (as these structures are located quite superficially), enhancing spread. Finally, other authors[6,8] have postulated the scenario of irradiated BCC entrapped within scar tissue for long periods of time, then suddenly breaking free, with a much more aggressive and invasive growth pattern than the original tumor.

The effects of radiotherapy on neighboring host tissue may extend to deep subcutaneous tissue, as well as the more closely neighboring dermis, fascia and muscle. This is particularly plausible in the midface region, where the relatively superficial location of deep subcutaneous tissue renders it susceptible to radiation damage. Generally, cartilage and bone are felt to be natural barriers to tumor, with invasion by malignancy a rare event. However, the hypothesis has been advanced that radiation damage to these tissues may compromise this protective ability. Such an effect, combined with the aforementioned deep diversion of residual tumor by scar tissue, could help explain the significantly increased deep subcutaneous invasion seen with our group of postradiation BCCs.

The data from our study allow for other observations. The average preoperative size

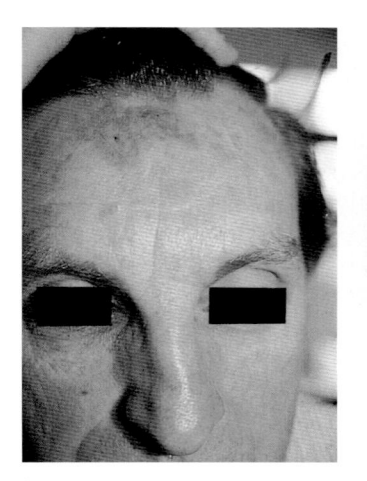

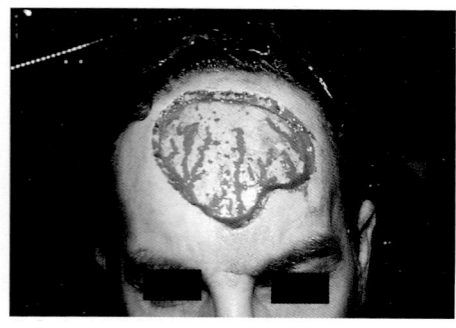

Figure 11.1
(A) Preoperative clinical appearance of large basal cell carcinoma of the forehead recurring following radiotherapy. (B) Postoperative defect of large basal cell carcinoma of the forehead recurring following radiotherapy.

of the postradiation BCCs in our series was 2.1 cm. These data support the concept that recurrent BCCs tend to be larger, on average, than primary lesions (Figure 11.1).[18,19] In their series of 97 recurrent BCCs, Sakura and Calamel[17] found an average size of 1.9 cm. Roenigk et al[20] noted that 33.2% of their 214 recurrent BCCs were over 2.0 cm. Of 33 horror BCCs reported by Jackson and Adams,[7] 28 (84.8%) were also larger than 2.0 cm. Postradiation BCCs would be expected to have a relatively large size, due to their status as recurrent tumors, and the increased horizontal and vertical extension we have shown them to display *vis-á-vis* other treatment subclasses of recurrent BCC.

The series also demonstrated 19 of 27 (70.4%) of the tumors to be located in the mid-third of the face (Figure 11.2). According to the literature, a disproportionately high number of recurrent BCCs develop in this region relative to the number of primary BCCs located there. In reviewing 3054 BCCs, Koplin and Zarem[21] found 50% of recurrences to occur in the nasal and periorbital zones, while only 39.5% of primary BCCs were located there. Roenigk et al[20] noted that 41% of their recurrent BCCs were within the nasal zone, as opposed to 22% of primary BCCs. In addition, there may be an increased tendency toward destructive behavior tumors of the midface region. All four incurable BCCs described by Hirshowitz and Mahler[6] occurred in this region. Twenty-one of 33 BCCs described by Jackson and Adams[7] and 29 of 33 'living death' BCCs chronicled by Pierce et al[8] also arose in the midface zone. Possible explanations for the location and behavior of these tumors were discussed earlier.

TREATMENT RECOMMENDATIONS

As was illustrated previously, the recurrence rates for repeat irradiation or standard surgical excision of BCC recurring after radiotherapy are unacceptably high. Several factors suggest that MMS is the treatment of choice for this entity. The large size and midface location of the majority of the postradiation recurrences in our series are independent indications for treatment with Mohs surgery. Numerous studies have clearly shown that MMS is the treatment of choice for large tumors, especially those of the head and neck.[18,20,22–24] In terms of more specific

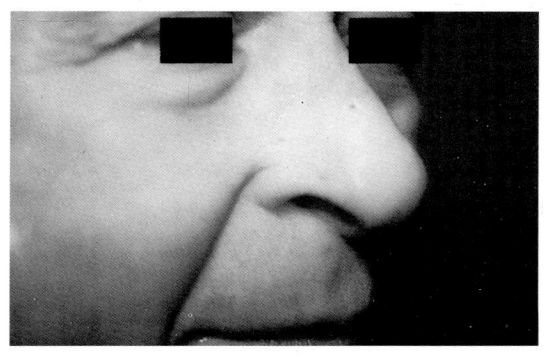

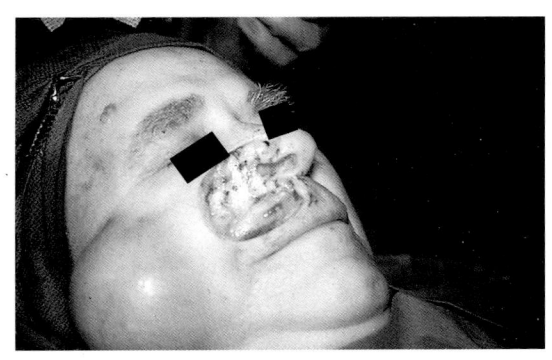

Figure 11.2
(A) Preoperative clinical appearance of basal cell carcinoma of the midface recurring following radiotherapy. (B) Postoperative defect of basal cell carcinoma of the midface recurring following radiotherapy (note extensive subclinical extension of the tumor).

tumor location, BCCs of the midface may track along deep subcutaneous tissue planes and between embryonic fusion planes. Basal cell carcinomas recurring following irradiation often manifest sclerotic and/or infiltrating architectures, making them especially capable of such movement. This type of tumor extension is ideally suited to treatment by MMS, with its unique abilities to examine the entire surgical margins and map tumor spread precisely. Mohs micrographic surgery also achieves tumor eradication with maximal tissue conservation, another reason for its use in this region of foremost cosmetic concern.

Although MMS seems the treatment of choice for BCC recurring after irradiation, the special nature of this entity raises the issue of the use of modified or adjuvant therapy to minimize risk of recurrence. One possibility is resection of an additional MMS layer beyond the initial tumor-free margin, as may be done for other aggressive, difficult tumors such as dermatofibrosarcoma protuberans and Merkel cell carcinoma. Such resection could prove beneficial in cases with discontinuous tumor spread, which might well be a relatively common scenario following radiotherapy, owing to the postulated scar formation and consequent residual tumor entrapment. The disadvantage to such a technique would be larger resultant defects at sites that are often cosmetically critical.

When considering adjuvant therapy, the question also arises of additional radiation following MMS. There are potential difficulties with this approach. If one assumes initial radiotherapy was administered properly, recurrence implies an inherent or acquired 'radiation resistance' among these BCCs. The usefulness of further radiation on such a tumor population is dubious. Furthermore, additional radiotherapy of previously irradiated tissue often results in chronic radiation dermatitis. Hansen and Jensen[5] found that 61% of BCCs recurring following irradiation and radiated again displayed poor cosmetic results, as opposed to only 17% of similarly recurrent BCCs subsequently treated by surgical excision. Similar results could be anticipated with adjuvant radiotherapy, since primary BCCs generally receive 3000–4500 rads as a treatment course, while significant chronic radiation damage may be seen after as little as 4000–5000 rads of total radiation.[25,26]

Conclusion

Our recent quantitative findings firmly support the already strong historical evidence that BCC recurring after radiotherapy is a unique subset of recurrent BCC. These tumors often manifest aggressive, invasive behavior evidenced by both the high recurrence rates and large numbers of incurable and metastasizing lesions described in the literature, as well as the heightened horizontal and vertical extension seen in our series. We have found them to be large, with the majority developing in the mid-third of the face. Cutaneous oncologists should be sensitive to recurrence of these tumors. Early diagnosis and treatment, as well as awareness of the characteristic prominent extension and deep subcutaneous invasion of these malignancies, is important. Mohs micrographic surgery offers the unique advantages of precise tumor mapping and maximal tissue conservation in the eradication of these difficult BCCs.

References

1. Cobbett JR, Recurrence of rodent ulcers after radiotherapy, *Br J Surg* (1965) **52**:347–9.
2. Hayes H, Basal cell carcinoma: the East Grinstead experience, *Plas Reconstr Surg* (1962) **30**:273–80.

3. Rank B, Wakefield A, Surgery of basal cell carcinoma, *Br J Surg* (1958) **45**:531–47.

4. Churchill-Davidson I, Johnson E, Rodent ulcers: an analysis of 711 lesions treated by radiotherapy, *Br Med J* (1954) **1**:1465–8.

5. Hansen PB, Jensen MS, Late results following radiotherapy of skin cancer, *Acta Radiol (Ther) (Stockholm)* (1968) **7**:307–19.

6. Hirshowitz B, Mahler D, Incurable recurrences of basal cell carcinoma of the mid-face following radiation therapy, *Br J Plast Surg* (1971) **24**:205–11.

7. Jackson R, Adams RH, Horrifying basal cell carcinoma: a study of 33 cases and a comparison with 435 non-horror cases and a report on four metastatic cases, *J Surg Oncol* (1973) **5**:431–63.

8. Pierce GW, Klabunde EH, Brobst HJ, Preliminary report on improper selection of treatment for basal cell epithelioma in the region of the orbit and the nose, *Plast Reconstr Surg* (1953) **11**:147–53.

9. Rowe DE, Carroll RJ, Day CC, Mohs surgery is the treatment of choice for recurrent (previously treated) basal cell carcinoma, *J Dermatol Surg Oncol* (1989) **15**:414–31.

10. Smith SP, Foley EH, Grande DJ, Use of Mohs micrographic surgery to establish quantitative proof of heightened tumor spread in basal cell carcinoma recurrent following radiotherapy, *J Dermatol Surg Oncol* (1990) **16**:1012–16.

11. Smith SP, Grande DJ, Basal cell carcinoma recurring after radiotherapy: a unique, difficult treatment subclass of recurrent basal cell carcinoma, *J Dermatol Surg Oncol* (1991) **17**:26–30.

12. Dzubow LM, Rigel DS, Robins P, Risk factors for local recurrence of primary squamous cell carcinomas, *Arch Dermatol* (1982) **118**:900–2.

13. Menn H, Robins P, Kopf AW et al, The recurrent basal cell epithelioma: a study of 100 cases of recurrent, re-treated basal cell epitheliomas, *Arch Dermatol* (1971) **103**:628–31.

14. Freeman RG, Duncan WC, Recurrent skin cancer, *Arch Dermatol* (1973) **107**:395–9.

15. Levine H, Cutaneous carcinoma of the head and neck: management of massive and previously uncontrolled lesions, *Laryngoscope* (1983) **93**:87–105.

16. Mora RG, Robins P, Basal-cell carcinomas in the center of the face: special diagnostic, prognostic and therapeutic considerations, *J Dermatol Surg Oncol* (1978) **4**:315–21.

17. Sakura CY, Calamel PM, Comparison of treatment modalities for recurrent basal cell carcinoma, *Plast Reconstr Surg* (1979) **63**:492–6.

18. Robins P, Chemosurgery: my 15 years of experience, *J Dermatol Surg Oncol* (1981) **7**:779–89.

19. Von Essen CF, Roentgen therapy of skin and lip carcinoma: factors influencing success and failure, *Am J Roentgenol* (1960) **83**:556–70.

20. Roenigk RK, Ratz JL, Bailin PL et al, Trends in the presentation and treatment of basal cell carcinomas, *J Dermatol Surg Oncol* (1986) **12**:860–5.

21. Koplin L, Zarem HA, Recurrent basal cell carcinoma, *Plast Reconstr Surg* (1980) **65**:656–63.

22. Mohs FE, *Chemosurgery: microscopically controlled surgery for skin cancer* (Charles C Thomas: Springfield, Illinois 1978) 154.

23. Swanson NA, Mohs surgery: technique, indications, applications

and the future, *Arch Dermatol* (1983) **119**:761–3.
24. Roenigk RK, Mohs micrographic surgery, *Mayo Clinic Proc* (1988) **63**:175–83.
25. Prasad KN, *Human radiation biology* (Harper and Row: Hagerstown, Maryland 1974) 240–56.
26. Rubin P, Casarett GW, *Clinical radiation pathology* (WB Saunders: Philadelphia 1968) 62–119.

Chapter 12

METASTATIC BASAL CELL CARCINOMA

Jacob S. Lo
Stephen N. Snow
Frederic E. Mohs

INTRODUCTION

Although basal cell carcinoma (BCC) is a common malignancy affecting man, metastatic basal cell carcinoma (MBCC) is a very rare clinical and pathological entity. The primary tumor in MBCC typically begins as a neglected, large, ulcerated, locally invasive and destructive neoplasm that recurs despite repeated surgery or radiotherapy.[1] Metastatic basal cell carcinoma has been reported in four patients with basal cell nevus syndrome.[2-5] It has also been associated with secondary[6] and systemic[7] amyloidosis, AIDS-related complex (ARC),[8] AIDS[9] and other cell-mediated immunodeficiency states.[10] A total of 205 cases of MBCC were reported in the literature up until 1980 although only 175 of these cases fulfill the criteria for the diagnosis of MBCC.[11] Since then, approximately 60 more cases have been reported.

CRITERIA FOR DIAGNOSIS OF METASTATIC BASAL CELL CARCINOMA

The criteria for making the diagnosis of MBCC have been established by Lattes and Kessler in 1951 and Cotran in 1960.[12,13] Three conditions must be met in order to make the diagnosis of MBCC. They point out that: (1) the primary tumor must be of the skin and not of mucous membrane or glandular tissue; (2) both the metastasis and primary lesion must show identical pathology proved by microscopic sections; and (3) metastasis must be demonstrated at a site distant from the primary lesion and cannot be a result of direct extension.

Direct implantation and proliferation in bronchi secondary to aspiration has been reported.[14-16] However, such cases do not fulfill the criteria for the diagnosis of MBCC as defined by Lattes and Kessler.[12] Although fine-needle aspiration of lymph nodes may yield results consistent with the diagnosis of MBCC, this technique may not be adequate to establish a firm diagnosis.[11] In general, histological confirmation is required to establish a diagnosis of MBCC.

INCIDENCE

The reported incidence of MBCC ranges from 0.0028% to 0.55%[13,17-24] as tabulated in Table 12.1. The smallest incidence of MBCC in the literature, 0.0028%, was reported by Paver et al,[17] who reviewed records of 50 000 patients in Australia and

Table 12.1
Reported incidences of MBCC

Authors	Incidence (%)
Paver et al[17]	0.0028
Weedon and Wall[18]	0.01
Lo et al[19]	0.03
Cotran[13]	0.1
Lakshmipathi and Hunt[20]	0.1
Scanlon et al[21]	0.2
Conley[22]	0.25
Wronkowski[23]	0.5
Cade[24]	0.55

New Zealand. Among pathological specimens, the incidence of MBCC has been reported to be 0.01%.[18] A higher incidence of 0.1% was reported by Cotran.[13] This figure was based on 9 cases of MBCC found among 9050 cases of BCC evaluated at the Memorial Hospital in New York. However, this figure may reflect a preselected referral population.[16] We reported an incidence of MBCC of 0.03%.[19] This figure was based on 12 cases of MBCC found among 36 000 consecutive cases of BCC evaluated at the University of Wisconsin Mohs Surgery Clinic from 1936 to 1988. The clinical data from each of the 12 cases of MBCC that we reported in our series are summarized in Table 12.2. Findings of these 12 patients as a series are summarized in Table 12.3.

Table 12.2
Clinical data of 12 patients with MBCC

Case	Sex	Age of onset (years)	Age at metastasis (years)	Age at death	Pathological size (cm) of primary tumor	Location of primary BCC	Number of recurrences
1	M	36	70	70	5.0 × 9.0	Ear	Many
2	M	38	55	Alive (+25 years)	9.2 × 7.4	Temple	Many
3	M	45	55	59	3.0 × 3.6	Nasal bridge	Many
4	M	52	69	75	10.0 × 10.0	Lower eyelid	1
5	M	<10	52	53	3.0 × 4.0	Back	3
6	M	51	61	62	8.0 × 8.0	Cheek (below ear)	3
7	M	39	81	81	8.0 × 8.0	Upper lip	Many
8	M	61	69	69	7.0 × 20.0	Upper arm	0
9	M	44	50	52	5.0 × 5.0	Cheek and lip	1
10	M	71	85	86	4.0 × 5.0	Temple	0
11	M	37	58	Alive (+6.75 years)	7.0 × 9.2	Upper neck	Many
12	M	47	67	69	5.8 × 3.8	Lateral canthus	11

M, male; BCC, basal cell carcinoma; 5-FU, 5-fluorouracil; MBCC, metastatic basal cell carcinoma

Lakshmipathi and Hunt,[20] Scanlon et al,[21] Conley,[22] Wronkowski[23] and Cade[24] have reported higher incidences. However, their figures are based on smaller groups of patients.

AGE OF ONSET OF PRIMARY TUMOR

The median age of onset of the primary tumor in MBCC is 45.[11] This figure is appreciably lower than that reported for nonmetastatic BCC.[25] A possible explanation for this is that elderly patients with recent-onset BCCs may not survive long enough to develop metastasis. A long period of time may be required between the beginning of a tumor and metastasis. An alternative explanation is that BCCs occurring at an earlier age may exhibit more aggressive behavior.[11] The median age at the first sign of metastasis has been reported to be 59.[11] In a series of 12 patients reported by us, the mean and median ages at the first sign of metastasis were 64.3 and 64 years, respectively.[19]

INTERVAL FROM ONSET OF PRIMARY TUMOR TO METASTASIS

The median interval from onset of the primary tumor to the time of metastasis has been reported to be 9 years.[11] This figure is in accord with the calculated intervals of

Table 12.2 contd

Location of metastases	Treatment of metastases	History of radiation	Other BCCs	Other carcinoma	Cause of death
Cervical lymph nodes, dura	None	None	None	None	MBCC
Cervical lymph nodes, common carotid artery	Neck dissection, carotid artery resection, cobalt radiation	For teenage acne	31	SCC	Alive 25 years after diagnosis of MBCC
Submaxillary and cervical lymph nodes, lung	Radiation and neck dissection	None	None	SCC	Unknown
Lung	Pneumonectomy	None	1	SCC	Myocardial infarct
Axillary and supraclavicular lymph nodes, lung recurrent laryngeal nerve	Adriamycin, cytoxan, CCNU, 5-FU, bleomycin	None	None	None	MBCC
Skin, cervical lymph nodes	Fixed tissue excision of	None	2	None	MBCC
Lung	None	For acne	>42	SCC	MBCC
Lung, lymph nodes	Velban, bleomycin, CCNU	None	1	None	MBCC
Cervical lymph node and bone	Chemotherapy	None	2	None	MBCC
Cervical lymph nodes	Radical neck dissection	None	3	None	MBCC
Cervical lymph nodes and skin	Radical neck dissection	None	>36	None	Alive
Lymph nodes, esophagus	Palliative surgery, gastrectomy	None	>4	None	MBCC

Table 12.3
Summary of series of 12 patients with MBCC

Sex	12 males, 0 females
Time of onset of primary tumor	
Range (years)	<10 to 71
Mean age (years)	47.4
Median age (years)	45
Age at first sign of metastasis	
Range (years)	50 to 85
Mean age (years)	64.3
Median age (years)	64
Interval from onset of primary tumor to time of metastasis	
Range (years)	7 to 34
Mean (years)	18.6
Median (years)	14
Age at death (n = 10)	
Range (years)	52 to 86
Mean (years)	67.6
Median (years)	69
Interval from time of diagnosis of MBCC to death (n = 9)	
range (years)	<1 to 6
Mean (months)	23.4
Median (months)	14
Histological findings of the primary tumor	
Morpheaform variant in at least part of the tumor	11 patients
Adenocystic variant in at least part of the tumor	2 patients
Metatypical variant in at least part of the tumor	4 patients
One histological variant only in primary tumor	8 patients
Two histological variants in primary tumor	3 patients
Three histological variants in primary tumor	1 patient
Perineural extension	5 patients
Sites of metastases	
Lymph node	10 patients
Lung	5 patients
Skin	2 patients
Bone	1 patient
Dura	1 patient
Carotid artery	1 patient
Esophagus	1 patient
History of skin graft at site of primary tumor	3 patients
History of radiation treatment for primary tumor	6 patients
History of radiation treatments for acne	2 patients

11 and 9.6 years reported by Mikhail et al[26] and Farmer and Helwig,[27] respectively. The interval from onset of the primary tumor to the time of metastasis ranges from 0 to 45 years.[11] An interval of 6–10 years from onset of the primary tumor to the time of metastasis is not uncommon.[28] The mean and median intervals from onset of the primary tumor to the time of metastases were 18.6 and 14 years (n = 11), respectively, in our series.[19] Since our patients were all treated by Mohs micrographic surgery, it is possible that the longer interval from the time of the primary tumor to the time of metastasis may be directly proportional to the completeness of initial tumor excision. Most cases of MBCC show active disease at the primary and metastatic site.

Gender

Most series of MBCC show a predominance of male patients. In a review of the literature, the male to female ratio was 2:1 for those reported cases of MBCC that mentioned gender of the patient.[11] In our series of patients with MBCC, all 12 were men.[24] Whether or not being male is a risk factor for developing MBCC remains to be elucidated.

SKIN COLOR

It appears that almost all cases of MBCC have occurred in patients with light complexions, since there have been only five cases of MBCC occurring in black patients to date.[29-33] It is interesting to note that in four of these five cases of MBCC occurring in black patients, the primary tumors were not in the head and neck regions.[30-33] Given the rarity of BCCs in blacks in general, the occurrence of MBCC in these patients appears to be disproportionately high. It is also interesting to note that several cases of MBCC have been reported in the Japanese literature, including three with lung metastases.[34]

LOCATION OF PRIMARY TUMOR

Of primary tumors in MBCC 85% occur on the head and neck region, with the remaining 15% occurring on the trunk and extremities.[16,26,27,32] This distribution is also similar to that for nonmetastasizing primary BCC.

Certain sites of the primary tumor are associated with increased risk for metastasizing. Primary BCCs of the nose are less prone to metastasize while those on the scalp have a slightly increased tendency to metastasize more often.[11] Moreover, Dzubow reported that BCCs occurring on the skin overlying the superficial lobe of the parotid gland may be at risk for metastasizing if tumor penetration is deep.[35] Some sites that are atypical for nonmetastasizing BCCs but have been reported as the site of the primary lesion in MBCC include abdomen,[36] scrotum,[28,37-39] vulva,[31,40-42] nipple,[43] axilla[44] and anus.[45] In general, the occurrence of large ulcerated genital tumors should prompt the consideration of requesting a preliminary metastatic work-up because of the rarity of primary genital BCCs and possible increased incidence of metastasis involving genital BCCs.

MULTIPLE PRIMARY TUMORS

Although the primary tumor is usually solitary, multiple sites have also been reported.[12,46] Since some patients may present with more than one BCC at the time of metastasis, it may be difficult to tell which specific BCC metastasized. In some cases, it may be helpful to review the microscopic slides of the primary BCCs to determine their morphological type and match it with the corresponding morphological pattern of the MBCC. Whether or not multiple primary tumors can metastasize remains to be proved and is controversial.

SMALL PRIMARY TUMORS

The typical primary tumor in MBCC is large, ulcerative, deeply penetrating, and recurrent after previous surgery or radiotherapy.[27] In our series of patients with MBCC, 9 out of 12 patients had primary tumors that were 20 cm^2 larger. However, it is important to appreciate that small BCCs can also give rise to metastases, especially if they involve deep subcutaneous tissue. Presently, there is no universally accepted size criterion for calling a BCC 'small'. Kord et al reported three cases of MBCC associated with 'small' primary tumors ranging in size from 3.0×3.0 cm to 4.4×6.0 cm.[47]

There are a few reports of MBCCs developing from apparently smaller primary BCCs. Steiner et al[48] reported a case of MBCC in a woman with a history of four BCCs that were all 1.0 cm or smaller. This patient first developed BCC during childhood and died at 29 years of age.

More recently, Menz et al reported a case of MBCC in a 45-year-old man who had a history of several BCCs that were all 1 cm in diameter or smaller.[49] Their case was interesting in that the primary lesion was not only small but absent at the time of metastasis. Although metastasis can occur in small, minimally invasive BCCs, this event is exceptionally rare.

SURVIVAL

Survival after primary signs of metastasis has been reported to range from less than 1 month to 192 months.[11] However, approximately 20% of patients with MBCC survive 1 year and approximately 10% survive 5 years.[27] The median survival after primary signs of metastases is 8 months.[11] This figure was based on a review of the literature of 79 cases that mentioned survival. The route of metastasis, the interval before the first sign of metastases, the age at first sign of metastases, and the age of onset of BCC do not correlate with survival.[11] Moreover, although most reported patients with MBCC are male, gender has no influence on survival.[11]

The mean and median survival of the series of patients with MBCC reported by us were 23.4 months ($n = 9$) and 14 months, respectively.[19] In calculating mean and median survival, we included only those patients who died of MBCC. One of our patients is still alive after developing MBCC 6 years previously. This patient's primary tumor was 3.4 × 3.7 cm and developed on the left side of his neck (Figure 12.1) when he was 37 years old. He was subsequently treated with Mohs micrographic surgery. Perineural spread of BCC was noted histologically. The final defect was 7.0 × 9.2 cm (Figure 12.2). He developed MBCC 21 years later, at which time he presented with two subcutaneous nodules on the left side of his neck (Figure 12.3). Radical neck dissection demonstrated MBCC involving 6 of 27 left cervical lymph nodes and skin.

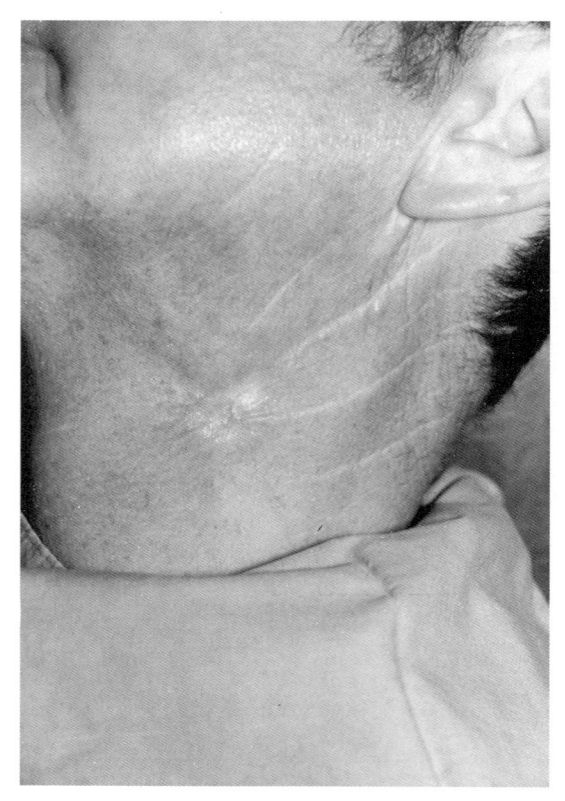

Figure 12.1
Primary morpheaform basal cell carcinoma (3.4 × 3.7 cm) on the left upper neck (Case 11).

More remarkable is another patient in our series of patients with MBCC who is still alive after developing MBCC 25 years ago. To our knowledge, this patient is the longest surviving patient with a history of MBCC. Hence, the course of MBCC may not be universally a rapid downhill course. Other cases of MBCC with survival beyond 10 years have also been reported.[11]

HISTOLOGY

Some patients exhibit more than one histological variant of BCC in their primary

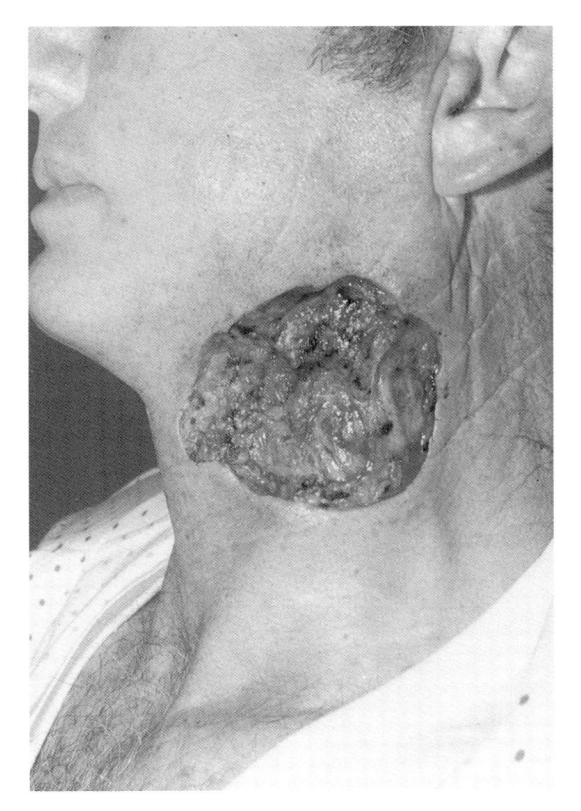

Figure 12.2
Defect (7.0 × 9.2 cm) after completion of Mohs micrographic surgery.

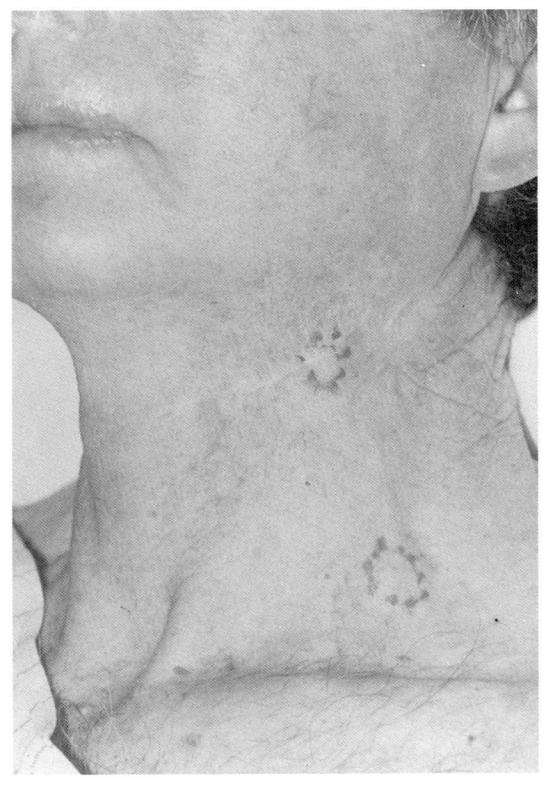

Figure 12.3
Two subcutaneous nodules on the left side of the neck 21 years after excision of the primary basal cell carcinoma.

tumor.[19] The morpheaform histological variant of BCC is present in at least part of the primary tumor in 11 of 12 patients in our series of MBCC patients.[19] However, it was difficult to tell with certainty whether the spindle strands of basophilic cells were due to a true morpheaform pattern or to an extrinsic focus of fibrous reaction around the primary tumor.

The predominance of the morpheaform pattern of BCC in a series of patients with MBCC reported by us may be due to the fact that this pattern of BCC is more difficult to detect clinically since the lesions are usually flat and may be more likely to be overlooked during a skin examination than other histological variants. The other histological variants of BCC are easier to detect and were treated by Mohs micrographic surgery. The completeness of excision of the tumor by this method may account for the relative scarcity of nonmorpheaform types of BCC in our series of MBCC patients.

Morpheaform and adenocystic types of BCC are more locally aggressive than other histological variants. They infiltrate microscopically into surrounding tissue far from the primary site.[50,51] The presence of sclerosis and irregular spiky outlines of basal cells one to three layers thick may indicate a potential locally aggressive lesion.[51,52]

However, others assert that the metatypical or basosquamous type of BCC is most likely to metastasize.[27] Farmer and Helwig examined 10 primary lesions of patients with MBCC and found that 8 exhibited features of metatypical BCC involving at least part of the tumor.[27] Moreover, recurrent tumors tended to exhibit a more metatypical appearance. Helwig et al believe that the metatypical appearance of the tumor may be a feature associated with the ability to metastasize. This conclusion was also previously stated by other authors.[53-57] However, some authors believe that no one histological type of BCC is more likely to metastasize than another.[1]

In a retrospective review of 36 000 cases of BCC treated at the Mohs Surgery Clinic between 1936 and 1988, there were 5500 cases of BCC with the invasive morpheaform pattern. Since our 12 patients with MBCC were all seen within this time frame and demonstrated the morpheaform pattern of BCC in at least part of the primary tumor, our metastatic rate for morpheaform BCC is thus 0.22% (12/5500). We believe that the deeply invasive morpheaform variant of BCC may be associated with a higher tendency to metastasize than other variants of BCC.

Mehregan[58] has identified some histological characteristics that locally aggressive BCCs on sun-protected skin exhibit. Palisading of nuclei at the periphery of tumor masses, retraction between the masses of basal cells and stroma, and variably dense mononuclear infiltrate in the area adjacent to the tumor were noted in these tumors. Other characteristics of aggressive tumors included: (1) involvement of the full thickness of the dermis; (2) involvement of the deep dermis or subcutaneous fat; (3) small nests and clumps of epithelial cells infiltrating between collagen bundles at the advancing border of lesions; and (4) perivascular and perineural tumor nests in the deep dermis. Full-thickness involvement of the dermis may include abnormal cells following the pathway of a hair follicle or eccrine sweat duct.

Although Farmer and Helwig stressed the metatypical features of the neoplastic epithelium, such as foci of squamous metaplasia as a possible histological marker for lesions with a tendency to metastasize,[27] Mehregan's series of aggressive BCCs did not show that these features were prominent. Mehregan feels that aggregation of small neoplastic cells and individual cells at the periphery of the lesion in the neoplasm may be a marker for highly invasive BCCs that have the ability to metastasize.[58]

Affinity of aggressive BCCs for perineural invasion was previously noted by Mohs and Lathrop in 1952.[59] However, it was not reported in MBCC until 1984 by von Domarus and Stevens.[11] Since then we have reported five cases of perineural invasion in 5 of our 12 patients with MBCC.[19] Perineural spread may be an important pointer to possible local recurrence and metastasis.

The metastatic tumor may occasionally show unusual histopathological features. Interestingly, Farmer and Helwig[27] reported shadow cells characteristic of pilomatricoma in two of five cases of MBCC with bony metastases.

Timing of repairs for large Mohs surgery defects

Mikhail et al[26,60] believes that immediate placement of skin grafts after surgical resection of BCCs may cause residual tumor to penetrate deeper tissue. A thick scar may form under the skin graft which would prevent residual BCC from reaching the surface of the skin graft. This, in turn, may promote tumor invasion of blood vessels and also obscure early detection of recurrent tumors. He recommends that reconstructive surgery be deferred for at least 6 months while evidence of recurrent tumor is looked for. Although we prefer to allow defects created by Mohs micrographic surgery for large or recurrent BCCs to heal by second intention for the same reasons as mentioned by Mikhail, we also take other factors (that is, ability of the patient to care for a wound, risk factors for infection, exposed cartilage, and patient's preference) into consideration when deciding whether or not immediate reconstructive surgery will be performed.

HISTORY OF RADIATION THERAPY AS A RISK FACTOR

Although radiation therapy is a treatment modality for BCC, it may also be a risk factor for developing MBCC. Six of our 12 patients with MBCC had history of radiation treatment for their primary tumor.[19] In addition, two other patients had history of radiation treatment for acne. Some authors postulate that radiation therapy as primary treatment of BCC may transform a low-grade tumor into a highly malignant one.[61,62]

HEMATOLOGENOUS VERSUS LYMPHATIC SPREAD

Hematologic and lymphatic spread are reportedly equally frequent in MBCC.[11] Since metastatic squamous cell carcinoma spreads to lymph nodes in 80–90% of cases, the even distribution of the route of metastasis in MBCC argues against squamous differentiation as the determining factor for lymph node metastasis in a BCC.[11]

SITES OF METASTASES

Lymph nodes are the most common organs containing metastatic tumor. The lung is the second most common site for metastatic tumor. Lung metastases account for 18–20% of cases. Liver and bone involvement vary from 15 to 18% in occurrence.[27] Other sites of metastases include spleen, kidney, pancreas, pleura, diaphragm, vena cava, adrenal glands, thyroid gland, pituitary gland and heart.[5,11,19,27] Rare sites of metastases found in our series of patients include the dura, esophagus and common carotid artery.[18] Although cutaneous metastasis has been reported,[19,26,37] it is also considered extremely rare.

IMMUNE DEFICIENCY STATES AS POSSIBLE RISK FACTOR

Metastatic basal cell carcinoma has been reported in various cell-mediated immune deficiency states.[9,10] Some authors[10,16] suggest that deficient cell-mediated immunity may contribute in some way to the metastasis of BCC. Patients with severe immunologic deficit may tolerate distant implants of a neoplasm that usually only survives on the skin.[16] One group believes that patients with AIDS have a higher risk of developing cutaneous neoplasms.[63] However, only one case of MBCC involving a patient with AIDS[8] and another case involving a patient with ARC[9] have been reported. Further support for an etiologic role of deficient cell-mediated immunity in the pathogenesis of MBCC may be derived from case reports.

Staley et al[39] reported a case of MBCC with multiple primary tumors on the scrotum. This patient was nonreactive to immediate hypersensitivity testing. Negative results were obtained with purified protein derivative (PPD), mumps, *Candida* and streptokinase/streptodornase at 48 h. Moreover, testing with *Trichophyton–Dermatophyton*-O-extract and histoplasmosis was also negative. The in vitro assay of cell-mediated immunity using phytohemagglutinin-stimulated lymphocyte transformation was virtually nonreactive. The patient was treated with weekly bacillus Calmette–Guerin immunotherapy administered by scarification with resultant regression of lesions and development of a positive reaction to PPD and other antigens. Moreover, he developed a normal result with lymphocyte transformation tests. Treatment later with combination chemotherapy (cisplatin, bleomycin, and 5-fluorouracil (5-FU)) every 3 weeks results in smaller right groin lymph nodes, healed scrotal lesions, and marked regression of pulmonary metastasis.

Histological findings have also implied that a defect in the host immune response may play an etiologic role in the development of MBCC, as Farmer and Helwig described a paucity of inflammatory cells, particularly around recurrent tumors.[27] Decreased numbers of circulating T lymphocytes have been described in a series of patients with nonmetastasizing BCCs. The number of T lymphocytes directly correlated with tumor size, being lower with large tumors.[64] The large tumors on histological examination also exhibited a paucity of lymphocytic infiltrate around the tumor. This may serve as additional evidence that a cellular immunity may play an etiologic role in the development of large BCCs and their potential to metastasize.

Mikhail et al[26] has also described one patient with MBCC that exhibited normal delayed hypersensitivity. Hence, additional factor(s) may be necessary in the pathogenesis of MBCC. Safai and Good speculated that a combination of stromal independence and immunodeficiency is needed in order for successful metastasis to occur.[10] Further investigation is needed to define the role, if any, of deficient cell-mediated immunity in the pathogenesis of MBCC.

Treatment

The main treatment modalities for MBCC are radiation, surgery and chemotherapy. However, the treatment of MBCC is difficult to evaluate because of the rarity of this entity. Since there are no controlled trials of treatment modalities in the literature, we can only draw information about treating MBCC from scattered case reports.

It is generally thought that all treatment modalities are ineffective in prolonging survival when bone metastases are demonstrated.[65] However, there are rare exceptions. Hartman et al reported a case of MBCC with cervical vertebral and epidural metastasis that was treated with radiotherapy which initially resulted in a remission interval of 3-years.[66] A relapse was treated with laminectomy and chemotherapy. The patient remained asymptomatic for 54 months after the diagnosis of bone metastasis was made.

Surgical treatment of MBCC has resulted in several cases of long-term survival.[27,67,68] An aggressive surgical approach to management of MBCC, where feasible has been recommended by Chandler and Lee.[69] Resection of lymph node[27,67] and pulmonary metastases[68,70] with subsequent long-term survival have been reported. One patient has survived 25 years to date after resection of pulmonary metastases.[19]

Various chemotherapeutic agents such as cyclophosphamide, actinomycin D, nitrogen mustard, 6-mercaptopurine, bleomycin, 5-FU and methotrexate have been used alone and in combination with little or no success.[28,31,61,71–73] However, one patient who underwent treatment with 5-FU reportedly survived for more than 2 years.[27] Adjunctive agents such as parahormone, methadone, prednisone, mithramycin and L-dopa can provide symptomatic relief and may be warranted when metabolic aberrations compromise the patient.[61]

Bleomycin, used as a single drug, was possibly effective in one patient with MBCC who died shortly after the second course of bleomycin.[10] This patient also developed a squamous cell carcinoma of the lungs with widespread metastases. Bleomycin, used in combination chemotherapy, has also demonstrated only minimal success in the treatment of MBCC.[34,74]

There are several case reports that suggest cisplatin (*cis*-diamminedichloroplatinum II) has activity in BCC.[75-79] Two cases resulted in complete remission, although the follow-up was less than 1 year.[76,79] One case of MBCC with lung metastases failed to respond to cisplatin;[69] however, the treatment failure may have been secondary to use of a lower dosage as compared to other authors. However, this patient showed no evidence of BCC 22 months after resection of lung metastases. The patient did not react to testing with PPD and could not be sensitized to DNCB. It is attractive to speculate that the success or failure of chemotherapy in the treatment of MBCC may be a function of the integrity of the host immune system.

Work-up for Suspected MBCC

There is little in the literature regarding the work-up of patients suspected to have MBCC. Mikhail et al[26] suggests that a chest radiograph, a bone radiograph and a serum alkaline phosphatase level be obtained in any patient with a history of BCC who complains of weight loss, pulmonary symptoms or bone pain. Radionuclide radiography and bone biopsy may also be helpful. When patients present with large BCCs and metastatic tumor is suspected, we prefer to obtain a regional CT scan before performing Mohs micrographic surgery since it provides us with information regarding tumor size and whether there are metastatic lesions in the lymph nodes or bone. Regional lymph node dissection should be performed only if there is evidence of clinical involvement.[36]

Since successful treatment of MBCC is rare and life expectancy after metastasis is usually short early and adequate treatment of the primary BCC is very important. The most expedient preventive measure is complete surgical extirpation of the primary tumor. According to Conley et al, Mohs micrographic surgery is the treatment of choice to accomplish adequate surgical treatment of the primary BCC.[61]

Metastatic Potential

The low metastatic potential of BCC has been attributed to its stromal dependence. Some authors have stressed that other factors may determine the metastatic potential of BCCs. Blewitt hypothesized that BCCs metastasize rarely because there must be a critical mass or depth before metastasis can occur.[80] He also conjectured that metastatic potential may be related to the probability of a tumor contacting a large-caliber vessel. Yet we have observed microscopic intravascular BCC without evidence of metastasis documented by chest radiographs and regional examination. This observation was also noted serendipitously by Dzubow[35]. Yet others believe that metastatic potential of BCCs may be related to certain histological features,[58,61] as presented in our discussion on histology. In general, it is plausible that all these factors contribute to the metastatic potential. However, it is the degree to which each of these factors contributes to the metastatic potential that remains to be determined.

Acknowledgments

We wish to thank Philip L. Bailin (Cleveland, Ohio) for donating the photographs used in Figures 12.1 and 12.2. We also wish to thank Rachel Caruso for the tremendous amount of work she did in compiling our data.

References

1. Amonette RA, Salasche SJ, Chesney TM et al, Metastatic basal cell carcinoma, *J Dermatol Surg Oncol* (1981) **7**:397–400.
2. Goldberg HM, Pratt-Thomas HR, Harvin JS, Metastatic basal cell carcinoma, *Plast Reconstr Surg* (1977) **59**:750–3.
3. Murphy KJ, Metastatic basal cell carcinoma with squamous appearances in the naevoid basal cell carcinoma syndrome, *Br J Plast Surg* (1975) **28**:331–4.
4. Taylor WB, Anderson DE, Howell JB et al, The nevoid basal cell carcinoma syndrome, *Arch Dermatol* (1968) **98**:612–14.
5. Winkler PA, Guyuron B, Multiple metastases from basal cell naevus syndrome, *Br J Plast Surg* (1987) **40**:528–31.
6. Beck HI, Andersen JA, Birkler NE et al, Giant basal cell carcinoma with metastasis and secondary amyloidosis. *Acta Derm Venereol (Stockholm)* (1983) **63**:564–7.
7. Lichenstein HL, Lee JC, Amyloidosis associated with metastatic basal cell carcinoma, *Cancer* (1980) **46**:2693–6.
8. Sitz KV, Keppen M, Johnson DF, Metastatic basal cell carcinoma in acquired immunodeficiency syndrome-related complex, *JAMA* (1987) **257**:340–3.
9. Steigleder GK, Metastasizing basalioma in AIDS, *Z Hautkr* (1987) **62**:661.
10. Safai B, Good RA, Basal cell carcinoma with metastasis: review of literature, *Arch Pathol Lab Med* (1977) **101**:327–31.
11. von Domarus H, Stevens PJ, Metastatic basal cell carcinoma. Report of five cases and review of 170 cases in the literature, *J Am Acad Dermatol* (1984) **10**:1043–60.
12. Lattes R, Kessler RW, Metastasizing basal cell epithelioma of the skin — a report of two cases, *Cancer* (1951) **4**:866–78.
13. Cotran RS, Metastasizing basal cell carcinoma, *Cancer* (1961) **14**:1036–40.
14. Pickren JW, Katz AD, Aspiration metastases from basal cell carcinoma, *Cancer* (1958) **11**:183–9.
15. Guillan RA, Johnson RP, Aspiration metastases from basal cell carcinoma — the 92nd known case, *Arch Dermatol* (1978) **114**:589–90.
16. Wermuth BM, Fajardo LF, Metastatic basal cell carcinoma: a review, *Arch Pathol* (1970) **90**:458–62.
17. Paver K, Poyzer K, Burry N et al, The incidence of basal cell carcinoma and their metastases in Australia and New Zealand, *Australas J Dermatol* (1973) **14**:53.
18. Weedon D, Wall D, Metastatic basal cell carcinoma, *Med J Aust* (1975) **2**:177–9.
19. Lo JS, Snow SN, Reizner GT et al, Metastatic basal cell carcinoma: report of twelve cases with a review of the literature, *J Am Acad Dermatol* (1991) **24**:715–19.
20. Lakshmipathi T, Hunt KM, Metastasizing basal cell carcinoma, *Br J Dermatol* (1967) **79**:267–70.
21. Scanlon EF, Volkmer DD, Oviedo MA et al, Metastatic basal cell carcinoma, *J Surg Oncol* (1980) **15**:171–80.
22. Conley J, Cancer of the skin of the nose, *Ann Otol Rhinol Laryngol* (1974) **83**:2–8.
23. Wronkowski Z, Metastases in dermal basal cell carcinoma, *Nowotwory* (1968) **18**:51–5.
24. Cade S, *Malignant disease and its treatment by radium* (The Williams & Wilkins Co.: Baltimore 1940) 1070–85.
25. Kopf AW, Computer analysis of 3531 basal cell carcinomas of the skin, *J Dermatol (Tokyo)* (1979) **6**:267–81.

26. Mikhail GR, Nims LP, Kelly AP et al, Metastatic basal cell carcinoma: review, pathogenesis and report of two cases, *Arch Dermatol* (1977) **113**:1261–9.

27. Farmer ER, Helwig EB, Metastatic basal cell carcinoma: a clinicopathologic study of seventeen cases, *Cancer* (1980) **46**:748–57.

28. Cieplinski W, Combination chemotherapy for the treatment of metastatic basal cell carcinoma of the scrotum — a case report, *Clin Oncol* (1984) **10**:267–72.

29. Schwartz RA, De Jager RI, Janniger CK et al, Giant basal cell carcinoma with metastases and myelophthisic anemia, *J Surg Oncol* (1986) **33**:223–6.

30. Binkley GW, Rauschkolb RE, Basal cell epithelioma metastasizing to lymph nodes, *Arch Dermatol* (1962) **86**:332–5.

31. Jiminez HT, Fenoglio CM, Richart RM, Vulvar basal cell carcinoma with metastasis: a case report, *Am J Obstet Gynecol* (1975) **121**:282–6.

32. Lanehart WH, Sanusi ID, Migra RP et al, Metastasizing basal cell carcinoma originating in a stasis ulcer in a black woman, *Arch Dermatol* (1983) **119**:587–91.

33. Lambert WC, Kasznica J, Chung HR et al, Metastasizing basal cell carcinoma developing in a gunshot wound in a black man, *J Surg Oncol* (1984) **27**:97–105.

34. Akiyama S, Imaizumi M, Sakamoto J et al, Basal cell carcinoma with lung metastasis, *Japan J Surg* (1985) **15**:215–20.

35. Dzubow LM, Metastatic basal cell carcinoma originating in the supraparotid region, *J Dermatol Surg Oncol* (1986) **12**:1306–8.

36. El Ferzli G, Ozuner G, Worth MH Jr, Diffuse metastatic basal cell carcinoma, *Contemp Surg* (1988) **33**:25–32.

37. Hughes JM, Metastatic basal cell carcinoma: a report of two cases and a review of the literature, *Clin Radiol* (1973) **24**:392–3.

38. Richter G, Subpleural lung metastases from basal cell carcinoma, *Hautarzt* (1957) **8**:215–19.

39. Staley TE, Nieh PT, Ciesielski TE et al, Metastatic basal cell carcinoma of the scrotum, *J Urol* (1983) **130**:792–4.

40. Hoffman MS, Roberts WS, Ruffolo EH, Basal cell carcinoma of the vulva with inguinal lymph node metastases, *Gynecol Oncol* (1988) **29**:113–19.

41. Sworn MJ, Hammond GT, Buchanan R, Metastatic basal cell carcinoma of the vulva-case report, *Br J Obstet Gynaecol* (1979) **86**:332–4.

42. Perrone T, Twiggs LB, Adcock LL et al, Vulvar basal cell carcinoma: an infrequently metastasizing neoplasm, *Int J Gynecol Pathol* (1987) **6**:152–65.

43. Shertz WT, Balogh K, Metastasizing basal cell carcinoma of the nipple, *Arch Pathol Lab Med* (1986) **110**:761–2.

44. Hazen HH, Basal cell cancers of the skin, *South Med J* (1917) **10**:241–6.

45. White WB, Schneiderman H, Sayre JF, Basal cell carcinoma of the anus: clinical and pathological distinction from cloacogenic carcinoma, *J Clin Gastroenterol* (1984) **6**:441–6.

46. Hirschowitz B, Mahler D, Unusual case of multiple basal cell carcinoma with metastasis to the parotid lymph gland, *Cancer* (1968) **22**:654–7.

47. Kord JP, Cottel WI, Proper S, Metastatic basal cell carcinoma, *J Dermatol Surg Oncol* (1982) **8**:604–8.

48. Steiner I, Rothrockel P, Sich J et al, Metastasizing basilioma at an early age, *Cesk Patol* (1984) **20**:246–51.

49. Menz J, Sterrett G, Wall L, Metastatic basal cell carcinoma associated with a

small primary tumour, *Australas J Dermatol* (1985) **26**:121–4.

50. Dellon AL, Host-tumor relationships in basal cell and squamous cell cancer of the skin, *Plast Reconstr Surg* (1978) **62**:37–48.
51. Pickering PP, Nickel WR, Classifications of basal cell carcinoma, *Plast Reconstr Surg* (1957) **19**:218–23.
52. Sloane JP, The value of typing basal cell carcinomas in predicting recurrence after surgical excision, *Br J Dermatol* (1977) **96**:127–32.
53. Jacobs GH, Rippey JJ, Altini M, Prediction of aggressive behaviour in basal cell carcinoma, *Cancer* (1982) **49**:533–7.
54. Borel DM, Cutaneous basosquamous carcinoma, *Arch Pathol* (1973) **95**:293–7.
55. Montgomery H, Basal squamous cell epithelioma, *Arch Dermatol Syphiol* (1928) **18**:50–73.
56. Helwig EB, Thomas CC, Basal cell carcinoma of the left leg with metastasis to the left inguinal lymph nodes, multiple skin metastases and involvement of the bone marrow, *Arch Dermatol* (1968) **97**:597.
57. Graham JH, Urbach F, Alkek DS, Metastatic basal cell carcinoma, *Arch Dermatol* (1969) **99**:778.
58. Mehregan AH, Aggressive basal cell epithelioma on sun-protected skin: report of eight cases, one with pulmonary and bone metastases, *Am J Dermatopathol* (1983) **5**:221–9.
59. Mohs FE, Lathrop TG, Modes of spread of cancer of skin, *Arch Dermatol* (1952) **66**:427–39.
60. Mikhail GR, Kelly AP Jr, Elmquist JG, Metastatic basal cell epithelioma discovered by chemosurgery, *Arch Dermatol* (1972) **105**:103–4.
61. Conley J, Sachs ME, Romo T et al, Metastatic basal cell carcinoma of the head and neck, *Otolaryngol Head Neck Surg* (1985) **93**:78–85.
62. Conway M, Hugo NE, Metastatic basal cell carcinoma, *Am J Surg* (1965) **110**:620–4.
63. Slazinski L, Stall JR, Mathews CR, Basal cell carcinoma in a man with acquired immunodeficiency syndrome, *J Am Acad Dermatol* (1984) **11**:140–1.
64. Dellon AL, Potvin C, Chretien PB et al, The immunobiology of skin cancer, *Plast Reconstr Surg* (1975) **55**:341–54.
65. Thackray AC, Histological classification of rodent ulcers and its bearing on prognosis, *Br J Cancer* (1951) **213**:216.
66. Hartman R, Hartman S, Green N, Long-term survival following bony metastases from basal cell carcinoma: report of a case, *Arch Dermatol* (1986) **122**:912–14.
67. Christensen M, Briggs RM, Coblentz MG et al, Metastatic basal cell carcinoma: a review of the literature and report of two cases, *Am Surg* (1978) **44**:382–7.
68. Borel DM, Cutaneous basosquamous carcinoma. Review of the literature and report of 35 cases, *Arch Pathol* (1973) **95**:293–7.
69. Chandler JJ, Lee L, Lymph node metastases from basal cell carcinoma, *NY State J Med* (1982) **82**:67–9.
70. Icli F, Omer U, Erdogan Y et al, Basal cell carcinoma with lung metastases: a case report, *J Surg Oncol* (1986) **33**:57–60.
71. Assor D, Basal cell carcinoma with metastasis to bone, *Cancer* (1967) **20**:2125–37.
72. Chien WL, Basal cell carcinoma with metastases to bones and lung, *Va Med Mon* (1966) **93**:14–17.
73. Hall TE, Tappan WM, Decker JW, Basal cell carcinoma with metastases:

report of two cases, *Rocky Mt Med* (1970) **67**:39–40.
74. Yamagami T, Araki S, Aiko Y et al, Examination of metastatic basal cell carcinoma, *Kurume Med J* (1974) **21**:83–6.
75. Wieman TJ, Shively EH, Woodcock EM, Responsiveness of metastatic basal cell carcinoma to chemotherapy, *Cancer* (1983) **52**:1583–5.
76. Salem P, Hall SW, Benjamin RS et al, Clinical phase I-II study of cis-diamminedichloroplatinum (II) given by continuous infusion, *Cancer Treat Rep* (1978) **62**:1553–6.
77. Guthrie TH, Porubsky ES, Successful systemic chemotherapy of advanced squamous and basal cell carcinoma of the skin with diamminedichloroplatinum II and doxorubicin, *Laryngoscope* (1982) **92**:1298–9.
78. Coker DD, Elias EG, Viravathana T et al, Chemotherapy for metastatic basal cell carcinoma, *Arch Dermatol* (1983) **119**:44–50.
79. Woods RL, Stewart JF, Metastatic basal cell carcinoma: report of a case responding to chemotherapy, *Postgrad Med J* (1980) **56**:272–3.
80. Blewitt RW, Why does basal cell carcinoma metastasize so rarely? *Int J Dermatol* (1980) **19**:144–6.

Chapter 13

MOHS MICROGRAPHIC SURGERY: EUROPEAN EXPERIENCE

António Picoto
Francisco Camacho
Neil P.J. Walker
Alejandro Camps-Fresneda

THE BEGINNING IN GERMANY

Dr Günter Burg was probably the first European to perform Mohs micrographic surgery in Germany. He was trained in New York by Dr Perry Robins for four months and then spent several weeks with Dr Frederick Mohs. He returned to the Department of Dermatology at the University of Munich and, under the leadership of Professor Braun Falco, started practicing the technique. The fixed-tissue technique, chemosurgery, was initially performed. Later, Dr Birger Konz started to practice the frozen technique. This pioneering work resulted in publications in the German literature.[1-7] When Dr Burg dedicated his efforts to other areas of dermatology, Dr Konz continued performing Mohs micrographic surgery in Europe. Later, Dr Burg became chairman at Wurzburg and again introduced the Mohs micrographic method to that region. A variation of the Mohs technique was developed in Germany by Dr Helmut Breuninger, the so-called 'cake technique', and is still widely used.[8,9]

PORTUGAL

Dr António Picoto became involved in Mohs micrographic surgery after meeting Dr Perry Robins when the International Society for Dermatologic Surgery was founded in Morocco in 1978. Dr Robins invited Dr Picoto to learn the Mohs technique in 1979. In 1980, Dr Picoto began the practice of Mohs micrographic surgery, fresh-tissue technique, in Lisbon at the Centro de Dermatologia Médico Cirurgica de Lisboa, as part of the network of the National Health Service in Portugal. A Section of Mohs micrographic surgery was established. Today, the procedure is performed daily in Portugal and a training program has begun for new physicians.

Dr Alejandro Camps-Fresneda trained in Portugal for several weeks and then went to the USA with Dr Rex Amonette of Tennessee. After his training, Dr Camps-Fresneda established a Section of Mohs Micrographic Surgery at the Hospital del Sagrado Corazon in Barcelona with the enthusiastic support of Dr Pablo Umbert, head of the Department of Dermatology.

Other students of the training program in Portugal have been successful in establishing practices in Mohs micrographic surgery all over the world, such as Dr Eugénio Pimentel, head of the Mohs Surgery Section of the Hospital das Clinicas de San Paulo, Brazil, and Dr Richard Motley in Cardiff, UK, with the enthusiastic support of his department chairman, Professor Ronald Marks.[10–13] The practice in Portugal expanded with the addition of Dr José Manuel Labareda.

Spain

In Spain some physicians had the fortune of studying with Professor Felipe de Dulanto and Dr Antonio Picoto among others. Professor de Dulanto paid great attention to surgical advances. He was trained in Germany but did not lose sight of the 'birth of American surgery'. In 1969, with the support of Professor de Dulanto, Francisco Camacho began chemosurgery with zinc chloride paste in Granada. Its use was limited to recurrent basal cell carcinomas in specific locations such as the inner canthus.

The International Society for Dermatologic Surgery was founded in 1978, and at the meeting in Marrakesh, Drs Perry Robins, George Popkin and Günter Burg and other Europeans were among the founding members. However, only the Americans presented material on Mohs micrographic surgery. That meeting served as the first international link between America and Europe in dermatologic surgery, and because of that, yearly meetings followed. In February 1980, the first Spanish course of dermatologic surgery took place in Granada, Spain, and Dr Robins was invited, providing his experience during the four-day meeting. By that time, Mohs micrographic surgery had become an established technique in Granada.

In October of 1980, Professor Camacho went to the chemosurgery unit at New York University to spend time with Dr Robins. In 1981, Professor Camacho became chairman of the Department of Dermatology at Seville, Spain. There were difficulties introducing dermatologic surgery in a department that had been heavily medically oriented. Mohs micrographic surgery began in a small operating theatre built for that purpose.

The relationship between the Department of Dermatology at the University of Seville and the chemosurgery unit at NYU became much more evident in 1982 when the Course for Dermatologic Surgery took place in Seville. Dr Robins was invited to explain the basics of Mohs micrographic surgery at this course and met further with Professor Camacho's collaborators. In October of 1982, Drs José Carlos Moreno and Julián Sanchez-Conejo-Mir went to the chemosurgery unit at NYU for further training. Dr Sanchez-Conejo-Mir had a particularly strong interest in this technique and was therefore named head of the teaching unit of micrographic surgery. His doctorial thesis was on the application of this technique to non-melanoma cutaneous cancer.[14] At first the authors started performing Mohs micrographic surgery without a cryostat, and therefore renamed the technique 'demorate Mohs micrographic surgery' (DMMS). A year later, a cryostat was bought enabling the performance of Mohs micrographic surgery by the fresh-tissue technique. This also led to the comparison of DMMS and the value of paraffin-embedded margins with the fresh-tissue technique.

The United Kingdom

The development of micrographic (Mohs) surgery in the UK has been slow but sure. Dr E Crouch from Gloucester and Dr W Bowers from Truro both spent some time with Dr Mohs and were able to develop the technique locally in the early and mid-1980s. In Newcastle, Dr Mike Dahl and colleagues have evolved successfully a system of fixed section Mohs to compliment their departmental work pattern.

In 1984 Dr Neil Walker from London spent one year as a Fellow with Dr Philip Bailin at the Cleveland Clinic and in 1985 Dr Christopher Zachary also from London, spent a year with Dr Neil Swanson in Ann Arbor. Shortly after his return Dr Walker moved into full-time laser research although he had started operating on a few cases in Cambridge. Dr Zachary returned to his post at St John's Hospital, London in 1986 and initiated the technique there. In May 1987 he returned to the United States and Dr Walker was asked to continue his work, finally being appointed as a Senior Lecturer at the Institute of Dermatology in 1988. This unit now operates on 860 cases annually and has close links with the Department of Plastic Surgery, St Thomas Hospital and with Moorfield's Eye Hospital. Dr Richard Motley from Cardiff has since trained with Dr Picoto and Cardiff together with other centres are gradually developing expertise in the technique.

EUROPEAN SOCIETY FOR MICROGRAPHIC SURGERY

The Spanish have made regular contributions to the body of knowledge of Mohs micrographic surgery at Spanish and European meetings. Through these meetings and after much discussion with people like Dr Picoto, Dr Camps-Fresneda and other experts in Mohs micrographic surgery, it was decided that there was a need to create a European society of Mohs surgery in order to promote the Mohs method in Europe, document the success achieved in treating these tumors, publish results, establish standards, and begin training programs.[15-27] Progress was slow because many dermatologists felt that the Mohs technique was time-consuming and that the same results could be achieved more expeditiously with classical surgical methods. But an enthusiastic group of founding members thought the time had come for the European Society for Micrographic Surgery to be established on 6 and 7 April 1990, in Estoril, Portugal. The founding members were: Helmut Breuninger, Germany; Francisco Camacho, Spain; Costa Galvão, Brito, Maria Celeste, Portugal; Patrick Dierick, Belgium; Birger Konz, Germany; Ölle Larko, Sweden; Günter Burg, Germany; Alejandro Camps-Fresneda, Spain; Arlette de Coninck, Belgium; Alexandro Gimburg, Israel; José Manuel Labareda, Portugal; Leonard Marini, Italy; Richard Motley, UK; António Picoto, Portugal; A.F. Ribas dos Santos, Portugal; Julian Sanchez-Conejo-Mir, Spain; Pablo Umbert, Spain; Martino Neumann, Netherlands; Paulo Santos, Portugal; Diane Roseeuw, Belgium; Bo Stenquist, Sweden; Neil Walker, UK; Giorgio Landi, Italy.

After the meeting in Estoril, it was decided to meet annually together with the Congress of the ISDS. These were in Florence (1990), Munich (1991) and Paris (1992). Members of the European Society for Micrographic Surgery (A Picoto, A de Coninck, D Roseeuw, L Marini, H Breuninger, A Camps-Fresneda, P Umbert, J Sanchez-Conejo and F Camacho) also cooperated with Dr Fred Mohs and Dr Perry Robins to write chapters on the 'Introduction to the technique' and 'Historical evolution' of Mohs micrographic surgery.[28]

During the Second Congress of the European Academy of Dermatology and Venerology in Athens (1991), the Society made a large contribution to the dermatosurgical program. This participation and its reception helped to establish the practice of Mohs micrographic surgery in departments of dermatology such as the University Hospital in Seville. We informed Dr

Mohs of the founding of the Society and of efforts to expand in Europe. The Society has been very encouraged by Dr Mohs' support.

Mohs micrographic surgery in Europe

Mohs micrographic surgery is performed in Europe in the following countries: Portugal, Spain, Belgium, Germany, Italy, UK and Sweden. The procedure will soon be established in Greece by Dr George Sgouros, who trained with Dr Mohs, and his associates Drs Paul Larson and Steve Snow. The procedure is also performed in Israel. It is hoped that new countries will soon adopt this technique.

The European Society for Micrographic Surgery now has 23 members with new applicants waiting to join. It is interesting that in Munich, Germany in 1967 the American College of Chemosurgery was founded by Drs William Bush, Roger Lanbenheimer, Roy Seeper, Perry Robins, George Vavruska and Frederic Mohs.[28] Now, after 23 years, a European Society has been born, this time in Portugal. The seed finally grew!

References

1. Burg G, Robins P, Chemochirurgie, chirurgis entfernung chemisch fixierten tumorgewebes mit mikroskopischer kontrolle, *Der Hautarzt* (1972) **23**:16–20.
2. Burg G, Braun-Falco O, Chemochirurgie des basalioms, chirurgische entfernung chemish fixiesten tumorgewebes mit mikroskopischer kontrolle, *Dtsch Arzteblatt Heft* (1973) **36**:2303–12.
3. Burg G, Hiresch RD, Konz B, Braun-Falco O, Histographic surgery: accuracy of visual assessment of the margins of basal-call carcinoma, *J Dermatol Surg* (1975) **1**:21–4.
4. Burg G, Mikroskopisch kontrollierte (histographische) chirurgie. In: Konz B, Burg G, eds, *Dermatochirurgie in klinik and praxis* (Springer: Heidelberg 1977).
5. Burg G, Perwein C, Konz B, Kristische bewertung der mikroskopisch kontrolliesten chirurgie, *Z Haut Geschlechs Krankh* (1982) **148**:237.
6. Weissman I, Konz B, Burg G, Bönninger-Beckers F, Mikoroskopisch kontrollieste (histrighische) chirurgic der basaliome: operatives vorgehen und behandlungser—gegebrisse—In: Eichmenn F, Schnyder V, eds, *Das basaliom* (Springer: Heidelberg 1981).
7. Konz B, Die operative therapie der basaliom aus der sicht der dermatologen. In: Eichmann F, Schnyder U, eds, *Das basaliom* (Springer: Heidelberg 1981).
8. Breuninger H, Histologic control of excised tissue edges in the operative treatment of basal-cell carcinomas, *J Dermatol Surg Oncol* (1984) **10**:724–8.
9. Breuninger H, Schaumburg-Lever G, Control of excisional margins by conventional histopathological techniques in the treatment of skin tumours. An alternative to Mohs technique, *J Pathol* (1988) **154**:167–71.
10. Picoto A, Quimiocirurgia pelo método de Mohs (primeiros dois anos de experiência), *Trab Soc Port Derm Ven* (1983) **41**:15–31.
11. Picoto AM, Picoto A, Technical procedures for Mohs fresh tissue surgery, *J Dermatol Surg Oncol* (1986) **12**:134–8.
12. Camps-Fresneda A, *Cirugia Micrográfica de Mohs*, Doctoral thesis, Barcelona, 1990.
13. Motley RJ, Holt PJ, A simple device for optimal tissue preparation for

Mohs micrographic surgery, *Br J Dermatol* (1992) **126**:57–9.

14. Sanchez-Conejo-Mir J, *Cirurgia Controlada al Microscopio. Evaluación Terapéutica en el Cancer Cutáneo no Melanoma*, Doctoral thesis, Sevilla, 1986.

15. Umbert P, Camps A, Primer año de experiencia en cirugia de Mohs en fresco, *Acta Dermo-Sifiliograficas* (1983) (74); 9–10:400.

16. Camps A, Umbert P, Epiteliomas recidivantes y de alto riesgo: cirugia de Mohs en fresco. *Tecnica Oncologia* (1984) **80**:VIII/50.

17. Umbert P, Camps A, Cirugie en frais de Mohs. Traitement de choix des epiteliomas recidivant et de haut risque. 2 ans d'experience, *Rev Med* (1984).

18. Camps A, Umbert P, Seleccion de tumores para cirugia de Mohs. Indicaciones para el processo de reconstruccion, *Monografias de Dermatologia* (1990) **III**:239.

19. Umbert P, Dificultades histopathologicas durante la lectura de la cirugia micrografica de Mohs (CMM), *Arch Dermatol* (1990) 364–5.

20. Garces et al, Carcinomas de pene. Tratamiento mediante cirugia micrográfica de Mohs, *Med Cila D Prensa* (1992).

21. Stenquist B, Gisslén H, Hersle K et al, Mikroskopisk kontrollerad kirurgi för operation av komplicerad hudcancer. Program-Och Abstractbok, Svensk Kirurgisk Förenings 2:A Kongress I Göteborg 1986 F 89 (Abst in Swedish).

22. Stenquist B, Gisslén H, Hersle K et al, Kirurgi vid komplicerad hudcancer, *Hygiea* (1986) **95**:136 (abst in Swedish).

23. Stenquist B, Gisslén H, Gunnarsson G et al, Mikroskopiskt kontrollerad kirurgi vid komplicerad hudcancer, *Läkartidn* (1988) **85**:3471–3 (Swedish).

24. Stenquist B, Baum H, Gisslén H et al, The effect of intralesional interferon on aggressive basal cell carcinoma (BCC) verified by Mohs surgery. In: *Book of Abstracts*, Xth International Congress of Dermatologic Surgery, Brussels 1989, 0 30 (abst).

25. Wennberg A-M, Baum H, Larkö O et al, Behandling av komplicerade basaliom med intralesionellt Interferon, *Hygiea* (1989) **98**:142 (abst in Swedish).

26. Stenquist B, Gisslén H, Wennberg A-M et al, Treatment of aggressive basal cell carcinoma with intralesional interferon—evaluation of efficacy by Mohs surgery, *Short Abstracts IV*, World Congress on Cancers of the Skin, New York 1991 (abst).

27. Stenquist B, Wennberg A-M, Gisslén H et al, Treatment of aggressive basal cell carcinoma with intralesional interferon—evaluation of efficacy by Mohs' surgery, *J Am Acad Dermatol* (1992) in press.

28. Camacho Martinez F, ed., Cirugia micrográfica de Mohs, *Monografias de Dermatologia* (1990) **III**:200–256.

Chapter 14

IMMUNOHISTOCHEMICAL DIAGNOSIS OF SKIN TUMORS

Ken Hashimoto
Mitsuru Setoyama
Eugene Hashimoto

In the practice of dermatologic surgery histopathological diagnosis of the lesion is important to select the method of treatment and to determine the extent of the excision according to the degree of malignancy. In most cases definitive diagnosis has already been made prior to the surgery and the responsibility of making accurate diagnosis falls on the dermatopathologist and not on the surgeon. However, the interpretation of immunostains, which are employed frequently today, is usually not provided adequately and it is often left to the surgeon to correlate these to the clinical findings. The following case will serve as an example. Skin biopsy showed that multiple deep subcutaneous nodules with some ulceration showed pleomorphic nonpigmented, nongranular cells. S-100 stain was positive. Pathology reported metastatic amelanotic melanoma. In the absence of a primary lesion and because of the nonspecificity of S-100 for melanoma, the surgeon requested an HMB-45 stain, usually positive in most types of melanomas, which was negative. Finally, electron microscopy was ordered and it revealed dense granules typical of granular cell Schwannoma. The final diagnosis of malignant granular cell Schwannoma was established. In this case the surgeon had knowledge that HMB-45 stain is more specific for melanoma, S-100 stains Schwann cells, and the S-100(+)/HMB-45(−) situation warrants electron microscopic exploration for neurogenic tumors. He could have ordered additional nerve-related stains (Table 14.1) instead of electron microscopy. If the surgeon becomes familiar with available immunostains, he could specify the types of stains which promise the best results.

Many monoclonal antibodies work only on fresh frozen tissue and, therefore, the surgeon, anticipating utilization of such stains should preserve the specimen in normal saline-soaked gauze and store in the freezer in a small air-tight bottle or Petri dish, instead of in formalin or alcohol preservative. In Table 14.1 the most commonly used immunostains and their specificities are listed. References to these stains are published elsewhere.[1]

In Mohs micrographic surgery, the tumor cells or masses are often difficult to differentiate from normal cells or structures. Since fresh frozen tissue sections are routinely used to define the extent of tumor invasion, all immunostains are readily applicable except S-100 stain which requires formalin fixation. If melanoma cells are similar to

Table 14.1
Immunostains for various tumors

Antibodies	Tumor
	Melanoma
S-100[a]	Schwann cell and its tumors: neurofibroma, nevus, granular cell Schwannoma
	Langerhans cells and its tumors: histiocytosis-X
	Phagocytes and epithelioid cells
HMB-45[a]	Spindle cell melanoma (−); all other melanomas (+)
MEL-5[a]	Amelanotic melanoma (+/−); all other melanomas (+)
	Normal melanocyte (+)
	Epithelial tumors
Cytokeratin	Whole keratin antibodies such as Dako antikeratin stain most epithelial tumors such as basal cell epithelioma and squamous cell carcinoma
MA903, 904[a]	Keratin-derived amyloid (+)
AE1–3	Well-characterized antibodies for research
	Langerhans cell and its tumors (histiocytosis-X)
S-100[a]	Also positive in nevus cell, melanomas (see Melanoma)
HLA-DR	Also positive in dermal histiocytes and blood vessels
CD1 (OKT-6)	Most specific
	Blood vessel and its tumors
Factor VIII-related antigen[a]	
B-15	
Desmin[a]	Large vessels with smooth muscle coat
	Connective tissue tumors
Vimentin	Also positive in myoepithelial cells of eccrine and apocrine glands, hair muscle, leiomyoma, melanoma, etc.
Factor XIIIa	Dermal dendritic cells (phagocyte) in dermatofibroma, Kaposi's sarcoma
	Histiocyte/Phagocyte
α_1-antitrypsin and α_1-antichymotrypsin	
Lysozyme[a]	
	Monocyte
HLA-DR	See Langerhans cell
MO5	
	Nerve and its tumors
Myelin basic proteins[a]	
Neurofilament	
Neuron-specific enolase (NSE)[a]	Also positive in melanoma
S-100[a]	See Langerhans cell

melanophages at the margin of the excision or spindle cells of grade IV squamous cells carcinoma are similar to reactive connective tissue cells, a number of antimelanoma and antikeratin immunostains are applicable to frozen sections (Table 14.1). The only disadvantage would be the time required to perform these stains, which is approximately 30–60 min. With some experience and familiarity with each antibody (dilution of antibody, incubation time, etc.) the procedure time could be shortened. If immunostains become popular among Mohs micrographic surgeons and demand for certain antibodies increases, direct conjugates will be commercially produced at a reasonable price and this should shorten

Table 14.1 contd

Antibodies	Tumor
	Merkel cell carcinoma
Simple epithelium keratin CAM 5.2, CK5[a]	
Epithelial membrane antigen	Also positive in sweat glands
Chromogranin A	
Neuron-specific enolase (NSE)[a]	Also positive in melanoma
Metenkephalin	
	Sweat gland tumors, skin metastasis of breast carcinoma and GI cancers, Paget disease
Carcinoembryonic antigen (CEA)[a]	
Epithelial membrane antigen (EMA)	
Vimentin[a]	If myoepithelial cells (smooth muscle cells) are included in the tumor
	Lymphoma and myelogenic leukemia
Leukocyte common antigen[a]	All types of leukemia
CD2 (Leu5), CD3 (Leu4)	All T cells
CD4 (Leu3, OKT4)	T-helper cells
CD8 (Leu 2a, OKT8)	Suppressor/cytotoxic T cell
CD19 (Leu12), CD20(Leu16)	B cell
	Mitotic cell marker
Ki67	All types of cells in mitotic cycle
	Basal membrane
Type IV collagen	
Laminin	
β_4 integrin	
	Muscle and its tumor (leiomyoma)
Desmin[a]	
Actin[a]	
Myoglobin	Striated muscle and its tumor

[a]Applicable to formalin-fixed, paraffin-embedded tissue sections.

the procedure significantly. Availability of a fluorescence microscope will further shorten the processing time because this eliminates peroxidase stain. For example, in the case of melanoma differentiation, the removed tissue will be sectioned at 6–10 µm in a cryostat, placed on a glass slide, air dried for 2 min, incubated for 15–30 min with properly diluted antimelanoma antibody (HMB-45, MEL-5, etc.) which is conjugated with fluorescein, rinsed with normal saline, and examined under the fluorescence microscope. The total time would be 20–30 min. The key to this highly specific, one-step staining method is the availability of reasonably priced fluorescein conjugates of antimelanoma antibodies.

SURGICAL DERMATOLOGY

BASAL CELL CARCINOMA VERSUS HAIR FOLLICLE

In Mohs micrographic surgery of basal cell carcinoma (BCC) of the face, vellus hair follicles often resemble tumor strands. This may result in unnecessary extension of the excisional margin and larger defects. The expression of cell surface glycoproteins is often different in transformed malignant cells from that of their matrix cells. This difference has been observed in 130-kDa glycoprotein expressed in BCC and normal hair follicles.[2] As illustrated in Figures 14.1 and 14.2A,B, a monoclonal antiglycoprotein, TNKH-1, can differentiate normal hair follicles which express this cell surface substance only on the basal cells of outer root sheath, whereas the surface of entire tumor cells of BCC is TNKH-1 positive.[2] A similar pattern of differential staining between normal hair follicle and BCC could be obtained by the use of cell surface adhesion molecules, β_1 and α_3 integrin.[3]

Desmoplakin is a desmosome-associated protein and, therefore, is present in epithelial tissues[4] and their tumors such as BCC, squamous cell carcinoma and metastatic breast carcinoma. It is absent from melanoma cells, histiocytic tumor cells and vascular tumors. When applied to a BCC versus hair follicle differentiation problem, it has an additional useful feature. Desmoplakin antibody stains the outer layers of the hair follicle as TNKH-1, but often the tumor cells in the inner portion of the BCC islands are strongly labeled and peripheral cells are negative or weakly reactive (Figures 14.2C and 14.2D). In some specimens, this pattern is reversed.

BASAL CELL CARCINOMA VERSUS SWEAT GLANDS

Eccrine and apocrine glands and their ducts are often confused with BCC in frozen sections. Carcinoembryonic antigen (CEA) is only expressed in sweat gland and duct structures (Figure 14.3).

BASAL CELL CARCINOMA VERSUS CONNECTIVE TISSUE CELLS

In recurrent BCC, stromal reaction and fibrosis often make it difficult to distinguish tumor cells from reactive cells. In this situation cytokeratin is positive in BCCs and negative in stromal cells. On the other hand vimentin is positive in stromal cells and negative in BCCs. If clustered cells are diffi-

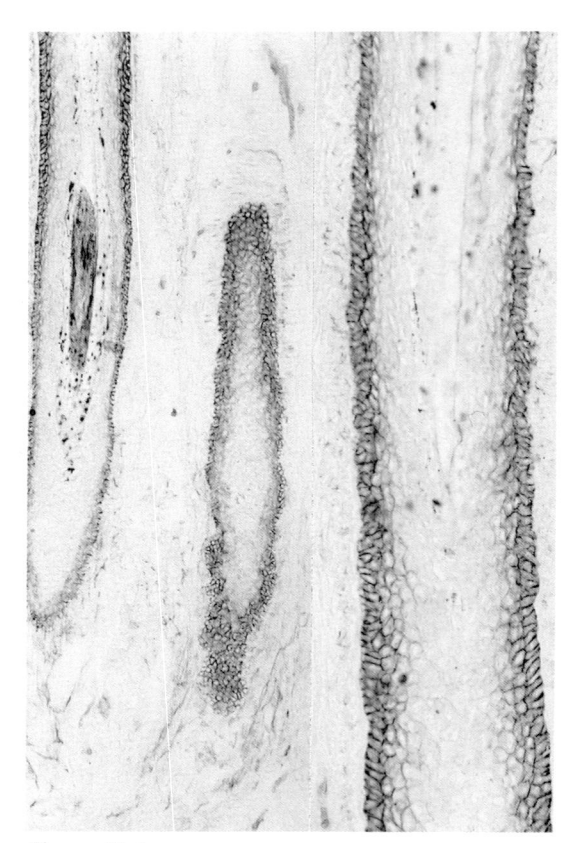

Figure 14.1
TNKH-1 stain of normal hair follicle. Notice that only the basal layer of the outer root sheath is positively labeled. Left: ×50. Right: ×100.

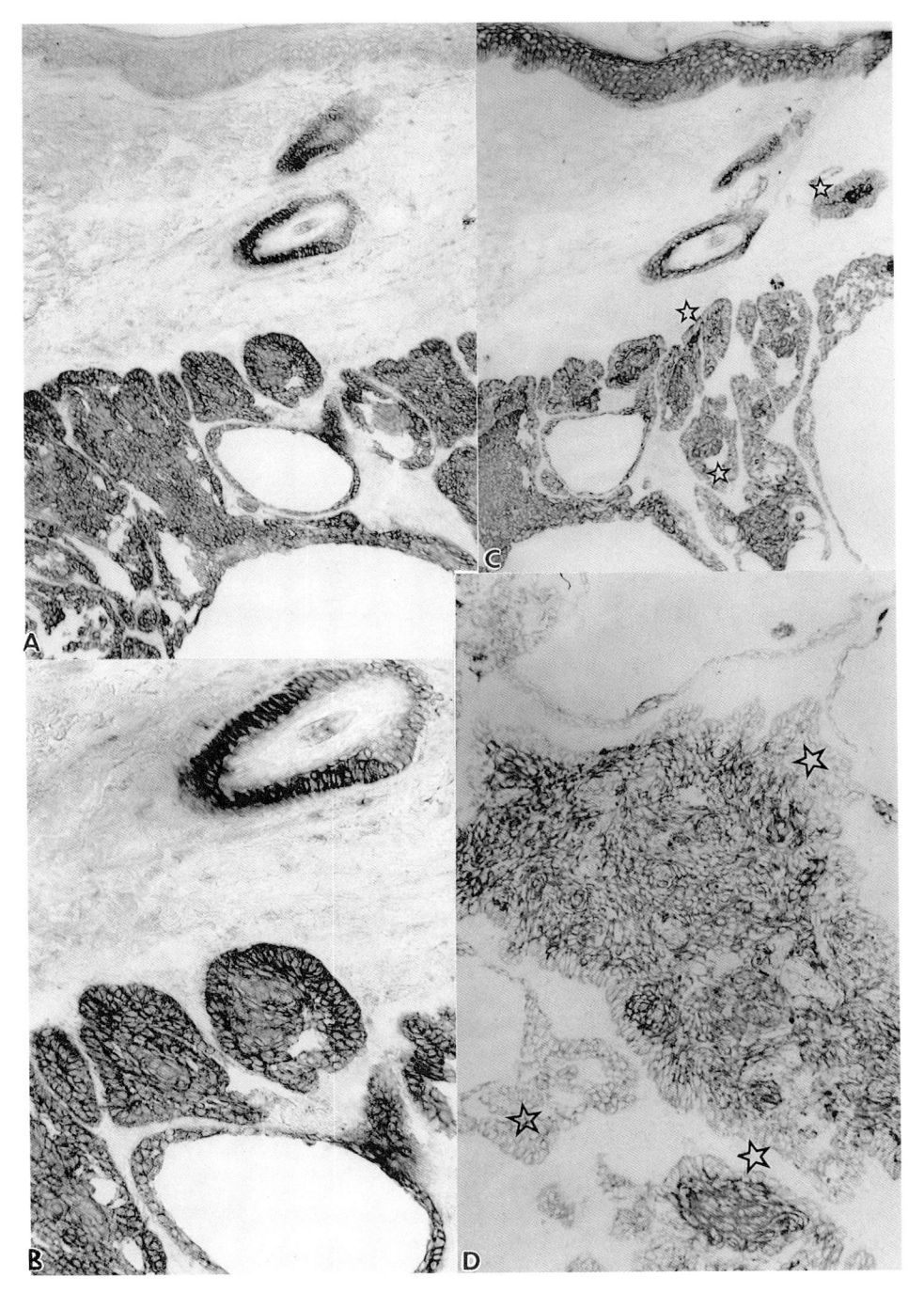

Figure 14.2
(A,B) TNKH-1 stain of hair follicles is limited to the outer layer, while BCC islands are stained in toto. (C,D) Desmoplakin stains the epidermis, and outer layers of hair follicles, while BCC islands are stained positive only in their center portion and negatively in their periphery (☆). A and C: ×25. B and D: ×90.

SURGICAL DERMATOLOGY

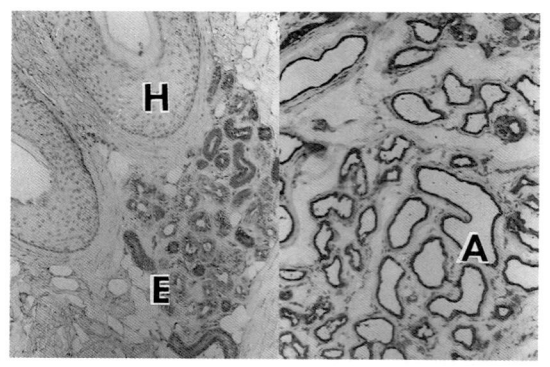

Figure 14.3
Carcinoembryonic antigen is strongly positive in eccrine (E) and apocrine (A) glands and ducts. It is negative in hair follicle (H). BCC (not included) is also negative. ×50.

cult to identify with BCC because aggregated connective tissue cells appear similar, basement membrane components such as type IV collagen and laminin are useful because they surround BCCs (Figure 14.4), while they are absent around the reactive connective tissue cell mass.

MELANOMA DIAGNOSIS

There is no melanoma-specific antibody; all monoclonal antibodies currently available are melanoma-associated antibodies, meaning that they also stain nonmelanomas such as neurogenic tumors and nevus cell nevus.[5] However, when applied to primary melanoma of the skin, the only nonspecific stains one should worry about are related to normal skin such as epidermis, hair follicles, sebaceous glands and sweat glands which are usually negative with antimelanoma antibodies. To be commercially marketable, such antibodies should be applicable to formalin-fixed, paraffin-embedded tissue sections. There are only a few good monoclonal antimelanoma antibodies which work on fixed tissue (Table 14.1).

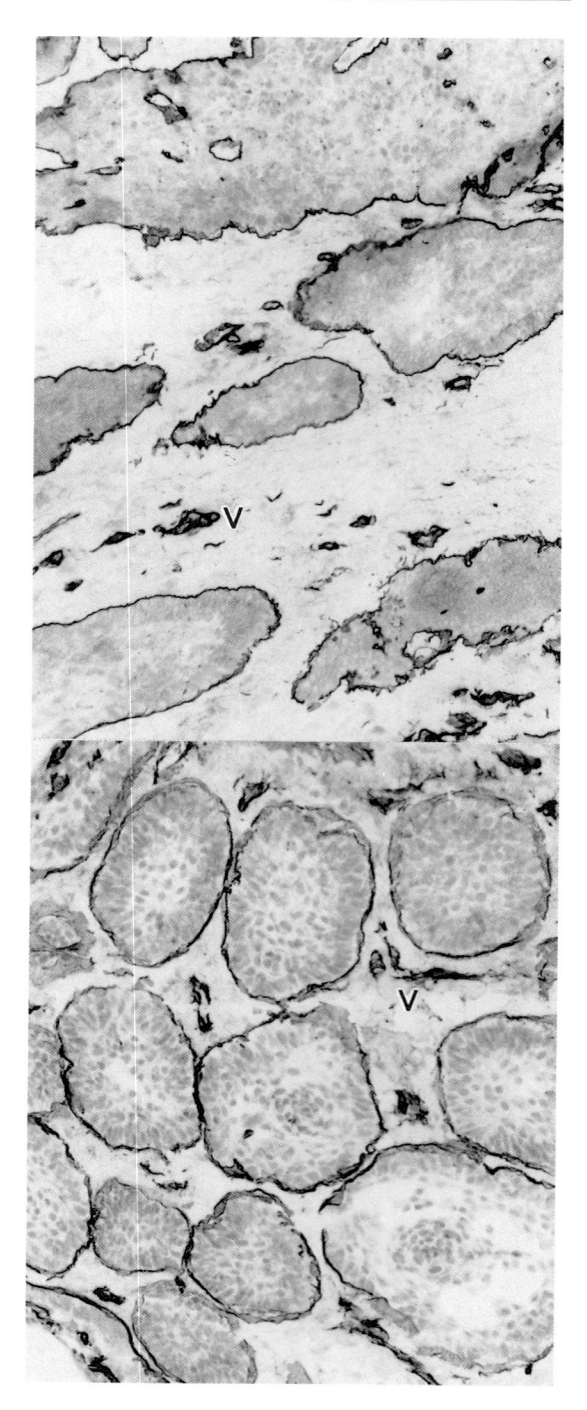

Figure 14.4
Laminin delineates the periphery of tumor islands of BCC. Blood vessels (V) are also stained. None of the stromal cells is positive. Upper: ×50. Lower: ×70.

S-100 is a mixture of polyclonal antibodies used on formalin-fixed tissue. However, it is nonspecific, staining positively Langerhans cells, epithelioid cells and phagocytes. HMB-45 is fixation tolerant and is more specific for melanocytes in the skin.[6] It is, however, often negative in spindle cell and desmoplastic melanoma. Since there is no perfect antibody, one must run a battery of several different stains as listed in Table 14.1.

Differentiating malignant melanoma from dysplastic nevus or early invasive junctional nevus has been helped by the use of TNKH-1[7] in frozen section which labels cell surface glycoprotein of differentiated melanocytic cells including benign nevus cells. Once the cell becomes malignant it loses this antigen and becomes TNKH-1 negative. Unfortunately, TNKH-1 is fixation intolerant. Detection of malignant transformation of melanocytic cells has been done with various combinations of antibodies against gangliosides and oncogenes.[8]

Mitotic index of skin tumors

An estimate of mitotic activity based on the number of mitotic figures in H&E sections has routinely been done by conventional histopathology. A new antibody, Ki-67 detects mitotic cells and is commercially available.[9] This antibody labels the nucleus of any cell undergoing mitosis (late S, M and G_2 phases). When it is applied to frozen sections, one can count Ki-67-positive cells and get an idea about the degree of tumor proliferation (Figure 14.5).

Unfortunately, Ki-67 cannot differentiate malignant cell division from benign or pseudomalignant proliferation such as keratoacanthoma. Therefore, it is essential to use this information only to estimate malignancy based on cell turnover given other diagnostic information about the tumor.

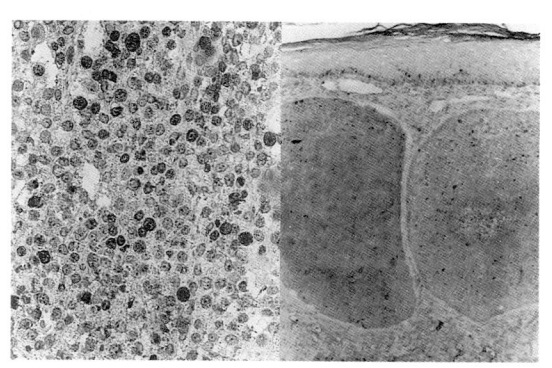

Figure 14.5
Ki-67 stains many cells (nuclei) in the lesion of nodular melanoma (left), whereas only scattered stains are seen in the tumor islands of BCC (right). Left: ×100. Right: ×30.

References

1. Mehregan AH, Hashimoto K, *Pinkus guide to dermatopathology*, 5th edn (Appleton & Lange: Norwalk, CT 1991) 65–78.

2. Setoyama M, Hashimoto K, Dinehart SM et al, Immunohistochemical differentiation of basal cell epithelioma from cutaneous appendages using monoclonal anti-glycoprotein antibody TNKH1. Its application in Mohs' micrographic surgery, *Cancer* (1991) **66**:2533–40.

3. Peltonen J, Larjava H, Jaakkola S et al, Localization of integrin receptors for fibronectin, collagen, and laminin in human skin, *J Clin Invest* (1989) **84**:1916–23.

4. Setoyama M, Choi KC, Hashimoto K et al, Desmoplakin I and II in acantholytic dermatoses: preservation in pemphigus vulgaris and pemphigus erythematosus and dissolution in Hailey-Hailey's disease and Darier's disease, *J Dermatol Sci* (1991) **2**:9–17.

5. Fukaya T, Hashimoto K, Eto H et al, Mouse monoclonal antibody (FKH1) detecting human melanoma-associated antigens, *Cancer Res* (1986) **46**:5195–200.

6. Wick MR, Swanson PE, Rozamora A, Recognition of malignant melanoma by monoclonal antibody HMB-45: an immunohistochemical study of 200 paraffin-embedded cutaneous tumors, *J Cutan Pathol* (1988) **15**:201.
7. Nakanishi T, Hashimoto K, The differential reactivity of benign and malignant nevo-melanotic lesions with mouse monoclonal antibody, TNKH1, *Cancer* (1987) **59**:1340–4.
8. Yamamura K, Mishima Y, Antigen dynamics in melanocytic and nevocytic melanoma oncogenesis: anti-ganglioside and anti-ras p21 antibodies as markers of tumor progression, *J Invest Dermatol* (1990) **94**:174–82.
9. Gerdes J, Lemke H, Baisch H et al, Cell cycle analysis of a cell proliferation-associated human nuclear antigen defined by the monoclonal antibody, *J Immunol* (1984) **133**:1710–15.

Chapter 15

SURGICAL MARGINS FOR NONMELANOMA SKIN CANCERS

David G. Brodland

One of the most hotly debated issues in the dermatologic and oncologic literature in the past decade has been the optimal margins of excision for malignant melanoma. Of central importance in this debate is the question of how wide is wide enough and are 5-cm margins unnecessary. These same questions should be asked with regard to nonmelanoma skin cancers (NMSCs). While the stakes may be higher in melanoma, there is still much at stake from the patient's perspective in the treatment of basal cell and squamous cell carcinoma of the skin. At stake is cure versus recurrence of the tumor. It is implicit in recurrence not only that subsequent therapy will cause sacrifice of more skin, but that the chance of successful eradication of the tumor decreases with each subsequent treatment.[1-3] In the case of both basal cell carcinoma (BCC) and squamous cell carcinoma (SCC), the chance of metastasis increases.[1-6] On the other hand, since the majority of nonmelanoma skin cancers occur upon the head and neck, it is important for the patient that tissue is maximally conserved so as to minimize the functional and cosmetic consequences of the excision. Therefore, it is incumbent upon the cutaneous surgeon to perform effective and efficient excisions. Mohs micrographic surgery is ideally suited for maximizing cure rates while minimizing tissue loss and is widely available across the USA. Therefore, it is important that standard excisions be carefully planned and executed with rational guidelines for margins that result in highly efficacious removal of NMSCs.

While there are several studies addressing the issue of optimal surgical margins for BCC,[7-12] none of these studies was designed prospectively to provide specific guidelines. The literature regarding SCC includes recommended margins of excision ranging from 2 mm to more than 2 cm, often based on anecdotal, arbitrary and often unsubstantiated data.[1,13-17] No guidelines for the margin of resection of SCC have been based on prospective data measuring the subclinical tumor extension. Recently, two prospective studies defining appropriate margins for excision of BCC and SCC have been reported.[18,19] In these studies, the subclinical lateral tumor extension and, in the case of the SCC, the depth of tumor invasion were evaluated. Based on these data, guidelines were proposed for the margin of excision that would provide a 95% histological tumor clearance rate.

The guidelines recommended for BCC are based on the results of a study of 106 clinically well-defined tumors that are 2 cm or less in diameter (Figure 15.1). The width of the surgical margins that would provide histologically tumor-free margins in 95% of the lesions was estimated to be 3.79 mm, which gives a 95% confidence interval between the 89th and 98th percentile (these percentiles correspond to 3.21 mm and 4.86 mm, respectively). This study did not include BCCs with any ill-defined clinical borders or which had been previously treated. In addition, all tumors greater than 2 cm in size were excluded from the study. The margins studied were lateral margins only. The depths of basal cells were not specifically addressed; however, none of the BCCs in the study group exhibited extension beyond the superficial subcutaneous layer. Therefore, it was recommended that excisions be carried down to the mid-subcutaneous fat in areas with abundant fatty tissue. In areas of thinner subcutaneous tissue, the excision should extend to the fascia, perichondrium, or periosteum. In summary, this study proposed guidelines of 4 mm clinically tumor-free margins for primary BCCs that are 2 cm or smaller in size and which have well-defined clinical margins.

The study of subclinical tumor extension in primary cutaneous SCCs was similar to the study of BCCs in that the method used to determine the maximal lateral subclinical tumor extension was the Mohs micrographic surgery technique. One hundred and forty-one tumors from 111 patients were studied. The minimum lateral margin required for tumor clearance was determined for each lesion. Four-millimeter margins were required to achieve a greater than 95% tumor clearance rate in the 141 tumors studied. This result does not take into account the individual characteristics of each tumor. Therefore, minimal lateral margins for clearance were determined for various subgroups of these tumors based on the characteristics of the tumors. Size was found to significantly influence the subclinical lateral extension of the tumor. Tumors were grouped according to maximum diameters of 0–9 mm, 10–19 mm, and 20 mm or larger. Four-millimeter margins were adequate to clear 95% or more of the tumors in the first two groups; however, 6-mm margins were necessary for tumors 20 mm or larger.

The histological grade of all tumors was determined and evaluated for its influence on the subclinical tumor extension. There was a greater than 95% tumor clearance rate with 4-mm margins in tumors that were grade 1. However, grades 2 and 3–4 tumors required 6-mm margins to attain the 95% histological clearance standard. This finding suggests that higher grade tumors are more likely to extend further beyond clinical margins.

The relative risks for tumor recurrence according to its location[20,21] have been suggested to be highest for the scalp, ears, eyelids, nose and lips, and tumors in these locations were therefore classified as high-risk tumors. All other locations were

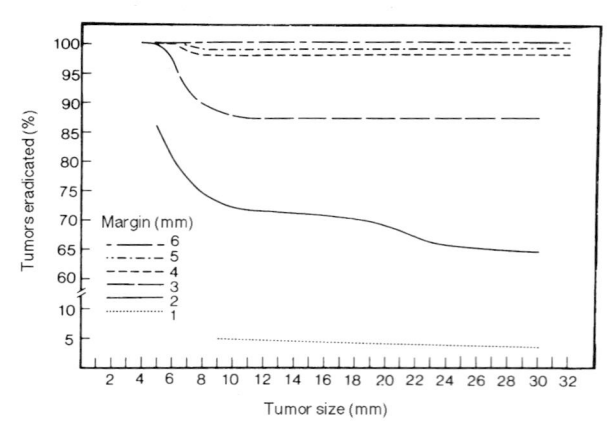

Figure 15.1
Percentage of tumors of different sizes that would have been eradicated by given size of margin (1–6 mm). Each tumor size (horizontal axis) includes population of tumors less than or equal to size specified. (Reproduced with permission from Arch Dermatol (1987) 123:340–4, Copyright 1987, American Medical Association.)

considered low risk. Tumors in high-risk locations were found to extend further beyond the clinical borders than tumors in all other locations. Squamous cell carcinomas from low-risk sites were adequately cleared with 4-mm margins whereas those in high-risk locations required 6-mm margins.

The relationship of tumor size to subclinical tumor extension was evaluated within the group of tumors in high-risk locations. The 0–9-mm SCCs located in the high-risk areas were all cleared with 4-mm margins. However, the group of tumors 10–19 mm in size required 6-mm margins to achieve a 95% histological clearance rate. There were 10 tumors in high-risk areas which were 2 cm or larger and a 9-mm margin was needed to achieve the 95% clearance rate. However, due to the small numbers, this did not attain statistical significance.

The depth of invasion was documented based on the histological presence or absence of tumor extending to the subcutaneous tissue. Thirty percent of the 141 tumors were documented histologically to extend into the subcutaneous tissue plane though none extended beyond the mid-subcutis. These invasive tumors were compared with the less deeply infiltrating tumors to determine whether the invasive tumors also had greater lateral tumor extension. In fact, we found that the invasive tumors did have greater lateral subclinical extension and required a 6-mm margin to attain a 95% histological clearance rate. This is in contrast to the less deeply invasive tumors, which required only a 4-mm margin.

The deeply invading subset of lesions was studied for factors that might predict subcutaneous invasion such as histological grade and tumor size. The histological grade was significantly related to tumor invasiveness. In addition, larger tumor size was associated with a greater tendency to invade the subcutaneous tissue. Of interest is the fact that despite the relationship of invasiveness to histological grade and tumor size there was a greater than anticipated percentage of low-grade and small tumors which extended into the subcutaneous fat. For these reasons, we recommend that excisions of SCCs include the entire underlying subcutaneous tissue.

The proposed margins of standard excision for primary cutaneous SCC are a minimum of 4 mm beyond the clinical borders of SCCs except in those tumors which have characteristics which were found to be at high risk for greater subclinical extension. These high-risk tumors require at least 6-mm margins and include those with diameters of 2 cm or larger, histological grades 2, 3 or 4, location on the scalp, ears, eyelids, nose or lips, and histological evidence of invasion into the subcutaneous tissue (Table 15.1).

Table 15.1
Guidelines for surgical margins of primary cutaneous squamous cell carcinoma

Surgical margins	Size	Histological grade	Anatomical location	Depth of invasion
4 mm	<2 cm	1	Low risk[a]	Dermis
6 mm	≥2 cm	2,3,4	High risk[b]	Subcutaneous tissue

[a]Indicates tumors ≤1 cm located in high-risk locations.
[b]Scalp, ears, eyelids, nose, and lips.

DISCUSSION

Nonmelanoma skin cancers are the most common malignancies in the Caucasian population of the USA. Despite the fact that NMSC is 18 times more common than melanoma, little attention has been paid to the development of statistically defensible guidelines for efficacious margins of excision. While deaths attributable to NMSC are less than for melanoma, it is projected that there will be at least 2000 deaths in the USA attributable to NMSC annually. Naturally, the goal of the cutaneous surgeon in the treatment of NMSC is the complete removal of the tumor. The tendency for these contiguous tumors to extend subclinically beyond the apparent margins has been well documented. The importance of successfully extirpating the entire tumor at the time of initial treatment is underscored by the fact that subsequent treatment modalities for recurrent tumors are much less likely to be curative.[1-3,20,22] Furthermore, even though metastasis for cutaneous SCC and BCC is uncommon, failure of the initial therapy may put those patients at greater risk for metastasis of both BCC and SCC.[1-5] The distress and concern that a patient experiences with recurrent tumor is also an important consideration mandating efficacious therapy.

Implicit in efficacious removal of tumor is minimizing unnecessary tissue loss. The majority of skin cancers occur on the head and neck, making the preservation of function and appearance following treatment a significant factor in efficacious tumor removal. The results of two prospective studies which accurately estimate the subclinical tumor extension of BCC and SCC have been presented. Guidelines for clinically tumor-free margins that will result in histological clearance of 95% of the tumors have been proposed. Although surgical margins which are histologically clear of tumor can be expected to provide a high cure rate, it must be emphasized that because this group of patients did not have long-term follow up, the proposed guidelines do not imply cure rates. Rather, they are intended to allow the dermatologic surgeon to anticipate the subclinical tumor extension with at least 95% confidence. These guidelines are intended for therapeutic modalities which rely on visual delineation of tumor margins and the inclusion of a margin of normal-appearing skin. These guidelines are optimally suited for excisional surgery since the only variables affecting the efficacy of the treatment are the lateral and deep margins. It is recommended that the depth of the excision always extend down to and include the subcutaneous tissue, leaving only the lateral margins in question. The guidelines for lateral margins are not directly applicable for electrodesiccation and curettage since the effectiveness of this technique is very technician sensitive. Another variable that must be considered is the histological subtype of a tumor since, for example, BCCs of the sclerosing variety are much more difficult to 'feel' and thus to effectively extirpate by electrodesiccation and curettage.

In conclusion, guidelines are proposed for the surgical margins in excisions of primary nonmelanoma skin cancer. Primary BCCs less than 2 cm in diameter with well-defined clinical margins should be excised with a minimum margin of 4 mm of normal-appearing skin. The depth of the excision should be to the mid-subcutis in skin with abundant fatty tissue, whereas deeper excision to the fascia, perichondrium or periosteum is indicated where the subcutaneous layer is scant.

Margins for excision of cutaneous SCCs should be no less than 4 mm for those tumors without high-risk characteristics. However 6-mm margins are necessary for tumors with any of the following high-risk characteristics: 2 cm in diameter or larger; histological grade 2, 3 or 4; location on the scalp, ears, eyelids, nose or lips; and invasion into the subcutaneous tissue. For BCCs and SCCs that occur in sites where tissue conservation is essential, Mohs micrographic surgery may be the treatment of choice. In addition, all recurrent lesions should be excised with 100% microscopically controlled margins.

REFERENCES

1. Popkin GL, DeFeo CP Jr, Basal cell epithelioma. In: Andrade R, Gumport SL, Popkin GL et al, eds, *Cancer of the skin* (WB Saunders Co.: Philadelphia 1976) 821–44.
2. Sage HH, Casson PR, Squamous cell carcinomas on the scalp, face, and neck. In: Andrade R, Gumport SL, Popkin GL et al, eds, *Cancer of the Skin* (WB Saunders Co.: Philadelphia 1976) 899–915.
3. Mohs FE, *Chemosurgery: microscopically controlled surgery for skin cancer* (Charles C Thomas: Springfield, Illinois 1978).
4. Amonette RA, Salache SJ, Chesney TM et al, Metastatic basal cell carcinoma, *J Dermatol Surg Oncol* (1981) **7**:397–400.
5. Lo JS, Snow SN, Reizner GT et al, Metastatic basal cell carcinoma: report of 12 cases with review of literature. *J Amer Acad Dermatol* (1991) **24**:715–19.
6. Ames FC, Hickey RC, Metastasis from squamous cell skin cancer of the extremities, *South Med J* (1982) **75**:920–3.
7. Weatherly-White RCA, Lesavoy MA, The integument. In: Hill GJ, ed. *Outpatient surgery* (WB Saunders Co.: Philadelphia 1980) 322.
8. Goodnight JE, Tumors of the skin. In: Walcott MW, ed. *Ambulatory surgery and the basis of emergency surgical care* (JB Lippincott Co.: New York 1981) 221.
9. Macomber WB, Wang MKH, Sullivan JG, Cutaneous epithelioma, *Plast Reconstr Surg* (1959) **24**:545–62.
10. Pillsbury DM, Shelly WB, Ligman AM, *Dermatology* (WB Saunders Co.: Philadelphia 1956) 1141–52.
11. Bart RS, Schrager D, Kopf AW et al, Scalpel excision of basal cell carcinomas, *Arch Dermatol* (1978) **114**:739–42.
12. Albright SD, Treatment of skin cancer using multiple modalities, *J Am Acad Dermatol* (1982) **7**:143–71.
13. Macomber WB, Wang MKH, Sullivan JG, Cutaneous epithelioma: a study of 853 lesions, *Plast Reconstr Surg* (1959) **24**:545–62.
14. Ratzer ER, Strong EW, Squamous cell carcinoma of the scalp, *Am J Surg* (1967) **114**:570–6.
15. Bumsted RM, Ceilley RI, Auricular malignant neoplasms: identification of high-risk lesions and selection of method of reconstruction, *Arch Otolaryngol* (1982) **108**:225–31.
16. Albright SD III, Treatment of skin cancer using multiple modalities, *J Am Acad Dermatol* (1982) **7**:143–71.
17. Glass RL, Spratt JS Jr, Perez-Mesa C, The fate of inadequately excised epidermoid carcinoma of the skin, *Surg Gynecol Obstet* (1966) **122**:245–8.
18. Wolf DJ, Zitelli JA, Surgical margins for basal cell carcinoma, *Arch Dermatol* (1987) **123**:340–4.
19. Brodland DG, Zitelli JA, Surgical margins for excision of primary cutaneous squamous cell carcinoma, *J Amer Acad Dermatol* (1992) **27**:241–8.

20. Roenigk RK, Ratz JL, Bailin PL et al, Trends in the presentation and treatment of basal cell carcinomas, *J Dermatol Surg Oncol* (1986) **12**:860–5.
21. Mohs FE, Zitelli JA, Microscopically controlled surgery in the treatment of carcinoma of the scalp, *Arch Dermatol* (1981) **117**:764–9.
22. Robbins P, Reyes B, Cure rates of skin cancer treated by Mohs micrographic surgery. In: Roenigk RK, Roenigk HH Jr, eds, *Dermatologic surgery: principles and practice* (Marcel Dekker, Inc.: New York 1989) 855.

Chapter 16

THE ROLE OF EMBRYOLOGIC STRUCTURAL DEVELOPMENT IN THE SPREAD OF CUTANEOUS CARCINOMA

J. Michael Wentzell
June K. Robinson

INTRODUCTION

An understanding of embryologic development is critical to the analysis of the spread of cutaneous carcinoma. Tumor spread is affected by various physical planes which arise and demarcate during embryologic development. Tumor has been noted to be limited by or to track along dermis, fascial planes, periosteum, perichondrium, nerve sheath and vessels.[1] It has been a commonly held belief that planes of embryologic fusion act in a similar manner to direct or limit tumor spread. Authors have spoken of 'deep invasion' and 'limitation of spread' associated with fusion planes, but there have been no statistical studies comparing relative depths or breadths of invasion to confirm this impression.

This chapter will analyze in detail the evolution of the fusion plane/tumor spread concept. Though the theory that tumor spreads along lines of embryologic fusion was ultimately proven invalid,[2] that theory led to a more thorough understanding of how tumor spreads along other developmental planes. Let us now study in detail the concept, evolution and implications of the fusion plane/tumor spread theory to gain a better understanding of how embryologic structural development can influence the growth of cutaneous carcinoma.

If fusion planes do direct tumor spread, two criteria should be met: (1) if fusion planes exist, they should be identifiable. That is, there should be some histologic or biochemical evidence that the 'memory' of the fusion site still exists within the tissues of the site. (2) If fusion planes limit or direct tumor spread, then, other things being equal, tumors arising directly adjacent to an embryologic fusion plane should demonstrate statistically greater growth away from the plane than across it.

Neither of these criteria has ever been documented. Until these criteria are met, it is not possible to assert that embryologic fusion planes exist as a limiting influence in the spread of cutaneous carcinoma. Obviously, criterion (2) is dependent upon criterion (1). Fusion planes must be proven to exist before their influence upon tumor spread can be measured. Finally, after 40 years of discussion, our knowledge of embryologic development has expanded enough to suggest that fusion planes cannot exist as modulators of tumor spread in normally developed individuals.[2]

Since embryologic development is so critical to our understanding of tissue planes and tissue composition, it is important to review the processes involved.

REVIEW OF EMBRYOLOGIC DEVELOPMENT

In order to understand the potential implications of 'embryologic fusion planes' we will briefly review the pertinent normal embryonic development of the head and neck.[3-9]

With the progressive development of the embryo from week 4 to week 8, it grows from approximately 3.5 to 28 mm in length (Figure 16.1). During this time various anatomical regions expand in size and begin to grow together. First, their respective epithelium-covered surfaces meet. Then follows regression of the apposing epithelial surfaces. Epithelium migrates across the outside surface of the original junction site.[10,11] This sequence is termed *fusion*, and must be differentiated from *merging* (Figure 16.2). *Merging* results as mesenchymal development creates swellings or hillocks which push overlying epithelium outward (as during cartilage or

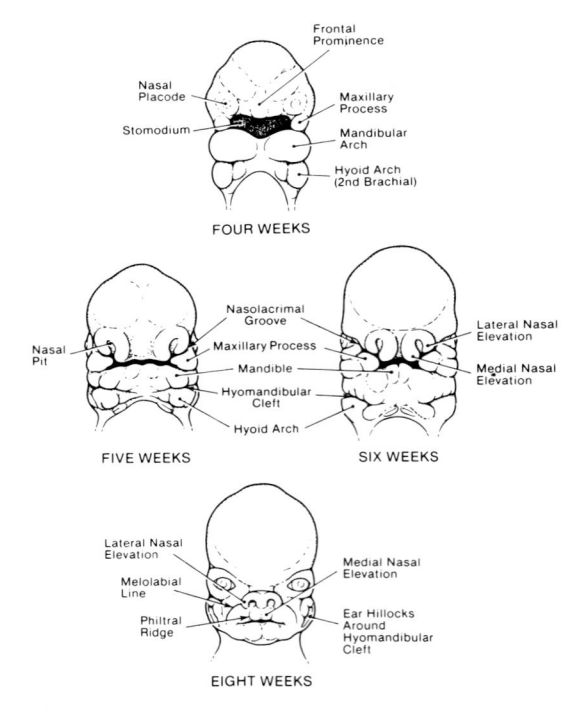

Figure 16.1
Embryonic development of the face from 4 to 8 weeks gestation. (Reprinted by permission of Elsevier Science Publishing Co., Inc. from J Dermatol Surg Oncol (1990) **16**:1001.[2])

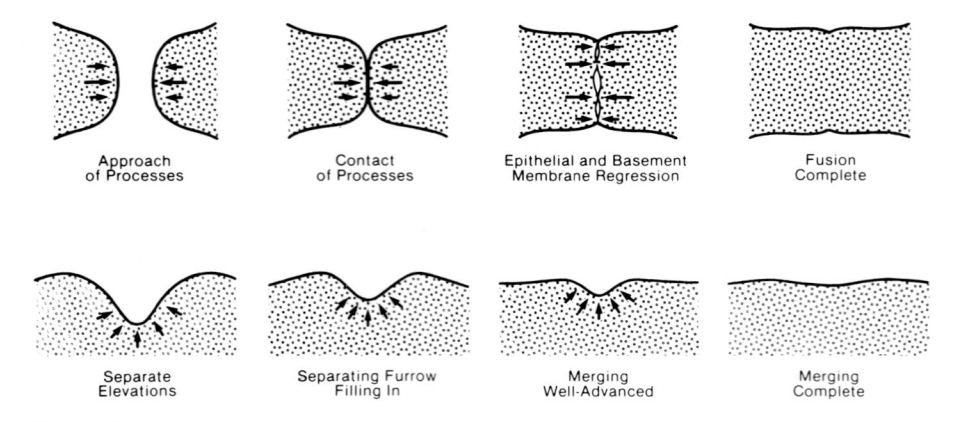

Figure 16.2
Schematic comparison of fusing and merging. (Reprinted by permission of Elsevier Science Publishing Co., Inc. from J Dermatol Surg Oncol (1990) **16**:1002.[2])

bone development). Photomicrographs document that certain sites of merging on the nose and ear lack any sort of identifiable 'planes of fusion' between hillocks.[12] This chapter does not address the already well-documented spread of tumor along surfaces like cartilage and bone which are involved in merging.

Information regarding mechanisms of fusion is still incomplete.[10] Imprecise use of nomenclature in the literature has added to the confusion. In the 3-mm embryo at day 22 the right and left mandibular prominences merge[3,7] or possibly fuse[10] to form the mandibular arch (first branchial arch) which will become the lower lip and chin. Rostral to the mandibular arch the prominent depression called the stomodium eventuates in the oral cavity as surrounding tissues grow forward. Above this the forebrain prominence becomes the frontal (or frontonasal) prominence with its medial and lateral nasal elevations which eventually fuse at the posterior aspect of the nares. The frontonasal prominence is separated from the medially advancing maxillary processes by the lacrimal groove. The frontonasal prominence and the maxillary process fuse in a line which extends from the medial canthus along the nasofacial sulcus and nasolabial groove down each philtral ridge. As the fusion is taking place along the nasolacrimal groove, the maxillary and mandibular prominences are merging[4] (or possibly fusing[10]) to form the oral commissures.

It is important to note that the melolabial line (often called the nasolabial line) is not a line of embryonic fusion. Rather, it develops over the surface of the maxillary process and actually crosses the line of fusion over the former nasolacrimal groove.

During the sixth week the ear takes shape as three hillocks develop along the mandibular arch. Three similar swellings develop along the hyoid arch (second branchial arch). These hillocks or swellings are developmentally analogous to the aforementioned medial and lateral nasal elevations. While the knowledge of the development of the auricle is less precise than was once thought,[7] a general scheme is presented in Figure 16.3 with the mandibular arch components becoming the tragus and helix (together with a contribution from the auricular fold) and the hyoid arch components becoming the lobule, antitragus and antihelix. If a true fusion site exists in the ear, it is between the tragus and the antitragus along the hyomandibular cleft (first branchial groove).

Focal mesenchymal proliferations create the various hillocks and elevations previously mentioned. Mesenchyme eventually differentiates into dermis, muscle, cartilage and associated structures.

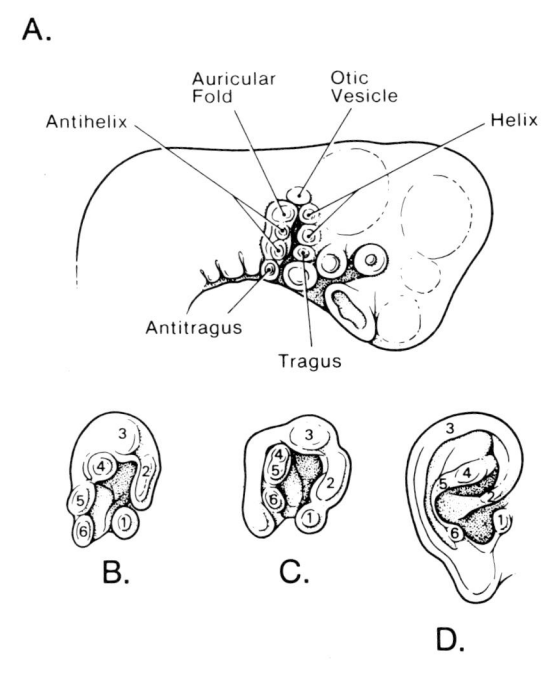

Figure 16.3
Embryonic development of the auricle. (Reprinted by permission of Elsevier Science Publishing Co., Inc. from J Dermatol Surg Oncol (1990) **16**:1002.[2])

The dermis of a 7-week embryo is an open cellular network which by light microscopy is devoid of intercellular fibrous matrix. At this stage there is no apparent inferior boundary separating dermis from hypodermis. Electron microscopy reveals fibers only beginning to form at the mesenchymal cell (fibroblast) surface and at the rudimentary basement membrane zone.[13,14]

Once fusions have taken place, the path is cleared for further mesenchymal development. The facial nerve and muscles of facial expression (which arise in the second branchial arch) grow across former fusion sites as they come to occupy positions about the head and neck. Muscles of mastication, innervated by the trigeminal nerve, likewise cross former fusion sites. Blood vessels arise segmentally from mesenchymal differentiation within each region, each developing segment joining up with the adjacent developing segment.

Thus the nasofacial sulcus, nasolabial groove, posterolateral nares and philtral rims as well as the palate are some of the sites of embryologic fusion. Sites of merging are innumerable and are represented by such structures as the glabella which develops over the nasion and the medial and lateral nasal elevations which eventuate in the dorsal and lateral nose, the columella and the philtrum. Merging hillocks form the auricle of the ear while fusion or merging may be the mechanism by which the tragus and antitragus come together along the hyomandibular cleft. Merging is probably the mechanism of formation for the oral commissures and the midline of the lower lip, though fusion is not clearly excluded as a possible mechanism.

Failure of the various prominences to properly fuse results in well-recognized clefting syndromes.[5,7,8,15] Failure of merging of mesenchymal derivatives also results in recognizable craniofacial malformations.[16]

Since the fusion plane theory has so dominated our concepts of tumor spread for over 40 years, it is important to explore the origins and expansion of that theory.

TUMOR SPREAD AND FUSIONS: ORIGINS AND DEVELOPMENT OF THE THEORY

In 1952 Frederic Mohs and Theodore Lathrop stated that epitheliomas arising over sites of embryologic fusion may invade to an unexpected depth.[1] They felt that this was due to invasion of and subsequent spread along condensed connective tissue planes oriented perpendicularly to the skin surface. In 1978 Mora and Robins reviewed 848 cases of basal cell carcinoma and similarly felt that embryologic fusion planes of the midface allowed malignant cells easy passage for invasion.[17] In 1979 Panje and Ceilly reviewed 150 cases of midface cancers. These authors concluded that the spread of epithelial carcinomas was 'markedly influenced by embryologic fusion planes'.[18] Levine et al concluded that deep midfacial extension of tumor was probably due to embryologic lines of fusion.[19] Similar conclusions have been made about tumor arising on the auricle.[20,21] Subsequent authors have cited various of these articles in support of the view that tumors invade deeply along fusion planes and have less of a tendency to cross them.[22–34]

Each of the above studies was anecdotal in nature. Each depended upon the respective authors' empirical assessments. Statistical significance was not sought until 1986 when Granstrom et al analyzed 23 recurrences along 171 basal cell carcinomas of the head and neck. They found a significant statistical association between recurrences and the perceived proximity of tumor to fusion planes.[30] However, certain sites which they identified as sites of fusion clearly are not. Others similarly failed to make the distinction between sites of fusion and regions of merging.[18,20,21,27] As reviewed above, the two concepts represent two very different developmental processes.

While the fusion plane theory was being explored, factors other than fusion planes were increasingly being implicated in the recurrence and spread of midfacial and auricular tumors. These factors include the higher density of nerves or presence of perichondrium and periosteum in close proximity to dermis,[1] high density of midfacial sebaceous glands[22] and conservative nature of previous treatment attempts.[35] None of the fusion plane studies attempted to correct for such factors as confounding variables which might have impacted on the study of tumor spread and fusion planes.

The midface and ear have several sites of skeletal muscle insertion directly into dermis (Figure 16.4). For example, skeletal muscle can be demonstrated to insert into the papillary dermis of the philtrum.[2] Dermal muscle insertion is independent of fusion. It occurs after fusion has taken place. Muscle derived from the second branchial arch migrates across former fusion sites uninhibited. Its insertions are irrespective of the former fusion sites. However, many sites of central facial muscle insertion coincide with or exist near many fusion sites. Thus muscle insertion is another confounding variable for which fusion plane/tumor spread studies should have accounted.

Studies show that the behavior of epidermal components is dependent upon the character of subjacent connective tissue stroma.[28,36,37] This could account for the often repeated observation that nasal tumors tend to invade deeply along the alar labial fold. Tumor may be spreading along the deeply diving alar fibromuscular stroma over which it developed, quite independently of the nearby fusion site. Recall that the alar musculature derives

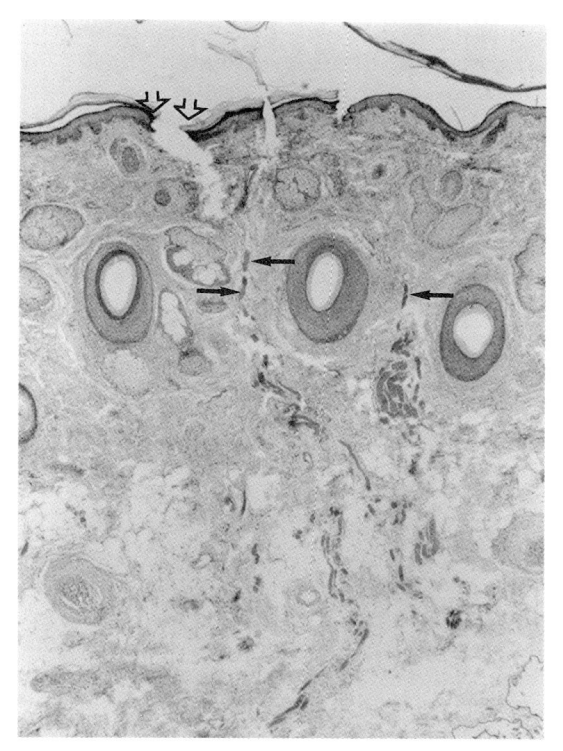

Figure 16.4
*In a section from the philtral ridge of an adult, skeletal muscle bundles (closed arrows) extend almost to the papillary dermis at the fusion site. The philtral ridge was scored with a surgical incision prior to taking the specimen. This score is indicated by the open arrows. Masson trichrome stain, ×40. (Reprinted by permission of Elsevier Science Publishing Co., Inc. from J Dermatol Surg Oncol (1990) **16**:1004.[2])*

from the second branchial arch, not from the derivatives of the frontal process where it is ultimately found. If tumor is tracking along and is influenced by that particular stroma, by definition it is not being influenced by the fusion site but by second branchial arch derivatives which came from a region distant to it.

Despite the apparent general support for the fusion plane concept, several points of confusion exist in the literature. In one case the melolabial line was erroneously interpreted as a fusion plane, this being offered as a reason for tumor limitation.[1] Since the melolabial line is not a fusion site, limitation of tumor to one side of that line is probably due to a change in stromal character. The fibromuscular upper lip is very different from the adjacent cheek, though they both originate from the maxillary process.[38]

Thus, we may postulate that when stroma changes, the character of tumor spread responds. From the above illustrations and from our own studies we have seen that stromal change does not necessarily correspond to a site of fusion.

After the various embryologic processes fuse, mesodermal structures (muscles, nerves and associated connective tissues) subsequently migrate across the plane of fusion. This raises two important questions: (1) How can 'fusion planes' persist after this migration of structures across the former boundary? (2) If fusion planes do exist as boundaries to tumor growth, why aren't they boundaries to normal growth of muscle and nerve?

Though authors seem to differ in their views as to what actually occurs when tumor cells encounter a fusion plane,[1,18,30] there is general agreement that tumor would rather invade deeply than cross a fusion plane. Through much empirical evidence, fusion planes' influence on tumor spread gained almost mythic proportions. There is even suggestion that fusion planes are more impervious to invasion, for example, than is muscular fascia or even periosteum or bone.[18]

If in theory it is the stroma of the fusion plane which is responsible for such influence on tumor spread, of what is this stroma made? At the fifth week of gestation, fine collagen fibrils drape over mesenchymal cells.[39] The transition from a primary cellular dermis to a primarily fibrous phase occurs after fusion takes place, after 12 weeks gestation.[13] While fusion is occurring in the embryo, basement membranes are only rudimentary (though type IV collagen is detectable).[40] If epithelial behavior corresponds to stromal character, it is likely that as fusion occurs and epithelium regresses between the two fusing processes, there will also be regression of the corresponding basement membrane. This fusion-related basement membrane disintegration has been documented.[41-44] Unfortunately, the catabolism of basement membranes is still poorly understood.[45] There was no microscopic evidence of persistent basement membranes or structural changes of any kind at fusion sites in our own studies.[2]

If the epithelium at the fusion site has regressed and the basement membranes have disintegrated, of what then can a residual 'fusion plane' be composed? When the epithelium between fusing processes does dissolve, there is mesenchymal ingrowth from either side.[11,44-46] With this ingrowth there is initial condensation of cellular mesenchyme at the site. However, the mesenchyme then becomes homogeneous and there is loss of histologic distinction of the original fusion site.[12] The mesenchymal tissue at this stage is composed of loosely arranged stellate cells.[47] Thus, there is no evidence of epithelial, basement membrane or mesenchymal 'memory' of the fusion site.

All of this is not to say that vertically oriented fascial planes do not exist. On the face, for example, the fibrous component of the superficial fascia originates from the dermis where it forms a reticulated septal network permeating the panniculus.[48] But this network does not appear to be dependent upon fusion planes. We encountered septae from this network, as mentioned above.

Our own studies and those cited above indicate that in the normally developed human, there are no fusion plane remnants. Fusion plane remnants may well exist only in individuals with anatomical and developmental abnormalities such as epithelial pearls on the palate, cleft lips, etc.[46,49]

Thus it would seem that despite general support in the literature, careful study does not support the concept that embryologic fusion planes exist as factors in tumor spread. This in no way negates the important clinical observations made by authors over the past 40 years. There can be no doubt that tumors arising in certain locations have a great propensity for spread and recurrence.[50] Some of these locations include central fascial and auricular tumors. Cancers arising in these locations require meticulous attention. For 40 years the fusion plane theory has encouraged us to focus careful attention on these tumors, helping us to recognize their relative virulence. Now that embryologic fusion cannot be held responsible for the behavior of these tumors, new theories and new studies will promote a more exact understanding of the spread of cutaneous cancer.

REFERENCES

1. Mohs FE, Lathrop TG, Modes of spread of cancer of skin, *Arch Dermatol* (1952) **66**:427–39.
2. Wentzell JM, Robinson JK, Embryologic fusion planes and the spread of cutaneous carcinoma: a review and reassessment, *J Dermatol Surg Oncol* (1990) **16**:1000–6.
3. Johnston MC, Sulik KK, Development of the face and oral cavity. In: Bhaskar SN, ed., *Orban's oral histology and embryology* (CV Mosby: St Louis 1986) 1–23.
4. Johnston MC, Sulick KK, Embryology of the head and neck. In: Serafin D, Georgiade NG, eds, *Pediatric plastic surgery* (CV Mosby: St Louis 1984) 184–215.
5. Johnston MC, Hassel JR, Brown KS, The embryology of cleft lip and cleft palate, *Clin Plast Surg* (1975) **2**:195–203.
6. Patten BM, Developmental anatomy. In: Anson BJ, ed., *Morris' human anatomy* (McGraw-Hill: New York 1966).
7. Patten BM, The normal development of the facial region. In: Pruzansky S, ed., *International symposium on congenital anomalies of the face and associated structures* (Charles C Thomas: Springfield 1961) 11–45.
8. Arey LB, *Developmental anatomy* (WB Saunders: Philadelphia 1965).
9. Blechschmidt E, *The stages of human development before birth* (WB Saunders: Philadelphia 1961).
10. Millicovsky G, Johnston MC, Active role of embryonic facial epithelium: new evidence of cellular events in morphogenesis, *J Embryol Exp Morph* (1981) **63**:53–66.
11. Smiley GR, Koch WE, The fine structure of mouse secondary palate development *in vitro*, *J Dent Res* (1971) **50**:1671–7.
12. Vargas VI, Palatal fusion *in vitro* in the mouse, *Arch Oral Biol* (1967) **12**:1283–8.
13. Smith LT, Holbrook KA, Development of dermal connective tissue in human embryonic and fetal skin, *Scan Electron Microsc* (1982) **4**:1745–51.
14. Smith LT, Holbrook KA, Byers PH, Structure of the dermal matrix during development and in the adult, *J Invest Dermatol* (1982) **79**:93s–104s.
15. Kawamoto HK, The kaleidoscope world of rare craniofacial clefts, *Clin Plast Surg* (1976) **3**:529–47.
16. van der Meulen JC, Mazzola R, Vermey-Keers C et al, A morphogenic classification of craniofacial malformations, *Plast Reconstr Surg* (1983) **71**:560–72.
17. Mora RG, Robins P, Basal-cell carcinomas in the center of the face:

special diagnostic, prognostic and therapeutic considerations, *J Dermatol Surg Oncol* (1978) **4**:315–21.
18. Panje WR, Ceilly RI, The influence of embryology of the midface on the spread of epithelial malignancies, *Laryngoscope* (1979) **89**:1914–20.
19. Levine H, Bailin P, Wood B et al, Tissue conservation in the treatment of cutaneous neoplasms of the head and neck, *Arch Otolaryngol* (1979) **105**:140–4.
20. Ceilly RI, Bumsted RM, Smith WH, Malignancies on the external ear: methods of ablation and reconstruction of defects, *J Dermatol Surg Oncol* (1979) **5**:762–7.
21. Bailin PL, Levine HL, Wood BG et al, Cutaneous carcinoma of the auricular and periauricular region, *Arch Orolaryngol* (1980) **106**:692–6.
22. Salasche SJ, Currettage and electrodesiccation in the treatment of midfacial basal cell epithelioma, *J Am Acad Dermatol* (1983) **8**:496–503.
23. Salasche SJ, Status of currettage and electrodesiccation in the treatment of primary basal cell carcinoma, *J Am Acad Dermatol* (1984) **10**:285–7.
24. Levine H, Cutaneous carcinoma of the head and neck: management of massive and previously uncontrolled lesions, *Laryngoscope* (1983) **93**:87–105.
25. Levine HL, Bailin PL, Basal cell carcinoma of the head and neck: identification of the high risk patient, *Laryngoscope* (1980) **90**:955–61.
26. Bumsted RM, Ceilly RI, Panje WR et al, Auricular malignant neoplasms, *Arch Otolaryngol* (1981) **107**:721–4.
27. Stanley RB, Burres SA, Jacobs JR et al, Hazards encountered in management of basal cell carcinomas of the midface, *Laryngoscope* (1984) **94**:378–85.
28. Pollack SY, Goslen BJ, Sherertz EF et al, The biology of basal cell carcinoma: a review, *J Am Acad Dermatol* (1982) **7**:569–77.
29. Lang PG, Osguthorpe JD, Indications and limitations of Mohs micrographic surgery, *Dermatol Clin* (1989) **7**:627–8.
30. Granstrom G, Aldenborg F, Jeppson P-H, Influence of embryonal fusion lines for recurrence of basal cell carcinoma in the head and neck, *Otolaryngol Head Neck Surg* (1986) **95**:76–82.
31. Mohs F, Larson P, Iriondo M, Micrographic surgery for the microscopically controlled exision of carcinoma of the external ear, *J Am Acad Dermatol* (1988) **19**:729–37.
32. Rapini RP, Pitfalls of Mohs micrographic surgery, *J Am Acad Dermatol* (1990) **22**:681–6.
33. Dzubow LM, Chemosurgical report: recurrence (persistence) of tumor following excision by Mohs surgery, *J Dermatol Surg Oncol* (1987) **13**:27–30.
34. Robinson JK, Mohs chemosurgery in the management of skin tumors. In: Moosa AR, Robson MC, Schimpff SC, eds, *Comprehensive textbook of oncology* (Williams and Wilkins: Baltimore 1986) 278–89.
35. Robins P, Albom MJ, Recurrent basal cell carcinoma in young women, *J Dermatol Surg Oncol* (1975) **1**:49–51.
36. Martin GR, Kleinman HK, Terranova VP et al, The regulation of basement membrane formation and cell matrix interactions by defined supramolecular complexes. In: *Basement membranes and cell movement*, Ciba Foundation Symposium 108 (Pitman: London 1984) 197–212.
37. Billingham RE, Silvers WK, Dermoepidermal interactions and epithelial specificity. In: Fleischmajer R, Billingham RE, eds, *Epithelial–mesenchymal interactions*,

18th Hahneman Symposium (Williams and Wilkins: Baltimore 1968) 252–66.

38. Walker LR, Mudrovich S, Epker BN, The nasolanial fold: applied surgical anatomy and histology, *Am J Cos Surg* (1991) **8**:217–21.

39. Smith LT, Holbrook KA, Madri JA, Collagen types I, III, and V in human embryonic and fetal skin, *Am J Anat* (1986) **175**:507–21.

40. Fine J-D, Smith LT, Holbrook KA et al, The appearance of four basement membrane zone antigens in developing human fetal skin, *J Invest Dermatol* (1984) **83**:66–9.

41. Vermeij-Keers C, *Transformations in the facial region of the human embryo* (Springer-Verlag: Berlin 1972) 7–30.

42. Ferbman AI, Electron microscope study of palate fusion in mouse embryos, *Dev Biol* (1968) **18**:93–116.

43. Tryggvason K, Pihlajaniemi T, Salo T, Studies on the molecular composition and degradation of type IV procollagen. In: *Basement membranes and cell movement*, Ciba Foundation Symposium 108 (Pitman: London 1984) 117–29.

44. Barry A, Development of the branchial region of human embryos with special reference to the fate of epithelia. In: Pruzansky S, ed., *International symposium on congenital anomalies of the face and associated structures* (Charles C. Thomas: Springfield 1961) 46–62.

45. Tondury G, On the mechanism of cleft formation. In: Pruzansky S, ed., *International symposium on congenital anomalies of the face and associated structures* (Charles C. Thomas: Springfield 1961) 85–101.

46. Kitamura H, Epithelial remnants and pearls in the secondary palate in the human abortus: a contribution to the study of palate formation, *Cleft Palate J* (1966) **3**:240–57.

47. Moriarty TM, Weinstein S, Gibson RD, The development in vitro and in vivo of fusion in the palatal processes of rat embryos, *J Embryol Exp Morph* (1963) **11**:605–19.

48. Dzubow LM, The fascia of the midface: an anatomic and histologic analysis. *J Am Acad Dermatol* (1986) **14**:502–7.

49. Schendel SA, Pearl RM, DeArmond SJ, Pathophysiology of cleft lip muscle, *Plast Reconstr Surg* (1989) **83**:777–84.

50. Whitaker DC, Unresectable primary facial cutaneous carcinoma, *J Dermatol Surg Oncol* (1992) **18**:125–9.

Chapter 17

TREATMENT AND PREVENTION OF BASAL CELL CARCINOMA WITH ORAL ISOTRETINOIN

Gary L. Peck
John J. DiGiovanna
Kenneth H. Kraemer
Joseph A. Tangrea
Earl G. Gross

While there are many excellent methods for the effective treatment of isolated basal cell carcinomas,[1] patients with numerous lesions may be difficult to manage even with currently available therapies. Patients with xeroderma pigmentosum, the nevoid basal cell carcinoma syndrome, skin severely damaged by sunlight or with a history of arsenic or irradiation exposure may develop dozens or hundreds of basal cell carcinomas throughout their lives. These patients with multiple primary tumors could benefit from safe and effective, topical or systemic, chemotherapy and chemoprevention.

Other factors also argue for the development of effective agents for skin cancer chemoprevention. For example, in spite of currently available therapies, approximately 2000 deaths/year occur in the USA due to nonmelanoma skin cancer. Patients with large skin cancers may be significantly disfigured by curative therapy. Finally, many patients do not discontinue sunbathing until significant photodamage of the skin, including the development of precancerous or cancerous lesions, has occurred. Since the detrimental effects of a lifetime of sunlight are progressive, these patients, in spite of ceasing sunlight exposure, are destined to develop more skin cancers unless effective chemopreventive measures are taken.

This chapter summarizes several studies describing chemotherapeutic or chemopreventive effects of isotretinoin in skin cancer. The initial study describes the evaluation of isotretinoin at high dose as a chemotherapeutic agent for basal cell carcinoma and at lower doses for chemoprevention.[2] The second study, based on the beneficial chemopreventive results from the first study, examines the chemopreventive effects of isotretinoin in xeroderma pigmentosum, an autosomal-recessive, precancerous genodermatosis characterized by defective DNA repair, which predisposes patients to the development of multiple

---

Based in part on a presentation subsequently published in DePalo G, Sporn M, Veronesi U (eds), *Progress and Perspectives in Chemoprevention of Cancer* (Serono Symposia Publications from Raven Press, Volume 79: New York 1992) 149–59.

skin tumors.[3] The last study describes a double-blind, placebo-controlled, multicenter trial using isotretinoin at very low dosage in patients with a history of at least two basal cell carcinomas related to chronic sunlight exposure.[4,5]

PILOT STUDY OF ISOTRETINOIN FOR BASAL CELL CARCINOMA

Oral isotretinoin was first used in patients with multiple basal cell carcinomas in a two-stage trial. In the first treatment stage high doses were employed as chemotherapy. The second phase used lower doses for chemoprevention.[2]

Chemotherapy

Twelve patients with a total of 270 basal cell carcinomas due to chronic sunlight exposure, irradiation or arsenical insecticide exposure, and nevoid basal cell carcinoma syndrome received an average maximum dosage of 4.5 mg/kg per day oral isotretinoin. Mean treatment duration at these dosages was approximately 8 months. In this series there was complete clinical remission in 43 tumors (16%). Of these 43 tumors, 35 underwent biopsy: 21 specimens were free of tumor, but 14 were not. Thus approximately 10% of tumors underwent complete clinical and histological remission. A marked individual variation in therapeutic response was evident. For example, one patient had 15 of 37 lesions undergo complete clinical regression, whereas another had none of his 8 lesions completely disappear clinically. This variation in therapeutic response did not seem to vary with dosage, location of tumors, etiology of tumors, duration of therapy, or age or sex of the patient.

In some patients treated with high-dose isotretinoin, inflammation developed in the tumors but not in the adjacent skin which was clinically free of tumor. After treatment was discontinued and the inflammatory reaction subsided, an objective reduction in tumor mass was noted in those tumors in which an inflammatory reaction had occurred. However, other patients demonstrated clinical involution of their tumors without signs of inflammation, which indicated that regression need not be mediated by inflammation. In some patients therapy with isotretinoin inflamed previously undetected lesions, similar to what is observed with topical 5-fluorouracil in the treatment of solar keratoses. Smaller tumors responded better to high-dose isotretinoin; 23% of 3–5-mm tumors achieved a complete response, in contrast to only 7% of tumors 10 mm or larger. Lower doses (0.5–1.5 mg/kg per day) were ineffective as chemotherapy since there were no complete regressions and only one tumor underwent partial regression. No tumors became inflamed at these dose levels. Because these results compared unfavorably with standard therapy, the use of oral isotretinoin as a chemotherapeutic agent for basal cell carcinoma was abandoned.

Chemoprophylaxis

This lower-dose phase included only three of the 12 patients involved in the chemotherapy phase. Initially, an average oral isotretinoin dosage of 1.5 mg/kg per day was used for a mean duration of 34 months. Subsequently, the dosage was lowered to 40 mg per day (0.5 mg/kg per day). While each of the three previously studied patients had varying percentages of complete response (3%, 12%, 45%) to isotretinoin during chemotherapy, none developed new tumors within the next 2–8 years. One of these patients, who had the nevoid basal cell carcinoma syndrome, developed 25 new tumors/year for many years prior to therapy, but only one tumor/year during his 7-year treatment period with isotretinoin. After cessation of therapy due to skeletal toxicity, he developed 29 tumors in the first year. Another of these patients, whose skin cancers were secondary to arsenical insecticide exposure, averaged five tumors/year for 6 years prior to isotretinoin, but no new tumors during the 8 years of therapy. However, this patient is unique in that he had developed only one new tumor in the first 4 years after discontinuation of therapy. Similarly, among patients who withdrew from the trial because they could not tolerate the mucocutaneous toxicities observed at high dosage, it was noted that pre-existing lesions enlarged and new tumors began to appear at varying intervals after therapy ceased. This indicates that the chemopreventive effects of retinoids would require maintenance therapy.[6]

Toxicities

The toxicities observed were dose dependent and were more frequent and severe during the initial high-dose, chemotherapeutic phase of this study. Side-effects at high dose observed in at least 50% of patients included mucocutaneous toxicity (cheilitis, facial dermatitis, xerosis with itching, dryness of the nasal mucosa with minor nosebleeds, stratum corneum fragility), systemic toxicity (arthralgias/myalgias, fatigue) and laboratory abnormalities (hyperlipidemia, abnormal liver function tests (SGPT, SGOT)). Radiographic abnormalities of the spine (retinoid hyperostosis: anterior spinal ligament calcification with osteophyte and bony bridge formation) were observed in four of eight patients with multiple basal cell carcinomas treated with high-dose isotretinoin (2 mg/kg per day or more) for a minimum of 2 years.[7] In addition, calcification of peripheral tendons and ligaments, especially in the foot, was observed.[8] The radiographic abnormalities represent the only chronic toxicity of high-dose isotretinoin observed in these patients.

PREVENTION OF SKIN CANCER IN XERODERMA PIGMENTOSUM WITH ISOTRETINOIN

Xeroderma pigmentosum is an extremely rare, autosomal-recessive disorder with an incidence of about one per million and characterized by sun sensitivity and a deficiency in the repair of ultraviolet-damaged DNA.[9] Skin cancers develop in this disease at a frequency more than 1000 times that in the general population. Thus, patients with xeroderma pigmentosum are ideal candidates for studies of cancer prevention in humans.

A controlled prospective study was conducted to determine whether high-dose oral isotretinoin (2 mg/kg body weight per day), given for 2 years, was effective in preventing the development of new skin cancers in patients with xeroderma pigmentosum.[3] Control was achieved by comparing the frequency of tumors in each patient during treatment with the 2-year period before treatment and a 1-year period after treatment.

Seven patients with xeroderma pigmentosum were enrolled in the protocol; five completed the study as outlined without dose modification. Two patients were unable to complete the protocol because of persistent laboratory test abnormalities during treatment. The total number of tumors in the five patients decreased from 121 (mean, 24; range, 8–43) in the 2 years before treatment to 25 (mean, 5; range, 3–9) in the 2 years of therapy, with a mean reduction in the tumor rate of 63% ($P = 0.019$). In four of the five patients there was a reduction in the number of tumors during treatment as compared with that before treatment. In these four patients, the onset of improvement was noted within 2 months of the start of treatment, and the reduction in tumor frequency persisted so that during the 2-year treatment interval there was a 70–93% decrease in the frequency of skin cancers ($P = 0.006$). The one patient who did not have a decrease in tumor frequency during treatment had eight histologically documented tumors in the 2 years before treatment and nine during the 2 years of treatment.

During the posttreatment observation period, which lasted a minimum of 9 months, an increase in the frequency of skin cancers was observed in all five patients. This increase usually became apparent within 3 months of stopping treatment. A mean 8.5-fold increase in the annual rate of tumor occurrence (range, 2–19-fold) was observed in the posttreatment period as compared with the treatment period ($P = 0.007$).

Posttreatment tumor rates were at least as high as those in the pretreatment interval. Three patients had an increase in tumor-removal rate after treatment of about two-fold, as compared with the pretreatment rate. Thus, the treatment may have suppressed an acceleration in tumor formation in these patients. Alternatively, there may have been a temporary rebound in tumor incidence after the withdrawal of therapy (Figure 17.1).

The best response to therapy was observed in the patients who had had the highest frequency of tumors before treatment. The decrease in tumor frequency during treatment compared to the tumor incidence observed during the pretreatment period, and the increase in tumor frequency compared to the 2-year treatment period seen in four of five patients, were significant ($P = 0.045$ by the nonparametric generalized sign test).

Side-effects of oral isotretinoin at 2 mg/kg per day included moderate to severe mucocutaneous toxicities (cheilitis, xerosis, conjunctivitis), and systemic toxicities (arthralgias, hypertriglyceridemia, abnormal liver function tests) in the majority of patients. In addition, poor wound healing, secondary infection with *Staphylococcus aureus* and pyogenic granulomas

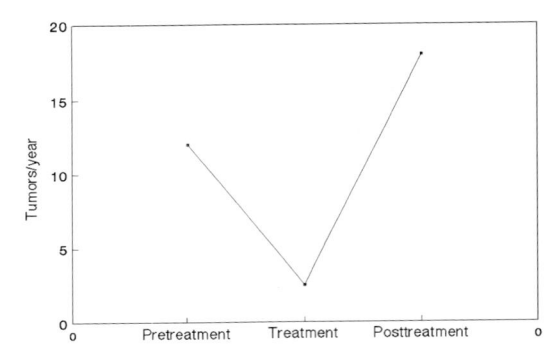

Figure 17.1
Mean annual tumor incidence in five patients with xeroderma pigmentosum before, during and after treatment with oral isotretinoin (2 mg/kg body weight per day). The duration of the pretreatment and treatment periods was 2 years. The mean posttreatment observation period was 12 months (range 9–14).

were noted. Two patients developed skeletal toxicity resembling diffuse idiopathic skeletal hyperostosis, including vertebral bony bridging and extraspinal involvement, such as calcification of the Achilles tendons and plantar ligaments in the feet. We consider these toxicities to be substantial and excessive for long-term therapy with isotretinoin at 2 mg/kg per day for nonmelanoma skin cancer prevention. Therefore, we are currently exploring the use of lower doses (0.5–1.5 mg/kg per day) of oral isotretinoin for the prevention of skin cancer in the patients who completed the high-dose study.

All seven patients who were enrolled in the high-dose phase of this study were included in the subsequent low-dose trial of isotretinoin.[10] The five patients who completed 2 years of isotretinoin at 2 mg/kg per day without dose modification were included, as were the two patients whose dose had to be lowered due to toxicity. Patients were treated with oral isotretinoin at 0.5 mg/kg per day for 1 year and monitored for the incidence of new tumors and toxicity. In comparison to the interval without treatment, the frequency of skin cancers occurring during the low-dose treatment decreased in most patients. In some patients, there was an apparent dose response. Furthermore, mucocutaneous toxicity and laboratory abnormalities were less severe with the low-dose treatment. This study is continuing in an effort to better define the chemopreventive effect and observed toxicities relative to the dose of isotretinoin.

This study indicates that high-dose (2 mg/kg per day) isotretinoin is effective in preventing the formation of new skin cancers in patients with xeroderma pigmentosum. Furthermore, the withdrawal of therapy resulted in a rapid reversal of the chemoprophylactic effect with a significant increase in tumor rates compared to the treatment period. This finding firmly links isotretinoin therapy with tumor suppression. Our data suggest that isotretinoin suppresses tumor promotion or progression, perhaps by either preventing the conversion of premalignant to malignant lesions or by arresting the growth of existing malignant lesions that were too small to be identified clinically. The length of time required for the tumorigenic process to progress from the initial sun injury to the formation of a malignant skin tumor in patients with xeroderma pigmentosum is thought to be several years. In our patients, isotretinoin seemed to act as a switch, rapidly turning off the appearance of tumors within 2 months of the onset of therapy and quickly losing effectiveness within 3 months of the withdrawal of treatment. The speed at which this preventive effect can be switched on and off is probably too rapid to result from alterations in the initial mutational steps in tumor formation, since such alterations would not be expected to prevent tumors for several years.

MULTICENTER TRIAL OF LOW-DOSE ISOTRETINOIN FOR BASAL CELL CARCINOMA

Based on the results of the above studies, the chronic administration of low-dose isotretinoin (10 mg/day or 0.14 mg/kg per day) was evaluated for efficacy in the prevention of new basal cell carcinomas in patients with a history of at least two basal cell carcinomas in the 5 years prior to entry into the study.[4,5] Patients in this study were also monitored for the development of acute and chronic toxicity.

Careful attention was given to choosing the dose used in this trial. Consideration was given to patient acceptability, given the drug's chronic dosing schedule and expected side-effects, and the possible unmasking of the trial by isotretinoin's characteristic mucocutaneous toxicity. Isotretinoin, at this dose level, has been clinically useful with minimal morbidity in the treatment of benign dermatoses.[11,12] This study was a randomized, double-masked, placebo-controlled trial with a sample size of 981 patients coordinated by the National Cancer Institute and conducted at eight clinical centers in the USA. Analyses were made of the cumulative incidence curves (drug versus placebo) of the first new basal cell carcinoma over the 3-year treatment period and of the multiplicity of basal cell carcinomas between treatment groups by comparing tumor rates (defined as the total number of basal cell carcinomas for all visits divided by the number of person-years of follow-up).

The results indicate no significant difference between treatment groups ($P = 0.72$) in the comparison of the 3-year cumulative incidence curves for new basal cell carcinomas. At the end of 3 years of intervention, 327 patients in the isotretinoin group and 327 patients in the placebo group had developed at least one new basal cell carcinoma. Isotretinoin also had no effect on multiplicity as measured by rate of basal cell carcinoma formation. The tumor rate was 0.94 tumors per patient per year in the isotretinoin group as compared to 0.96 per patient per year in the placebo group ($P = 0.83$). While cumulative incidence rates and tumor rates were highest in males, older patients, patients with the greatest prior solar damage, and, most strongly, in patients with the greatest number of basal cell carcinomas in the 5 years prior to entering the study, there was no indication of a protective effect of isotretinoin in any of these subgroups.

Adverse reactions, reported both in the isotretinoin group (76% of patients) and in the placebo group (43% of patients), were mild in nature and dose modification was considered necessary for fewer than 20% of the reactions. Significant differences in observed side-effects were noted between treatment groups for mucocutaneous toxicities, hypertriglyceridemia, and in the development and progression of cervical and thoracic hyperostotic vertebral abnormalities. At the end of the 3-year treatment period, the mean total serum triglycerides was 1.63 mmol/l in the isotretinoin group and 1.45 mmol/l in the placebo group ($P < 0.001$). Mean total serum cholesterol did not differ between groups. Upon comparing baseline versus end-of-treatment (3-year) radiographs of the cervical and thoracic spine in a subsample of 269 patients, 40.3% of isotretinoin patients and 18.5% of placebo patients exhibited progression of pre-existing hyperostotic vertebral abnormalities ($P < 0.001$), while 8.6% of isotretinoin patients and 1.5% of placebo patients developed new hyperostotic involvement of previously unaffected vertebral levels ($P = 0.015$).[5] These mild to moderate radiographic changes appeared to be a continuation of a pre-existing process rather than a unique or distinct pathological change and were not productive of clinical symptoms.

The lack of benefit observed in this trial differs from the results of previous studies, probably because of the much lower dose of isotretinoin used. It should be mentioned, however, that even at the low dose of 10 mg/day, isotretinoin produced measurable systemic toxicity. This finding should be considered in the risk–benefit analysis of the chronic use of isotretinoin and must be considered in planning future chemopreventive studies. For otherwise healthy patients, such as those in this multicenter trial, it may be difficult to justify testing much higher doses of isotretinoin due to the likelihood of producing more toxicity. However, for patients with precancerous genodermatoses (nevoid basal cell carcinoma syndrome, xeroderma pigmentosum) who may develop several dozen skin cancers per year, the potential benefit of moderately higher doses of isotretinoin may outweigh the expected detriment of increased toxicity.

Discussion

The synthetic retinoids, isotretinoin and etretinate, have been used in the treatment and prevention of cutaneous malignancy in patients with multiple basal cell carcinomas due to chronic sunlight exposure, the nevoid basal carcinoma syndrome, or xeroderma pigmentosum; multiple actinic keratoses; multiple keratoacanthomas (Ferguson-Smith); solitary large keratoacanthomas; porokeratosis of Mibelli with malignant degeneration (squamous cell carcinoma, Bowen's disease); malignant eccrine poroma; epidermodysplasia verruciformis; oral leukoplakia; cutaneous metastases of malignant melanoma; and cutaneous T cell lymphoma (mycosis fungoides and Sezary syndrome).[14,15] Except for the few reports describing complete responses of actinic keratoses, solitary keratoacanthomas, and approximately 10% of basal cell carcinomas, the synthetic retinoids usually do not cure the cutaneous tumors listed above. Instead, they produce variable degrees of partial regression when given at high dosage.

The data from this report indicate that: (1) high-dose (mean: 4.5 mg/kg per day) isotretinoin can cause complete clinical and histological regression in approximately 10% of basal cell carcinomas—in view of the small percentage of complete therapeutic responses and the toxicities seen at these dose levels, high-dose isotretinoin is not recommended as chemotherapy for patients with multiple basal cell carcinomas; (2) lower doses of isotretinoin (0.5–1.5 mg/kg per day) are ineffective as chemotherapy but are partially effective in the chemoprevention of new basal cell carcinomas in patients with precancerous genodermatoses (xeroderma pigmentosum, nevoid basal cell carcinomas syndrome) as well as in patients with sporadic basal cell carcinomas; and (3) low-dose isotretinoin (10 mg/day or 0.14 mg/kg per day) is ineffective for chemoprevention of basal cell carcinoma, but productive of minor mucocutaneous toxicities, mild hypertriglyceridemia, and mild to moderate radiographic abnormalities of the vertebrae.

These results also indicate that long-term administration of isotretinoin is usually needed for successful chemoprevention. However, the need for continuous, rather than intermittent, chemoprevention therapy and the lowest effective dose necessary for this purpose may vary from patient to patient.

Because of the apparent need for chronic, if not lifetime, maintenance therapy for cancer chemoprevention, the lowest effective dosage should be determined and employed not only to minimize acute toxicity, but also to minimize the risk for chronic toxicity. In this report, chronic toxicities of isotretinoin did develop, namely radiographic abnormalities resembling diffuse idiopathic skeletal hyperostosis and calcification of extraspinal tendons and ligaments. This toxicity may be dose-dependent with higher doses (1.0–2.0 mg/kg per day), resulting in more extensive radiographic change than that observed with chronic, low-dose regimens. However, lowering the dose of isotretinoin, in an attempt to minimize the risk of retinoid hyperostosis, may reduce its cancer chemopreventive effect.

Recently, isotretinoin has been reported to cause regression of squamous cell carcinoma. Complete and partial regressions occurred in four patients with large, recurrent or metastatic squamous cell carcinomas treated with oral isotretinoin, 1.0 mg/kg per day.[16] The authors suggest that retinoid activity correlates directly with the degree of differentiation of transformed cells and, therefore, the well-differentiated nature of squamous cell carcinomas may have been a factor in the excellent therapeutic responses observed. Isotretinoin, given as a chemopreventive agent, was also found to lower the rate of second primary squamous cell carcinomas among patients with previously treated head and neck cancers.[17] Although chemoprevention of potentially lethal cancer was observed, the high dose of isotretinoin used (50–100 mg/m^2) resulted in significant participant toxicity, with 33% of subjects dropping out over the 12-month treatment period. Skeletal changes were not monitored in this study.

Current goals are to determine which tumors are retinoid-responsive either for chemotherapy or for chemoprevention, to determine the lowest effective doses in order to minimize acute toxicity and the risk of chronic toxicity, and to test newer retinoids which may be more efficacious but, more importantly, may lack some or all of the more troublesome toxicities observed with isotretinoin and etretinate (Table 17.1). It would be a major advance,

Table 17.1
Skin cancer chemoprevention trials: suggested methods

1. Select patients with a high pretreatment yearly tumor incidence.
   A. This facilitates detection of a chemopreventive effect.
   B. The risk of developing a new tumor is directly related to number of prior tumors.[18–20]
2. Biopsy and treat each existing lesion prior to initiating the trial.
   A. This establishes an accurate pretreatment incidence rate.
   B. Eliminating pre-existing lesions facilitates diagnosis of new lesions.
3. Select chemopreventive agents, such as retinoids, which have higher therapeutic indices based on screens for efficacy and toxicity.
4. Perform dose-finding studies.
   A. Determine dose dependency of efficacy.
   B. Determine dose dependency of acute toxicity and resulting patient compliance.
   C. Determine lowest effective dose to minimize risk of acute and chronic toxicity.

indeed, if new retinoids were found to be equal in efficacy to existing agents but markedly less toxic. In fact, some of the more recently synthesized retinoids are less likely to produce the systemic toxicities that are so well known for isotretinoin and etretinate, such as alterations in liver function tests and serum lipids, bone toxicity, and even teratogenicity.[21,22]

REFERENCES

1. Sarnoff DS, Peck GL, Basal cell carcinoma. In: Magrath I, ed., *New directions in cancer treatment* (Springer-Verlag: New York 1989) 541–5.
2. Peck GL, Gross EG, Butkus D et al, Chemoprevention of basal cell carcinoma with isotretinoin, *J Am Acad Dermatol* (1982) **6**:815–23.
3. Kraemer KH, DiGiovanna JJ, Moshell AN et al, Prevention of skin cancer in xeroderma pigmentosum with the use of oral isotretinoin, *N Engl J Med* (1988) **318**:1633–7.
4. Tangrea J, Edwards B, Hartman A et al, Isotretinoin-basal cell carcinoma prevention trial—design, recruitment results, and baseline characteristics of the trial participants, *Controlled Clin Trials* (1990) **11**:433–50.
5. Tangrea JA, Edwards BK, Taylor PR et al, Long-term therapy with low dose isotretinoin for prevention of basal cell carcinoma: a multicenter clinical trial, *J Natl Cancer Inst* (1992) **84**:328–32.
6. Peck GL, Long-term retinoid therapy is needed for maintenance of cancer chemopreventive effect, *Dermatologica* (1987) **175** (supplement 1):138–44.
7. Gerber LH, Helfgott RK, Gross EG et al, Vertebral abnormalities associated with synthetic retinoid use, *J Am Acad Dermatol* (1984) **10**:817–23.
8. DiGiovanna JJ, Helfgott R, Gerber LH et al, Extraspinal tendon and ligament calcification after long-term isotretinoin therapy, *J Invest Dermatol* (1987) **88**:485.
9. Kraemer KH, Lee MM, Scotto J, Xeroderma pigmentosum: cutaneous, ocular, and neurologic abnormalities in 830 published cases, *Arch Dermatol* (1987) **123**:241–50.
10. Kraemer KH, DiGiovanna JJ, Peck GL, Oral isotretinoin prevention of skin cancer in xeroderma pigmentosum: individual variation in dose response, *J Invest Dermatol* (1990) **94**:544.
11. Farrell LN, Strauss JS, Stranieri AM, The treatment of severe cystic acne with 13-cis–retinoic acid. Evaluation of sebum production and the clinical response in a multiple–dose trial, *J Am Acad Dermatol* (1980) **3**:602–11.
12. Jones DH, King K, Miller AJ et al, A dose response study of 13-cis retinoic acid in acne vulgaris, *Br J Dermatol* (1983) **108**:333–43.

13. Tangrea JA, Kilcoyne RF, Taylor PR et al, Skeletal hyperostosis in patients receiving long-term, very-low-dose isotretinoin, *Arch Dermatol* (1992) **128**:921–5.

14. Mahrle G, Retinoids in oncology, *Curr Probl Dermatol* (1985) **13**:128–63.

15. Peck GL, Therapy and prevention of skin cancer. In: Saurat JH, ed., *Retinoids: new trends in research and therapy* (Karger: Basel 1985) 345–54.

16. Lippman SM, Meyskens FL Jr, Treatment of advanced squamous cell carcinoma of the skin with isotretinoin, *Ann Intern Med* (1987) **107**:499–501.

17. Hong WK, Lippman SM, Itri LM et al, Prevention of second primary tumors with isotretinoin in squamous cell carcinoma of the head and neck, *N Engl J Med* (1990) **323**:795–801.

18. Epstein E, Value of follow-up after treatment of basal cell carcinoma, *Arch Dermatol* (1973) **108**:798–800.

19. Bergstresser PR, Halprin KM, Multiple sequential skin cancers. The risk of skin cancer in patients with previous skin cancer, *Arch Dermatol* (1975) **111**:995–6.

20. Robinson JK, Risk of developing another basal cell carcinoma: a 5-year prospective study, *Cancer* (1987) **60**:118–20.

21. Gollnick H, New indications and new retinoids, *Dermatologica* (1987) **175** (supplement 1):182–95.

22. Steele CE, Marlow R, Turton J et al, In vitro teratogenicity of retinoids, *Br J Exp Pathol* (1987) **68**:215–23.

Chapter 18

INTERFERON FOR SKIN CANCER

Hubert T. Greenway

INTRODUCTION

Interferons (IFNs) consist of a class of low molecular weight glycoproteins which possess the ability to transfer intracellular messages. They were first discovered in 1957 by Isaacs and Lindenmann[1] and initially raised interest because of their antiviral properties. The antitumor effects of IFNs were realized thereafter and may play an important role in the treatment of certain skin cancers. The antitumor effects may include direct action against tumor cells, decreased proliferation, cellular differentiation, decreased oncogene expression and the development of tumor-associated antigens. In addition, a number of immune functions including the activation of natural killer cells may also play a role in the treatment of cutaneous neoplasms.

At the present time there are three main types of IFN: alpha IFN; beta IFN; and gamma IFN. The three types of IFN proteins have molecular weights ranging from 16 000 to 45 000 daltons and differ both structurally and antigenically. IFN alpha, or leukocyte IFN, can be induced by a number of stimuli including tumor cells. Both recombinant and natural alpha IFNs are available for clinical use. While up to sixteen subtypes of alpha IFNs exist, recombinant alpha IFNs each contain only one subtype of alpha IFN and differ from each other by only one amino acid. Natural alpha IFN is produced by either cultured lymphoblastoid cells or peripheral blood mononuclear cells and contains multiple subtypes of alpha IFN. IFN beta, or fibroblast IFN, currently has only one known subtype and shares some cell surface receptors with alpha IFN. IFN gamma, or immune IFN, has several unusual properties including a relatively greater immunomodulatory activity. IFN gamma is structurally and antigenically different from alpha and beta IFN. The different types of IFN are listed in Table 18.1.

Table 18.1
Types of interferon

Type	Subspecies	Main Action
Alpha (α)	16	Antiviral, antitumor
Beta (β)	1	Antiviral, antitumor
Gamma (γ)	1	Immune enhancer

BASAL CELL CARCINOMA

Basal cell carcinoma is the most common neoplasm in man with approximately 500 000 new cases developing each

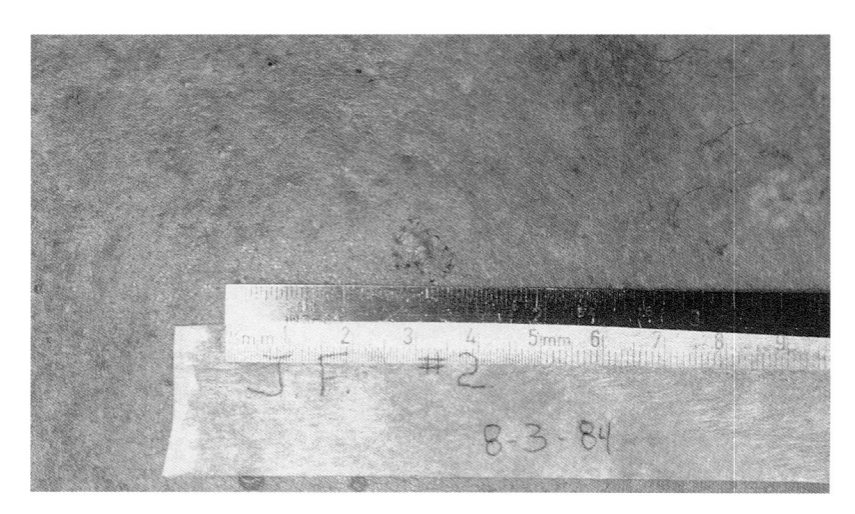

Figure 18.1
Superficial basal cell carcinoma of the back, pre-interferon.

year. Most cases occur in areas of maximum sun exposure including the face and neck. Basal cell carcinomas are locally invasive and have the potential of destroying significant amounts of tissue. Metastasis is rare. The most common forms of basal cell carcinoma are nodular and superficial in type; however, various other forms including pigmented, morphea-like and fibro-epithelioma may occur. Surgical and non-surgical treatments include standard excision, shave excision electrodesiccation and curettage, cryosurgery, laser surgery and radiation therapy. Mohs micrographic surgery is the technique that may be utilized in certain tumors where maximum cure rate and preservation of surrounding tissue are required.

Basal cell carcinomas were first treated in 1985 with intralesional recombinant alpha-2b IFN. A series of eight patients, each with one basal cell carcinoma, were injected intralesionally with 1.5 million international units (IU) 3 times a week for 3 weeks for a total of nine injections.[2] The unit volume was 0.15 ml with the total consisting of 13.5 million units. Lesions consisted either of primary nodular (three cases) or primary superficial (five cases) basal cell carcinoma located on the back, shoulders, arms and neck. The lesion size was a minimum of 6 mm with the largest lesion treated being 14 mm. Prior to treatment an incisional punch biopsy confirmed the diagnosis but removed less than 25% of the original lesion. Side-effects to IFN occurred in all patients and were mild to moderate in each case. Fever, lightheadedness, muscle and joint aches, malaise, headaches, chills, and gastrointestinal discomfort were common systemic effects, with itching and pain at the site of injection being common local side-effects. Systemic side-effects were treated with acetaminophen (paracetamol) with good results and local side-effects were treated with cool water compresses. A decreased white blood cell count was noted in three patients with a return to normal in each patient either during or shortly after treatment. Clinical evaluation continued for a period of 8 weeks after completion of the 3-week treatment period. At the end of the evaluation period an excisional biopsy was performed on the treatment site with no residual basal cell carcinoma found in any of the eight cases (Figures 18.1–18.4). Clinically, the nodular component in those

INTERFERON FOR SKIN CANCER

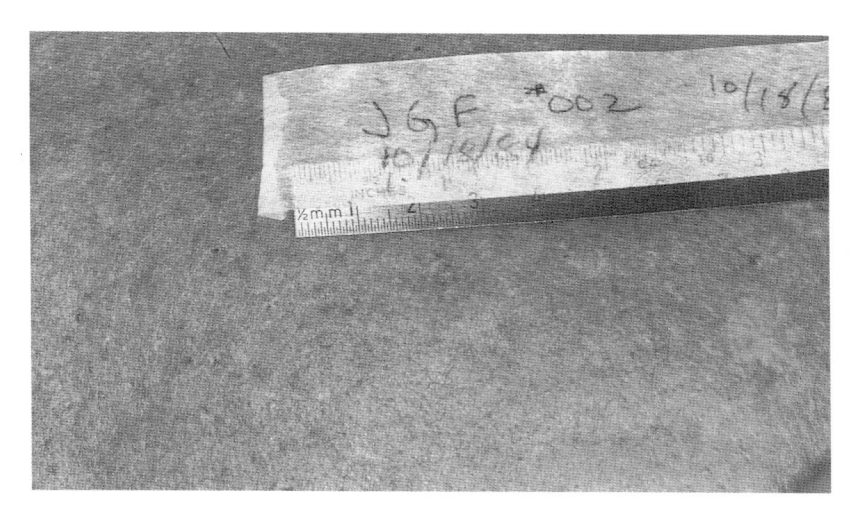

Fitgure 18.2
Superficial basal cell of the back 8 weeks after completion of a series of injections 3 times a week for 3 weeks (nine injections, 13.5 million IU of alpha 2-b). No evidence of residual tumor on excisional biopsy (same case as in Figure 18.1).

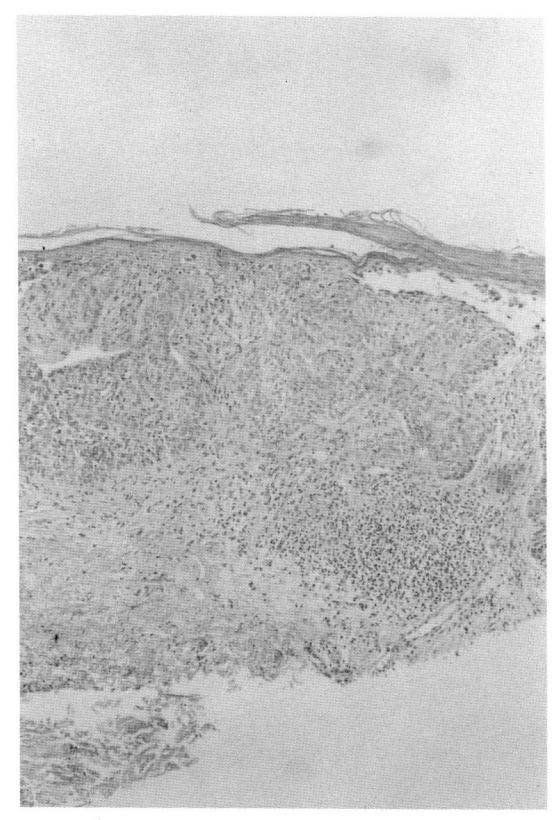

Figure 18.3
Basal cell carcinoma incisional biopsy (less than 25% of overall lesion).

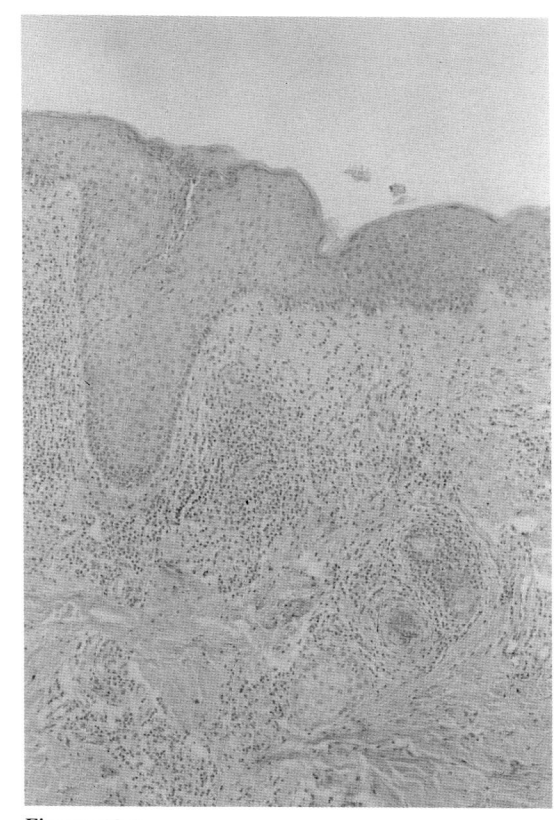

Figure 18.4
No evidence of residual tumor post-interferon alpha 2-b therapy. (Same case as in Figure 18.3.)

167

cases decreased during the follow-up period with an increase in erythema noted in both the nodular and superficial cases.

Because of the short follow-up period and the single regimen a series of four dosing regimens were then evaluated for comparison.[3] Regimens consisted of: (1) 2.25 million IU 3 times a week for 2 weeks; (2) 4.5 million IU 3 times a week for 1 week; (3) 1.5 million IU 3 times a week for 1 week; and (4) one injection of 4.5 million IU. All treatments were given by intralesional injection, with a total of 82 patients being evaluated at Scripps Clinic and Research Foundation, La Jolla, California and the University of Texas Medical School, Houston, Texas. Cure rates were less than with the 3-week regimen, with those patients receiving six injections of 2.25 million IU achieving a 74% cure rate (14 out of 19) (Figures 18.5 and 18.6); those patients receiving a three-injection regimen of 4.5 million IU achieving a cure rate of 38% (8 out of 21); those patients receiving

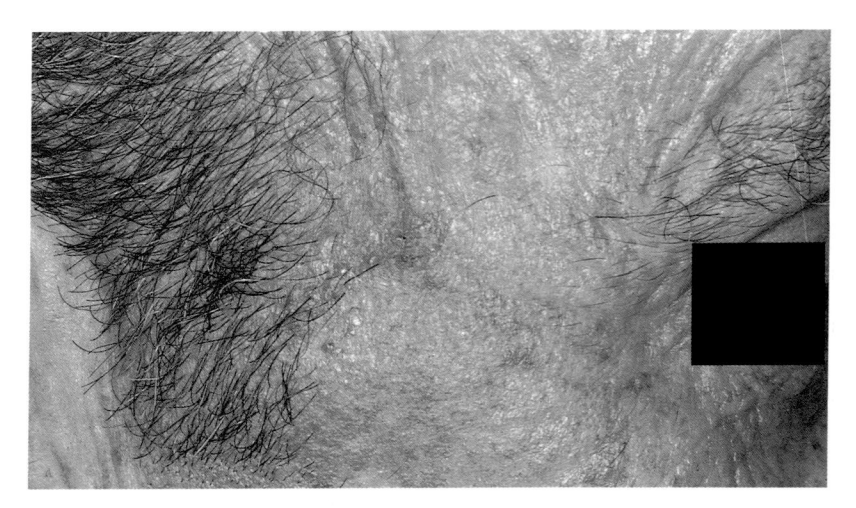

Figure 18.5
Basal cell carcinoma right temple, pre-alpha 2-b interferon therapy.

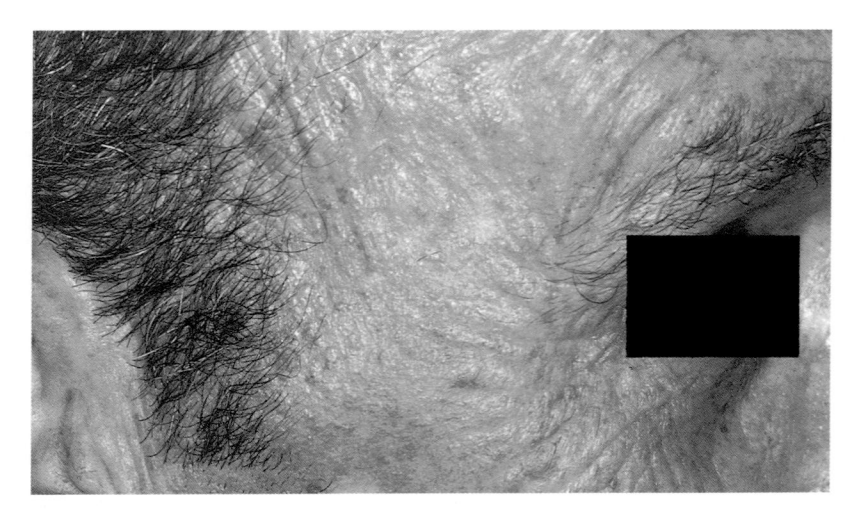

Figure 18.6
Basal cell carcinoma right temple, post-alpha 2-b interferon therapy. No residual tumor.

Table 18.2
Cure rates—therapeutic trials: interferon alpha 2-b intralesional therapy for basal cell carcinoma

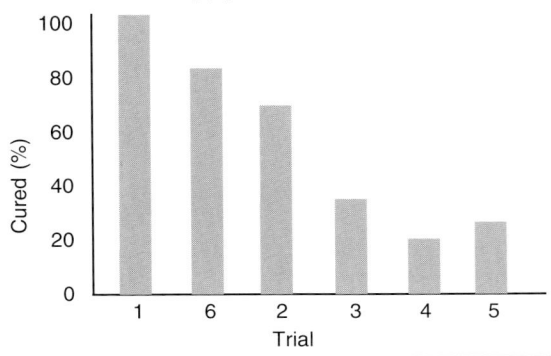

Trial	Dose Alpha 2b Interferon	Schedule	No Patients	Cured (%)
*1	1.5 million IU	3× wk × 3 wks	8/8	100
2	2.25 million IU	2× wk × 2 wks	14/19	74
3	4.5 million IU	3× wk × 1 week	8/21	38
4	1.5 million IU	3× wk × 1 week	5/21	24
5	4.5 million IU	Single Dose	6/21	29
*6	1.5 million IU	3× wk × 3 wks	96/118	81

*Preferred regimen.

three injections of 1.5 million IU over 1 week achieving a 24% cure rate (5 out of 21); and those patients receiving a single injection of 4.5 million IU achieving a 29% cure rate (6 out of 21) (Table 18.2). Results indicated that a 3-week period of injections was required in order to achieve the best results and modifications and shortening of the regimen, even while increasing the amount of IFN, did not offer significant improvement.

Following this study, the long-term effects of IFN in the treatment of basal cell carcinoma required further evaluation. While the initial 3-week regimen had achieved significant success, that success was based on evaluation of the treatment sites 8 weeks after completion of therapy. Long-term evaluation of those treated was instituted with a large, multi-center, double-blind trial of 172 patients, each with one primary nodular or superficial basal cell carcinoma.[4] Treatment consisted of alpha 2-b IFN versus a placebo injected into a biopsy-proven primary nodular or superficial basal cell carcinoma 3 times a week for 3 weeks. Intralesional therapy consisted of 1.5 million IU given with a volume of 0.15 ml for a total cumulative dose of 13.5 million IU, or treatment with a placebo of the same volume with the placebo consisting of the vehicle for the IFN preparation, containing phosphate buffers, glycine, and human albumin. The double-blinded study involved a 3:1 ratio of IFN-treated to placebo-treated lesions. Only primary nodular and superficial basal cell carcinomas were studied with deep lesions and central facial lesions being excluded. Because of the set volume of IFN injected, lesion sizes ranged from 0.5–2 cm for superficial tumors, and 0.5–1.5 cm for nodular ulcerative tumors. Prior to treatment each basal cell carcinoma was confirmed by a small punch biopsy removing less than 25% of the total lesion. Side-effects common to IFN were again noted, with flu-like symptoms and local reactions being more common in IFN-treated patients (Table 18.3). Systemic side-effects were again treated with acetaminophen and for the most part decreased as the treatment progressed. A decrease in white blood cell count was noted in 15% of IFN-treated patients and 12% of placebo-treated patients, with a slight increase in SGOT levels in two patients from both the IFN and placebo-treated groups. All laboratory parameters returned to normal following treatment. Clinically the raised component of the nodular lesions was again noted to flatten shortly after completion of therapy. An increase in erythema reflecting an early transient inflammatory response was noted in those patients receiving IFN. Patients were followed for 1 year and, at that point, the entire treatment site was excised and evaluated histologically. There was no histologic evidence of disease in 81% of patients who were treated with IFN and 20% of patients who were treated with the

Table 18.3
Adverse effects of intralesional interferon

Arthralgia*
Cardiac dysfunction
Chills*
Confusion
Fever*
Headache*
Laboratory abnormalities
Malaise*
Myalgia*
Nausea
Vomiting
Weakness*

*, Most common.
All side-effects were mild to moderate at dosage of 1.5 million IU.

placebo. While the 81% cure rate for patients receiving IFN did not equal the published cure rates for various surgical modalities it did demonstrate a significantly effective response as measured by an absolute histologic cure rate as opposed to clinical evaluation. The cure rate for those patients receiving the placebo was surprising and may be in part related to the human albumin present in the placebo solution.

Basal cell carcinomas of the central face can be more of a concern because of the possibility of scarring associated with surgery. In addition, tumors may extend deep in certain locations, perhaps related to embryonic fusion planes. Nodular basal cell carcinomas of the central face were evaluated in a study of 10 patients at Scripps Clinic and Research Foundation. Nine of the 10 patients completed the study with each patient having one nodular basal cell carcinoma treated with intralesional IFN. Again, a small pretreatment punch biopsy established the diagnosis and removed less than 25% of the original lesion. Patients received either 1.5 million IU 3 times a week for 3 weeks or 3.0 million IU 3 times a week for 3 weeks. Seven of the nine patients had no evidence of residual disease and the difference in dose, ie, 1.5 versus 3 million units, did not result in an increase in cure. A 75–80% cure rate was achieved in each dosage regimen.

Lower dose regimen in the treatment of basal cell carcinoma failed to show any significant results. Wickramasinghe et al[5] treated basal cell carcinoma in 11 cases with a lower dosage of 0.9 million IU, resulting in a lack of cure in any of the patients. The dosage and concentration of alpha 2-b IFN appears to play an important role in the final cure rate.

A single intralesional injection of IFN would be an ideal treatment for basal cell carcinoma.[6] Several sustained-release formulations of alpha 2-b IFN have been evaluated.[7] Cure rates ranged from 50% in patients receiving one injection to 80% in patients receiving three intralesional injections. While this three-injection regimen roughly equates with the cure rate achieved with the previous nine-injection modality, patients suffered significant side-effects. With the sustained-release formulations 82% of patients had at least one severe reaction which prevented them from continuing their normal daily activities. Thus, at the present time these regimens are limited by the increased side-effects encountered with higher dosages of intralesional IFN.

Variations in dosage may be required in the treatment of large basal cell carcinomas. Larger sized lesions may require an increased amount of IFN or, in certain cases, the lesion may be divided into quadrants with only one portion of the lesion being treated at any one time. Dr S Tucker and colleagues at the University of Texas Medical School in Houston (personal communication), found they were able to achieve an 80% cure rate by modifying the dosage and treating portions of the tumor at separate times. Side-effects were mild to moderate and correlated with the amount of IFN given. Alpha 2-b IFN appears to be a safe and effective treatment for primary nodular and superficial basal cell carcinomas.

Other types of IFN have also been evaluated in the treatment of basal cell carcinoma. Alpha 2-c recombinant IFN and human natural leukocyte IFN were utilized to treat basal cell carcinomas in 106 patients. Twenty patients received alpha 2-c recombinant IFN and 86 patients received natural human leukocyte IFN. Patients were followed clinically with treatment consisting of 2–5 million IU units daily of alpha 2-c recombinant IFN given 5 times weekly for 4 weeks. The total dosage was 40–100 million IU. Of the 20 patients, 14 had no evidence of residual basal cell carcinoma based on a follow-up clinical evaluation. Human natural leukocyte IFN-treated patients received dosages of 400 000 to 1.2 million IU for a period of 3–6 weeks with a total dose range of 8–30 million IU. Determination of cure was by clinical findings and associated post-treatment incisional punch biopsies indicating cures in 61 out of 86 patients.[8] Gamma IFN when given intralesionally failed to provide an effective treatment for basal cell carcinoma.[9,10] At the present time it would seem that alpha 2-b IFN appears to be the IFN of choice for intralesional treatment of basal cell carcinoma.

Histologically, the two most difficult forms of basal cell carcinoma for which to provide treatment are the sclerotic basal cell carcinoma and recurrent basal cell carcinoma with the associated scar. These lesions may occur on the central face and treatment with intralesional alpha 2-b IFN provides cure rates in only the 50% range. In both of these subtypes of basal cell carcinoma the difficulty is delivering the active drug to the individual tumor cells and IFN treatment has proved to be not nearly as effective as in primary nodular and superficial basal cell carcinomas.

Side-effects have been related to the amount of IFN given for therapy. The dosage regimen of 1.5 million units of alpha 2-b IFN intralesionally 3 times a week for 3 weeks causes only mild to moderate systemic and local side-effects. These are of the type expected with the use of IFN and consist most frequently of fever, arthralgias and muscle aches (see Table 18.3). Acetaminophen is used for treatment of the systemic side-effects and the frequency and severity of these side-effects may be blocked by the use of oral acetaminophen given 30 min prior to treatment. Additionally, oral acetaminophen (650 mg) is given at 4 h and 8 h post-treatment regardless of symptoms. The use of acetaminophen results in the elimination of systemic side-effects in a number of patients and significantly decreases them in the vast majority of others. Because the side-effects most commonly occur 4–8 h after intralesional therapy, patients benefit by receiving their injections late in the day as opposed to an early morning treatment. Cool tap water compresses may be utilized for any local side-effects. The currently recommended dose for intralesional therapy with alpha 2-b IFN is 1.5 million IU 3 times a week for 3 weeks. Most commonly, a 30 gauge needle and tuberculin syringe are appropriate with a Luer–Lok syringe occasionally being required. Dermatologists are most familiar with intralesional therapy and injection directly into the tumor with a fan-type approach to distribute the 1.5 million IU (volume 0.15 ml) of the drug throughout the entire tumor. Intralesional therapy requires the 10 million unit vial of alpha 2-b IFN mixed with 1 ml of dilutant. Treatment is directly intralesional into the tumor and not given in the underlying subcutaneous fat. Because the treatment is not yet approved for this indication in the United States, it is suggested that a small, 2–3 mm punch biopsy be obtained from the treated area 2–3 months post conclusion of therapy. Thus, not only is the site followed clinically but it is histologically evaluated as well without requiring a significant scar. Neutralizing antibodies have been shown to develop in some patients, although occurring infrequently with alpha 2-b IFN.[11] Accordingly, consideration may be given to evaluation of neutralizing antibodies in patients receiving IFN therapy.

SQUAMOUS CELL CARCINOMA

In addition to local invasions, squamous cell carcinomas also have a metastatic potential which may be higher in certain patients who are immunosuppressed. Some effectiveness in the treatment of squamous cell carcinoma with intralesional IFN was demonstrated by Blanchet-Barden et al,[12] and Berman et al.[13] The effect of intralesional alpha 2-b IFN was evaluated by Edwards, ourselves and others[14] (Figures 18.7 and 18.8) in 36 patients with cutaneous squamous cell carcinomas arising in actinically damaged skin. Lesion size ranged from 0.5–2 cm and

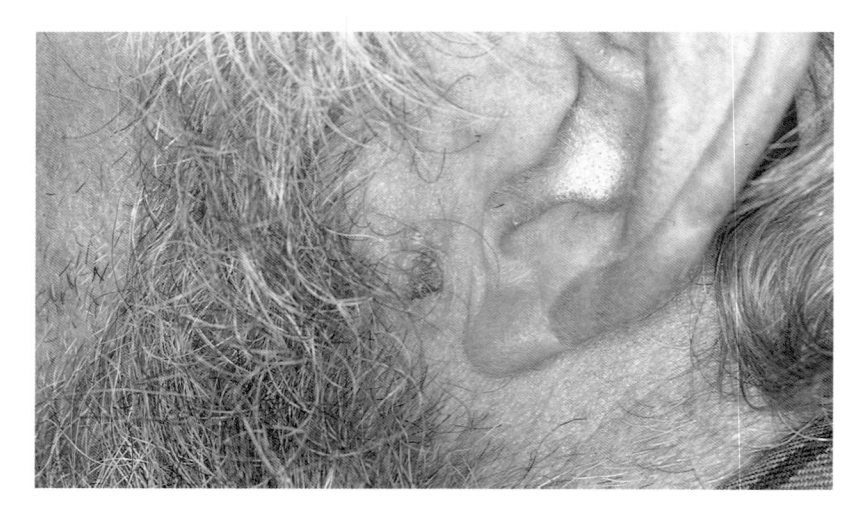

Figure 18.7
Invasive squamous cell carcinoma, left pre-lobular cheek, pre-interferon treatment.

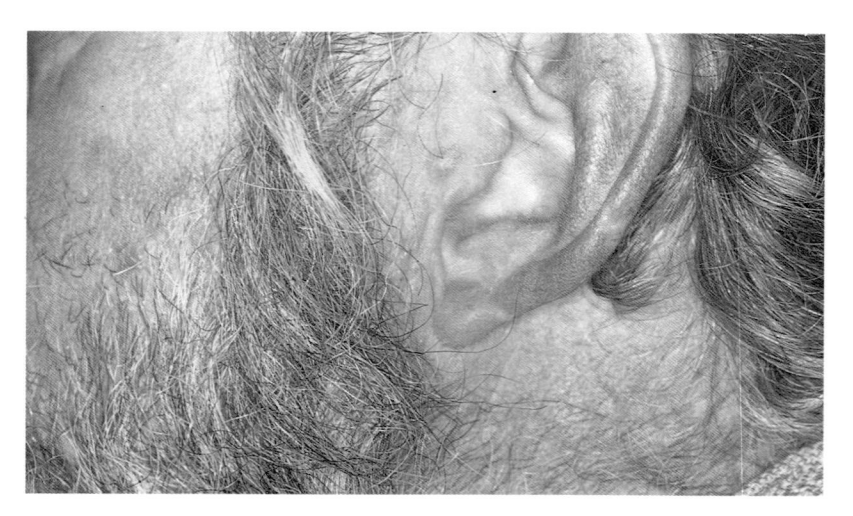

Figure 18.8
Invasive squamous cell carcinoma, left pre-lobular cheek. Complete elimination of tumor with interferon alpha 2-b injected at a dose of 1.5 million IU 3 times a week for 3 weeks. Post-treatment prior to excision of area 18 weeks after completion of therapy. (Same case as in Figure 18.7.)

there was no evidence of lymphadenopathy or metastatic spread prior to treatment. Primary invasive squamous cell carcinomas were present in 27 patients and in situ squamous cell carcinomas in the remaining seven. Treatment consisted of alpha 2-b IFN in a dosage of 1.5 million IU injected intralesionally 3 times a week for 3 weeks up to a total of 13.5 million IU. The entire treatment site was excised and evaluated histologically 18 weeks after completion of therapy. No residual squamous cell carcinoma was noted in 33 out of 34 patients who could be evaluated resulting in a cure rate of 97.1%. Side-effects were again mild or moderate and occurred in approximately two-thirds of patients. Three patients had a decreased white blood cell count and seven patients had mild elevation of one or more tests of liver function with all laboratory values returning to normal after therapy.

Ikic' et al treated 10 patients with squamous cell carcinoma via intralesional alpha 2-c IFN.[8] Treatment of dosages ranging from 2 to 5 million IU given several times a week for 4 weeks (total dose 40–100 million IU). Clinically no evidence of tumor was noted in four of 10 patients post-treatment with five patients noting a reduction of tumor and one patient failing to respond. Additionally, Ikic' et al[8] treated squamous cell carcinoma with intralesional human natural leukocyte semipurified concentrated IFN in 45 patients. Dosages ranged from 0.4 to 1.2 million IU given several times a week for 3–6 weeks. Total dosages ranged from 5 to 22 million IU. Clinically there was no evidence of residual squamous cell carcinoma in 29 out of 45 patients with 13 patients demonstrating a decrease of their tumor and three patients showing no clinical improvement.

Alpha 2-a IFN has been combined with 13-cis retinoic acid for the treatment of squamous cell carcinoma. Lippman et al[15] treated 32 patients with advanced squamous cell carcinoma of the skin and noted an overall response of 68% (19 out of 28 cases which could be evaluated). Treatment consisted of subcutaneous alpha 2-a IFN (3 million IU per injection) and oral 13-cis retinoic acid (1 mg per kg), with the duration of treatment being 2 months. Complete response was noted in 25% of patients with a 93% response rate noted in those with only local disease as compared to a lesser response rate in those having regional or metastatic disease. Median response duration was greater than 5 months and, while no life threatening side-effects were noted, 18 patients required dose reduction related to significant side-effects.

Actinic keratoses may be considered precancerous solar-induced lesions that may progress in certain cases. Edwards et al[16] treated actinic keratosis with alpha 2-b IFN and were able to effectively cure a majority of lesions. Treatment consisted of multiple injections and because of this, this modality did not provide advantages over current, standard therapeutic approaches. Current research continues, in order to provide a topical IFN that might be of value in actinic keratoses.

Malignant melanoma

Alpha IFN has been evaluated extensively in multiple clinical trials in patients with metastatic melanoma[17–19] with response rates in the 16–22% range. Side-effects are dose-related and in light of the higher required dosages have been more significant. Some patients have been able to treat themselves at home in the evening and continue daily activities. Figure 18.9 demonstrates a lentigo malignant melanoma of the left forehead in an elderly gentleman with a level of invasion of 0.42 mm. Initial metastatic evaluation was negative but within 2 years the patient developed multiple lung metastases which were treated with systemic alpha 2-b IFN, which resulted in decrease in the size of

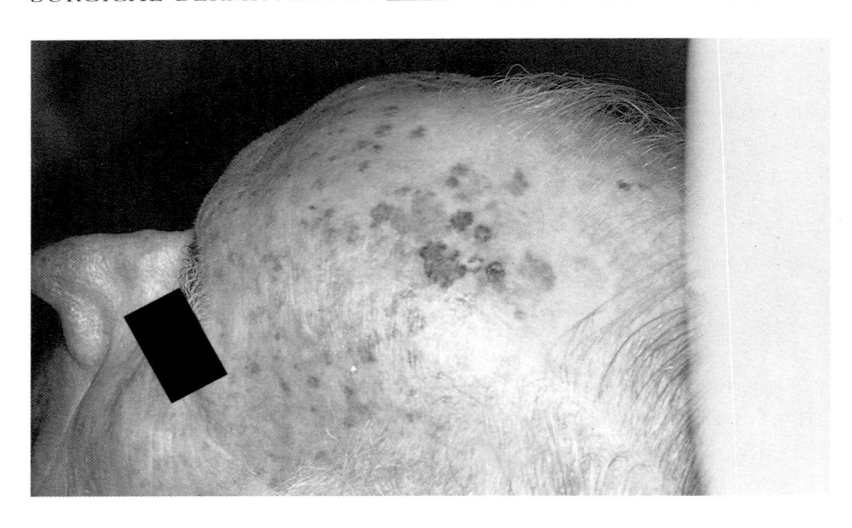

Figure 18.9
Lentigo malignant melanoma, left forehead, with one solitary focus of invasion to a thickness of 0.42 mm. Lung metastases treated with alpha 2-b interferon.

the lung metastases for a period of 18 months.

Interferon has also been utilized in the treatment of multiple satellite lesions in patients with malignant melanoma. Van Wussow et al[20] noted a partial or local response in 24 out of 51 patients with cutaneous metastasis when the drug was given intralesionally. Unfortunately, there was no increase in overall survival. Natural beta IFN was injected into skin metastases of one patient who noted complete clearing of 101 cutaneous leg skin metastatic lesions. The patient remained clear for 5 years.[21] Intralesional therapy in a patient with multiple satellite metastases of the left forehead and temple who had previously undergone several surgical attempts as well as post-surgical radiation of his invasive malignant melanoma has recently been completed at the Scripps Clinic and Research Foundation. Treatment began with 1.5 million IU given intralesionally and was gradually increased to 6 million IU. Treatments continued over a 4-week period and at the present time the patient is 6 months post-treatment with no evidence of residual satellites or further disease.

The use of IFN prophylactically in the treatment of patients with malignant melanoma remains controversial. Patients with an initial tumor thickness greater than 1.5 mm (Clark's Level III) may be at higher risk and, thus, may be candidates for IFN adjunctive therapy. In one 2-year follow-up study patients in this category receiving IFN were 91% tumor free compared to 75% tumor free for those patients not receiving IFN.[22-24] IFN may offer a role in adjunctive therapy in those patients more at risk of developing metastatic disease.

KAPOSI'S SARCOMA

Alpha IFN has shown activity for Kaposi's sarcoma in patients with AIDS. A clear dose response effect has been demonstrated[25] where patients receiving higher dosages (20–50 million IU) demonstrated more activity than those receiving lower dosages (1–3 million IU). Patients who failed to respond to low-dose therapy subsequently demonstrated some activity to higher dosages. Current treatments are in the range of 30–36 million IU with either alpha 2-a or 2-b IFN, utilized by being given intramuscularly or subcutaneously. Most patients also receive zidovudine or other combination therapy. Patients who do not manifest a profound immunosuppression at the time of their presentation for Kaposi's sarcoma appear to respond more effectively than those patients who have full-blown immunosuppression.

Conclusion

Interferon offers promise in the treatment of various cutaneous neoplasms, most notably primary nodular and superficial basal cell carcinoma and primary squamous cell carcinoma. The treatment offers a non-surgical regimen which may be important in certain patients. Work continues on a sustained-release as well as on a topical formulation.

Acknowledgments

Studies involving alpha 2-b IFN in the treatment of basal cell carcinoma and squamous cell carcinoma were supported by grants from Schering-Plough Corporation.

References

1. Isaacs A, Lindenmann J, Virus interferences: I. The interferon, *Proc Soc Lond (Biol)* (1957) **147**:258–67.
2. Greenway HT, Cornell RC, Tanner DJ et al, Treatment of basal cell carcinoma with intralesional interferon, *J Am Acad Dermatol* (1986) **15**:437.
3. Greenway HT, Yount A, Interferon therapy for basal cell carcinoma, *Skin Cancer Foundation Journal* (1991) **IX**:43 and 93.
4. Cornell RC, Greenway HT, Tucker SB et al, Intralesional interferon therapy for basal cell carcinoma, *J Am Acad Dermatol* (1990) **23**:694–700.
5. Wickramasinghe L, Hudson T, Wacks H et al, Treatment of neoplastic skin lesions with intralesional interferon, *J Acad Dermatol* (1989) **93**:572.
6. Greenway HT, Cornell RC, Current status: interferon therapy for basal cell carcinoma (editorial review), *Arch Derm* (1990) **126**:8.
7. Edwards L, Tucker SB, Reredina D et al, The effect of an intralesional sustained release formulation of interferon alpha 2-b on basal cell carcinoma, *Arch Dermatol* (1990) **126**:1029.
8. Ikic' D, Padovan I, Pipic N et al, Interferon therapy for basal cell carcinoma and squamous cell carcinoma, *Int Clin Pharm* (1991) **29**:324.
9. Edwards L, Whiting D, Roger RN et al, The effect of intralesional interferon gamma on basal cell carcinoma, *J Am Acad Dermatol* (1990) **22**:496.
10. Tank B, Werner-Habets JM, Naafs et al, Intralesional treatment of basal cell carcinoma with low-dose recombinant interferon gamma, *J Am Acad Dermatol* (1989) **21**:731.
11. Antonelli G, Correnii M, Turrisiani O et al, Neutralizing antibodies to interferon alpha: relative frequency in patients treated with different interferon preparations, *Inf Dis* (1991) **163**:882.
12. Blanchet-Barden C, Puissant A, Lutzner M et al, Interferon treatment of skin cancer in patients with epidermodysplasia verruciformis, *Lancet* (1981) **1**:274.
13. Berman B, Whiting D, Edwards L et al, Efficacy of interferon alpha 2-b for cutaneous squamous cell carcinoma, *J Invest Dermatol* (1989) **93**:541.
14. Edwards L, Berman B, Greenway H et al, Eradication of squamous cell

carcinoma by intralesional interferon alpha 2-b therapy, *Arch Derm* (1992) (submitted); abstract, *J Interferon Res* (1991) **11**(1):594.

15. Lippman SM, Parkinson DR, Itri LM et al, 13-cis Retinoic acid and interferon alpha 2-a: effective combination therapy for advanced squamous cell carcinoma of the skin, *J Natl Cancer Inst* (1992) **84**:235–41.

16. Edwards L, Levine N, Weidner M et al, Effects of intralesional alpha 2 interferon on actinic keratoses, *Arch Dermatol* (1986) **122**:779.

17. Creagen ET, Ahmann DL, Frytak S et al, Three consecutive phase II studies of recombinant interferon alpha 2-a in advanced malignant malenoma. Updated analysis, *Cancer* (1987) **57**:638.

18. Legha SS, Interferons in the treatment of malignant melanoma, *Cancer* (1987) **59**:638.

19. Creagen ET, Schaid DJ, Ahmann DL et al, Interferon strategies in malignant melanoma: promises, perils, and perspectives, *J Invest Dermatol* (1989) **93**:546.

20. Von Wussow P, Block B, Hartmann F et al, Intralesional interferon alpha therapy in advanced malignant melanoma, *Cancer* (1988) **61**:1071.

21. Ishihara K, Hayasaka K, Yamazaki N et al, Current status of melanoma treatment with interferon, cytokines and other biologic modifiers in Japan, *J Invest Dermatol* (1989) **92**:326.

22. Kokoschka EM, Trautinger F, Mischksche M et al, Long-term adjuvant therapy of high risk malignant melanoma with recombinant interferon alpha 2-b, *J Invest Dermatol* (1989) **93**:560.

23. Landthaler M, Braun-Falco O, Adjuvant therapy of high-risk malignant melanoma patients with gamma interferon, *J Am Acad Derm* (1989) **20**:687.

24. Baron S, Tyring SK, Fleischmann WR et al, The interferons: mechanisms of action and clinical applications, *JAMA* (1991) **266**:1375.

25. De Witt R, Schutterkerk JK, Boucher CA et al, Clinical and virological effects of high dose recombinant interferon-alpha in disseminated AIDS-related Kaposi's sarcoma, *Lancet* (1988) **ii**:1214.

Chapter 19

THE RISK OF DEVELOPING ANOTHER SKIN CANCER

Michael M. Schreiber

Incidence rates for melanoma and nonmelanoma skin cancers have been frequently published and are continuously being updated.

What has not been widely studied is the risk of developing two or more primary cutaneous malignant melanomas (CMM) and nonmelanoma skin cancers (NMSC). It is believed that patients with a first primary skin cancer are at a higher risk than individuals in the general population of having a second similar primary malignancy, either concurrently or metachronously (Table 19.1).

Table 19.1
Risk for subsequent primary skin cancers[1]

Cancer type		Risk (%)
Melanoma	(in 10 years)	0.486–3.95
Nonmelanoma	(in 1 year)	36.39 (1 new)
		16.15 (2 new)
		8.61 (3 new)
	(in 3 years)	49.98 (1 new)
		30.08 (2 new)
		19.37 (3 new)
Squamous cell	(in 3 years)	17.34 (1 new)
		5.06 (2 new)
		1.64 (3 new)
Basal cell	(in 3 years)	46.90 (1 new)
		26.83 (2 new)
		16.93 (3 new)

CUTANEOUS MALIGNANT MELANOMA

At the Fourth World Congress on Cancers of the Skin in 1991, Rigel stated that the lifetime risk (cumulative incidence) of an American developing a CMM is now 1 in 105 (0.0095).[2] He projected this lifetime risk to be 1 in 75 (0.0133) by the year 2000. According to published data,[3–7] individuals with a CMM have a risk of between 0.0128 and 0.0390 of developing a second primary CMM in their remaining life. Thus, the risk of a second CMM may be at least four times higher than for the primary.

A study by Beardmore and Davis[3] of 1444 patients with a primary CMM found that 57 patients (0.0395) developed another primary melanoma in 0–240 months of follow-up. Of these 44, 77% had two and one patient had six. Most of these tumors developed within 5 years of the first; 56% were in males, and most were in different parts of the body than the index CMM. They observed that the older the patient and the longer the survival after the first CMM, the greater the chances of developing another primary CMM.

Other published articles rate the risk of another CMM at 0.0128,[4] 0.034,[5] 0.036[6] and

0.038,[7] either concurrently or in 10 years of follow-up.

A personal communication from Thomas Moon of the Arizona Cancer Center, University of Arizona Health Sciences Center, stated that between January 1985 and September 1991 there were 822 patients diagnosed with CMM from southeast Arizona. Only four of the patients had a secondary primary CMM diagnosed and the tumors were in the same general areas as the index CMM. The rate of a second primary was 0.00486 with an average follow-up of 3.3 years. The annual incidence rate was constant (0.002) during the first 3 years after the primary CMM. What may account for this low incidence compared to other studies was that second primaries were not counted unless occurring 6 months after the first CMM.

There are pre-existing disorders in which there is a predisposition to develop CMM and thus multiple primary CMM. Titus-Ernstoff et al[8] found that in melanoma kindreds of patients with the dysplastic nevus syndrome, 30% developed a second primary CMM. They concluded that the increased relative risk of developing multiple primary CMM was six-fold. This increased relative risk was also found by Wallace.[9] A report by Green and Fraumeni[10] found a risk of 0.027 for multiple primary CMM in 7233 hereditary melanoma patients. They observed that subsequent primaries are more frequent in females and occur at a younger age than in males. Another published study of 357 patients with atypical mole syndrome by Tiersten et al[11] found that 64% of the patients who developed a CMM had a previous personal history of a CMM.

Other conditions at risk for developing multiple CMM include seropositivity for human immunodeficiency virus,[12] immunosuppression due to malignancies,[13] organ transplant,[14] xeroderma pigmentosa,[15] levodopa administration[16] and giant pigmented nevi.[17]

NONMELANOMA SKIN CANCERS (BASAL CELL AND SQUAMOUS CELL)

As with malignant melanomas, multiple primary NMSCs are not rare. Indeed they are quite common. Epidemiological studies on the chances of developing more than one primary NMSC are few.[1,17,18] A recent published report, using standards and procedures recommended by NCI-SEER, was from southern Arizona on data collected from January 1985 through June 1988.[1] This study involved 6310 patients with an index NMSC. As would be expected, the median age of these patients was 69 years. The greatest risk of developing new NMSCs was during the first 12 months after the index NMSC was removed. This first-year risk was 36.39% for one new, 16.15% for two new and 8.61% for three new NMSCs. Over the 3½-year period of the study, 49.98% developed one (72.8% in first year), 30.08% had two and 19.37% had three new NMSCs. The risk varied according to whether the primary NMSC was a basal cell carcinoma (BCC) or a squamous cell carcinoma (SCC).

With primary SCC, the risk of developing a second primary over the period of the study was 17.34% and all of these occurred in the first year. A higher risk was found for patients with a primary BCC, with 46.9% developing a second primary over the 3½-year period. Most (70.73%) were diagnosed during the first year.

MELANOMA WITH NONMELANOMA SKIN CANCERS

Recently, Lindelof et al[20] found an increased relative risk of developing a second CMM (four- to six-fold) after the occurrence of a primary BCC. They also observed an increased risk of other NMSCs both before (four- to five-fold) and after (three- to six-fold) a BCC was discovered.

In Southern Arizona, studies at the Arizona Cancer Center between January 1985 and 1988 found that a patient with one type of skin cancer was at increased risk of developing other primary skin cancers. Age-adjusted relative risks were 3.29 for BCC occurring in patients with CMM, 1.48 for SCC and CMM and 0.85 for SCC, BCC and CMM occurring in the same patient.

Conclusion

The risk of developing a second skin cancer exists and is very high. Awareness of this fact should alert physicians to the importance of thorough and frequent total skin scrutiny for new malignancies in skin cancer patients.

References

1. Schreiber MM, Moon TE, Fox SH et al, The risk of developing subsequent non-melanoma skin cancers, *J Am Acad Dermatol* (1990) **23**:1114–18.
2. Friedman RJ, Rigel DS, Silverman WK et al, Malignant melanoma in the 1990s: the continued importance of early detection and the role of physician examination and self-examination of the skin, *CA* (1991) **41**:201–26.
3. Beardmore GL, Davis NC, Multiple primary cutaneous melanomas, *Arch Dermatol* (1975) **111**:603–9.
4. Pack GT, Scharnagel IM, Hillyer RA, Multiple primary melanoma: a report of 16 cases, *Cancer* (1952) **5**:1110–15.
5. Bellet RE, Vaisman I, Mastrangelo MJ et al, Multiple primary malignancies in patients with cutaneous melanoma, *Cancer* (1977) **40**:1974–81.
6. Allen AC, Spitz S, Malignant melanoma: a clinicopathologic analysis of the criteria for diagnosis and prognosis, *Cancer* (1953) **6**:1–45.
7. Casemelli N, Fontoma V, Cataldo I et al, Multiple primary melanoma, *Tumari* (1975) **61**:481–6.
8. Titus-Ernstoff L, Duran DH, Ernstoff MS et al, Dysplastic nevi associated with multiple primary melanoma, *Cancer Res* (1988) **48**:1016–18.
9. Wallace DC, Beardmore GL, Exton LA, Familial malignant melanoma, *Ann Surg* (1973) **177**:15–20.
10. Green MH, Fraumeni JF, The hereditary variant of malignant melanoma. In: Clark WH Jr, Goldman LI, Mastrangelo MJ, eds, *Human malignant melanoma* (Grune and Stratton: New York 1979) 143–4.
11. Tiersten AD, Caron MG, Kopf AW et al, Prospective follow-up for malignant melanoma patients with atypical mole (dysplastic-nevus) syndrome, *J Dermatol Surg Oncol* (1991) **17**:44–8.
12. Rivers JK, Kopf AW, Postel AH, Malignant melanoma in a man seropositive for human immunodeficiency virus, *Am Acad Dermatol J* (1989) **20**:1127–8.
13. Bery JW, The incidence of multiple primary cancers. Development of further cancers in patients with lymphomas, leukemias and myeloma, *J Natl Cancer Inst* (1967) **38**:741–52.
14. Greene MH, Young TI, Malignant melanoma in renal transplant recipients, *Lancet* (1981) **1**:1196–9.
15. Tullis BD, Lynde CW, McLean DI, Multiple melanomas occurring in a patient with xeroderma pigmentosa, *Am Acad Dermatol J* (1984) **11**:364–7.
16. Bernstein JE, Medencia M, Soltani K et al, Levodopa administration and multiple primary cutaneous melanomas, *Arch Dermatol* (1980) **116**:1041–4.
17. Reed WB, Becker SW Sr, Becker SW Jr, Nickel WR, Giant pigmented nevi,

melanoma and leptomeningeal melanocytosis, *Arch Dermatol* (1965) **91**:100–19.

18. Scotto J, Fears TR, Fraumeni JF Jr, Incidence of non-melanoma skin cancer in the United States, Bethesda, Md, National Institutes of Health Publication No. 83-2433, 1983.

19. Goldberg LH, Carter-Campbell S, Yiannion JA, The risk of acquiring a new skin cancer in patients with a previously diagnosed skin cancer, *Skin Cancer Found J* (1988) **25**:6.

20. Lindelof B, Sigurgeirsson B, Wallberg P et al, Occurrence of other malignancies in 1973 patients with basal cell carcinoma, *Am Acad Dermatol J* (1991) **25**:245–8.

Chapter 20

METASTASIS: BASIC MECHANISMS AND APPLICATIONS IN DERMATOLOGY

David G. Brodland

Dermatologists have assumed an active role in the diagnosis and treatment of skin malignancy. Many types of cutaneous malignancies have the potential to metastasize so it is inevitable that we will encounter metastatic disease. In assuming greater responsibility for diagnosis, management and treatment of potentially metastatic disease, the dermatologist should pursue expertise in cutaneous oncology. Understanding the basic mechanisms of metastasis is essential.

Metastasis is defined as a neoplastic lesion arising from another neoplasm with which it is no longer in contact.[1] It is important to distinguish between tumorigenesis and metastasis. Tumorigenesis can and often does occur without metastasis. However, metastasis does not occur without tumorigenesis. Tumorigenesis may occur in nonmalignant and nonmetastatic neoplasias such as warts.[2] However, some malignant neoplasms can give rise to metastasis. The term 'metastatic potential' refers to the likelihood of a tumor system developing the necessary mechanisms to metastasize. Basal cell carcinoma has a very low metastatic potential while malignant melanoma has a very high metastatic potential. Squamous cell carcinoma has an intermediate metastatic potential.

Metastasis is complex. It is not simply tumor cells separating from the primary neoplasm and passively floating down the bloodstream and lodging in distant tissue. Although complex, when viewed simplistically metastasis has a predictable sequence of steps. These steps are accomplished in different ways by different tumors, which accounts for the multiplicity of patterns of metastasis.

There are several key biological properties that cells must acquire and effectively express before metastasis can occur. These properties make it possible for a particular cell to progress through the steps of metastasis. Although it is an oversimplification of a complex and dynamic process, it is useful to think of six steps in the sequence of metastasis. These include: (1) detachment from the primary tumor; (2) local invasion and intravasation of the cell into a vessel; (3) passage through the blood or lymphatic circulatory system; (4) stasis in a vessel at the recipient site; (5) extravasation through the vessel wall and invasion of the recipient tissue bed; and (6) proliferation within the tissue.

Even tumor cells within the same primary tumor have been shown to be phenotypically heterogeneous, adding to the complexity of this process.[3–5] Therefore, even tumor cells from the same cell line are not equal with regard to their metastatic potential.

In order to understand the metastatic sequence, we will review the basic steps in this process as well as some of the biological mechanisms used by the tumor cell in the process of metastasis. Finally, the way in which these sequential steps relate to the clinical pattern of metastasis will be discussed.

THE STEPS OF METASTASIS

A prerequisite for metastasis is the acquisition of a tumorigenic phenotype.[6] While tumorigenesis is necessary for metastasis, metastasis does not invariably follow tumorigenesis. Such is the case in basal cell carcinomas and verrucae, in which tumorigenesis is rarely or never followed by metastasis.

If metastasis is to occur after tumorigenesis, the tumor cell must acquire the ability to detach from the primary tumor and maintain homeostasis without normal cell–cell interactions. The mechanisms for tumor cell detachment are poorly understood but it is felt that the ability to readily detach favors a more highly metastatic phenotype.[7,8] It is generally thought that tumor cells are more easily separable from one another than normal cells. The key feature for viable metastasis, however, is functional autonomy after separation.

Invasiveness is a property which is also essential for tumor cells to separate from the primary tumor and to pass into, and eventually out of, the bloodstream. A three-step hypothesis of tissue invasion has been proposed.[9] These steps include attachment to the tissue matrix or basement membrane, enzymatic degradation of the intervening tissue, and locomotion into this tissue (Figure 20.1).

Tumor cell attachment appears to be a specific interaction of the tumor cell with specific components of the tissue or blood vessel it is invading. Attachment sites for many invading tumors are the stromal fibronectin of the tissue matrix or the laminin from the basement membrane zone of blood vessels. Specific receptors on the tumor cell surface selectively interact with these components of the tissue matrix or vessel. The experimental evidence supporting attachment of tumors by specific receptors includes studies of highly aggressive and invasive tumors which express laminin receptors in numbers which are 50 times normal.[10] It has been shown that blocking these receptors attenuates these tumors' tendency to metastasize.[11,12] In fact, an experimental model using melanoma cells showed metastasis inhibition in association with pretreatment with fibronectin receptor blocking peptides.[13]

Once a tumor cell is adherent to the tissue to be invaded, various hydrolytic enzymes are secreted to focally degrade this intervening tissue. Hydrolytic enzymes which have been identified include metalloproteinases, cathepsin B, type IV collagenase, elastase, heparitinase, and plasminogen activator. These have been noted to be released in significant quantities by metastatic cells but not by nonmetastatic cells.[14] In the tumors with metalloproteinases, metalloproteinase blocking antibodies abolish invasive action of the tumor cells.

When the way is prepared for the tumor cell, directed motility is the third essential step for invasion. An interesting new class of cytokines, the autocrine motility factors, have been recently characterized.[7,15] These are chemical mediators produced by the tumor cells that stimulate their movement into the area of hydrolytic degradation. This seems to be a very important factor in invasiveness. Another mechanism which has been previously characterized is cell movement by chemotaxis in which degradation products of extracellular matrix molecules serve as chemotaxins to the tumor cell.

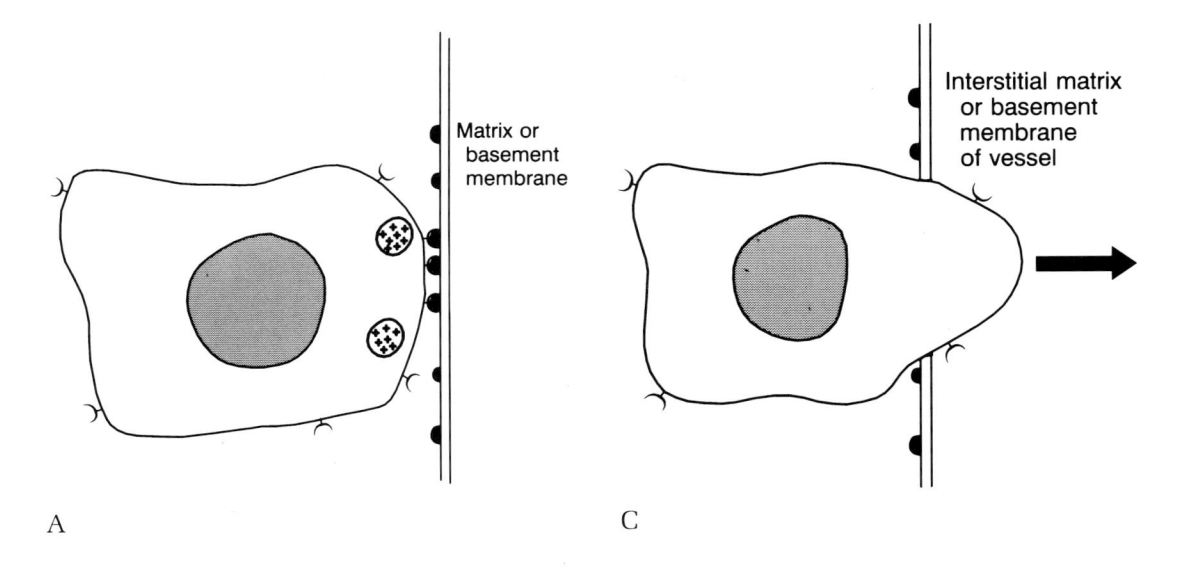

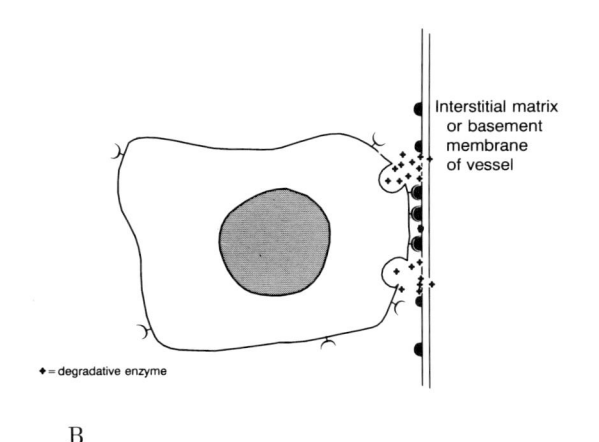

Figure 20.1
(A) Attachment of tumor cell by specific receptor interaction with interstitial matrix or basement membrane of vessel. (B) Enzymatic breakdown of interstitial matrix or basement membrane of vessel. (C) Movement through degraded interstitial matrix or basement membrane.

Intravasation is the second step of metastasis and utilizes the invasion sequence to accomplish intravasation. The invasive tumor cell attaches to specific molecules of the subendothelial matrix such as fibronectin, laminin, and collagen types IV and V.[10,16,17] Degradation of the basement membrane is followed by movement of the cell into the blood vessel. Again, there is experimental evidence that the ability to degrade basement membranes is seen to a greater degree in more aggressive metastatic cells.[18]

Other factors relating to the ease of intravasation are tumor-induced recruitment of capillaries or tumor-directed angiogenesis.[19] When vessels are readily available, intravasation is more likely. In addition, the blood vessels associated with tumors have endothelium that is often defective and more permeable and susceptible to tumor invasion.[20,21]

Once successful intravasation occurs and the tumor cell is circulating, it is tempting to think that metastasis is likely to occur. However, circulation of tumor cells alone does not constitute metastasis.[22,23] In fact, the chance of an embolized cell successfully establishing a distant colony is exceedingly small. Survival estimates of embolized cells range from 1 in 1000 to 1 in 1 000 000.[1,13] One of the reasons that cell survival is so low is that the bloodstream constitutes a mechanical and immunologic barrier to the circulating tumor cell.[24] Most cells are destroyed within the bloodstream before distant implantation can occur.[12,25] Cell rupture and demise is most frequently a result of mechanical trauma resulting from intravascular turbulence, shearing force, and cell shape transitions. Cells that manage to survive these insults must also avoid detection by the immune system, which, of course, has a very important antitumor effect.[26] Successfully metastasizing tumors often display properties which are protective against mechanical and immunologic destruction (Figure 20.2). Homotypic aggregation is an example of one such protective mechanism.[25] Tumor cells aggregate into multicellular embolic units, the outer layers of which serve as a protective cushion for the centrally located tumor cells.[9] Heterotypic aggregation is characterized by deposition of fibrin around the tumor cells after they lodge in a recipient tissue bed.[27] Other forms of heterotypic aggregation are with platelets, lymphocytes and soluble blood components. Again, this insulative coating serves as protection from the mechanical and immunologic damage.[28] These protective mechanisms have been shown to be important in metastasis since the inhibition of homotypic and heterotypic aggregation has been shown to prevent metastasis in some tumor models.[29] Another adaptive technique

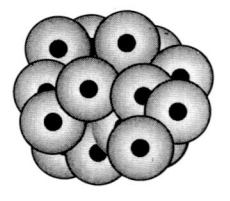

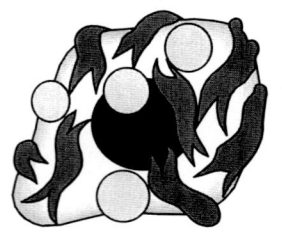

Figure 20.2
Homotypic aggregation characterized by multicellular conglomerations of tumor cells. Heterotypic aggregation occurs when tumor cells become coated with various proteins and cells such as platelets and fibrin.

which metastatic tumor cells have been shown to utilize to escape immunologic detection relates to genetic alternation.[6] The loss of expression of major histocompatibility antigens in a highly metastatic murine tumor model has been shown to attenuate immune responses to the cell. When genetic manipulations experimentally reinstate the expression of this antigen, the metastatic properties of the tumor cells are abrogated.

A common misconception is that a tumor cell intravasates into either the blood or lymphatic circulatory system and remains within it until implantation. Anatomically, it has been shown that the disseminating tumor cell can pass freely through communications between lymph and blood vessels.[30] Therefore, lymphatic and hematogenous metastasis can and often does occur in parallel.[31] The view that tumors which tend to metastasize to the lymphatics or hematogenously do so because they preferentially invade lymph vessels or blood vessels is simplistic, and the explanation must involve some other mechanisms since the blood and lymphatic circulations are so extensively interconnected. It is more likely that preferential metastasis to a lymph node or a specific organ is a form of site-specific metastasis rather than selective invasion of a particular circulatory system.

The next step in metastasis involves the stasis of embolic cells in the recipient tissue. It is this step that is the most important in determining the pattern of metastasis for a given tumor line. Stasis of a tumor cell may be a nonspecific mechanical event such as random tumor cell thrombosis. Alternatively, there may be site-specific attachment in which the tumor cell selectively adheres to a specific organ's vessel wall while bypassing nontarget organs. Regardless of the mechanism, in order to successfully achieve stasis, the cells must remain resistant to further mechanical and immunologic damage so that the processes of extravasation and proliferation can occur.

Achieving stasis enables extravasation, the next step in metastasis. Again, the three-step sequence of invasion is believed to occur, that is the tumor attaches to the vessel wall and subsequently the parenchymal tissue, the intervening tissue is degraded and the cell advances into the area which has been appropriately prepared.

Once the tumor has successfully extravasated and invaded the recipient parenchymal tissue tumor cell proliferation, the final step of metastasis begins. It is felt that this step may also play an important role in determining whether metastasis will be site-specific or not. For example, if a growth factor critical to the survival of a given tumor cell is found in sufficient concentration in only one organ, then it can be expected that metastasis will appear directed at or specific to this particular organ. Regardless of site specificity, tumor cell proliferation in any foreign environment requires the presence of certain local growth factors or the acquisition by the tumor of special adaptive mechanisms. Various mechanisms that facilitate proliferation in foreign environments include: (1) the presence of organ-specific growth factors to which tumor cells are responsive; (2) the increased or decreased sensitivity of the tumor cells to growth factors or growth inhibitors; (3) the production of autocrine growth factors; and (4) the production of angiogenic factors. The availability of organ-specific growth factors that are mitogenic to the tumor cells in concentrations sufficient to promote tumor proliferation[14] is an important determinant of successful metastasis. The presence of organ-specific growth factors used by metastatic tumor cells has been confirmed experimentally. Another mechanism which enables colonization of tumor cells in distant tissue is altered sensitivity to normal growth factors[14] and normal growth inhibitors.[6] A specific example of altered sensitivity is noted in one study where transforming growth factor beta resulted in a stimulatory response in growth rather than the normal inhibitory response.[32]

A third quality that can enhance the proliferation of tumors in a foreign environment is the ability of the tumor cells to produce their own growth factors. These substances are known as autocrine growth factors.[33,34] Autocrine growth factors are of great advantage to metastatic tumor cells since they enable them to grow in distant organs regardless of local availability of growth factors. Squamous cell carcinoma cell lines have been shown to secrete their own transforming growth factor alpha in addition to overexpressing epidermal growth factor receptors, which is believed to confer a proliferative advantage.[35] This same cell line has been shown to produce insulin-like growth factor I, which is also a mitogen.

The ability of the tumor to evoke angiogenesis is another property that enhances successful proliferation of metastatic colonies.[1] The ingrowth of a rich new vascular supply makes possible the growth of micrometastases, and, subsequently, the establishment of tumor colonies. In fact, angiogenic factors have been found experimentally in metastatic tumors.[36]

CLINICAL PATTERNS OF METASTASIS

There are three basic patterns of distribution seen in metastatic cancer. This distribution is most closely related to the mechanism of cellular stasis.[37] The distribution pattern may be solely determined by the anatomical proximity and lymphatic drainage in the region of the primary tumor (that is mechanical tumor stasis). Alternatively, the pattern of metastasis may be governed by an intriguing phenomenon seen in some tumors and recognized as site-specific metastases. Selective attachment of the tumor cell to a specific organ constitutes specific or selective metastasis. Finally, a pattern of distribution may be independent of mechanical and organ-specific factors (nonselective tumor stasis).

The mechanical tumor implantation pattern is characterized by tumor stasis in the first capillary bed encountered by a circulating tumor cell (Figure 20.3). This pattern is seen in 50–60% of metastases.[31] A tumor characteristic that favors mechanical implantation is the formation of multicellular emboli such as seen in homotypic tumor aggregation, since these large aggregates are more likely to arrest in a capillary bed due to their size. Heterotypic aggregation of tumor cells with platelets, lymphocytes, and soluble blood components may also favor regional patterns of metastasis.

Cancers which metastasize predominantly on a mechanical basis to the lymphatics in the region are head and neck cancers,[38] particularly squamous cell carcinomas. Some melanomas are also known to be limited to a mechanical pattern involv-

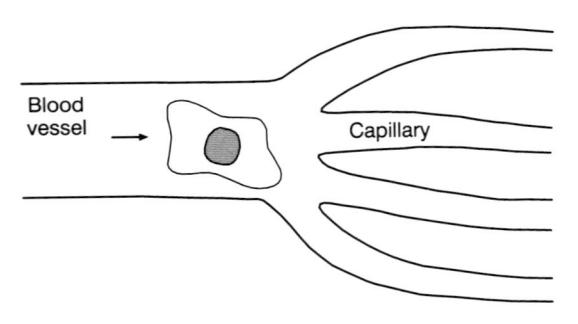

Figure 20.3
Tumor cell lodged in capillary bed leads to mechanical pattern of metastasis.

ing only the regional lymph nodes. However, melanomas are also known to have the capacity to metastasize in all clinical patterns.

The concept of site-specific tumor metastasis is more than a century old.[39] Clearly some tumors have a mysterious propensity to selectively implant in specific distant organs while bypassing nearby organs (Figure 20.4).[40,41] These site-specific tumors have a capacity to select specific recipient organs and selectively adhere and invade the endothelia of these organs. No tumor type is purely site specific in all situations. However, some types are known to have a great propensity to metastasize to certain organs such as the prostate to the axial spine[42] and melanoma to the brain.

One important factor in the selectivity of site-specific metastasis is preferential adhesion to organ-specific adhesion molecules[7] located within the vessel wall. Preferential adhesion of metastatic tumors to both organ-specific endothelial cells[43] and subendothelial components of blood vessels has been demonstrated.[27] This basic mechanism for site-specific metastasis is illustrated by the fact that some malignant cells with a higher affinity for laminin than for fibronectin tend to metastasize to the lung, which has a laminin-rich basement

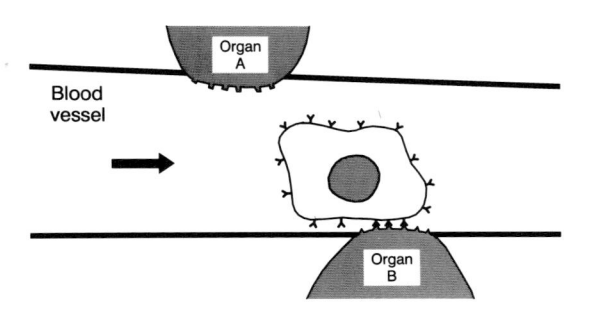

Figure 20.4
Organ-specific tumor cell–receptor interaction results in site-specific metastasis.

membrane. In contrast, the cells with higher affinity for fibronectin are preferentially metastatic to the liver, which has less laminin and a greater fibronectin content.[27] Organ-specific receptors on tumor cell membranes that may function as adherence sites specific for that organ have also been identified. The leukocyte-function-associated antigen is one such adhesion molecule[44] and has been shown to be important in site-specific metastasis of lymphoma cells. These cells show a predilection for liver metastasis and, when incubated with the leukocyte-function-associated antigen antibodies, fail to adhere to the liver cells.[45] Those lymphoma cells which lack this antigen do not tend to metastasize to the liver.[46]

Another organ homing mechanism which has been proposed and suggested experimentally is chemotaxis. Degradation products of extracts prepared from the organ for which a particular tumor cell line is selective induce migration of tumor cells whereas extracts from other organs do not.[47] Many of the substances which have been found to be chemotaxic to organ-specific tumors are fragments of extracellular matrix molecules that may be produced by the action of a tumor-derived enzyme. Examples of these chemotaxins include fragments of fibronectin, laminin, collagen and elastin, and byproducts of resorbing bone. Thus, it is possible that tumor enzymes break down extracellular matrix, causing release of chemotactic factors, which draws more tumor cells to the specific site in which a tumor cell has already established a colony. Theoretically, molecules released during tissue injury or normal physiological breakdown of tissue could also provide a chemotactic gradient and metastasis. This situation is suggested by studies which have shown that tumor cells preferentially metastasizing to elastin-rich lung tissue are usually able to degrade elastin and to migrate in response to elastin fragments.[48,49]

Yet another way of promoting site-specific metastasis is when a tumor cell's proliferation is specifically enhanced within a given organ. Tumor emboli most likely disseminate to many organs[1,23,50,51] but successful implantation and proliferation often only occur in select organs. Both organ-selective and nonselective proliferation may be due in part to the local environment. For example, metastatic cells may have a growth factor requirement that is adequately fulfilled in a particular organ. An example of this is in murine melanoma cells that preferentially colonize the lung. In vitro, they exhibit lung-extract-stimulated growth. Conversely, growth inhibition occurs when these cells are exposed to extracts from other organs.

There are some tumors that are highly aggressive and high in metastatic efficiency and are biologically equipped to adhere to the vessel walls of many different organs and establish viable metastatic colonies in various tissues. This represents the nonselective metastasis pattern. Even tumors which are initially site specific may progress in metastatic efficiency and evolve the capability of nonselectively colonizing and growth in many different organs (Figure 20.5).[27] This ability gives rise to a nonspecific or random pattern of metastasis. There have been several biolog-

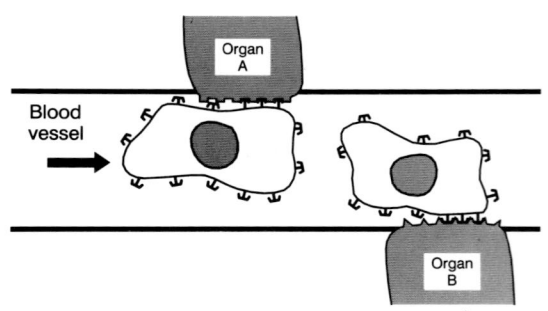

Figure 20.5
Nonspecific tumor cell–receptor interaction results in random pattern of metastasis.

ical properties shown to favor nonspecific metastasis. Autocrine growth factors strongly favor indiscriminate metastasis since they provide a stimulus for cell growth and proliferation regardless of the local environment. The presence and concentration of local growth factors are less important when the tumor cell can produce autocrine growth factors.

There are undoubtedly many other biological properties which are as yet uncharacterized which strongly influence the clinical patterns of metastasis. It is most intriguing that many of the biological properties that have been shown to influence the patterns of metastasis are relatively minor deviations from normal cell functions. This fact suggests that much can be learned about mechanisms of metastasis through better understanding of normal cell function. Continued elucidation and characterization of these biological determinants of clinical patterns of metastasis may ultimately have clinical application. If the likely site of metastasis for a given tumor could be characterized prior to metastasis, clinical monitoring and perhaps even prophylactic treatment could be improved. Therapeutic considerations will be affected by the understanding of the systemic significance of regional lymphatic metastasis versus a distant metastasis.

Unwarranted radical surgeries may be avoided when not beneficial to the patient. As they continue to expand our role in the diagnosis and management of potentially metastatic diseases, dermatologists are well advised to maintain a basic understanding of the mechanisms of metastasis.

REFERENCES

1. Poste G, Fidler IJ, The pathogenesis of cancer metastasis, *Nature* (1980) **283**:139–46.
2. Nicolson GL, Poste G, Tumor implantation and invasion at metastatic sites, *Int Rev Exp Pathol* (1983) **26**:77–181.
3. Fidler IJ, Hart IR, Biological diversity in metastatic neoplasms: origins and implications, *Science* (1982) **217**:998–1003.
4. Heppner GH, Tumor heterogeneity, *Cancer Res* (1984) **214**:2259–65.
5. Hart I, Fidler IJ, Implications of tumor heterogeneity for studies on the biology and therapy of cancer metastasis, *Biochem Biophys Acta* (1981) **651**:37–50.
6. Sobel ME, Metastasis suppressor genes, *JNCI* (1990) **82**:267–76.
7. Weiss L, Wart PM, Cell detachment and metastasis, *Cancer Metastasis Rev* (1983) **2**:111—27.
8. Cezeaux JL, Austin V, Hosseinipour MC et al, The effects of shear stress and metastatic phenotype on the detachment of transformed cells, *Biorheology* (1991) **28**:195–205.
9. Liotta LA, Tumor invasion and metastasis—role of the extracellular matrix: Rhoads Memorial Award Lecture, *Cancer Res* (1986) **46**:1–7.
10. Wewer LM, Taraboletti G, Sobel ME et al, Role of laninin in tumor cell migration, *Cancer Res* (1987) **47**:5691–8.

11. Barsky SH, Rao CN, Williams JE et al, Laminin molecular domains which alter metastasis in a murine model, *J Clin Invest* (1984) **74**:843–8.

12. McCarthy JB, Skubitz APN, Palm SL et al, Metastasis inhibition of different tumor types by purified laminin fragments and a heparin-binding fragment of fibronectin, *JNCI* (1988) **80**:108–16.

13. Humphries MJ, Olden K, Yamada KM, A synthetic peptide from fibronectin inhibits experimental metastasis of murine melanoma cells, *Science* (1986) **233**:457–70.

14. Zetter BR, The cellular basis of site-specific tumor metastasis, *N Engl J Med* (1990) **332**:605–12.

15. Liotta LA, Mandler R, Murano G et al, Tumor cell autocrine motility factor, *Proc Natl Acad Sci USA* (1986) **83**:3302–6.

16. McCarthy JB, Basara ML, Palm SL et al, The role of cell adhesion proteins—laminin and fibronectin—in the movement of malignant and metastatic cells, *Cancer Metastasis Rev* (1985) **4**:125–52.

17. Juliano RL, Membrane receptors for extracellular matrix macromolecules: relationship to cell adhesion and tumor metastasis, *Biochim Biophys Acta* (1987) **907**:261–78.

18. Liotta LA, Tryggvason K, Garbisa S et al, Metastatic potential correlates with enzymatic degradation of basement membrane collagen, *Nature* (1980) **284**:67–8.

19. Weidner N, Semple JP, Welch WR et al, Tumor angiogenesis and metastasis — correlation in invasive breast carcinoma, *N Engl J Med* (1991) **324**:1–8.

20. Warren BA, Tumor metastasis and thrombosis, *Thromb Diath Haemorr* (1974) **59** (supplement):139–56.

21. Fidler IJ, Balch CM, *Current problems in surgery: the biology of cancer metastasis and implications for therapy* (Mosby-Year Book Medical Publishers: St Louis 1987) 132–374.

22. Salsbury AJ, The significance of the circulating cancer cell, *Cancer Treat Rev* (1975) **2**:55–72.

23. Fidler IJ, Metastasis: quantitative analysis of distribution and fate of tumor emboli labeled with ^{125}I-5-iodo-2'-deoxyuridine, *JNCI* (1970) **45**:773–82.

24. Weiss L, Harlow JP, Elkin G et al, Mechanisms for the biomechanical destruction of 1210 leukemic cells: a rate regulator for metastasis, *Cell Biophys* (1990) **16**:149–59.

25. Fidler LJ, Bucana C, Mechanism of tumor cell resistance to lysis by syngenetic lymphocytes, *Cancer Res* (1977) **37**:3945–56.

26. Kreider JW, Barlett GL, Is there a host response to metastasis? In: Welch DR, Bhyan BK, Liotta LA, eds, *Cancer metastasis: experimental and clinical strategies* (Alan R. Liss: New York 1986) 61–75.

27. Nicolson GL, Organ specificity of tumor metastasis: role of preferential adhesion, invasion, and growth of malignant cells at specific secondary sites, *Cancer Metastasis Rev* (1988) **7**:143–88.

28. Dvorak HF, Seneger DR, Dvorak AM, Fibrin as a component of the tumor stroma: origins and biological significance, *Cancer Metastasis Rev* (1983) **2**:41–75.

29. Wagner HE, Thomas P, Wolf BC et al, Inhibition of sialic acid incorporation prevents hepatic metastases, *Arch Surg* (1990) **125**:351–4.

30. del Regata JA, Pathways of metastatic spread of malignant tumors, *Semin Oncol* (1977) **4**:33–8.

31. Liotta LA, Kohn E, Cancer invasion and metastasis, *JAMA* (1990) **263**:1123–6.
32. Schwarz LC, Gingras M-C, Goldberg G et al, Loss of growth factor dependence and conversion of transforming growth factor-E$_1$ inhibition to stimulation in metastatic H-ras-transformed murine fibroblasts, *Cancer Res* (1988) **48**:6999–7003.
33. Sporn MB, Todaro GJ, Autocrine secretion and malignant transformation of cells, *N Engl J Med* (1980) **303**:878–80.
34. Sporn MB, Roberts AB, Peptide growth factors and inflammation, tissue repair, and cancer, *J Clin Invest* (1986) **78**:329–32.
35. Reiss M, Stash EB, Villucci VF et al, Activation of the autocrine transforming growth factor alpha pathway in human squamous cell carcinoma cells, *Cancer Res* (1991) **51**:6254–62.
36. Folkman J, Greenspan HP, Influence of geometry on control of cell growth, *Biochim Biophys Acta* (1975) **417**:211–36.
37. Hart IR, 'Seed and soil' revisited: mechanisms of site-specific metastasis, *Cancer Metastasis Rev* (1982) **1**:5–16.
38. Schirrmacher V, Cancer metastasis: experimental approaches, theoretical concepts, and impacts for treatment strategies, *Adv Cancer Res* (1985) **43**:1–73.
39. Paget S, The distribution of secondary growths in cancer of the breast, *Lancet* (1889) **1**:571–3.
40. Willis RA, *The spread of tumours in the human body*, 3rd edn (Butterworths: London 1973).
41. Sugarbaker EV, Patterns of metastasis in human malignancies, *Cancer Biol Rev* (1981) **2**:235–303.
42. Chackal-Roy M, Niemeyer C, Moore M et al, Stimulation of human prostatic carcinoma cell growth by factors present in human bone marrow, *J Clin Invest* (1989) **84**:43–50.
43. Auerbach R, Lu WC, Pardon E et al, Specificity of adhesion between murine tumor cells and capillary endothelium: an in vitro correlate of preferential metastasis in vivo, *Cancer Res* (1987) **47**:1492–6.
44. Springer TA, Dustin ML, Kishimoto TK et al, The lymphocyte function-associated LFA-1, CD2 and LFA-3 molecules: cell adhesion receptors of the immune system, *Annu Rev Immunol* (1987) **5**:223–52.
45. Roos E, Roossien FF, Involvement of leukocyte function-associated antigen-1 (LFA-1) in the invasion of hepatocyte cultures of lymphoma and T-cell hybridoma cells, *J Cell Biol* (1987) **105**:553–9.
46. Roossien FF, de Rijk D, Bikker A et al, Involvement of LFA-1 in lymphoma invasion and metastasis demonstrated with LFA-1-deficient mutants, *J Cell Biol* (1989) **108**:1979–85.
47. Hujanen ES, Terranova VP, Migration of tumor cells to organ-derived chemoattractants, *Cancer Res* (1985) **45**:3517–21.
48. Yusa T, Blood CH, Zetter BR, Tumor cell interactions with elastin: implications for pulmonary metastasis, *Am Rev Respir Dis* (1989) **140**:1458–62.
49. Blood CH, Sasse J, Brodt P et al, Identification of a tumor cell receptor for VGVAPG, an elastin-derived chemotactic peptide, *J Cell Biol* (1988) **107**:1987–93.
50. Fidler IJ, Gersten DM, Hart IR, The biology of cancer invasion and metastasis, *Curr Probl Cancer* (1982) **7**:4–8.
51. Poste G, Experimental systems for analysis of malignant phenotype, *Cancer Metastasis Rev* (1982) **1**:141–201.

Chapter 21

DERMATOFIBROSARCOMA PROTUBERANS

Edmund R. Hobbs

Dermatofibrosarcoma protuberans (DFSP) is a relatively uncommon soft tissue fibrohistiocytic tumor of intermediate malignancy. While DFSP seldom metastasizes, it frequently 'recurs' or persists because of inadequate resection, even when this is carried out with wide margins. Evidence is accumulating that Mohs micrographic surgery provides a significantly higher cure rate than does wide excision, with or without standard margin control. This chapter describes the clinical and histological presentations of DFSP and its variants, the tumor's biological behavior, and the Mohs technique as applied to DFSP. Published accounts of DFSP cases treated by the Mohs method are reviewed.

CLINICAL APPEARANCE

Dermatofibrosarcoma protuberans appears initially as a dusky indurated plaque which often escapes recognition by both patient and physician. Cases have been reported in all races and ages, but appear to be most common in early to middle adult life, with a slight male preponderance. Lesions are most common on the trunk, but can occur anywhere. Sometimes a history of antecedent trauma is obtained. Initial lesions are often flat or even depressed,[1] yellowish, and sclerotic, resembling morphea, and may progress as such;[2] more commonly, one or more nodules develop with time. These may be flesh colored or dusky blue–red, or red–brown, and may become quite large. They progress slowly, with relentless subcutaneous infiltration well beyond the surface component. The incidence of DFSP has been estimated at 0.8 cases per one million persons per year.[3] A recent population study in Rochester, Minnesota disclosed a significantly higher incidence of five cases per million.[4]

HISTOLOGY

Dermatofibrosarcoma protuberans is characterized microscopically by a storiform or reed-mat-like array of slender fibroblasts around hypocellular hubs, imparting a cartwheel or whirligig appearance (Figure 21.1). Collagen fibers are thin, delicate and nonpolarizable;[5] pre-existing collagen is wavy and infiltrated by spindle cells. Peripherally, the tumor is less cellular. Mitotic activity is usually low, and the amount of stromal mucin is variable. Inflammatory infiltrates, foamy histiocytes, multinucleated cells and hemosiderin deposits are uncommon.[6] The overlying epidermis is usually thin or ulcerated.

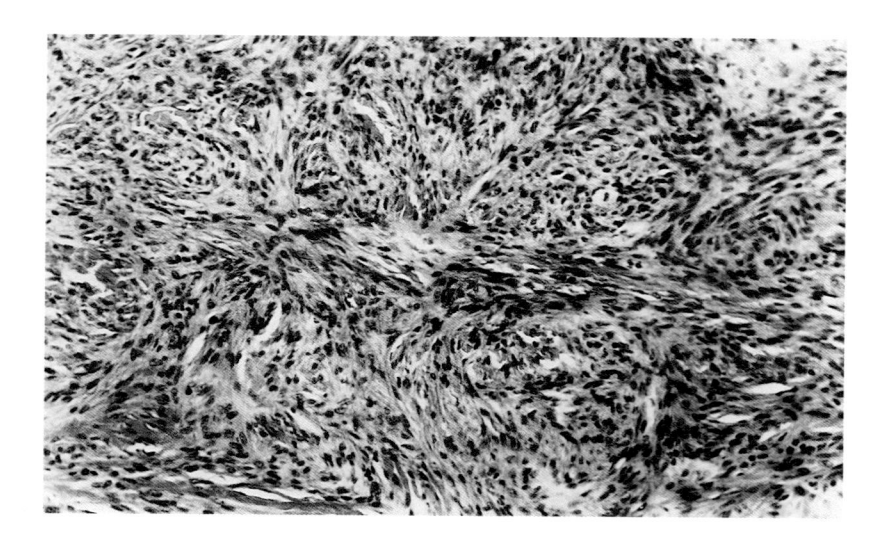

Figure 21.1
Interlacing bands and whorls of fibroblasts result in a storiform pattern characteristic of dermatofibrosarcoma protuberans (hematoxylin and eosin, original magnification ×10).

Hemorrhage and cystic changes are sometimes seen, but necrosis is rare.[7]

Kamino and Jacobson[6] described two patterns of extension into subcutaneous tissue. In 12 of 40 cases (30%) they observed the classic extension of spindle-shaped cells along septae and between fat cells in a honeycomb or lacelike pattern. In 24 cases (60%) there was a distinct multi-layered pattern in which bundles of slender spindle-shaped cells exhibited an orientation predominantly parallel to the skin surface. This pattern of subcutaneous involvement has not been described previously, and was found more commonly in early lesions.

VARIANTS

The Bednar tumor is a pigmented form of DFSP occurring predominantly in blacks and representing less than 5% of all DFSP.[8] The admixture of small melanin-containing dendritic cells probably represents secondary melanocyte colonization from the epidermis.[9,10] Insufficient data regarding Bednar tumors exist to allow comparison of their biological behavior with that of other forms of DFSP,[7,8] though there are some data suggesting that they may have a lower recurrence rate.[11] Onada et al[12] reported a Bednar tumor which recurred twice and metastasized widely to many organs. The recurrent and metastatic lesions appeared fibrosarcomatous and lacked pigment production and a storiform pattern.

Myxoid DFSP is characterized by the interstitial accumulation of hyaluronic acid ground substance,[7,13] rendering the usual storiform pattern less pronounced, and a nonpatterned array of vessels more apparent. These tumors can resemble myxoid liposarcoma,[7] and are said to share clinical features with the myxoid variant of malignant fibrous histiocytoma.[13] Tumors with a monotonously haphazard arrangement of spindle or stellate tumor cells with little variation in cellularity from field to field should be closely examined for foci of subtle radial arrangement and peripheral web-like patterns of infiltration,[13] which permit the correct diagnosis. Focal areas of myxoid change appear to be more prevalent in recurrent DFSP.[14]

Giant cell fibroblastoma is a rare mesenchymal tumor occurring predominantly in the first decade of life, showing a unique combination of spindle cell patterns, myxoid areas, pleomorphic and multinucleated giant cells, and distinctive sinusoid-like spaces.[15] Misdiagnosis as sarcoma is not unusual. Local recurrence is common, but metastasis unreported. The tumor is classified as a DFSP variant because of shared clinical and morphological characteristics, its biological behavior and storiform pattern, and tentacular infiltration of adjacent adipose tissue.[15] Most convincing is the occasional finding of sinusoid-like spaces at the periphery of some cases of adult DFSP,[15] and a case of giant cell fibroblastoma in an 8 year old which recurred locally 15 years later as a typical case of DFSP.[16]

There is no general agreement regarding the histogenesis of DFSP. It has been classified as a fibroblastic, histiocytic or neural tumor. The bulk of evidence at this time appears to favor the fibroblast[17] or precursor mesenchymal stem cell.[14]

Occasionally, a case of DFSP may be found to contain foci indistinguishable from fibrosarcoma or malignant fibrous histiocytoma. If such areas comprise a significant portion of the tumor, not just microscopic foci, the tumor is best regarded as a fully malignant sarcoma and managed as such.[7]

Biological behavior

Dermatofibrosarcoma protuberans grows by direct extension, spreading outward and downward in tentacular fashion and tending to follow paths of least resistance. The tumor can invade muscle and bone, but such behavior is unusual in primary tumors, as these structures present relative barriers. When natural barriers are disrupted by a surgical procedure, extension into muscle and bone becomes more likely if the tumor is incompletely resected. Thus, recurrent tumors are more likely to involve these deeper structures. It follows that the best opportunity for cure, with the least disruption of uninvolved tissue, is the initial surgical procedure. (There is no suggestion, however, that biopsy alters DFSP behavior.)

Dermatofibrosarcoma protuberans metastasizes in less than 4% of cases.[7] Its metastatic capability is probably overestimated in older literature by virtue of the inclusion of other soft tissue malignancies, such as malignant fibrous histiocytoma, which were defined subsequently.[14,18,19] Although metastases are infrequent, they can occur nonetheless and, when they do, lung is the most frequent target organ, followed by lymph nodes.[7] Tumors with lesser degrees of cellularity and anaplasia, and low mitotic rates of 5–10 per high-power field, tend to follow a more indolent course.[20] However, lesions with low mitotic rates are also capable of metastasis.[21] Cases of DFSP which metastasize are almost always recurrent tumors, with a considerable interval between diagnosis and metastasis.[7]

Fibrosarcomatous foci have been considered to occur more frequently in recurrent DFSP,[7] and their significance is not well established. In the setting of recurrent lesions, their presence probably signals heightened metastatic potential.[7] Wrotnowski et al[22] recently reported finding fibrosarcomatous areas in the tumors in six DFSP patients, four of which were found on the initial excision. They believe that fibrosarcomatous change within DFSP represents the development of a separate, distinct second neoplasm, and recommend evaluation and follow-up for metastasis. In a series of nine patients subsequently reported by Ding et al,[23] five had fibrosarcomatous changes in the initial lesion, eight had recurrence in a time period they considered shorter than usual for DFSP, and one had a metastasis. However, the percentage of fibrosarcomatous change in both Wrotnowski's and Ding's initial lesion cases was so great—about 50% on average—that these tumors probably should not be classified as DFSP. Both series contained patients with nonfibrosarcomatous DFSP which transitioned with recurrence to lesions which were predominantly fibrosarcoma. But more interesting is that both reported patients who had initial lesions which contained a significant percentage of fibrosarcomatous change, but later recurred as pure DFSP.

The most singularly distinctive feature of DFSP is its propensity to recur, even after 'wide excision'. In 98 cases studied by Taylor and Helwig,[18] a 49% recurrence rate was found. In Hajdu's series[24] of 119 cases, 54% recurred after wide excision. Of 17 cases treated by Pack and Tabah,[25] 24% recurred. One-fourth of those treated by Burkhardt et al[26] recurred. Rowsell et al[27] reported five cases, all of which had to be returned to surgery when margins were found to be involved with tumor. Two of these patients required two additional surgical procedures each, and one required three additional surgical procedures, in spite of the authors' technique of taking an average 2.7-cm margin of clinically normal skin and subcutaneous tissue at the first re-excision. McPeak et al[21] reported an 11% recurrence rate in 27 patients treated with a 3-cm margin of clinically uninvolved skin, down to and including fascia. Roses et al[28] used 3-cm margins in 10 patients and reported a 20% recurrence rate. Bendix-Hansen et al[3] also took 3-cm margins in seven patients and reported no recurrences.

Most recurrences of DFSP are noted within 3 years. Most of Hajdu's recurrences were noted in the first year.[24] In McPeak's series,[21] 75% of recurrences were detected in the first 2 years. In Taylor and Helwig's series,[18] nearly 40% of recurrences were noted in the first year, and 75% within 3 years. One case recurred after 20 years, however. Pack and Tabah[25] also reported a delayed recurrence of 19 years. The ability of recurrent DFSP to escape detection for many years must be borne in mind when assessing treatment efficacy.

Recurrences are presumably the result of subtotal resection.[25] The nodular quality of DFSP can impart to the surgeon an erroneous impression of circumscription. Tentacular or web-like projections of tumor often extend more than 3 cm beyond the tumor's main body, infiltrating connective tissue both laterally and deep. These extensions cannot be detected visually and can be missed by any sectioning technique which does not examine the entire under-surface and lateral margins of the excised specimen. Failure to excise all of the finger-like projections results in recurrence.

TREATMENT

Treatment of DFSP is primarily surgical. Chemotherapy has no role, and radiation's role is limited. Cases of DFSP with fibrosarcomatous change have been reported after radiation therapy,[22] raising the possibility that radiation may induce increasingly malignant behavior. Dermatofibrosarcoma protuberans is relatively radioresistant, and radiation should be considered only when the tumor cannot be completely resected, either as a primary treatment modality, or as an adjunct to surgery.[29]

Current recommendations for the surgical treatment of DFSP call for wide excision with a 3-cm or greater margin, down to and including fascia.[3,21,28] Prophylactic lymph node dissection is not warranted. As indicated above, even after treatment of this type, recurrence rates are distressingly high. Moreoever, 3-cm margins are not always possible, such as when the tumor involves functionally or cosmetically important anatomical areas such as the hands and face. The 53% failure rate reported by Barnes and Coleman[30] on head and neck cases probably reflects inability to achieve such margins.

Evidence is accumulating that Mohs micrographic surgery achieves cure rates considerably higher than those reported with wide excision. Mohs surgeons consider the technique the treatment of choice.[31-33] While some who perhaps do not understand the technique regard it as 'cumbersome, time consuming, and expensive',[34] it appears that the procedure is gaining credence among others.[35]

Mohs surgery

Mohs micrographic surgery (Mohs surgery, histographic surgery, microscopically controlled excision, Mohs chemosurgery) has been shown to result in extremely high cure rates for tumors which grow by direct extension and which have low rates of metastasis. Its most frequent application is in the treatment of recurrent basal cell carcinomas, large or morpheaform basal cell carcinomas, and midfacial or periauricular basal cell carcinomas. It is also useful for Bowen's disease and squamous cell carcinoma, and a variety of less common cutaneous neoplasms. The precise margin control made possible by the Mohs procedure enables the removal of microscopic-sized tumor projections while conserving the maximum possible amount of normal tissue, and eliminates the guesswork inherent in treating tumors using arbitrary margin guidelines.

Technique

Prior to treatment by Mohs micrographic surgery, the diagnosis of DFSP is usually established by excision or by incisional biopsy. The Mohs procedure can be undertaken in the operating room using regional or general anesthesia, or in the office with local anesthesia, depending upon individual case circumstances. In the first stage, all clinically apparent tumor is resected and saved for subsequent permanent vertical sectioning. While not contributing to decision-making regarding margins, vertical sections of the main body of the tumor may reveal information of prognostic importance, such as the finding of fibrosarcomatous foci. A conservative lamellar excision is then undertaken, to include a rim of skin and subcutaneous tissue peripheral to and below the defect left by the debulking excision. To achieve a continuous plane around and below the defect and to prevent loss of continuity which might inadvertently lead to the omission of a piece of tumor, this resection is best carried out *en bloc*. Score marks are made on the skin surface to facilitate orientation, and a map of the specimen is drawn to reflect the anatomical position of the excised tissue. On a cutting board, the specimen is then divided into smaller pieces, the sizes of which are determined by the sizes of cryostat object disks and glass slides being used. The edges of these pieces are color-coded with dyes, and these markings are recorded on the map to permit orientation when the sections are viewed microscopically. The combination of skin score marks (or other aids such as temporary sutures), map and color-coding allows the Mohs surgeon to keep track of the precise anatomical location of each piece of tissue.

An alternative method of approaching the initial stage involves the simultaneous resection of all gross tumor together with a conservative margin of apparently normal tissue. To facilitate orientation, score marks on the periphery are extended onto the excised specimen. Then the tumor is debulked on the cutting board, with thin pieces of tissue carefully pared from the entire periphery of the excised tumor mass. Because of tissue mobility, this method tends to be somewhat more difficult, and great care must be taken both to maintain orientation and to preserve the continuity of a single plane peripheral to the tumor's main body, which is retained for subsequent study. Mapping and color-coding proceed as described.

A dressing is applied to the wound while frozen section specimens are prepared in the histology laboratory under the Mohs surgeon's supervision. On the object disks, the tissue is compressed or stretched as needed to permit planes of section which would not be possible were the tissue rigid. In contrast to the vertical sections which are cut in standard sectioning, the Mohs procedure results in slightly tangential—almost horizontal—sections which permit a simultaneous view of the lateral and deep margins (Figure 21.2). In the center of large, deep wounds, interior segments are truly horizontal and usually contain no skin elements at all. The sections are then stained with hematoxylin and eosin, and examined microscopically by the Mohs surgeon, who records on the map the precise locations of residual tumor found at the margins of resection. He then returns to the patient, identifies those locations in the defect, and conducts another lamellar excision at these sites, and maps, processes and examines those pieces microscopically. The procedure is repeated in this iterative fashion until no tumor is detected at the periphery. Such precise margin control allows the Mohs surgeon to be assured of achieving cure, yet minimizes the ultimate size of the wound, as the tumor is tracked to its full extent, and no extra tissue is taken. This tissue-sparing feature of Mohs surgery is a great advantage, as it minimizes the size of the defect, preserving reconstructive surgery options. Reconstruction can proceed immediately upon achievement of a tumor-free plane, or it can be delayed. Smaller wounds can even be closed primarily or allowed to heal by second intention.

The success of Mohs surgery hinges on a number of factors: its use for tumors which spread by direct extension; maintenance of a continuous plane around and below the tumor; meticulous mapping and attention to anatomical location; horizontal and tangential frozen sections which permit a 100% examination of all margins of resection, in contrast to standard vertical sections, which allow examination of only a fraction of the true resection margin; technical quality of slides; and the skill of the Mohs surgeon in differentiating the cancer from normal tissue. Because one individual excises, maps and examines the tissue histologically, possible orientation errors due to miscommunication are eliminated.

Some authors have remarked that soft tissue neoplasms, especially recurrent lesions,[30] can be more difficult to read histologically with tissue processed using frozen sections.[35–37] It must be kept in mind that the Mohs surgeon is not usually in the position of establishing the diagnosis, which normally has been done previously. Rather, he is tracking the tumor to its full extent. His task is to differentiate normal

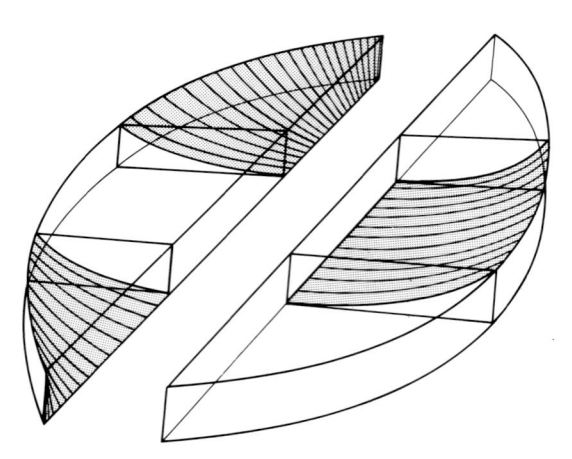

Figure 21.2
An excised piece of skin and underlying soft tissue is subdivided for histological examination by the Mohs method. The tissue is compressed and stretched as needed to establish planes of section allowing simultaneous examination of the entire deep and lateral margins. Three of the six tangential specimens which result are illustrated by the shaded areas.

benign tissue from abnormal cancerous tissue, which can usually be done quite handily with frozen sections in the case of DFSP. At times it may be difficult to reliably differentiate scar tissue from the less cellular tissue extensions which tend to occur at the periphery of DFSP. However, the finding of scar tissue implies that the plane of resection is not beyond and below the previous procedure, and if scar was left at the margin, the adequacy of resection would not be certain, as multifocal recurrence has not been excluded. Thus, the finding of scar at the resection margin justifies additional lamellar excision at that location.

Results

Frederic Mohs, who devised the procedure, reported seven cases of DFSP treated by the Mohs technique,[38] all without recurrence more than 5 years later. Five of these were treated by the fixed-tissue 'chemosurgery' technique, which is seldom used now, and two by the fresh-tissue technique described above. Robinson reported four cases, each without recurrence 5 years later.[36,39] Peters et al,[40] Hess et al[41] and Goldberg and Maso[33] reported Mohs procedures for facial DFSP, myxoid DFSP and DFSP in a child, respectively. Weber et al[42] used the Mohs technique to treat a 13 × 20 cm DFSP of the buttocks. Mikhail and Lynn[43] used Mohs surgery in two cases and had no recurrence in either more than 5 years later.[39] Recurrence of DFSP after a Mohs procedure has not yet been reported.

The largest series to date of patients treated by the Mohs technique was reported[32] by dermatologists and plastic surgeons from the Cleveland Clinic Foundation (Table 21.1). By the use of a team approach for tumor clearance and reconstruction, 10 patients were treated by the Mohs method between 1979 and 1986. One of these cases was subsequently reported in greater detail.[44] By November 1991, no recurrences had been detected in any of these 10 patients (Vidimos AT, personal communication).

In this series, two patients were female (cases 3, 7) and all patients but one were

Table 21.1
Summary of cases

Case no.	Year of birth	Tumor location	No. of prior excisions (excluding biopsies)	Mohs date	No of Mohs stages	Repair
1	1911	Chest/neck	2	10/1979	4	STSG, myocutaneous flap
2	1945	Back	4	03/1981	4	Primary closure
3	1945	Back	4	06/1983	2	Partial primary closure, STSG
4	1963	Chest	1	11/1983	3	None
5	1961	Scalp	2	02/1984	4	STSG
6	1941	Cheek	4	04/1984	4	STSG, then rectus abdominis free flap
7	1965	Shoulder	1	07/1984	4	STSG
8	1944	Hip	2	12/1984	2	Flap, STSG
9	1949	Thumb	1	05/1985	2	None
10	1980	Back	2	02/1986	2	Primary closure

STSG, split-thickness skin graft.

less than age 37 at the time of initial onset of the tumor. One patient was 5 years old at the time of surgery (case 10). Eight were caucasians, one black (case 2), and one oriental (case 7). Seven tumors occurred on the trunk, one on the cheek, one on the scalp, and one on the thumb. All 10 had prior excisional surgical treatment, with an average of two surgical excisions, excluding biopsies. Six were referred because of recurrence, while the remainder were sent because of the finding of positive margins at surgery. Median duration of illness prior to referral was 5 years.

Seven patients were treated under general anesthesia, and three received local anesthesia (cases 2, 4, 9). An average of three Mohs stages (lamellar excisions) was required. Muscle was invaded by tumor in four cases; in two of these, tumor extended to periosteum, but did not involve bone. The unusually high percentage of cases with muscle invasion (40%) reflected an advanced state of disease in this series of patients with persistent or recurrent tumors. Two patients were allowed to heal by second intention, two wounds were closed primarily, two received split-thickness skin grafts only, and four were repaired with combinations of split-thickness skin grafts and flaps or partial primary closure.

The follow-up period for this series of patients exceeds that period in which recurrences of DFSP are most likely. Because residual tumor can occasionally escape detection for many years, it is not possible to say yet that each of these patients has been cured. The successes reported by the Cleveland Clinic group and others together reflect a significantly higher cure rate than is typically reported with conventional surgical procedures, including 'wide excision'. The American College of Mohs Micrographic Surgery and Cutaneous Oncology has begun a registry of patients with DFSP. This data base will become an important source of information regarding Mohs surgery as treatment for this cancer.

While certainly no one believes that the Mohs procedure will always result in cure each time it is used for this difficult tumor, the results reported to date appear to indicate that the Mohs procedure should be regarded now as the treatment of choice.

References

1. Page EH, Asaad DM, Atrophic dermatofibroma and dermatofibrosarcoma protuberans, *J Am Acad Dermatol* (1987) **17**:947–50.
2. Lambert WC, Abramovits W, Gonzalez-Sevra A et al, Dermatofibrosarcoma non-protuberans: description and report of five cases of a morpheaform variant of dermatofibrosarcoma, *J Surg Oncol* (1985) **28**:7–11.
3. Bendix-Hansen K, Myhre-Jensen O, Kaae S, Dermatofibrosarcoma protuberans. A clinico-pathological study of nineteen cases and review of world literature, *Scand J Plast Reconstr Surg* (1983) **17**:247–52.
4. Chuang TY, Su WP, Muller SA, Incidence of cutaneous T cell lymphoma and other rare skin cancers in a defined population, *J Am Acad Dermatol* (1990) **23**:254–6.
5. Barr RJ, Young EM Jr, King DF, Non-polarizable collagen in dermatofibrosarcoma protuberans: a useful diagnostic aid, *J Cutan Pathol* (1986) **13**:339–46.
6. Kamino H, Jacobson M, Dermatofibroma extending into the subcutaneous tissue. Differential diagnosis for dermatofibrosarcoma protuberans, *Am J Surg Pathol* (1990) **14**:1156–64.
7. Enziger FM, Weiss SW, *Soft tissue tumors*, 2nd edn (CV Mosby: St Louis 1988) 252–68.

8. Dupree WB, Langloss JM, Weiss SW, Pigmented dermatofibrosarcoma protuberans (Bednar tumor). A pathologic, ultrastructural, and immunohistochemical study, *Am J Surg Pathol* (1985) **9**:630–9.

9. Fletcher CD, Theaker JM, Flanagan A et al, Pigmented dermatofibrosarcoma protuberans (Bednar tumor): melanocytic colonization or neuroectodermal differentiation? A clinicopathological and immunohistochemical study, *Histopathology* (1988) **13**:631–43.

10. Lambert MW, Lambert WC, Schwartz RA et al, Colonization of normelanocytic cutaneous lesions by dendritic melanocytic cells: a simulant of acral-lentiginous (palmar-plantar-subungual-mucosal) melanoma, *J Surg Oncol* (1985) **28**:12–18.

11. Ding JA, Hashimoto H, Sugimoto T et al, Bednar tumor (pigmented dermatofibrosarcoma protuberans). An analysis of six cases, *Acta Pathol Jpn* (1990) **40**:744–54.

12. Onada N, Tsutsumi Y, Kakudo K et al, Pigmented dermatofibrosarcoma protuberans (Bednar tumor). An autopsy case with systemic metastasis, *Acta Pathol Jpn* (1990) **40**:935–40.

13. Frierson HF, Cooper PH, Myxoid variant of dermatofibrosarcoma protuberans, *Am J Surg Pathol* (1983) **7**:445–50.

14. Fletcher CD, Evans BJ, MacArtney JC et al, Dermatofibrosarcoma protuberans: a clinicopathological and immunohistochemical study with a review of the literature, *Histopathology* (1985) **9**:921–38.

15. Shmookler BM, Enzinger FM, Weiss SW, Giant cell fibroblastoma. A juvenile form of dermatofibrosarcoma protuberans, *Cancer* (1989) **64**:2154–61.

16. Alguacil-Garcia A, Giant cell fibroblastoma recurring as dermatofibrosarcoma protuberans, *Am J Surg Pathol* (1991) **15**:798–801.

17. Lautier R, Wolff HH, Jones RE, An immunohistochemical study of dermatofibrosarcoma protuberans supports its fibroblastic character and contradicts neuroectodermal or histiocytic components, *Am J Dermatopathol* (1990) **12**:25–30.

18. Taylor HB, Helwig EB, Dermatofibrosarcoma protuberans: a study of 115 cases, *Cancer* (1962) **15**:717–25.

19. Weiss SW, Proliferative fibroblastic lesions: from hyperplasia to neoplasia, *Am J Surg Pathol* (1986) **10**(supplement 1):14–25.

20. Chattopadhyay TK, Singh MK, Arunabh, Dermatofibrosarcoma protuberans—a clinicopathological study of ten cases, *Jpn J Surg* (1986) **16**:435–8.

21. McPeak CJ, Cruz T, Nicastri AD, Dermatofibrosarcoma protuberans: an analysis of 86 cases—five with metastasis, *Ann Surg* (1967) **166**:803–16.

22. Wrotnowski U, Cooper PH, Shmookler BM, Fibrosarcomatous change in dermatofibrosarcoma protuberans, *Am J Surg Pathol* (1988) **12**:287–93.

23. Ding J, Hashimoto H, Enjoji M, Dermatofibrosarcoma protuberans with fibrosarcomatous areas. A clinicopathologic study of nine cases and a comparison with allied tumors, *Cancer* (1989) **64**:721–9.

24. Hajdu SI, *Pathology of soft tissue tumors* (Lea and Febiger: Philadelphia 1979) 60, 83.

25. Pack GT, Tabah EJ, Dermatofibrosarcoma protuberans: a report of thirty-nine cases, *Arch Surg* (1951) **63**:391–411.

26. Burkhardt BR, Soule EH, Winkelmann RK, Dermatofibrosarcoma protuberans: study of 56 cases, *Am J Surg* (1966) **111**:638–44.
27. Rowsell AR, Poole MD, Godfrey AM, Dermatofibrosarcoma protuberans: the problem of surgical management, *Br J Plast Surg* (1986) **39**:262–4.
28. Roses DF, Valensi Q, LaTrenta G et al, Surgical treatment of dermatofibrosarcoma protuberans, *Surg Gynecol Obstet* (1986) **162**:449–52.
29. Marks LB, Suit HD, Rosenberg AE et al, Dermatofibrosarcoma protuberans treated with radiation therapy, *Int J Radiat Oncol Biol Phys* (1989) **17**:379–84.
30. Barnes L, Coleman JA, Dermatofibrosarcoma protuberans of the head and neck, *Arch Otolaryngol* (1984) **110**:398–404.
31. Sagi A, Ben-Yakar Y, Mahler D, A ten year old boy with dermatofibrosarcoma protuberans of the face, *J Dermatol Surg Oncol* (1987) **13**:82–3.
32. Hobbs ER, Wheeland RG, Bailin PL et al, Treatment of dermatofibrosarcoma protuberans with Mohs micrographic surgery, *Ann Surg* (1988) **207**:102–7.
33. Goldberg DJ, Maso M, Dermatofibrosarcoma protuberans in a 9-year-old child: treatment by Mohs micrographic surgery, *Pediatr Dermatol* (1990) **7**:57–9.
34. Woods JE, Jackson IT, Treatment of dermatofibrosarcoma protuberans with Mohs micrographic surgery, *Ann Surg* (1988) **208**:669.
35. Snyderman NL, ed., Controversies: dermatofibrosarcoma protuberans, *Head Neck Surg* (1990) **12**:178–81.
36. Robinson JK, Dermatofibrosarcoma protuberans resected by Mohs surgery (chemosurgery). A 5-year prospective study, *J Am Acad Dermatol* (1985) **12**:1093–8.
37. Weimar VM, Ceilley RI, Chemosurgical reports: a myxoid variant of malignant fibrous histiocytoma: report of a case treated by Mohs technique with a slight modification, *J Dermatol Surg Oncol* (1979) **5**:16–18.
38. Mohs FE, *Chemosurgery: microscopically controlled surgery for skin cancer* (Charles C Thomas: Springfield IL 1978) 251.
39. Rockley PF, Robinson JK, Magid M et al, Dermatofibrosarcoma protuberans of the scalp: a series of cases, *J Am Acad Dermatol* (1989) **21**:278–83.
40. Peters CW, Hanke CW, Estes NC et al, Chemosurgery reports: myxoid dermatofibrosarcoma protuberans, *J Dermatol Surg Oncol* (1985) **11**:268–71.
41. Hess KA, Hanke CW, Estes NC et al, Chemosurgery reports: myxoid dermatofibrosarcoma protuberans, *J Dermatol Surg Oncol* (1985) **11**:268–71.
42. Weber PJ, Gretzula JC, Hevia O et al, Dermatofibrosarcoma protuberans, *J Dermatol Surg Oncol* (1988) **14**:555–8.
43. Mikhail GR, Lynn BH, Dermatofibrosarcoma protuberans, *J Dermatol Surg Oncol* (1978) **4**:81–4.
44. Hobbs ER, Ratz JL, Dermatofibrosarcoma protuberans of the hand: report of a case treated with Mohs micrographic surgery, *Cleve Clin J Med* (1988) **55**:252–6.

Chapter 22

ATYPICAL FIBROUS XANTHOMA AND MALIGNANT FIBROUS HISTIOCYTOMA

Marc D. Brown

INTRODUCTION

Fibrohistiocytic tumors are a heterogeneous group of soft tissue neoplasms composed of cells which resemble fibroblasts and/or histiocytes. Historically, fibrohistiocytic tumors were designated as such to imply their tissue origin from a pleuropotential tissue histiocyte that could assume fibroblastic properties. To date, the histiogenesis of fibrohistiocytic tumors remains uncertain, although more recent immunohistochemical studies provide evidence that the fibroblast is the probable mesenchymal cell of origin.[1,2]

Fibrohistiocytic tumors can be classified according to their malignant potential. For example, the most common fibrohistiocytic neoplasm is the benign dermatofibroma, which has no invasive or malignant potential and rarely requires surgical intervention. The dermatofibroma is considered to be a cutaneous form of the benign fibrohistiocytoma. There is a deeper fibrohistiocytoma which is seen less commonly but at times does exhibit a more locally aggressive growth pattern.[1] It does not metastasize but can show a higher incidence of local recurrence. The dermatofibrosarcoma protuberans (DFSP) is considered to be a fibrohistiocytic sarcoma of intermediate malignancy. It has histologic similarity to the benign fibrohistiocytoma, but grows in a more infiltrative fashion and has a marked tendency for local recurrence. In rare instances, a DFSP can metastatize.[3] The diagnosis and management of this tumor is considered in more detail in Chapter 21. The malignant fibrohistiocytoma (MFH) is the most aggressive of the fibrohistiocytic tumors, with a high local recurrence rate and a significant metastatic rate usually associated with a poor prognosis. Prognosis and survival appear in part to be related to tumor depth. For example, retroperitoneal and deeply situated skeletal muscle MFH tumors have a grave prognosis whereas MFH tumors confined to the subcutaneous tissue have a good prognosis. Fortunately, most cutaneous surgeons deal primarily with the more superficial of the MFH tumors. The atypical fibroxanthoma (AFX) represents the most superficial or limited form of a MFH tumor. Due to its more superficial intradermal location, the AFX pursues a relatively benign course with a relatively low recurrence rate and an excellent prognosis.

The scope of this chapter is to discuss the clinical diagnosis, histological appearance and surgical approach and management of the malignant fibrohistiocytoma as well as its superficial counterpart, the atypical fibroxanthoma.

ATYPICAL FIBROXANTHOMA

The atypical fibroxanthoma is probably best thought of as a superficial MFH or 'MFH in situ'. This tumor is histologically indistinguishable from pleomorphic forms of the MFH but it does not invade deeper subcutaneous tissue, fascia or muscle. Initially, AFX was interpreted as a benign reactive lesion but most dermatopathologists now view the AFX as a superficial or early form of the MFH.[4] Previously, AFX had been referred to as pseudosarcoma of the skin, pseudosarcomatous dermatofibroma and paradoxical fibrosarcoma.[1] The term AFX has been retained not only for historical reasons but also to distinguish it from the deeper, more invasive, MFH which necessitates a much more radical surgical approach. Due to the superficial location and usually small size (less than 2 cm) of the AFX, it pursues a relatively benign course.[5] However, in rare instances this tumor can metastasize to regional lymph nodes and an apparent AFX can progress to a MFH.[4,6,7] Thus, the AFX is best thought of as a fibrohistiocytic neoplasm of low-grade malignancy.

Clinically the AFX is typically seen on the actinically damaged skin of the elderly patient. It appears as an asymptomatic solitary nodule or nodular ulcer most commonly on the nose, cheek or ear (Figure 22.1). Typically an AFX tumor is less than 2 cm in size; its clinical appearance is not distinctive and it must be differentiated from a squamous cell carcinoma, basal cell carcinoma or necrotic pyogenic granuloma. As the tumor enlarges, it may erode, ulcerate and bleed. Less commonly, the AFX tumor will present on the extremities and trunk of younger persons.[8] These lesions are often larger, less well demarcated, and more nodular in appearance with extention into the subcutaneous tissue.

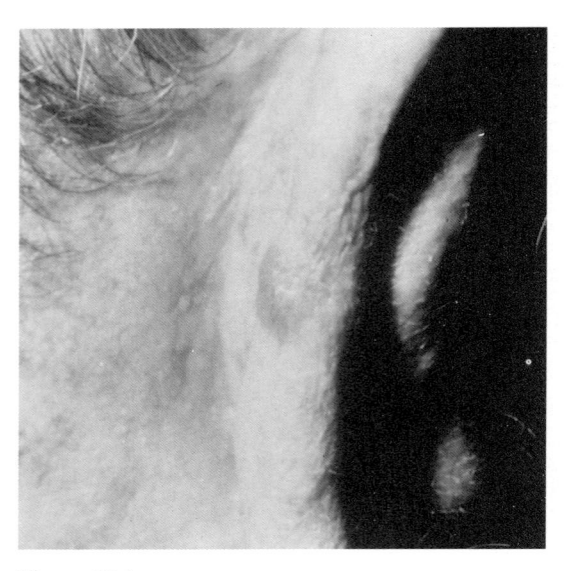

Figure 22.1
Atypical fibroxanthoma on mid-helical rim.

The etiology of the AFX is uncertain, but ultraviolet exposure has to be a prime consideration given the common occurrence of this tumor on the actinically damaged face of elderly persons. Other actinic-related neoplasms are often associated with an AFX. In some cases, previous radiographic therapy has been proposed as an etiologic factor[9] although this is not consistently documented. The AFX is thought to be a mesenchymal-derived neoplasm (like the MFH) rather than a spindled carcinoma.[1] Electron microscopic studies have demonstrated fibroblastic- and histiocytic-like cells and no features specifically suggesting epithelial differentiation.[10,11]

Microscopic findings under low-power magnification show an expansile dermal nodule that often abuts the epidermis. Dilated vessels are commonly seen adjacent to the tumor. Occasionally, dilatation of the subepidermal vessels may lead

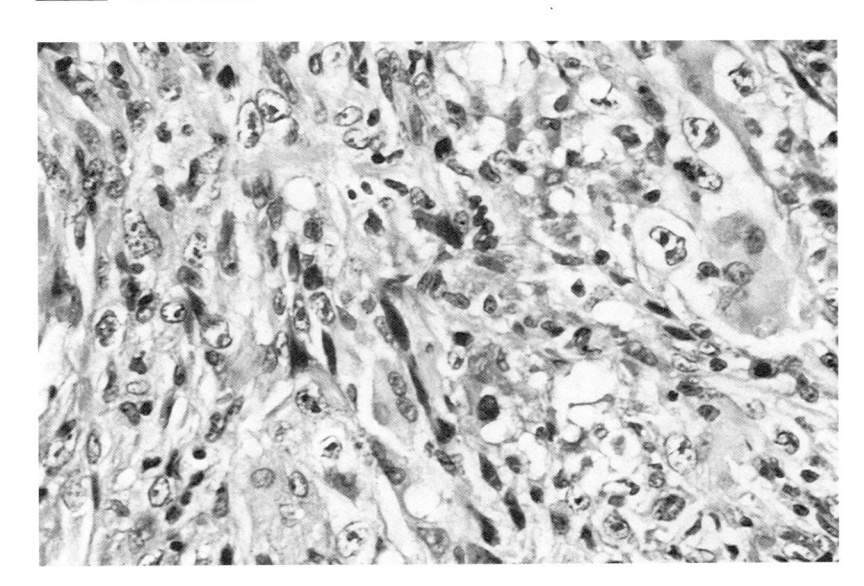

Figure 22.2
Atypical fibroxanthoma; note pleomorphism, spindle cells and giant cells.

to the separation of the epidermis from the underlying tumor. The AFX tumor can extend into the superficial subcutis but by definition does not invade more deeply.

Histologically the AFX resembles a pleomorphic MFH. There is a dense cellular infiltrate with pleomorphic hyperchromatic nuclei in an elongated irregular arrangement (Figure 22.2). A characteristic feature is that of large bizarre multinucleated cells arranged in a vague fascicular pattern. There can be marked nuclear atypicality with many mitoses. Cells will vary from plump spindled cells to large rounded cells. A scattered inflammatory infiltrate can sometimes be seen. The histological differential diagnosis of an AFX includes that of a spindle cell squamous cell carcinoma, melanoma or metastatic cancer. Mucin and melanin stains are helpful as are immunostains for cytokeratin and S-100 protein. The MFH differs from the AFX only by its deeper location in the subcutis or muscle and its often large size. Necrosis is also a prominent feature in MFH but is rarely seen in AFX. Because AFX is considered to be an early form of MFH the distinction of the two is somewhat arbitrary; nonetheless, it is important to distinguish them because of their differing natural histories and recommended surgical treatment. Deeper involvement, necrosis, and vascular or perineural invasion strongly suggest a diagnosis of MFH instead of AFX. An adequate biopsy is very important to distinguish AFX from MFH. If only a portion of the entire tumor is submitted for pathological interpretation, it may be difficult to assess the true depth and nature of invasion.

The AFX has a very good prognosis. Due to its 'in situ' dermal location, the risk of recurrence and/or metastatic disease is quite low. In one review, only nine out of 140 patients developed a recurrence and no metastatic lesions were found.[5] In rare instances the AFX tumor can metastasize to regional lymph nodes and an apparent AFX can progress to a MFH.[6,7]

Recommended surgical treatment of an AFX should be with a complete excision and margin control. Due to the possible extension into superficial subcutaneous tissue, curettage and electrodesiccation is not recommended. It wold seem unnecessary to utilize excisional margins of greater than 1 cm in order to achieve tumor-free peripheral margin control. Dissection should be carried well into the subcutaneous tissue in order to insure a free deep margin. Mohs micrographic surgery can also be utilized to treat AFX allowing for horizontal frozen section control. Brown and Swanson treated five patients with AFX.[12] All tumors were less than 2 cm in size, none were recurrent, and all were excised easily with only one stage of Mohs surgery. Although a conservative excision may be sufficient treatment for AFX, Mohs surgery does offer the advantage of tissue conservation in important facial areas as well as assurance of tumor-free margins at the time of surgery. If an AFX does recur in a deeper subcutaneous location, then it should be considered a MFH and treated accordingly.

Malignant fibrohistiocytoma

The malignant fibrohistiocytoma is the most common soft tissue sarcoma of late adult life.[13] Tumors previously described as pleomorphic variants of liposarcoma, fibrosarcoma or rhabdosarcoma were probably mislabeled examples of MFH. Malignant fibrohistiocytoma tumors can be classified as either superficial or deep. Superficial MFH tumors tend to be confined to the subcutaneous tissue but may be attached to the fascia. Most MFH tumors presenting to the dermatologic surgeon will be of this superficial type and overall will have a more favorable prognosis. However, the majority of MFH tumors are deeper lesions with approximately twice as many deeply situated tumors as superficial tumors.[14] The deep MFH tumors can extend from subcutaneous tissue through fascia and into muscle. At times the tumor can be situated entirely within the muscle; this is especially true when MFH involves limb skeletal muscles.[15]

Although there are several histological subtypes of MFH, the clinical features are relatively similar. This neoplasm typically appears between the ages of 50 and 70 years. The MFH tumor is extremely rare in patients under the age of 20.[1] The tumor is slightly more common in males, and Caucasians are affected more frequently than blacks or orientals. Clinically, the MFH presents as a painless enlarging mass of several months duration (Figure 22.3). At times, growth of the tumor may be rapid. Accelerated growth has been observed during pregnancy.[1] The tumor is usually solitary, can be multinodular, and may often be as large as 5–10 cm in size at the time of diagnosis (Figure 22.3). The more superficial of the MFH tumors are usually smaller at the time of diagnosis, in our series the average size was approximately 3 cm. The extremities are the most common site of involvement, especially the thigh, buttock and limb skeletal muscles.[13] The lower extremity is affected more commonly than the upper extemity. Any area of the body may be involved and approximately 10% of MFH tumors are on the head and neck region. Those MFH tumors located in the retroperitoneum are the largest because early diagnosis is difficult. If a malignant fibrohistiocytoma presents with evidence of metastatic disease, a primary source is usually readily diagnosable. This is in contrast to some other spindle cell tumors such as melanoma and spindle cell carcinoma where there may be an unknown primary.

Most patients with MFH are asymptomatic. On occasion there may be an associated fever and leukocytosis which seems to resolve after the tumor is removed.[1] Patients with retroperitoneal tumors may develop fatigue, weight loss, anorexia and abdominal pain. The etiology of the MFH

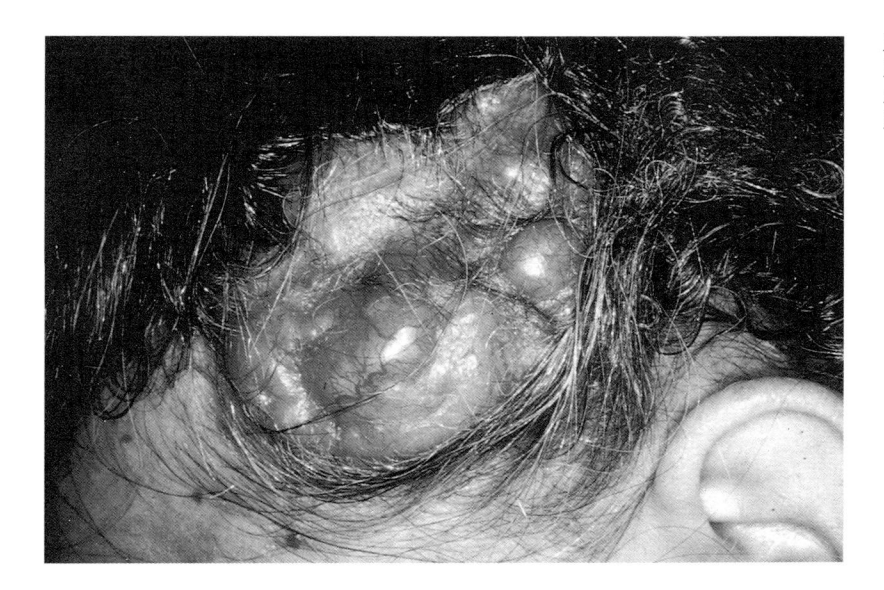

Figure 22.3
Large, multinodular malignant fibrous histiocytoma.

is unclear. There are sporadic reports suggesting that previous radiation exposure may be a predisposing factor but this would explain only a minority of cases. Unlike the case with AFX, sun exposure does not appear to be an important factor.

The MFH manifests a broad range of histological appearances and is divided into five subtypes which are not mutually exclusive (Table 22.1). The most common subtype is the *storiform-pleomorphic* type. This highly cellular tumor is composed of plump pleomorphic spindle cells, histiocytes, and frequent multinucleated giant cells. The morphological pattern is highly variable with frequent transitions from storiform to pleomorphic areas. Mitotic figures are common and often atypical. Although the storiform-pleomorphic MFH may resemble a DFSP, there are distinctive histological differences. The numerous atypical mitotic figures, less prominent storiform pattern, marked pleomorphism, and typical foamy giant cells seen with MFH are all key differential elements (Table 22.2). The storiform-pleomorphic pattern would be the most common subtype presenting to the dermatologic surgeon. This shows the closest resemblance to its superficial counterpart, the atypical fibroxanthoma.

Table 22.1
MFH: histological patterns

1. Storiform-pleomorphic
2. Myxoid
3. Giant cell
4. Inflammatory
5. Angiomatoid

Table 22.2
MFH: key histological features

1. Focal storiform pattern
2. Marked pleomorphism
3. Prominent atypical mitotic figures
4. Necrosis
5. Myxoid foci
6. Prominent foam cells and giant cells

The *myxoid variant* of MFH is the next most frequent subtype, comprising approximately 25%.[16] Histologically there is prominent myxoid change of the stroma. Large areas appear hypocellular with widely spaced bizarre spindle-shaped cells in a myxoid matrix rich in acid mucopolysaccharides. For unclear reasons, the myxoid variant can be a slower-growing tumor and has a slightly better prognosis. The last three histological subtypes are much less common. In the *inflammatory type* there is a diffuse neutrophilic infiltrate with numerous foam and xanthoma cells. The retroperitoneal MFH tumors are usually of the inflammatory type. The *giant cell* subtype shows osteoclastic-like giant cells.[17] The *angiomatoid* variant is the least common subtype. This tumor occurs in a younger population and combines features of both a fibrohistiocytic and a vascular neoplasm.[18] Patients are 20 years or younger and the tumor usually has a more superficial location in the subcutis. Gross examination of the angiomatoid MFH shows characteristic cystic areas of hemorrhage. Of all the histological subtypes, the angiomatoid has the best prognosis. The histological differential diagnosis of MFH includes pleomorphic variants of liposarcoma and rhabdomyosarcoma, pleomorphic carcinoma, histiocytic lymphoma, leiomyosarcoma and epithelioid sarcoma.[19]

Although the MFH has a clinical appearance of being a circumscribed tumor, it often spreads for considerable distance along fascial planes or between muscle fibers. Previously the MFH was considered a low-grade form of sarcoma; however, more recent understanding of this tumor shows it to be a fully malignant high-grade sarcoma. Invasive behavior of the MFH accounts for its high rate of local recurrence, estimated to be 40–50% even after wide local excision.[13,14] Unfortunately, the metastatic rate is also in the range of 40–45% with a high associated mortality. The 2-year survival is only about 60%. Metastatic disease occurs early (usually within the first 2 years after diagnosis) and most frequently affects the lung, liver, lymph nodes and bone.[13]

Prognosis appears to correlate best with the depth of the MFH tumor (not unlike other aggressive cutaneous tumors such as melanoma, squamous cell carcinoma and Merkel cell cancers). For example, less than 10% of MFH tumors confined entirely to the subcutis without deeper fascial or muscle involvement will metastasize.[1] When tumor does involve the fascia the rate of metastatic disease increases to almost 30%. Tumors involving the skeletal muscle will metastasize 40–45%. The size of the tumor also correlates with the risk of metastatic disease but this may be a covariable with tumor depth. Anatomical location of the tumor also correlates with prognosis. Distally located MFH tumors have a better prognosis than proximally located tumors.[14,15] Histological features, including degree of anaplasia and the number of mitoses, appear to have little prognostic value. However, the histological subtype of the myxoid and angiomatoid variant appear to do slightly better.[1] There is some evidence that tumors with a significant inflammatory response may have an improved prognosis but the metastatic rate for the inflammatory subtype is still in the range 30–35% (Table 22.3).

Surgical excision is the mainstay of therapy for MFH. Because this tumor can spread a considerable distance beyond the gross tumor margins, aggessive wide and deep local excision or even possible amputation have been recommended. Recurrence rates are directly related to the adequacy of the surgical treatment and establishment of tumor-free margins.[1] One of the major problems in dealing with this soft tissue sarcoma is adequate local control of the primary tumor. MFH tumors with local recurrence do have a much worse prognosis, so complete excision of

Table 22.3
Prognosis

Good	Poor
1. Superficial —intradermal —subcutis	1. Deep—skeletal muscle —retroperitoneal
2. Small tumor size	2. Large tumor size
3. Distal extremity	3. Proximal extremity
4. Myxoid or angiomatoid variant	

the primary tumor is important. Islands of tumor cells may extend well beyond what appears to be a well-encapsulated neoplasm. As with other aggressive cutaneous tumors, the MFH has a tendency to invade along fascial planes, muscle fibres, nerves and blood vessels. Wide excisional margins of 3–5 cm may still result in recurrence rates of 30–40%, depending somewhat on the previously described prognostic factors. Positive surgical resection margins will result in a local recurrence rate of 50–90%.[1] Recurrence will usually take place within the first 2 years after surgery of the primary tumor. More radical surgical procedures such as complete muscle compartment excision or limb amputation will give higher cure rates but with greater patient morbidity. Less radical surgery in conjunction with radiation and/or chemotherapy is becoming more popular for soft tissue sarcomas.[20] Even with adequate local control, metastatic disease will still occur. Only a minority of patients (less than 10%) will initially present with evidence of metastases. Because lymph node metastases are relatively infrequent, elective lymph node dissection of regional nodes is usually not recommended.[20] Lymph node dissection should be reserved for those patients with clinically suspicious nodes and/or a positive nodal biopsy.

For the more superficially located MFH tumors, Mohs micrographic surgery appears to be an excellent surgical modality. A more meticulous procedure, Mohs surgery is capable of tracing out the deepest and widest extensions of the MFH tumor as it spreads along anatomical planes. The MFH tumor is easily visualized with frozen section technology. We retrospectively looked at 17 patients with a total of 20 MFH tumors who underwent Mohs micrographic surgery.[12] Half of these patients already had local recurrence of their MFH from a previous non-Mohs procedure. All patients were treated in an outpatient setting. Standard tangential frozen sections were prepared in the usual manner after appropriate mapping and staining of the excised tissue. These tumors were widespread with an average preoperative tumor size of 3 cm. The patients required an average of 2.5 stages and 16 tissue sections to achieve tumor-free margins. The average postoperative defect size was 4.8 cm. The average follow-up was approximately 4 years. There was local recurrence of only one tumor and that patient subsequently underwent a second Mohs surgical procedure and remained tumor free. One patient developed probable metastatic disease to the lungs but an autopsy was not performed at the time of death. Thus, the overall success rate with Mohs surgery was excellent. These MFH tumors were primarily of the storiform-pleomorphic type with origin of the tumor in the dermis and subcutis. However, a number of these tumors did extend into the muscle. The more superficial location and relatively smaller size may have contributed to our higher success rate.

Table 22.4
Treatment

	Excisional margins	Mohs surgery	Adjuvant radiation/chemotherapy
AFX	1 cm	Tissue sparing for important cosmetic areas	No
MFH	3–5 cm	Yes (except for deep skeletal and retroperitoneal)	Yes, for high-risk tumors

Nonetheless for select MFH tumors, Mohs surgery offered a precise surgical approach with careful tracking of the tumor and clear definition of tumor-free margins. There was also the value of tissue sparing which becomes extremely important for the approximately 10% of MFH tumors located in the head and neck region. Table 22.4 summarizes the treatment options for MFH/AFX neoplasms.

The preoperative evaluation of patients with MFH is outlined in Table 22.5. It is important to note the size of the tumor, its anatomical location, and possible fixation of the tumor to deeper structures such as muscle. Careful palpation of regional lymph nodes should be performed. Clinically suspicious nodes should be biopsied. Because the lungs are the most common site of metastatic disease, a chest radiograph should be performed for all MFH tumors. For the higher risk deep and large MFH tumors, a CT of the chest should be undertaken. Evidence of metastatic disease may well alter the overall treatment plan. At times, resection of a solitary pulmonary metastasis can be peformed but only after a complete evaluation and staging of the metastatic disease. CT or MRI scans can also be helpful to assess the depth and extent of local spread of these MFH tumors.

Due to the high recurrence and metastatic rate of these soft tissue sarcomas, early consideration should be given to the use of adjuvant radiation therapy and/or chemotherapy. Occult micrometastases may respond to adjuvant therapy, although this has not been well studied specifically for MFH tumors. Soft tissue sarcomas do appear to respond to radiation therapy.[21,22] Radiation therapy is usually given postoperatively but also has been used preoperatively. The value of adjuvant chemotherapy remains controversial.[20] A prospective randomized study at the National Cancer Institute has shown improvement in disease-free and survival rates in patients with high-grade extremity sarcomas who underwent adjuvant chemotherapy.[23] Other studies have not shown a distinct advantage.[24,25] The drug that appears to be most efficacious is doxorubicin. Radiation and/or medical oncology should be consulted for the early aggressive management of these patients.

Table 22.5
Preoperative evaluation

1. Size and anatomical location
2. Fixation to deep structures
3. Lymph nodes
4. Chest radiograph
5. MRI to assess depth and extent of local spread
6. CT of chest for high-risk patients
7. Consultation with radiation and medical oncology

SUMMARY

AFX and MFH tumors are common soft tissue sarcomas which may present to the dermatologic surgeon for treatment and management. The AFX tumor is considered to be a limited, superficial MFH and is easily treated with a conservative excision with 1-cm margins to the level of the deep subcutaneous tissue. For tissue-sparing purposes in important cosmetic areas, Mohs surgery may be used. Most MFH tumors that the dermatologist will see are the more superficial lesions located in the subcutis with possible extension into fascia or muscle. Wide excision should be undertaken although the bias of this author is treatment with Mohs surgery. Mohs surgery offers a precise controlled excision with careful tracking of subclinical extension of the tumor. Local control with Mohs surgery appears to be excellent. The more superficial location and relatively smaller size may have contributed to the high success rate of Mohs surgery in our patient population. Nonetheless, for select MFH tumors Mohs surgery offers a precise surgical approach. Interpretation of the MFH tumor on frozen section histology is usually not difficult although having a dermatopathologist readily available for consultation is helpful. For larger (greater than 5 cm) and deeper (muscle compartment) MFH tumors, excision should be performed in an operating room setting. Radical excision with en bloc resection of the tumor in the entire compartment of origin is necessary to minimize risk of recurrence and metastatic disease. For high-risk tumors, adjuvant radiation therapy should be performed and consideration given to adjuvant chemotherapy. Combined treatment may well allow for limb-sparing surgery. For these high-risk tumors a multidisciplinary approach in a tertiary care center may well provide the best quality of care for the patients.

REFERENCES

1. Enzinger FM, Weiss SW, *Soft tissue tumors* (CV Mosby: St Louis 1988).
2. Fletcher CDM, McKee PH, Sarcomas—a clinicopathologic guide with particular reference to cutaneous manifestation, *Clin Exp Dermatol* (1984) 9:451–65.
3. McPeak CJ, Cruz T, Nicastv AD, Dermatofibrosarcoma protuberans: analysis of 86 cases—five with metastasis, *Ann Surg* (1967) 166:803–16.
4. Lever WF, Schaumburg-Lever G, Tumors of fibrous tissue. In: Lever WF, ed., *Histopathology of the skin* (JB Lippincott: New York 1983) 597–622.
5. Ivetzin DF, Helwig EB, Atypical fibrous xanthoma: a clinicopathologic study of 140 cases, *Cancer* (1973) 31:1541–52.
6. Helwig ED, May D, Atypical fibroxanthoma of the skin with metastases, *Cancer* (1986) 57:368.
7. Jacobs DS, Edwards WD, Ye RC, Metastatic atypical fibroxanthoma of the skin, *Cancer* (1975) 35:457.
8. Fretzin DF, Helwig EB, Atypical fibroxanthoma of the skin, *Cancer* (1973) 31:1541.
9. Hudson AW, Winkelmann RK, Atypical fibroxanthomas of the skin, *Cancer* (1972) 29:413.
10. Barr RJ, Wuerker RB, Graham JH, Ultrastructure of atypical fibroxanthoma, *Cancer* (1977) 30:736.
11. Weedon D, Kerr JFR, Atypical fibroxanthoma of skin: an electron microscopic study, *Pathology* (1975) 7:173.
12. Brown MD, Swanson NA, Treatment of malignant fibrous histiocytoma and atypical fibrous xanthomas with micrographic surgery, *J Dermatol Surg Oncol* (1989) 15:1287–92.
13. Weiss SW, Enzinger FM, Malignant fibrous histiocytoma—an analysis of 200 cases, *Cancer* (1978) 41:2250–66.
14. Kearney MD, Soule EH, Ivins JC, Malignant fibrous histiocytoma: a

15. Bertoni F, Capanna R, Biagini R et al, Malignant fibrous histiocytoma of soft tissue: an analysis of 78 cases located and deeply seated in the extremities, *Cancer* (1985) **56**:356.

retrospective study of 167 cases, *Cancer* (1980) **45**:167–78.

16. Weiss SW, Enzinger FM, Myxoid variant of malignant fibrous histiocytoma, *Cancer* (1977) **39**:1672.

17. Guccion JG, Enzinger FM, Malignant giant cell tumor of soft parts. An analysis of 32 cases, *Cancer* (1972) **29**:1518.

18. Enzinger FM, Angiomatoid malignant fibrous histiocytoma: a distinct fibrohistiocytic tumor of children and young adults simulating a vascular neoplasm, *Cancer* (1979) **44**:2147.

19. Headington JT, Niederhuber JE, Repola DA, Primary malignant fibrous histiocytoma of skin, *J Cutan Pathol* (1978) **5**:329–38.

20. Chang AE, Rosenberg SA, Clinical evaluation and treatment of soft tissue tumors. In: Enzinger FM, Weiss SW, eds, *Soft tissue tumors*, Chapter 2 (CV Mosby: St Louis 1988) 19–42.

21. McNeer GP, Cantin J, Chu F et al, Effectiveness of radiation therapy in the management of sarcoma of the soft somatic tissues, *Cancer* (1968) **22**:391–7.

22. Suit HD, Mankin JH, Schille AL et al, Results of treatment of sarcoma of soft tissue by radiation and surgery at Massachusetts General Hospital, *Cancer Treat Symp* (1985) **3**:43–7.

23. Rosenberg SA, Chang AE, Glatstein E, Adjuvant chemotherapy for treatment of extremity soft tissue sarcomas: review of National Cancer Institute experience, *Cancer Treat Symp* (1985) **3**:83–8.

24. Antman K, Amato D, Lerner H et al, Adjuvant doxorubicin for sarcoma, *Cancer Treat Symp* (1985) **3**:109–15.

25. Bramwell VHC, Rousse J, Santoro A et al, European experience of adjuvant chemotherapy for soft tissue sarcoma, *Cancer Treat Symp* (1985) **3**:99–107.

Chapter 23

SEBACEOUS CARCINOMA OF THE EYELID

Duane C. Whitaker

Sebaceous carcinoma (SC) of the eyelid is a rare malignancy which accounts for less than 1% of all eyelid tumors in Caucasian patients. This tumor may arise from the meibomian glands of the tarsal plate, the cilia-associated glands of Zeis of the eyelid margin, the caruncle, or the sebaceous glands of the periocular skin. Sebaceous carcinoma not only presents difficulties in recognition, diagnosis and treatment but is also perplexing in its etiology and spread. Because of its rarity many physicians are unaware of the entity. Ophthalmologists, dermatologists and pathologists (dermatologic or ophthalmic) should consider this tumor in the differential diagnosis of eyelid and conjunctival abnormalities. Its extreme clinical subtlety hinders prompt diagnosis and care. Though sebaceous malignancy of the eyelid is not usually a marker of Muir–Torre syndrome, patients should be examined for other cutaneous signs and questioned about visceral malignancy.[1]

INCIDENCE AND RISKS

A review of 20 patients diagnosed as having SC reported a mean age of 68.5 years at diagnosis with a range from 47 to 83 years, though younger ages are reported.[2,3] The most common skin cancers, basal cell carcinoma (BCC) and squamous cell carcinoma (SCC), occur largely in whites and have a higher incidence in males. However, as many as 57–77% of patients with SC are female. Sebaceous carcinoma accounts for 15–33% of eyelid tumors in some oriental populations.[4,5] Possible predisposing factors include irradiation, ultraviolet light (UV), and chronic inflammatory states of the lid or conjunctiva.[6]

Malignancy arising from skin usually presents as an indurated tumor mass but SC is often more subtle. When a nodule is present it tends to be yellow with telangectasia extending over the margin of the lesion. Sebaceous carcinoma occurs more frequently on the upper eyelid but can occur anywhere on the periocular and orbital tissues. Figure 23.1 shows a SC of the upper lid. Crusting or erosion may be present and hyperkeratosis may imply SCC. The patient may present with distortion of the normal lid–globe relationship, corneal exposure, or even orbital invasion. Chronic conjunctivitis or blepharoconjunctivitis may be part of the clinical picture and long-term treatment with topical medicaments or ophthalmic drops may have been tried. Previous biopsy may be

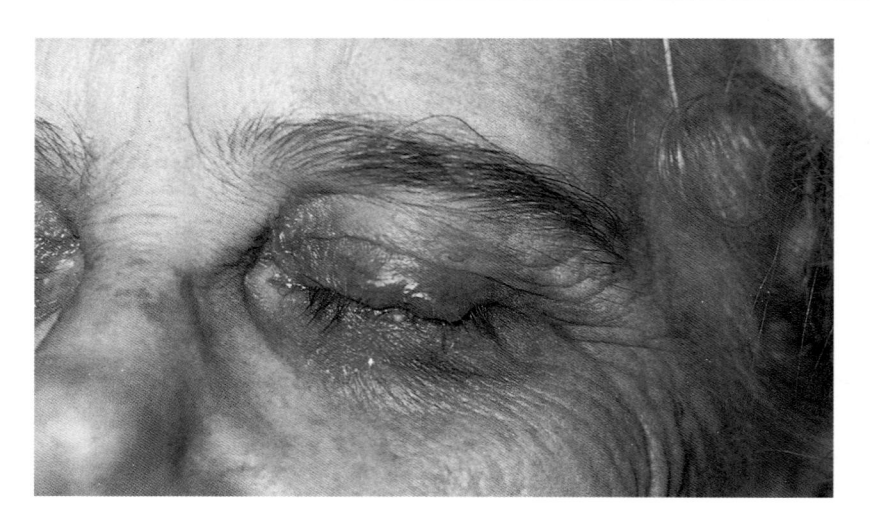

Figure 23.1
Sebaceous carcinoma of the upper lid with indistinct clinical margins.

read as nonspecific and patients' symptoms often include burning and puritus. There may be an abnormal appearance of the lid margin with a chronically injected conjunctiva. Clinical symptoms prior to diagnosis tend to be of long duration—frequently 10 years or more. Patients may carry a clinical diagnosis of recalcitrant chalazion if not biopsied. However, even biopsy does not assure correct diagnosis if the clinician and pathologist do not consider SC. Biopsy may be interpreted as actinic keratosis, Bowen's disease, a melanocytic lesion or inflammatory or granulation tissue. When pagetoid cells are seen in the epidermis, pathologists may interpret this as the atypical cells of an actinic keratosis of the eyelid. Some authors have advocated full-thickness biopsies of the lid at the margin to include conjunctiva, tarsal plate and skin.[2,7] While this type of biopsy may provide the highest yield, the tumor cells can still be missed due to sampling error and difficulty in adequate preservation of cellular detail. In fact, SC can mimic cicatricial pemphigoid or other bullous, inflammatory or proliferative conditions.[8] To make the diagnosis of SC, the treating physician must consider the diagnosis and obtain an adequate biopsy specimen.

HISTOPATHOLOGY

The most common histopathological picture of SC is a lobular pattern with architecture similar to normal sebaceous gland but less differentiated. Pleiomorphism, prominent nucleoli, mitotic figures and vacuolated cytoplasm with lipid droplets are seen (Figure 23.2). In some cases the tumor is primarily pagetoid or poorly differentiated and difficult to recognize as sebaceous in origin on hematoxylin and eosin (H & E). Variations in pattern may include papillary projections of sebaceous differentiation. Areas of central necrosis surrounded by sebaceous cells may also be seen. Frequently the papillary and lobular patterns are mixed within the same tumor. Oil-red-O stain on fresh frozen tissue may better demonstrate the foamy vacuolated cytoplasm than H & E and aid in diagnosis.[9] Either full-thickness or incisional biopsy at more than one site may be necessary to make the diagnosis. Clearly the tumor mass can arise from either side of the tarsal plate. It is a mistake to assume

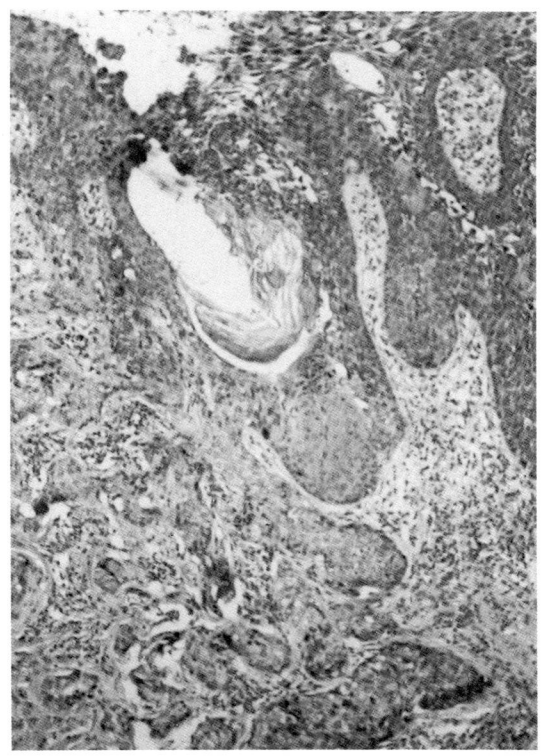

Figure 23.2
Hematoxylin and eosin biopsy of sebaceous carcinoma shows disorganized epithelium with mitotic figures and lipid droplets.

that a specimen of conjunctiva or skin alone will suffice. It has been suggested that tumors arising from the meibomian gland and those with conjunctival spread have a worse prognosis.[10,11] It may be necessary to obtain consultation with a pathologist who has made the diagnosis previously and is familiar with the difficulties in recognition of SC.

ETIOLOGIC CONSIDERATIONS

The etiology of SC is unknown. Ionizing radiation is an initiating factor for neoplasia in all tissues of the body. Therefore it is not surprising that several investigators have found irradiation to be a causative factor in SC.[6,12] Those patients with SC induced by irradiation had a poorer outcome than nonirradiated patients. It has been suggested that thiazide diuretics, when ingested, interact with nitrites in gastric acid medium, producing nitrosamines which could be carcinogenic in distant tissues.[6]

The role of the lacrimal canalicular apparatus in SC has been reviewed by Kahn and associates in detail. Pagetoid spread of tumor cells initially is an intraepithelial process. Subsequently the basement membrane is penetrated, with tumor invasion into underlying stroma. Pagetoid spread of SC can be seen in the canaliculus, in the lacrimal sac, and into the nasolacrimal duct with further intranasal spread. Tumor has also been seen within the lacrimal gland and ductuals. These observations document a predilection for this tumor to extend and invade along avenues of the lacrimal apparatus. Sebaceous carcinoma is thought to be of multifocal origin because there are skip areas interspersed amongst the tumor. It is plausible, however, that tear production and flow may play a role in the spread of tumor cells as well. Perhaps tumor cells from a single site of origin are showered onto healthy epithelium of the canalicular structures. These tissues may be resistant to tumor attachment and invasion for a period of time but ultimately tumor implantation occurs. Tumor cells may also move in a retrograde manner and enter the ductuals and parenchyma of the lacrimal gland. Perhaps once a site of malignancy develops, the lid, conjunctiva and lacrimal secretory and drainage apparatus become contaminated. This could in part account for recurrences of SC after apparent complete excision.

A related question is how surgeons and pathologists should interpret the clinical significance of pagetoid spread. It seems logical that atypical pleiomorphic cells are indeed an early extension of tumor. Yet one can also postulate that this may represent a reactive or metaplastic process and perhaps not all pagetoid cells need to be excised or obliterated. Unfortunately there is no convincing evidence to support either argument. Presently most tumor extirpation is guided by light microscopic diagnosis. Therefore nearly all authorities advocate removal of pagetoid cells where technically possible. There have been reports, however, of patients who have had long-term survival with no evidence of recrudescent disease even in the presence of positive pagetoid margins and no further treatment. Unfortunately, however, removing all atypical cells may necessitate exenteration of the involved eye. These considerations are reviewed in more detail below.

TREATMENT STRATEGIES

Sebaceous carcinoma is usually treated surgically. Because of the rarity of the tumor, it is difficult to gain a clear picture of the natural history of this disease. Risk to the patient falls into three categories: (1) local recurrence; (2) silent orbital invasion; and (3) lymph node or metastatic spread. Five-year survival rates range from 33 to 85%.[4] Tumors which recur may be seen at the lid margin or may be detected only later after orbital invasion. Such patients may not have obvious nodal or organ invasion. Spread to the regional lymph nodes is the most common mode of metastasis. Sebaceous carcinoma tends to spread to either preparotid, submandibular, cervical or supraclavicular nodes. Sebaceous carcinoma following presumed adequate therapy may recur with a single enlarged tumor-filled node at one of these sites. Though surgery is the treatment of choice, there are drawbacks and limitations to excision. All agree that histological monitoring of the surgical margins is important. However, if this tumor is multifocal in origin, then the logic of seeking clear margins diminishes. It may be that a wider field or regional therapeutic approach from the outset is necessary.

At the present time excision with the goal of obtaining clear margins is the standard of treatment. It is unclear what type of pathology is better, frozen or permanent paraffin sections. In general, paraffin sections will provide a higher quality microscopic view of cellular and architectural detail.[3] Clearly malignant cells and the tumor mass can generally be recognized with either mode of tissue processing. Paraffin sections may be the best medium to monitor and assess surgical margins when pagetoid spread is present. The drawback is delay in processing. Many patients have been treated with Mohs micrographic surgery for BCC and SCC of the eyelid. Frequently, very extensive defects result. However, with appropriate corneal protection measures, these patients are repaired several hours later or the next day with no loss in the quality of the surgery or complications related to a prolonged procedure. The high cure rates obtained by definite margin determination benefit the patient and outweigh the disadvantages of the extra time expended. Obtaining clear margins in SC, however, present additional difficulties. Some patients lack a tumor mass and have normal tissue interspersed with foci of tumor. Therefore a surgical mapping procedure coupled with delayed permanent sections may delay the procedure for days instead of hours. The goal of surgery is to obtain margins free of pagetoid cells. However, microscopic pagetoid cells may track into the orbit or onto the globe in the absence of clinical or imaging evidence or orbital invasion. In this setting it is very difficult to pursue surgery to the point of orbital exenteration. The management of pagetoid margins should be considered and treatment options reviewed with the patient prior to surgery. Cryotherapy has been recommended as adjunctive treatment to surgery for pagetoid cells.[13]

If tears play a role in the spread of the neoplastic cells of SC, this further complicates the dilemma. Some patients have long-term survival with apparent cure after surgical excision. There is probably individual tissue susceptibility to tumor invasion which may be related to duration of the lesion, characteristics of the lid and canalicular epithelium, or other factors. In SC it is often not possible to determine if orbital invasion has occurred. The more likely scenario is multiple tumor sites demonstrated on biopsy of some suspicious areas. These may extend into the canalicular system, or onto the palpebral conjunctiva or the caruncle without clear evidence of infiltration into the orbital fat, extraocular muscles or the globe itself. Neither the surgeon nor the patient wants to contemplate exenteration when there is no clear-cut evidence of orbital invasion. Often neither CT nor MRI definitely demonstrate invasion.

Specific surgical management should be tailored to the clinical and pathological presentation. The highest resolution imaging studies which show the orbit and its contents should be obtained. Even with an established diagnosis, biopsy of more than one site is recommended. If the tumor occurs in either canthus, there is risk of spread onto both lids. If there are any signs or symptoms on other periocular tissues aside from the primary tumor site, biopsy is recommended. When pagetoid spread is seen, one must suspect silent spread to other tissues. When surgical margins can be obtained by paraffin sections in 24 h or less, this may be the most suitable approach. When high-quality frozen sections are available, this method clearly can play a role in treatment. Tumor can be traced out and fully mapped with frozen sections. This can usually be accomplished in a single surgical session of 4 or 5 h or less. These 'clear margins' by frozen sections can then be conservatively re-excised and submitted for rush or permanent sections for a final check. Even when clear margins are obtained by this method, one cannot assume eradication. If well-chosen strategic biopsies have been taken prior to the surgical procedure, this increases the chance of complete excision. Close follow-up with a willingness to rebiopsy is critical.

There is no suitable method for staging SC based on its local presentation. Some authors have suggested that the presence of pagetoid spread in the lid indicates a worse prognosis. Patients who have had previous radiation to the eyelid skin and tumors which arise from the caruncle have a worse prognosis.[12] Patients with involvement of both upper and lower lids are at higher risk for local recurrence, orbital invasion and metastasis. Wide excision in the ocular region really has no meaning because eyelid excisions are either relatively narrow or involve an orbital exenteration. Most patients when diagnosed have difficulty accepting the fact that their problem of many years is now called cancer. It is difficult for them to make the mental transition from being followed for a presumed benign condition to the possible need for exenteration of an eye. Without obvious orbital invasion, patients should have treatment options explained to them to the best of their ability to understand. The fact that there is no one dogmatic and accepted method of treatment should be laid out for them. Most patients should be offered surgery with the most meticulous plan to obtain clear surgical margins but with the goal of preserving a functioning eye in the absence of clear orbital invasion. Patients should understand that frequent follow-up usually coupled with postoperative biopsies will be necessary.

Consultation with radiation therapy (RT) can be considered prior to surgery. The goal is not to embark on RT unless the patient refuses surgery. There is insufficient evidence that RT is efficacious in the treatment of SC other than as a salvage or adjunctive procedure, especially if the primary site of the tumor is the lid margin. However, the radiation therapist can obtain an image and photograph of the primary tumor field and be in a better position to offer RT should unresectable disease occur. Radiation therapy can play a role in the treatment of clinical stage II or III disease though some authors have advocated it as first-line treatment.[14] Radiation therapy is not our first-line choice for the treatment of SC of the eyelid.

Conclusions and Controversies

Therapy of SC will not advance until we understand the basic biology and origin of the tumor. Is it multifocal in origin or does it, like most malignancies, arise from a single cell line? Is the tumor spread further afield by the lacrimal secretion of tears and does it implant in distal sites earlier than can be clinically recognized? Are the atypical pagetoid cells seen in SC clear evidence of malignancy or possibly a reactive process which may not always signal tumor implantation? Even though these questions remain unanswered, it is still possible to recommend optimal therapy based on present knowledge. This should include thorough assessment, more than one biopsy and a surgical plan coupled with consideration of age, health and ocular status as well as patient mandates about what therapy they will accept. Excision should obtain clear surgical margins though in fact this may not be possible if all pagetoid cells are considered signs of the malignancy. Even orbital exenteration probably would not cure all such patients. Every effort to preserve a seeing eye should be expended. While RT is generally not a primary treatment it may be the only other option available when surgery has failed. Finally, regular follow-up for the first 5 years is critical and patients should be followed for at least 10 years.

References

1. Jakobiec FA, Zimmerman LE, La Piana F et al, Unusual eyelid tumors with sebaceous differentiation in the Muir-Torre syndrome, *Ophthalmologica* (1988) **95**:1543–8.
2. Kahn JA, Doane JF, Grove AS Jr, Sebaceous and meibomian carcinoma of the eyelid recognition, diagnosis, and management, *Ophthalmic Plast Reconstru Surg* (1991) **7**:61–6.
3. Folberg R, Whitaker DC, Tse DT et al, Recurrent and residual sebaceous carcinoma after Mohs excision of the primary lesion, *Am J Ophthalmol* (1987) **103**:817–23.
4. Kass LG, Hornblass A, Sebaceous carcinoma of the ocular adnexa, *Surv Ophthalmol* (1989) **33**:477–90.
5. Tan KC, Lee ST, Cheah ST, Surgical treatment of sebaceous carcinoma of eyelids with clinico-pathological correlation, *Br J Plast Surg* (1991) **44**:117–21.
6. Kahn JA, Grove AS Jr, Joseph MP et al, Sebaceous carcinoma diuretic use, lacrimal system spread, and surgical margins, *Ophthalmic Plast Reconstr Surg* (1989) **5**:227–34.
7. Loeffler M, Hornblass A, Characteristics and behavior of eyelid carcinoma (basal cell, squamous cell, sebaceous gland and malignant melanoma), *Ophthalmic Surg* (1990) **21**:513–18.
8. Grossnicklaus HE, Swerlick RA, Solomon AR, IgA and complement immunofluorescent pattern in sebaceous gland carcinoma of the eyelid, *Am J Ophthalmol* (1990) **109**:353–5.
9. Ratz JL, Luu-Duong S, Kulwin DR, Sebaceous carcinoma of the eyelid

treated with Mohs surgery, *J Am Acad Dermatol* (1986) **14**:668–73.
10. Yeatts RP, Waller RR, Sebaceous carcinoma of the eyelid: pitfalls in diagnosis, *Ophthalmic Plast Reconstr Surg* (1985) **1**:35–42.
11. Shields JA, Shields C, Sebaceous carcinoma of the glands of Zeis, *Ophthalmic Plast Reconstr Surg* (1988) **4**:11–14.
12. Hood IC, Qizilbash AH, Salama SS et al, Sebaceous carcinoma of the face following irradiation, *Am J Dermatopathol* (1986) **8**:505–8.
13. Lisman RD, Jakobiec FA, Small P, Sebaceous carcinoma of the eyelids: the role of adjunctive cryotherapy in the management of conjunctival pagetoid spread, *Ophthalmologica* (1989) **96**:1021–6.
14. Pardo FS, Wang CC, Albert D et al, Sebaceous carcinoma of the ocular adnexa: radiotherapeutic management, *Int J Radiat Oncol Biol Phys* (1989) **17**:643–7.

Chapter 24

MANAGEMENT OF NEOPLASMS IN THE NAIL

Robert Baran
Eckart Haneke

INTRODUCTION

Neoplasia of the nail area may be benign, benign but aggressive or malignant. Nail deformation most often denotes benignity, while partial or total nail destruction denotes malignancy.

A history of trauma, associated infection, the nail-screening effect, modifications of tumor behavior produced by the specialized nail anatomy, and variations in pigmentation are all factors which may mislead the clinician.

WARTS

Common warts are caused by human papilloma viruses of different DNA types. They are benign, weakly contagious, fibroepithelial tumors with a rough keratotic surface. Usually periungual warts are asymptomatic though fissuring may cause pain. Subungual warts initially affect the hyponychium, growing slowly towards the nail bed and finally elevating the nail plate. Subungual warts are painful and may mimic glomus tumor. The nail plate is not often affected, but surface ridging may occur, dislocation of the nail being exceptional.

Treatment of periungual warts is often frustrating. Saturated monochloroacetic acid may be applied sparingly, allowed to dry, and then covered with 40% salicylic acid plaster cut to the size of the wart and held in place with adhesive tape for 2–3 days. After 1–2 weeks most of the warts can be removed and this procedure repeated. However, this procedure may become more and more painful with each repetition. Subungual warts are treated similarly, after cutting away the overlying part of the nail plate. Recalcitrant warts may respond to diphencyprone. Some authorities recommend the use of cantharidin (0.007%). Cantharone is applied to the lesions and covered by a plastic tape for 24 h. The resultant blister should be retreated at 2-week intervals, three to four times if necessary. Shelley and Shelley[1] obtained elimination of 92% of a random series of 258 warts after a single treatment with a multiple puncture technique under local anesthesia with a bifurcated vaccination needle to introduce bleomycin sulfate (1 unit/ml sterile saline solution) into warts.

Surgical treatment should be reserved for difficult cases. Liquid nitrogen may cause blistering with the blister roof containing the epidermal wart component if the treatment succeeds. However, when the proximal nail fold is treated, freezing must not be prolonged since one may easily damage the matrix. This may result in circumscribed leukonychia or nail dystrophy. CO_2 laser treatment may also be successful. Since the incubation period of human warts may be up to several months, constant follow-up, even after seemingly successful therapy, is necessary to allow for early treatment of newly growing warts.

KERATOACANTHOMA

Subungual and periungual keratoacanthomas may occur as solitary or multiple tumors. They are rare benign, but rapidly growing, seemingly aggressive tumors usually situated below the edge of the nail plate or in the most distal portion of the nail bed.

The lesion may start as a small and painful keratotic nodule visible beneath the free edge, growing rapidly to a 1–2-cm lesion within 4–8 weeks. Its typical gross appearance, as a dome-shaped nodule with a central plug of horny material filling the crater, is not often seen subungually although histology of an adequate biopsy specimen will clearly show the characteristic pattern. Less frequently the tumor grows out from under the proximal nail fold, which becomes inflamed, and may cover or surround it with a cushion of swollen tissue. Spontaneous regression is uncommon in this area. The tumor soon erodes the bone, and this may be demonstrated radiologically as a fairly well-defined crescent-shaped lytic defect of the tuft adjacent to the overlying nail bed. Reconstitution of the bony defect can be expected. Diagnosis of subungual keratoacanthoma depends on the rapid growth, with bone erosion and characteristic histology. Its clinical differentiation from squamous cell carcinoma may be difficult.

Management of subungual keratoacanthoma ranges from conservative local excision to aggressive amputation. Mohs micrographic surgery may be the treatment of choice.[2] Ablative surgery for this benign condition should be discouraged. Systemic retinoids may be beneficial in keratoacanthoma. Eruptive keratoacanthomas have responded to oral etretinate 1 mg/kg per day with complete resolution. Recurrence can occur after cessation of treatment, requiring maintenance therapy (10 mg on alternate days); however, this mode of treatment is more effective as prophylaxis in multiple keratoacanthoma. 5-Fluorouracil has also been used, either injected into the lesion, or applied as a 20% ointment three times daily for 3–4 weeks. Intralesional bleomycin may be tried in the distal nail area as well as methotrexate.

IMPLANTATION EPIDERMOID CYST

Epidermoid cysts in the terminal phalanx of the digits are usually secondary to heavy trauma, with implantation of epidermis into subcutaneous tissue or even into the bone. The trauma may have been long ago (even decades) and may not always be recalled by the patient. Postoperative epidermoid cysts may occur in the proximity of scars. The distal phalanx gradually enlarges and clubbing becomes evident. Pain is of late onset.

Intraosseous cysts appear as round, osteolytic zones without trabecules and sclerosis. Treatment is by enucleation of the lesion, including its entire membrane. This can usually be achieved by a lateral L-shaped incision. Bone transplants are not necessary.

RADIODERMATITIS

Acute necrosis of the fingertip, nail apparatus and distal phalanx can occur as a result of massive radiation overdose. Chronic effects have been seen after the treatment of eczema, psoriasis and onychomycosis, and in health care workers before the institution of proper precautions.[3]

Ionizing radiation may cause loss of nails, and chronic radiodermatitis may lead to skin cancer up to 30 years after exposure. The earliest signs are longitudinal ridging and brittleness. Later, the surrounding skin appears sclerotic and atrophic with telangiectasia and hyperkeratosis.

The nail plates become dull and slightly opaque with a brownish hue. They may become variably thickened with splitting of the distal edges. The nail beds develop fine, red longitudinal striations which develop into punctate charcoal patches. A verrucous lesion appearing on the hyponychium or adjacent nail bed may herald the development of malignancy. Hyperkeratosis of the nail bed elevates the nail and causes pain. Paronychia-like flares are the rule.

Treatment depends on the size and location of the keratotic lesions. For small nail bed lesions, curettage may be efficient after a U-shaped piece of the distal nail has been excised. *En bloc* excision of the nail apparatus with healing by second intention or Mohs micrographic fresh-tissue technique which spares the normal surrounding tissue are treatments of choice. The defect can be covered with a free graft or a flap.

BOWEN'S DISEASE AND SQUAMOUS CELL CARCINOMA

Bowen's disease of the nail apparatus is a distinctive type of squamous cell carcinoma that differs from other variants. However, some authors prefer to avoid the use of the term Bowen's disease for in situ epidermoid carcinoma occurring beneath the nail plate, because: (1) it is not always easy to separate invasive from in situ carcinoma; and (2) it cannot be overemphasized that a biopsy specimen showing Bowen's disease does not exclude the possibility of invasive carcinoma in other areas of the lesions.

The malignant process may develop in the epithelium of the periungual area as well as in the subungual tissues. Periungual involvement includes: hyperkeratotic or papillomatous growth; erosions, scaling and fissuring of the nail folds; whitish cuticle; periungual swelling from deep tumor proliferation, with erythema caused by inflammation due to infection; and fissure or ulceration of the lateral nail groove, sometimes crusted with granulation-like tissue beneath the scab.

Subungual involvement was constant in the 12 cases of Guitart et al.[4] It may present with onycholysis, and nail clipping of the nonadherent portion of the nail plate shows hyperkeratosis or oozing ulceration of the nail bed. Appearance of normal pattern longitudinal melanonychia is a recent finding.[5,6] The nail plate may become dystrophic, even ingrown, or there may be partial or total nail loss, suggesting that the malignant process has developed in the nail matrix. Localized pain may be noted, for example, when the patient dials a phone number. The presence of nodularity, ulceration or bleeding indicates that the carcinoma has become invasive.[7] Bone involvement is seen in less than 20% of the patients. Metastases have been reported only in patients with hereditary ectodermal dysplasia.

The key to diagnosis is the histological examination. The picture is identical with that of Bowen's disease of other skin areas. The most important feature is the intact basement membrane. Bowen's disease has been reported in individuals between the ages of 20 and 90, the incidence being highest in the 50–69-year range. The tumor grows slowly and the duration of signs and symptoms from onset to the time of diagnosis has varied from several months to 18 years.

The etiology of subungual epidermoid carcinoma remains unclear. Arsenic cannot be excluded in old psoriatic patients, for example. Trauma and chronic paronychia have been cited as etiologic factors, but, above all, exposure to X-rays (physicians, dentists, patients). This may be followed by radiodermatitis which, along with HPV infection is the most common factor for the development of squamous cell carcinoma. HPV-16, -34 and -35 have been detected in epidermoid carcinoma in situ or invasive. The HPV genome was found in eight out of 10 periungual lesions by dot-blot analysis of frozen tissue and six of them were related to HPV-16.[8]

Using the polymerase chain reaction to detect HPV in formalin-fixed, paraffin-embedded specimens of periungual squamous cell carcinoma, Ashinoff et al[9] found that five of the seven periungual lesions contained HPV-16. In situ hybridization failed to identify HPV in any of these patients' tumors.

The need for complete removal of the lesion cannot be overemphasized. The best treatment is Mohs micrographic surgery, which allows adequate excision with maximal preservation of normal tissue and function. This can be performed with routine instrumentation as well as with the CO_2 laser in a focused-beam incisional mode, which ensures relatively minimal postoperative discomfort for the patient.

Excisional surgery may be used in some cases or for complete removal of the nail apparatus, with healing by second intention, grafting or flap, preferably cross-finger flap.

Electrosurgery is a therapeutic alternative in a very few selected cases. Liquid nitrogen may give good results in experienced hands; however, the excision margins cannot be controlled histologically.

EPITHELIOMA CUNICULATUM

Epithelioma cuniculatum is a rare, slow-growing, but locally destructive low-grade squamous cell carcinoma. Inflammatory features often accompanied by subungual purulent material may lead to disappearance of the nail plate. The nail bed may be covered with many 'holes' extruding toothpaste-like, foul-smelling, yellow–white material.[10] The radiographs of three patients showed erosion or disappearance of the distal third of the phalanx. Histology shows a verrucous surface and deep, blunt epithelial processes with large keratin cysts and sinuses. Successful treatment requires complete excision or Mohs micrographic surgery, because it is tissue-sparing; amputation should be avoided.

BASAL CELL CARCINOMA

Although basal cell carcinoma is the most common malignant skin tumor, it is exceptionally rare in the subungual region. The usual presentation is a chronic paronychia or a periungual eczematous process often associated with ulceration, granulation tissue, and pain. The diagnosis can only be confirmed by histological examination. Treatment of choice is complete surgical excision.

FIBROMOUS TUMORS
Fibrous dermatofibroma

True dermatofibromas are rare in the nail unit. They may arise superficially from the skin, subcutaneous tissues and nail bed, resembling cutaneous horns, fibrokeratomas or supernumerary digits; the latter, however, usually arise on the ulnar aspect of the fifth metacarpophalangeal joint. Dermatofibromas usually develop insidiously as nodular tumors which grow slowly. They are spherical or ovoid in shape and firm and elastic in consistency. They may be freely movable or fixed in position. The authors have observed a cherry-shaped distal subungual dermatofibroma lifting a great toenail up vertically.

Acquired periungual fibrokeratoma

Acquired periungual fibrokeratoma is probably identical to acquired digital fibrokeratoma and garlic clove fibroma.[11] They are acquired, benign, spontaneously developing, asymptomatic nodules with a hyperkeratotic tip and a narrow base, which occur mostly in the periungual area or elsewhere on the fingers. Most periungual fibrokeratomas emerge from the most proximal part of the nail sulcus, growing on the nail and causing a sharp longitudinal depression. Surgical treatment is the same as for Koenen's tumors and will depend on the size and location of the fibroma.

Koenen's tumor

Koenen's periungual fibromas develop in 50% of the cases of tuberous sclerosis (epiloia or Bourneville-Pringle disease) and are, consequently, as frequent as renal hamartomas. They usually appear between the ages of 12 and 14 years and increase progressively in size and number with age. Individual tumors are small, round, flesh-colored and asymptomatic, with a smooth surface.

The tip of the tumor may be slightly hyperkeratotic, resembling fibrokeratoma. It grows out of the nail fold, eventually overgrowing the nail bed and destroying the nail plate. Depending on its location, it may cause longitudinal depressions in the nail plate. Even tiny hyperkeratotic lesions in the cuticle area may produce identical longitudinal nail grooves and have the same significance as Koenen's tumor. Excessively large tumors are often painful and should be excised at their base.

In Koenen's tumor we have noted[12] that two portions can be distinguished: a small distal segment with loose collagen and many blood vessels, and a larger proximal part built up of dense collagen bundles and fewer capillaries. Koenen's tumors are cured by simple excision. Usually, no suture is necessary. Tumors growing out from under the proximal nail fold are removed after reflecting the proximal nail fold back by making lateral incisions down each margin in the axis of the lateral nail grooves. Subungual fibromas are removed after avulsion of the corresponding part of the nail plate.

Infantile digital fibromatosis (recurring digital fibrous tumors of childhood)[13] *(Synonym: benign juvenile digital fibromatosis)*

Recurring digital fibrous tumors (RDFT) are round, smooth, dome-shaped, shiny, firm dermal nodules, with reddish or livid red color, which are located on the dorsal and axial surfaces of the fingers and toes, characteristically sparing the thumbs and great toes. They may present at birth or develop during infancy. On reaching the nail unit, they may elevate the nail plate, leading to dystrophy but not to destruction. The tumor may cause considerable distortion of the digits. Often the tumor is multicentric, occurring on several digits. Ryman and Bale[14] reported 30 cases, seen in 36 years. The patients were 20 females and 10 males. The fingers and toes were equally affected. Multiple lesions occurred in 50% of patients, more often in the fingers, especially on adjacent fingers, and two patients had bilateral lesions.

Recurrence occurs in 60% after excision, so surgery should be attempted only if functional impairment occurs; however, excessive growth has been treated by amputation of the involved digit in some cases. Surgery necessitates going to the fascial and tendinous areas in an effort to avoid recurrences. It can be mutilating. As metastasis has never been recorded, the amputations sometimes performed in the past (38 of 115 cases to 1985) can no longer be justified.

Conservative treatment is best, since the lesions have a natural course; a tumoral stage followed by spontaneous resolution, explaining why they are not found in adults. Cryosurgery may accelerate this natural course.

Pyogenic granuloma (granuloma telangiectaticum, botryomycoma)

Pyogenic granuloma is a benign eruptive hemangioma typically following a minor penetrating skin injury. It starts with a minute red papule which rapidly grows. Its surface may become eroded by necrosis of the overlying epidermis. Crusting may mimic a malignant melanoma although the typical collarette can usually be seen. Pyogenic granuloma is commonly located at the proximal nail fold but may develop in the nail bed after a penetrating wound of the nail plate. Tenderness and a ready tendency to bleed are characteristic features. Extensive granulation tissue due to an ingrowing toenail is a variant of periungual pyogenic granuloma, and it also has been observed in patients treated with aromatic retinoids.[15] Differential diagnosis also includes cavernous angioma, pseudopyogenic granuloma, hemangiosarcoma and amelanotic melanoma. Histological documentation of the specimen is essential. Therapy should be as simple as possible to avoid disfiguring scars or nail deformity. Pyogenic granuloma may be removed by excision at its base followed by application of Monsel's or aluminum chloride solution. The use of lasers may also prove curative.

Glomus tumor

Seventy-five percent of glomus tumors occur in the hand, especially in the fingertips and particularly the subungual area. The glomus tumor is characterized by intense, often pulsating, pain that may be spontaneous or provoked by the slightest trauma. Changes in temperature, especially from warm to cold, may trigger pain radiating up to the shoulder. Sometimes the pain is worse at night. A tourniquet placed at the base of the digit stops the pain. The tumor is visible through the nail plate as a small bluish to reddish-blue spot several millimeters in diameter, rarely exceeding 1 cm in diameter. A nail with an erythematous focus that does not blanch totally with pressure and is associated with pain is a typical presentation. One-half of the tumors cause minor nail deformities, ridging and fissuring being the commonest. About 50% cause a depression on the dorsal aspect of the distal phalangeal bone or even a cyst visible on radiographs. If the tumor cannot be localized clinically or on radiographs, arteriography should be performed; this will reveal a star-shaped telangiectatic zone, useful for diagnosis and localization of the tumor.[16,17] Many patients give a history of trauma. The differential diagnosis include neuroma, causalgia, gout and arthritis.

The only treatment is surgical removal. Small tumors may be removed by punching a 6-mm hole into the nail plate, incising the nail bed, and enucleating the lesion. The small nail disk is put back in its original position as a physiological dressing. Larger tumors may be treated after removal of the proximal half of the nail plate; those in lateral positions are removed by an L-shaped incision parallel to and 4–6 mm on the volar side of the lateral nail fold. The nail bed is carefully dissected from the bone until the tumor is reached and extirpated. Extirpation is usually curative although the pain may take several weeks to disappear. Recurrences occur in 10–20% of cases and may represent either incomplete excision or new tumors. More extensive surgery initially may be warranted.

Exostosis

Subungual exostoses are not true tumors but rather outgrowths of normal bone or calcified cartilaginous remains. Whether or not subungual osteochondroma is a different entity is not clear. Subungual exostoses are painful osseous growths which elevate the nail. They are particularly frequent in young people and mostly located in the great toe, though subungual exostoses may also occur in lesser toes or less commonly thumb or index fingers. They start as small elevations of the dorsal aspect of the distal phalanx and may eventually emerge from under the nail edge or destroy the nail plate. If the nail is lost, the surface becomes eroded and secondarily infected, sometimes mimicking an ingrown toenail. Walking may be painful. The triad of pain (the leading symptom), nail deformation and radiographic features is usually diagnostic. The exostosis is an ill-defined trabeculated osseous growth with an expanded distal portion covered with radiolucent fibrocartilage.

Osteochondroma

Osteochondroma, commonly evoking the same symptoms as exostosis, is said to have a male predominance. There is also often a history of trauma. Its growth rate is slow. Radiography shows a well-defined circumscribed pedunculated or sessile bone growth involving the juxtaepiphyseal area of the phalanx with a hyaline cartilage cap.

Therapy consists of local curettage or excision of the excess bone under full aseptic conditions. The nail plate is partially removed and a longitudinal incision is made in the nail bed. The osseous growth with its cartilaginous cap is carefully dissected using fine skin hooks to avoid damage to the fragile nail bed and the tumor is removed with a fine chisel. Whenever possible, we prefer to remove the tumor by an L-shaped or a fish-mouth incision, in order to avoid avulsion of the nail plate.

Enchondroma

Solitary enchondroma of the distal phalanx is rare. It is a painful tumor which expands the tip of the finger. It may present clinically as paronychia or as clubbing with thickening, discoloration and longitudinal ridging of the nail. A nacar-white fungus-shaped tumor may lift the overlying nail plate.[18] Radiographs reveal a well-defined radiolucent defect with expansion of the distal phalanx or spotty calcifications. The enchondroma is typically located at the base of the distal phalanx abutting the articular surface. Pathological fractures may occur as a result of continuous thinning of the corticalis.

Treatment is required to prevent further enlargement of the enchondroma and because of its symptoms. The tumor is enucleated under full aseptic precautions. Histology shows hyaline cartilage proliferation with irregularly arranged cells. Bone grafts are not generally necessary.

Osteoid osteoma

Osteoid osteoma is a distinct clinical and pathological entity.[19] Its location in the distal phalanx is quite rare. The usual incidence is two males to one female. Osteoid osteoma usually evokes a 'nagging' pain, accentuated at night, which is poorly localized. Local tenderness is present in about one-half of the cases. There is no evidence of inflammation or systemic toxicity. Relief of pain by salicylates is characteristic. However, symptoms may vary considerably. Osteoid osteoma causes swelling of the distal phalanx or even enlargement of the entire tip. Clubbing, thickening or enlargement of the nail may occur. The skin is either normal in color or faintly violaceous. Increased sweating of the area has been described. Palpation with a blunt probe may help to localize the tender tumor on pressure. A nidus, characterized by a small area of rarefaction with surrounding sclerosis, is demonstrable radiologically in most cases; it is located in the medulla, in the cortex, or subperiosteally with a very thin covering of bone over the nidus. The hypervascularization, explaining the nail thickening, can be demonstrated by arteriography, thermography or scintigraphy. Young patients may have premature fusion of the adjacent epiphysis. Histologically, the nidus is a meshwork of osteoid trabeculae with varying degrees of mineralization in a background of vascular fibrous connective tissue.

Treatment is by *en bloc* resection through a 'fish-mouth' incision. Curettage may fail to eradicate the lesion. Radiography does not seem to be helpful in deciding whether the whole lesion has been removed. After therapy the swelling regresses, a normal nail regrows and the pain gradually disappears.

Giant cell tumor (benign synovioma, benign xanthomatous giant cell tumors, villonodular pigmented synovitis)

Giant cell tumor is a neoplasm derived from the tendon sheath or the joint synovia. It is the second most common subcutaneous tumor of the hand. It is more frequent in females than in males. On the digits, it usually occurs on the dorsum of the distal interphalangeal joint and usually appears as a solitary, often lobulated, slow-growing, skin-colored and smooth-surfaced nodule which tends to feel firm and rubbery. The tumor may enlarge to the size of a cherry and may cause pain on flexion by virtue of its dimensions. Only rarely does the tumor interfere with the nail unit. It may present in the region of the lateral nail fold and, in this location, periodic inflammation and drainage may occur. In contrast to malignant synovioma, no calcification is demonstrable on radiography. The tumor is composed of cell populations varying from groups of spindle-shaped cells to large numbers of histiocytic and multinucleated giant cells, some of which may contain hemosiderin or have a foamy cytoplasm, explaining some of the synonyms used for this condition.

Treatment is by careful surgical removal. An oblique incision along the greatest axis of the tumor enables the multilobulated lesion to be exposed.

Myxoid pseudocysts of the digits

Myxoid pseudocysts occur more often in women. They are typically found in the proximal nail fold of the fingers and rarely on toes. The lesions are usually asymptomatic, varying from soft to firm, and cystic to fluctuant, and may be dimpled, dome-shaped or smooth-surfaced. Transillumination confirms their cystic nature. They are almost always located to one side of the midline and rarely exceed 10–15 mm in diameter. The skin over the lesion is thinned and may be verrucous or may even ulcerate. Rarely, paronychial fistula may develop beneath the proximal nail fold and, exceptionally, under the nail plate. Longitudinal grooving results from pressure on the matrix. Subungual digital mucinous pseudocyst may produce a nail dystrophy and discoloration without abnormalities of the periungual skin. Degenerative, 'wear and tear' osteoarthritis, frequently with Herberden's nodes, is present in most cases. Spontaneous rupture or manipulation with a needle will release a thick, clear, gelatinous fluid. This decompresses the matrix and nail growth is normal until the cyst refills. Purulent drainage due to infection and development of septic arthritis of the distal interphalangeal joint has been reported. A multitude of treatments has been recommended, including repeated incision and drainage, simple excision, multiple needlings and expression of contents, radiotherapy (5 Gy, 50k, Al 1 mm, three times at weekly intervals), electrocautery, chemical cautery with nitric acid, trichloroacetic acid or phenol, massages or injection of proteolytic substances, hyaluronidase, steroids as flurandrenolone tape or intralesional injections, carbon dioxide laser vaporization and radical excision. Tomoda et al[20] reported a case that had had more than 20 recurrences, each treated by incision, the cyst eventually moving from the characteristic dorsal to a subungual position, producing an ulcer in the nail plate.

Kleinert et al[21] recommend the careful extirpation of the lesion. A tiny drop of methylene blue solution, diluted with a local anesthetic and mixed with fresh hydrogen peroxide, is injected into the distal interphalangeal joint at the volar joint crease. The joint will accept only 0.1–0.2 ml of dye.[22] This clearly identifies the pedicle connecting the joint to the cyst and also the cyst itself, which may look like a subcutaneous tenoarthrosynovial 'hernia'. This procedure sometimes reveals occult satellite cysts. The incision line is drawn on the finger, including a portion of the skin directly over the cyst and continuing proximally in a gentle curve to end dorsally over the joint. The lesion is meticulously dissected from the surrounding soft tissue and the pedicle traced to the joint capsule and resected. Dumbbell extension of cysts to each side of the extensor tendon is easily dissected by hyperextending the joint. Osteophytic spurs adjacent to the joint must be removed with a fine chisel or bone rongeur. Recently, Sonnex et al[23] used liquid nitrogen cryosurgery with an 86% cure rate. The field treated included the cyst and the adjacent proximal area to the transverse skin creases overlying the terminal joint.

Two freeze–thaw cycles were carried out, each freeze time being 30 s after the ice field had formed, and the intervening thaw times being at least 4 min; if this method is adopted then longer freeze times must be avoided or permanent matrix damage may occur. Salasche[24] suggested nail fold excision for posterior nail fold distal lesions. The injection of a sclerosing agent, such as 1% sodium tetradecyl sulfate (Sotradecol, Elkins Sinn, Cherry Hill, NJ), into mucoid cysts may well have superseded the previous treatments.[25] After the cyst has been pierced and its jelly-like material expressed, 0.10–0.20 ml is injected, painlessly. One single procedure may be enough. A second or third one can be performed at 1-month intervals.

METASTASES

Metastases to the fingertip or nail region are quite rare (about 70 cases reported)[26] and are often initially misdiagnosed as acute infection in and around the nail apparatus and treated as such by incisions. These lesions may be the first manifestation of an internal neoplasm.[27] Most metastatic tumors primarily affect the bone, with subsequent spread to soft tissues. Primary soft tissue metastases of the distal digit may secondarily involve the underlying bone. The symptoms and signs of metastases are very variable and include dusky red swelling painful or painless, expansile pulsation, pseudoclubbing, nail dystrophy, and changes simulating acute or chronic paronychia, a finger infection such as felon or osteomyelitis,[28] and even benign lesions such as glomus tumor and early rheumatoid arthritis. Whatever symptoms occur, the *signs increase out of proportion to the pain*, and in the absence of injury or infection this suggests the possibility of metastases. Radiographs usually show an osteolytic focus which may resemble spina ventosa or osteomyelitis. Bronchial carcinoma most frequently (half of the cases) produces phalangeal metastases. The other primary sites include breast (15% in female), kidney, colon, and rectum, parotid gland and seminoma.

Longitudinal Melanonychia and Subungual Melanocytic Lesions

Longitudinal melanonychia (LM) is characterized by a tan, brown or black longitudinal streak within the nail plate. Longitudinal melanonychia results from increased melanin deposition in the nail plate. This deposition may result from greater melanin synthesis by normally nonfunctional matrix melanocytes or from an increase in the total number of matrix melanocytes that synthesize melanin; in either instance, melanocytes may be normal or abnormal. Melanocytes in the distal portion of the nail matrix are more numerous and more strongly dopa positive than melanocytes in the proximal matrix. Probably as a result of greater melanocyte density and activity, LM usually originates in the distal matrix, a fortunate circumstance because permanent nail plate deformity is less common when surgery is performed in the distal (rather than in the proximal) matrix. Histology may identify the origin within the matrix of pigmentation in LM by the staining of nail plate clipping with Fontana–Masson's argentaffin reaction. The more proximal the origin, the more superficial is the melanin within the nail plate.

Periungual spread of pigmentation to the proximal and lateral nail folds is called Hutchinson's sign. It is the most important indicator of subungual melanoma (SM). When this sign is present, SM is the presumptive diagnosis. This sign, however, particularly when subtle, is not absolutely pathognomonic for SM. Occasionally, LM that is dark brown simulates pigmentation of the overlying cuticle and proximal nail fold. The pigmentation is visible because of the cuticle and proximal nail fold's relative transparency and not because of melanin deposition within these tissues. This sign, the pseudo-Hutchinson's sign, can be identified by careful inspection. In good lighting, it is usually possible to establish whether pigment is present *within* the periungual tissues or *beneath* them in the underlying nail plate.

Other clues to the diagnosis of SM can be important. The clinician should be suspicious when LM: (1) begins in a single digit of a person during the sixth decade of life or later—however, melanonychia due to subungual melanoma has even been observed in children; (2) develops abruptly in a previously normal nail plate; (3) becomes suddenly darker or wider; (4) occurs in either the thumb, index finger or great toe; (5) occurs in a person who gives a history of digital trauma; (6) occurs singly in the digit of a dark skinned patient, particularly if the thumb or great toe is affected; (7) demonstrates blurred, rather than sharp, lateral borders; (8) occurs in a person who gives a history of malignant melanoma; (9) occurs in a person in whom the risk for melanoma is increased (for example dysplastic nevus syndrome); (10) is accompanied by nail dystrophy, such as partial nail destruction or disappearance.

If the cause of LM is not apparent, it should be established by biopsy because the dangers of an error of judgment are two-fold:[29] (1) that the proper treatment of a malignant lesion will be delayed and so allow the disease to disseminate; and (2) that the treatment, correct for a malignant melanoma, will lead to severe, totally unnecessary, cosmetic disability if employed for a benign tumor. For these reasons, isolated pigmented streaks, involving any portion of the nail apparatus, necessitate biopsy, especially when the thumb or the great toe are involved. The only possible exceptions are in black and oriental patients, in whom it could represent a normal finding, in children when the band remains stable, and in Laugier–Hunziker–Baran's syndrome.[30]

Biopsy methods[31]

Various surgical approaches are available for nail biopsies in LM. The procedure that is ultimately selected will depend on: (1) the likelihood of subungual melanoma; (2) the need to select a procedure that will minimize the risk of postoperative dystrophy; (3) the location (medial or lateral) of the band within the nail plate; (4) the band width; and (5) the matrix origin (proximal or distal) of LM. The patient must be fully appraised of the risk of permanent postoperative dystrophy.

Periungual pigmentation present

When LM is accompanied by periungual pigmentation, the likelihood of subungual melanoma is high. Radiographs should be obtained and the patient examined for lymphadenopathy. If the risk of malignancy (according to the criteria outlined earlier) is great, if there is no history of previous nail surgery or ingestion of photosensitizing medications, and no evidence for a syndrome associated with hyperpigmentation, and if there is unequivocal evidence that the pigment is located within (and not beneath) the proximal and/or lateral nail folds, all affected portions of the nail apparatus (proximal and lateral nail folds, nail plate, nail bed, hyponychium and skin) are removed en bloc down to bone, with relative disregard for cosmetic appearance. To ensure complete biopsy and excision, 1 mm of normal tissue is included in the excision. The advantage of this method lies in completeness of excision. The pathologist is able to study the lesion in its entirety, render a precise diagnosis, and draw salient conclusions regarding prognosis. The conspicuous disadvantage of this approach is the potential for significant postoperative deformity.

Lateral third of the nail plate involved

Lateral longitudinal biopsy is the preferred method when LM involves the lateral third of the nail plate. Advantages of this technique include the following: (1) all affected tissue, including the matrix, proximal nail fold, cuticle, upper portion of the lateral nail fold adjacent to the proximal nail fold, nail bed, and nail plate, is completely removed; (2) the pathologist is able to examine the lesion in its entirety; (3) pigment recurrence or persistence is unlikely; and (4) postoperatively, the patient is left with a good cosmetic result with just a narrowed nail.

Midportion of the nail plate involved

When LM lies within the midportion of the nail plate, the potential dystrophy may be great and the selection of the optimum biopsy method is difficult. It is necessary to identify the origin (proximal or distal matrix) of pigmentation in LM. Pigment clinically localized within the dorsal half of the nail plate indicates a proximal matrix origin; pigment localized within the ventral nail plate indicates a distal matrix origin.

The level of pigment within the nail plate is defined microscopically with Fontana–Masson staining of clippings obtained from the free edge of the nail. When a distal matrix origin seems likely, the cuticle can be retracted proximally to confirm the distal origin of LM without excision of the proximal nail fold.

Thin band, less than 3 mm in width[32]

A thin melanotic band, represents a low risk for subungual melanoma. For example, in an 8-year-old patient with index nail involvement that originates in the distal two-thirds of the matrix, a 3-mm punch excision is indicated. Punch excision is performed through the nail plate with direct visualization of the band at its origin (Figure 24.1).

The origin of the band is exposed by reflecting the proximal nail fold with relaxing incisions, if necessary. With a 3-mm

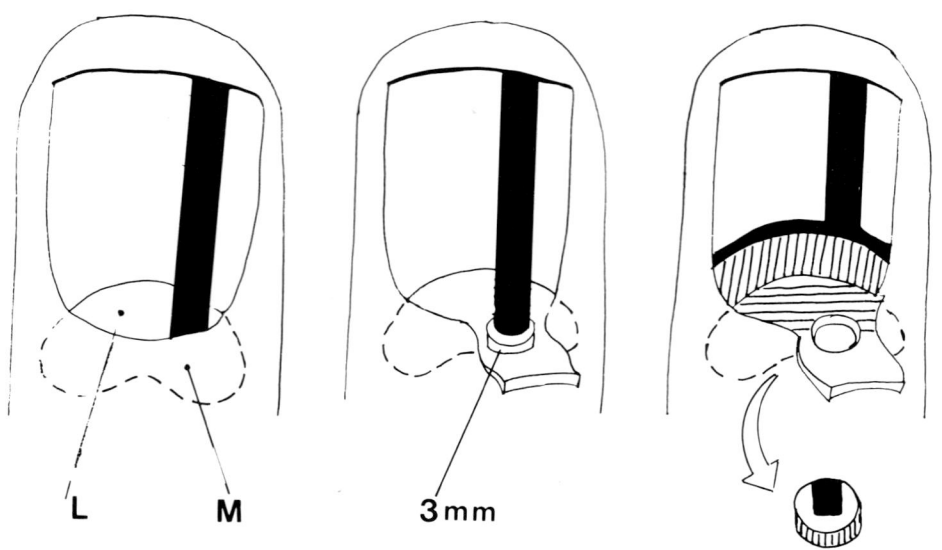

Figure 24.1
Punch biopsy of a band less than 3 mm in width and involving the midportion of the nail plate: L: lunula; M: matrix. (Adapted from Baran and Kechijian.[31])

punch, a circumferential incision is made around the origin of the band; *the cylinder of involved tissue is not removed at this time.* The next step is removal of the proximal (surrounding) third of the nail plate, leaving in place the cylinder of tissue containing the origin of LM. In the absence of the nail plate, the surgeon is able to inspect the surrounding nail matrix and bed with a head magnifier lens to determine whether pigment extends distally or laterally from the punch incision. The cylinder of tissue containing the origin of LM is then removed. Because the surrounding nail plate has been previously detached, the cylinder of tissue is completely accessible and excised with relative ease. The detached nail plate and cylinder of LM are submitted to the pathologist for sectioning through the band. With assistance from the surgeon, the pathologist is able to orient the specimens properly to ensure optimal sectioning and microscopic interpretation. The risk of postoperative dystrophy is minimal because only 3 mm of distal matrix is removed.

Biopsies of thin band less than 3 mm in width that originate in the proximal one-third of the matrix can also be performed with a 3-mm punch. The proximal nail fold must be reflected completely to ensure full exposure of the band. An attempt may be made to close the (proximal matrix) defect with 6-0 absorbable suture. Because the matrix is fragile and liable to tear easily, it is sufficient to achieve partial approximation rather than to attempt complete closure of the matrix biopsy margins. The risk of postoperative dystrophy is substantial in the nail surface.

Bands 3–6 mm in width
For bands between 3 and 6 mm wide that involve the distal two-thirds of the matrix, transverse elliptic excision is indicated (Figure 24.2). Although the potential for postoperative dystrophy is significant, an effort should be made, depending on the clinical circumstances, to excise completely the origin of the band, not only to prevent postoperative recurrence of LM

MANAGEMENT OF NEOPLASMS IN THE NAIL

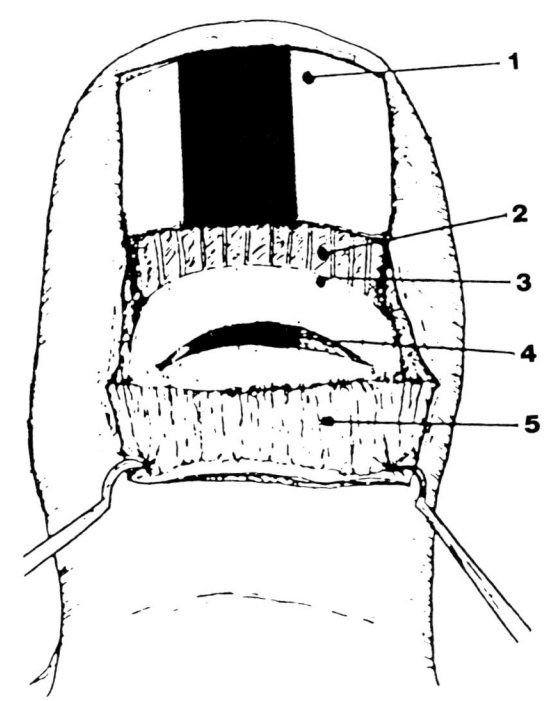

Figure 24.2
Transverse elliptic excision of a band 3–6 mm in width and involving the distal two-thirds of the matrix.

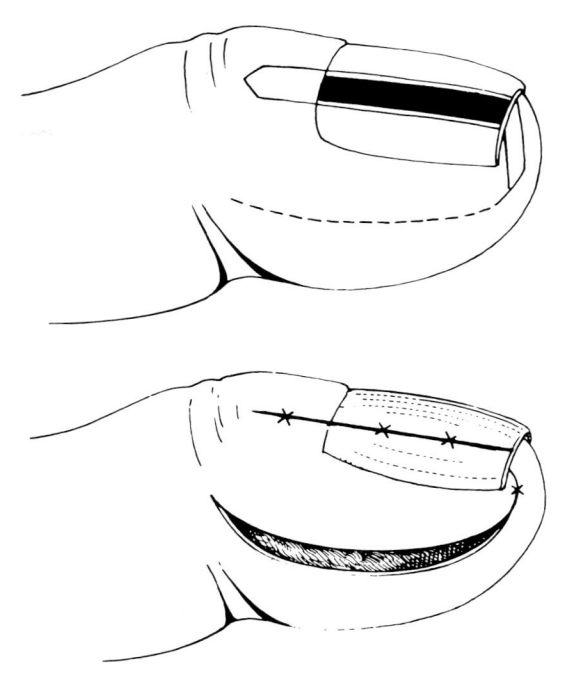

Figure 24.3
Releasing flap method indicated when 3–6-mm-wide bands involve the proximal third of the matrix.

but also to ensure that representative tissue is submitted for study. Because the proximal matrix remains intact, a thinned nail plate will regenerate postoperatively.

When 3–6-mm-wide bands involve the proximal third of the matrix, the releasing flap method of Schernberg and Amiel[33] is indicated (Figure 24.3). This technique enables removal of the proximal portion of the matrix with acceptable postoperative changes in the nail apparatus; the nail plate is diminished in width but is otherwise normal except for slight dystrophy, such as a longitudinal ridge. In this method, the pigmented band is completely excised in a rectangular monoblock comprising involved nail plate, bed, matrix and proximal nail fold nail plate, and proximal nail fold is delineated laterally by a curved incision running from the distal end of the monoblock incision to the proximal edge of the matrix. Inferiorly, the nail bed and matrix are separated from the underlying bony phalanx to provide complete mobility. The flap is rotated into position (abutting the incised medial portion of the nail plate, bed, matrix and proximal nail fold) and closed with 5-0 nylon sutures. The defect in the lateral nail fold is allowed to heal by second intention.

Bands wider than 6 mm

If the band is wider than 6 mm or if the full thickness of the nail is pigmented, a large portion of the matrix would necessarily be involved. Under these circumstances, the underlying disease process is unlikely to be benign. Depending on the clinical circumstances, partial longitudinal biopsy, transverse elliptic excision or punch biopsies from selected areas of the matrix can be performed or the entire portion of the involved nail apparatus can be excised *en bloc*.

MALIGNANT MELANOMA

Melanomas of the nail region are now better understood since the identification and analysis of acrolentiginous melanoma (ALM) as the most frequent type.[34] Superficial spreading melanoma (SSM) is rare. Appearance of nodular melanoma is debatable in the subungual area. Some cases are unclassifiable for two main reasons: (1) there may be a histological transition between SSM and ALM[35] indicating a close biological relationship between the two types; and (2) poor quality of the biopsy specimen.

Approximately 2–3% of melanomas in Caucasians, and 15–20% in blacks, are located in the nail apparatus.[36] However, since malignant melanoma is rare in blacks, the numbers of ungual melanomas in Caucasians and blacks do not differ significantly. In Caucasians, most patients have a fair complexion, light hair, and blue or hazel eyes. There is no sex predominance. The mean age is 60 years. Most tumors are located on the thumbs and great toes, but develop more commonly on the foot than on the hand.

Melanomas are often asymptomatic, pain and bleeding being rare. The clinical appearance of the tumor varies,[37] but half the patients note a mass below the nail, usually associated with the loss or partial destruction of the nail.

Periungual infection, ulceration of the nail bed, and granulation tissue occur in about one-third of the patients. In another third, discoloration of the nail area is the presenting sign. (1) Some lesions begin as a longitudinal melanonychia. This pigmented (brown or black) linear streak of variable width runs through the whole length of the visible nail. It was the first feature in 6 out of 10 patients with malignant melanoma.[38] After some months or years, the borders of the band widen and become blurred and ulceration appears. (2) A spot can appear in the matrix, nail bed or nail plate. This may vary in color from brown to black and may be homogeneous or irregular. It is seldom painful. (3) Less frequently, but almost pathognomonic, is the presence of Hutchinson's sign, a flat irregular brown black pigmentation of the matrix, nail bed, nail plate and surrounding tissues. It represents the radial growth phase of subungual melanoma and has proved to be a valuable clue to the clinical diagnosis of malignancy[32] after the pseudo-Hutchinson' signs have been ruled out. Its presence means that the entire nail apparatus must be removed (without prior incisional biopsy). This technique enables serial sections to be examined, which is particularly important in acral lentiginous melanoma in which histology may be difficult to interpret.

Approximately 25% of melanomas are amelanotic and may present as pyogenic granuloma, granulation tissue, ingrown nail and mycobacterial infections with nail dystrophy. The risk of misdiagnosis is therefore particularly high in these cases.

Subungual melanoma may also simulate subungual hematoma, which is not rare, and which may present without a history of severe trauma. It may follow repeated minor trauma which escapes the patient's attention, such as tennis toe or trauma from hard ski boots. Hematoma following a single trauma usually grows out in one piece rather than as a longitudinal streak. Subungual melanoma following a single injury to the digit was observed in eight cases after an interval of between 9 months and 7 years.[39] Repeated trauma may cause difficulties in differential diagnosis and nonmigrating hematoma should be ruled out.

References

1. Shelley WB, Shelley ED, Intralesional bleomycin sulfate therapy for warts; a novel bifurcated needle puncture technique, *Arch Dermatol* (1991) **127**:234–6.

2. Moreno Gimenez JC, Lerma Puerta E, Sanchez Conejo-Mir J et al, Queratoacantoma subungual, *Actas Dermo-Sif* (1987) **78**:561–4.

3. Guy RI, The etiologies and mechanisms of nail bed injuries, *Hand Clinics* (1990) **G6**:9–19.

4. Guitart J, Bergfeld WF, Tuthull RJ et al, Squamous cell carcinoma of the nail bed: a clinicopathological study of 12 cases, *Br J Dermatol* (1990) **123**:215–22.

5. Baran R, Gormley D, Polydactylous Bowen's disease of the nail, *J Am Acad Dermatol* (1988) **17**:201–4.

6. Baran R, Simon C, Longitudinal melanonychia: a symptom of Bowen's disease, *J Am Acad Dermatol* (1988) **18**:1359–60.

7. Mikhail G, Subungual epidermoid carcinoma, *J Am Acad Dermatol* (1984) **11**:291–8.

8. Moy RL, Eliezri Y, Nuovo GJ et al, Human papilloma virus type 16 DNA in periungual squamous cell carcinoma, *JAMA* (1989) **261**:2669–73.

9. Ashinoff R, Junli J, Jacobson M et al, Detection of HPV DNA in squamous cell carcinoma of the nail bed and finger determined by polymerase chain reaction, *Arch Dermatol* (1991) **127**:1813–18.

10. Magnin Ph, Label MG, Schroh R et al, Carcinoma cuniculatum localizado en el ledra subungual, *Rev Arg Dermatol* (1986) **67**:68–72.

11. Steel HH, Garlic-clove fibroma, *JAMA* (1965) **191**:1082–3.

12. Kint A, Baran R, Histopathologic study of Koenen tumors, *J Am Acad Dermatol* (1988) **18**:369–72.

13. Reye RDK, Recurring digital fibrous tumors of childhood, *Arch Pathol* (1965) **80**:228–31.

14. Ryman W, Bale P, Recurring digital fibromas of infancy, *Aust J Dermatol* (1985) **26**:113–7.

15. Baran R, Retinoids and the nails, *J Dermatol Treat* (1990) **1**:151–4.

16. Camirand P, Giroux JM, Subungual glomus tumor, *Arch Dermatol* (1970) **102**:677–9.

17. Priollet P, Pernes JM, Laurian C et al, Intérêt de l'artériographie dans l'exploration des tumeurs glomiques sous-unguéales, *J Mal Vascul* (1985) **10**:363–5.

18. Carvajal L, Uraga E, Garcia I et al, Tumours of the hallux: myxoma, osteochondroma and enchondroma, *Skin Cancer* (1987) **2**:197–201.

19. Aulicino PL, DuPuy TE, Moriarity RP, Osteoid osteoma of the terminal phalanx of finger, *Orthop Rev* (1981) **10**:59–63.

20. Tomoda T, Ono T, Ohyama K et al, Subungual myxoid cysts producing an ulcer in the nail plate, *Jap (Rinsho) J Dermatol* (1982) **9**:451.

21. Kleinert HE, Kutz JE, Fishman JH et al, Etiology and treatment of the so-called mucous cyst of the finger, *J Bone Jt Surg* (1972) **54A**:1455–8.

22. Newmeyer WL, Kilgore ES, Graham WP, Mucous cyst: the dorsal distal interphalangeal joint ganglion, *Plast Reconstr Surg* (1974) **53**:313–15.

23. Sonnex TS, Leonard J, Ralfs et al, Myxoid cysts of the finger: treatment by liquid nitrogen spray cryosurgery, *Br J Dermatol* (1982) **107**(supplement):21.

24. Salasche SJ, Myxoid cyst of the proximal nail fold, a surgical

approach, *J Dermatol Surg Oncol* (1984) **10**:35–9.

25. Audebert C, Treatment of mucoid cysts of fingers and toes by injection of sclerosant, *Dermatol Clin* (1989) **7**:179–82.

26. Wu KK, Guise ER, Metastatic tumors of the hand: a report of six cases, *J Hand Surg* (1978) **3**:241–6.

27. Camiel MR, Aron BS, Alexander LL et al, Metastases to palm, sole, nailbed, nose, face, and scalp from unsuspected carcinoma of the lung, *Cancer* (1969) **23**:214–20.

28. Marmor L, Horner RL, Metastasis to a phalanx simulating infection in a finger, *Am J Surg* (1959) **97**:236–7.

29. Sanderson KV, Mackie RM, Tumours of the skin. In: Rook A, Wilkinson DS, Ebling FJG, eds, *Textbook of Dermatology* (Blackwells Scientific: Oxford 1979) 2129–231.

30. Haneke E, Laugier–Hunziker–Baran-Syndrom, *Hautarzt* (1991) **42**:512–15.

31. Baran R, Kechijian P, Longitudinal melanonychia, *J Am Acad Dermatol* (1989) **21**:1165–75.

32. Kopf AW, Hutchinson's sign of subungual malignant melanoma, *Am J Dermatopathol* (1981) **3**:201–2.

33. Schernberg F, Amiel M, Etude anatomo clinique d'un lambeau ungueal complet, *Ann Chir Plast Esthet* (1985) **30**:127–31.

34. Clark WH, Bernardine EA, Reed RJ et al, Acral lentiginous melanomas. In: Clark WH, Goldman L, Mastranger, eds, *Human malignant melanoma* (Grune and Stratton: New York 1979) 109–29.

35. Sondergaard K, Tejan J, Subungual amelanotic melanoma: diagnostic pitfall, *Postgrad Med J* (1990) **66**:200–202.

36. Oropeza R, Melanomas of special sites. In: Andrade R, Gumpert SL, Popalin GL, Rees TD, eds, *Cancer of the skin* Vol 2 (Saunders: Philadelphia 1976) 924–87.

37. Patterson R, Helwig EB, Subungual melanoma: a clinical pathological study, *Cancer* (1980) **46**:2074–87.

38. Nogaret JM, André J, Parent D et al, Le melanome des extremités: diagnostic méconnu et traitement délicat. Revue des 20 observations, *Acta Chir Belg* (1986) **86**:238–44.

39. Roberts AHN, Subungual melanoma following a single injury, *J Hand Surg* (1984) **9**:328–30.

Chapter 25

EXCISIONAL BIOPSY AND WIDE EXCISION FOR MALIGNANT MELANOMA

Michael Landthaler

Surgical therapy is accepted worldwide as the therapy of choice for malignant melanoma, but a question of concern is the primary therapeutic approach to the tumor. In the USA excisional biopsy under local anesthesia with narrow margins and even incisional biopsy is done as the first procedure.[1] In many European countries excision of the suspected lesion under general anesthesia is recommended followed by cryostat section.[2] Recently, many studies have been published concerning this approach to the primary tumor and how much resection margin is needed.

REVIEW OF LITERATURE

As early as 1969 Epstein et al[3] analyzed the influence of nonradical first procedures on the prognosis of patients and could not find a negative effect. In this study, patients with incisional and excisional biopsies were not differentiated and important features such as tumor thickness were not taken into consideration.

In the more recent literature several studies have been published in which tumor thickness was partially taken into account. Eldh[4] could not detect statistically significant differences in the 5-year survival rate for patients with malignant melanoma and primary wide excision compared with patients who had excisional biopsies followed by delayed wide excision. This was valid for patients with malignant melanomas thinner than 2.25 mm and thicker lesions, more than 2.25 mm. Drzewiecki et al[5] analyzed the cumulative survival of 97 patients who had biopsies before radical surgery and 146 patients who had primary radical surgery. No difference in survival could be seen between the two groups of patients.

Griffiths and Briggs[6] followed 291 patients with malignant melanoma for a minimum of 10 years after primary surgical treatment. Sixty-three (23%) of these patients had received an incisional biopsy procedure prior to definitive wide margin excisional surgery. One-third of the lesions initially treated by incisional biopsy were rendered histologically unassessable on current histopathological criteria. Incisional biopsy significantly interfered with the accurate histopathological staging of the melanomas. When the incidences of local recurrences and death were related specifically to the thickness of the primary tumor, prognosis of patients was not significantly different between patients treated initially by either incisional biopsy,

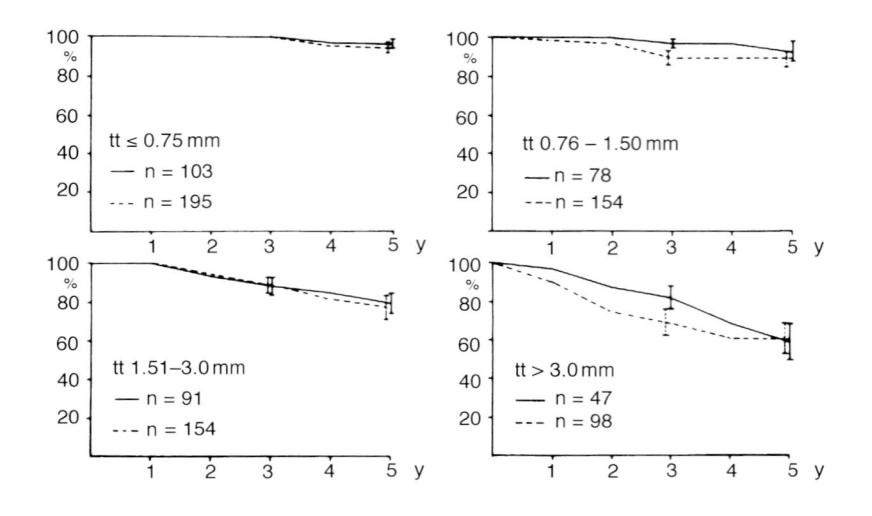

Figure 25.1
Survival in relation to tumor thickness and first procedure. (Reproduced with permission of JB Lippincott Co., Hagerstown, Md., from Cancer (1989) **64**:1615[8].)
—, Excisional biopsy and delayed wide excision.
---, Primary wide excision.

minimal margin excisional biopsy or primary wide excisional surgery.

Lederman and Sober[7] compared 5-year survival rates of 502 patients with clinical stage I melanoma. Thirty patients received wide excisional margin of 4–5 cm as the initial procedure. The second group of 472 patients had diagnostic incisional or excisional biopsy before wider therapeutic excision was performed within 2–4 weeks. Comparison of the outcome in both groups of patients did not show a statistically significant difference.

Landthaler et al[8] compared the 5-year disease-free rate and 5-year survival rate of 319 melanoma patients with a narrow excisional biopsy under local anesthesia as the first procedure followed by delayed wide excision with the 5-year disease-free rate and 5-year survival rate of 635 patients with primary melanomas excised radically with a safety margin of 3–5 cm. Five-year disease-free rate and 5-year survival rate did not differ in either group of patients. This was valid for thin (<0.75 mm), medium (0.76–3.0 mm) and thick (>3.0 mm) primary tumors (Figure 25.1). Additionally, the time interval between excisional biopsy and delayed wide excision had no influence on the outcome of the patients.

More recently, Evans and McCann[9] described a protocol which has been used in a prospective study of 806 patients with primary malignant melanoma. Excisional biopsies were performed as soon as possible and Breslow thickness and Clarks levels determined. Patients were assigned to low-, medium- and high-risk groups and definitive excision was carried out with a resection margin of 2, 20 and 50 mm respectively. Over 7 years no local recurrences have occurred thus far in the low- and medium-risk groups, suggesting that the protocol is safe.

The effect of the initial biopsy procedure on prognosis in stage I melanoma patients was investigated by Lees and Briggs.[10] One thousand and eighty-six patients were treated for primary clinical stage I cutaneous melanoma and followed for a minimum of 5 years from initial operation. Of these 96 (8.8%) were treated initially by incisional biopsy, 292 (26.8%) by narrow margin biopsy and 698 (64.3%) by wide margin excision. Logistic regression analysis was performed to assess the statistical significance of the association between the various factors. The method of initial biopsy was related to maximal tumor thickness, age and sex in comparing the biopsy techniques. Incisional biopsy rendered 38/96 (39.6%) of lesions not fully assessable on current histopathological criteria, significantly higher than for the other biopsy techniques ($P < 0.0001$). Incisional biopsy did not adversely affect prognosis in terms of local recurrence and mortality. Prognosis was related to tumor thickness and age and sex of the patient and not to biopsy technique. The authors therefore recommended that all suspicious lesions should be removed by excisional rather than incisional biopsy in order to avoid compromising the histological assessment, given the importance of maximal tumor thickness in determining treatment and prognosis.

The data from recent literature confirm that excisional biopsy of malignant melanoma followed by subsequent wide excision is a safe procedure for patients with malignant melanoma. Furthermore, excision of suspicious lesions under general anesthesia seems unnecessary, since a nonrandomized trial comparing the survival rate of melanoma patients treated under general anesthesia with survival of patients treated under local anesthesia did not demonstrate a negative effect of local anesthesia.[11]

Excisional Biopsy of Melanoma

An important advantage of excisional biopsy is that in the planning of definitive treatment, tumor thickness can be taken into account. This is important since recent studies have demonstrated that thin malignant melanoma does not necessarily require wide excision. Several retrospective studies concerning the influence of resection margin on disease-free survival and survival of melanoma patients have corresponding results.[12]

1. Increase of tumor thickness leads to an increase of local recurrences.
2. In thin melanomas a narrow resection margin is not followed by a higher local recurrence rate.
3. In thick melanomas treated with narrow resection margin, local recurrences increase.
4. Local recurrences do not influence overall survival.
5. A resection margin of 5 cm is unnecessary.

Tumor Thickness—Surgical Approach

Landthaler et al.[12] recently showed that the survival rate of 190 patients with a tumor thickness beyond 1.5 mm and a resection margin of less than 2.0 cm did not differ from the survival rate of 1150 patients with the same tumor thickness but a resection margin of more than 2.0 cm. A resection margin beyond 2.0 cm had no negative effect on survival of 75 patients with a tumor thickness of more than 1.5 mm, compared to a resection margin of more than 2.0 cm in 797 patients. But in the narrow resection group the disease-free survival was reduced due to local recurrences.

In a prospective and randomized WHO trial including patients with malignant melanoma with a tumor thickness of less than 2.0 mm it could be demonstrated that a wide excision margin of 1.0 cm is a safe procedure. Although in the narrow margin group more local recurrences were observed, the overall survival of patients with a margin of 1.0 cm was the same as that of patients with a margin of 3.0 cm.[13,14]

Incisional Biopsy of Melanoma

It must be emphasized that incisional biopsy of malignant melanoma is still controversial. Data from Rampen et al[15,16] indicate that incisional procedures may worsen the outcome of patients with malignant melanoma. Five-year survival of patients with incisional procedures was worse than that of patients with excisional procedures.

Van der Esch and Rampen[17] described a 46-year-old woman with melanoma of the leg from which a punch biopsy was taken. In the re-excision specimen two biopsy wounds were recognized, that were filled with tumor. The initial level III tumor had to be reported subsequently as a deep level IV melanoma because of increased tumor depth. In contrast, Penneys[18] could not confirm the concept that punch biopsy of a malignant melanoma brings tumor cells into the dermis. Punch biopsy was performed on 40 cases of malignant melanoma which were subsequently excised in their study.

In a study by Lederman and Sober,[19] statistically significant differences could not be found in the outcome of patients with incisional procedures compared with patients who had excisional biopsies. A total of 472 patients with clinical stage I melanoma were analyzed; 119 had an incisional biopsy and 353 an excisional biopsy. Patients were grouped by tumor thickness and the outcome compared between the two groups. Within each thickness group there was no statistically significant difference in survival between the two groups. None of the patients with primary tumors of less than 1.7 mm have died following incisional biopsy. In patients with medium tumor thickness and incisional biopsy the 5-year survival rate was 20% worse than in the control group. Therefore a negative effect of incisional biopsy cannot be excluded with certainty, even though multivariate analysis demonstrated that biopsy type was not a significant factor in this study.

Because an incisional procedure bears the additional risk that representative areas of a tumor may be missed, incisional biopsy in malignant melanoma should be avoided, and only performed in exceptional cases of large tumors which cannot easily be removed by excisional surgery. Since smear cytology is helpful, at least in eroded and ulcerated lesions, the indication for incisional biopsy is very rare in our experience. One must pay attention to the principle *primum nihil nocere* and reduce every risk for patients to the greatest extent possible.

REFERENCES

1. Koh HK, Medical progress: cutaneous melanoma, *N Engl J Med* (1991) **325**:171–82.
2. Braun-Falco O, Landthaler M, Hölzel D et al, Therapie und Prognose maligner Melanome der Haut, *Dtsch Med Wochenschr* (1968) **46**:1750–6.
3. Epstein E, Bragg K, Linden G, Biopsy and prognosis of malignant melanoma, *JAMA* (1969) **208**:1369–71.
4. Eldh J, Excisional biopsy and delayed wide excision versus primary wide excision of malignant melanoma, *Scand J Plast Reconstr Surg* (1979) **13**:341–5.
5. Drzewiecki KT, Ladefoged C, Christensen HE, Biopsy and prognosis for cutaneous malignant melanomas in clinical stage I, *Scand J Plast Reconstr Surg* (1980) **14**:141–4.
6. Griffiths RW, Briggs JC, Biopsy procedures, primary wide excisional surgery and long term prognosis in primary clinical stage I invasive cutaneous malignant melanoma, *Ann R Coll Surg Engl* (1985) **67**:75–8.
7. Lederman JS, Sober AJ, Does wide excision as the initial diagnostic procedure improve prognosis in patients with cutaneous melanoma? *J Dermatol Surg Oncol* (1986) **12**:697–9.

8. Landthaler M, Braun-Falco O, Leitz A et al, Excisional biopsy as the first therapeutic procedure versus primary wide excision of malignant melanoma, *Cancer* (1989) **64**:1612–16.

9. Evans J, McCann G, A new protocol for the treatment of stage I cutaneous malignant melanoma; interim results of the first 806 patients treated, *Br J Plast Surg* (1990) **43**:426–30.

10. Lees VC, Briggs JC, Effect of initial biopsy procedure on prognosis in stage I invasive cutaneous malignant melanoma: review of 1086 patients, *Br J Surg* (1991) **78**:1108–10.

11. Seebacher C, Heubaum F, Küster P et al, Vergleichende Analyse in Narkose und Lokalanästhesie operierter maligner Melanome der Haut, *Hautarzt* (1990) **41**:137–41.

12. Landthaler M, Braun-Falco O, Hölzel D et al, Der Sicherheitsabstand bei der primären operativen Versorgung des malignen Melanoms. In: Orfanos CE, Garbe K, eds, *Das maligne Melanom der Haut* (W Zuckschwerdt: München 1990) 209–13.

13. Veronesi U, Cascinelli N, Adamus J et al, Thin stage I primary cutaneous malignant melanoma. Comparison of excision with margins of 1 or 3 cm, *N Engl J Med* (1988) **318**:1159–62.

14. Veronesi U, Cascinelli N, Narrow excision (1-cm margin). A safe procedure for thin cutaneous melanoma, *Arch Surg* (1991) **126**: 438–41.

15. Rampen FHJ, van Houten WA, Hop WCJ, Incisional procedures and prognosis in malignant melanoma, *Clin Exp Dermatol* (1980) **5**:313–20.

16. Rampen FHJ, Spronk CA, How 'fine' is incisional biopsy of melanoma? *Ann Plast Surg* (1983) **16**:173–4.

17. Van der Esch EP, Rampen FHJ, Punch biopsy of melanoma, *J Am Acad Dermatol* (1985) **13**:899–902.

18. Penneys NS, Excision of melanoma after initial biopsy, *J Am Acad Dermatol* (1985) **13**:995–8.

19. Lederman JS, Sober AJ, Does biopsy type influence survival in clinical stage I cutaneous melanoma? *J Am Acad Dermatol* (1985) **13**:983–7.

Chapter 26

CURRENT MANAGEMENT OF THIN MELANOMA

Sandhya Yadav
Darrell S. Rigel

INTRODUCTION

The clinical management of thin cutaneous melanomas has become an important problem in the practice of medicine. In the 1930s, it was estimated that one in 1500 Americans would develop cutaneous melanoma during their lifetime.[1] During the 1980s, the incidence of melanoma doubled to one in 150. Currently, the rate continues to rise and the lifetime risk for Americans is now one in 105.

Early detection and treatment are crucial in cutaneous melanoma since surgical excision of a thin lesion results in a cure while metastatic disease responds poorly to available therapy. In fact, the death rate from melanoma continues to rise by approximately 2% per year. Paradoxically, the average thickness of melanomas presenting for treatment has decreased over the past 20 years.[2] Given the increasing incidence of melanoma, it follows that the absolute number of thin, early melanomas must also be rising dramatically, making their management even more relevant to the clinician (Figure 26.1).

DEFINITION OF THIN MELANOMAS

'Thin' melanomas are defined as in situ and invasive lesions less than 1.0 mm in Breslow's thickness. This corresponds to the definition given by the 1992 NIH Consensus Conference which discussed 'early' melanomas. Studies have shown that persons with in situ lesions have a 10-year survival rate that approaches 100% when treated surgically.[3-6] Patients with invasive melanoma less than 1 mm in thickness have a 95.5% probability of survival at 10 years (NYU Melanoma Cooperative Group, unpublished data) (Figure 26.2). The key,

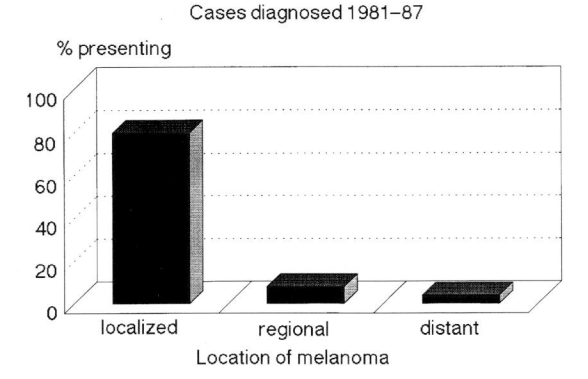

Figure 26.1
*Percent of cutaneous melanomas presenting by stage. (From Boring et al, CA (1992) **42**:23.)*

241

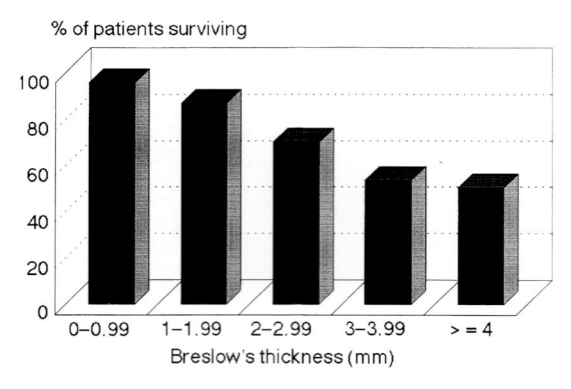

Figure 26.2
Ten-year survival rates of patients presenting with stage I melanoma grouped by Breslow's thickness. (From the NYU Cooperative Group data, 1992.)

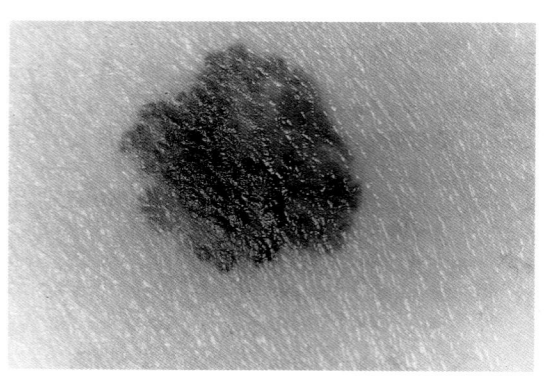

Figure 26.3
Early cutaneous melanoma showing the 'A,B,C and D' features.

therefore, to decreasing the melanoma death rate is to treat them while they are thin.

CLINICAL FEATURES OF THIN MELANOMAS

Before melanomas can be treated, they first must be diagnosed. Melanomas tend to grow radially for varying periods of time before becoming invasive. Patients with tumors in this radial-growth phase have a better prognosis than those with lesions in the vertical-growth phase.[7]

Fortunately, thin melanomas in a radial-growth phase have recognizable clinical characteristics (Figure 26.3). They often present as asymptomatic macules. Other features can be summarized using the mnemonic 'ABCD'.[8]

A — Asymmetry
B — Border irregularity
C — Color variegation
D — Diameter greater than 6 mm

Asymmetry refers to the inability to draw a line bisecting the melanoma that yields similar halves. In addition, thin melanomas tend to have a notched or indistinct border and contain multiple shades of browns and blacks haphazardly distributed within the lesion. In contrast, most benign pigmented lesions tend to be symmetric, with regular, distinct borders, and have uniform coloration. Any lesions with the A, B and C characteristics, having a diameter of greater than 6 mm, should be considered for biopsy.

HISTOLOGICAL FEATURES OF THIN MELANOMAS

The histology of a thin melanoma reflects the superficial nature of the lesion, with the majority of changes found in the epidermis (Figure 26.4). Single atypical melanocytes, sometimes in clusters, are present at all levels of the epidermis. Nests of melanocytes are irregularly distributed along the dermal–epidermal junction. In addition, if the melanoma is invasive, malignant cells will be found in the dermis. Pleomorphic nuclei with mitoses can also be present. A lymphocytic infiltrate with areas of fibrosis (that is regression) indicates a host immune response.[9,10]

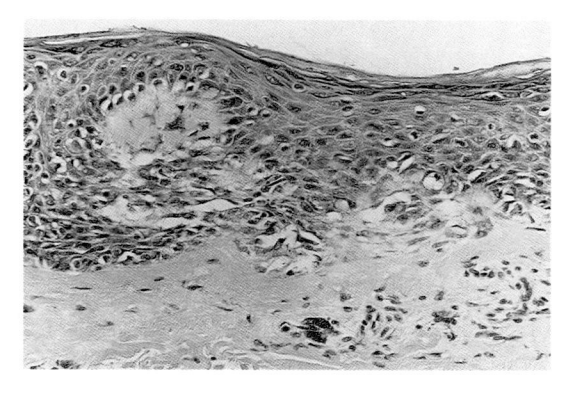

Figure 26.4
Photomicrograph of the histology of a thin melanoma. There are scattered melanocytes above the dermal–epidermal junction as well as an irregular nest and increased numbers of single melanocytes at the dermal–epidermal junction.

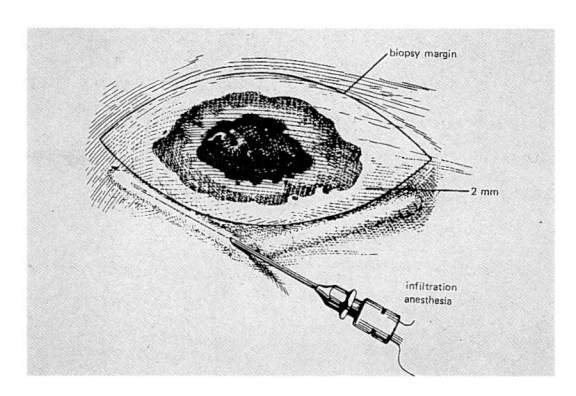

Figure 26.5
Recommended technique of excisional biopsy of a pigmented skin lesion.

Management

The management of patients with thin melanoma is staged:

1. Initial evaluation
2. Biopsy
3. Initial therapy
4. Follow-up evaluation

The focus of the initial evaluation of patients with a suspected melanoma is to identify other atypical skin lesions and their risk factors for melanoma. A complete personal and family history of melanoma should be obtained since a positive history increases the patient's subsequent melanoma risk. Other significant risk factors for cutaneous melanoma include red or blond hair, freckles, actinic keratoses, a history of three or more blistering sunburns prior to the age of 20, and a history of extensive exposure to sun as a child or teenager.[11,12]

The importance of a *total* cutaneous examination cannot be overstated. Melanomas, unlike other skin cancers, tend to occur in areas that are normally covered by clothing. The most frequent sites of melanoma development are on the superior trunk in men and on the legs in women.[13,14] These areas can easily be missed if a total cutaneous examination is not performed. In fact, there is a statistically significant increased chance of missing a melanoma when total cutaneous examination has not been performed.[15]

Biopsy technique

Once a suspicious lesion has been identified, it should be biopsied. A properly performed biopsy is essential to enhance the dermatopathologist's ability to diagnose a melanoma.

An excisional biopsy which includes 1–2 mm of normal-appearing skin is the best way to biopsy a melanoma (Figure 26.5). This gives the dermatopathologist the optimal specimen in which the parameters of size, symmetry and circumscription are easily evaluated; factors which are often important in diagnosis of pigmented lesions. In addition, important prognostic factors such as Breslow's thickness, ulceration, mitotic rate, regression, inflammation and blood vessel lymphatic involvement can be appropriately assessed.

While an excisional biopsy is ideal, it is not always practical in situations where the anatomic location or size of the lesion will not permit an easily obtainable primary closure. In these cases, an incisional biopsy may be performed.[16,17] The biopsy should be oriented to include the thickest portion of the melanoma, and, if possible, 1–2 mm of normal-appearing skin at the edge. Incisional biopsies do not adversely affect the 5-year survival rates of patients with melanoma if the entire melanoma is subsequently excised.[18–21]

A shave biopsy which transects the base of the melanoma or a punch biopsy that includes only a small portion of the lesion may not give the dermatopathologist an adequate specimen with which to make the diagnosis. Often, the true thickness of the lesion will be underestimated if the base of the melanoma has been transected.[22]

Most biopsies of malignant melanoma can be performed in an outpatient setting using local anesthesia. Local anesthesia should be administered in a field block surrounding the lesion. The incision should be placed, where possible, such that the long axis of the ellipse is oriented in a direction of probable lymphatic drainage for that anatomic site. The incision should reach into the subcutaneous fat but need not be carried to the level of the muscle fascia. Usually, the defect created can be closed primarily, with simple interrupted sutures. The specimen should be fixed in 10% formalin solution before being transported to the pathology laboratory.

Histopathological Evaluation

After the specimen is processed in the laboratory, the dermatopathologist should evaluate the lesion using permanent sections. Frozen section evaluation is not recommended for the diagnosis of malignant melanoma. If the lesion is a melanoma the pathology report should include the Breslow's thickness, and the status of the margins (for example, does the melanoma extend to any surgical margin?) to help assess the patient's prognosis and guide subsequent management. Additional pathological data useful in assessing patient prognosis include: subtype (for example superficial spreading, acral-lentiginous, nodular, or lentigo maligna), Clark's level, ulceration, regression, the presence of a precursor lesion, microscopic satellitosis (that is aggregates of neoplastic cells that are separated from the main bulk of the neoplasm by normal collagen), lymphatic invasion, mitotic rate, lymphocytic infiltrate and growth phase (that is radial- versus vertical-growth phase).[23]

Clinical Evaluation

Once a patient has been diagnosed as having a melanoma, further evaluation needs to take place. A comprehensive physical examination should be performed with particular emphasis on the total cutaneous examination to detect any other concurrent skin cancers or melanoma metastases. Other signs that are risk factors for melanoma should also be noted, such as the presence of atypical moles (formerly called 'dysplastic' nevi) or large number of nevi. In addition, careful palpation of the regional lymph nodes and skin surrounding the melanoma should be performed to detect any lymphatic spread. Palpable enlargement of the liver or spleen should also be documented. If a thorough medical history and careful physical examination do not reveal any abnormalities, routine screening laboratory studies for thin melanomas are not useful. Extensive diagnostic studies (CT scans, MRIs and nuclear scans) are not needed to stage these patients. There are no data to support the practice of obtaining baseline chest radiographs and liver function studies in asymptomatic persons with thin melanoma.[24] (Given the small, but significant, incidence of metastasis for thin melanoma, one cannot be critical of this practice, however.)

INITIAL SURGICAL THERAPY

The standard therapy for removal of a melanoma is surgical excision. For melanoma in situ, excision of the lesion with a 5-mm border of clinically normal-appearing skin is recommended. This approach should be curative.

Clinical trials have suggested that thin, invasive melanomas can be excised with narrower margins than have been traditionally recommended.[25-30] For melanomas less than 1 mm in thickness, a 1-cm margin of clinically normal-appearing skin and underlying subcutaneous tissue is recommended as an appropriate excision. Studies no longer indicate that the removal of the underlying muscle fascia increases survival or decreases the frequency of local recurrences. Therefore, it is recommended that the depth of the excision extend to the deep subcutis. The resulting surgical defect can often be closed primarily without the need for skin grafting or other more elaborate repairs.

The results of carefully designated studies are required before Mohs micrographic surgery can be recommended as a standard technique for melanoma removal.[31-33] Elective regional lymph node dissection is not recommended in patients with thin melanomas as defined above.[34]

FOLLOW-UP OF PATIENTS WITH THIN MELANOMAS

The prognosis for patients with thin melanomas is excellent. However, these patients should be followed for the rest of their lives for two reasons. First, there is a small but finite chance that the melanoma may recur. Second, the chance of a person developing another primary melanoma is approximately 4%.[35,36] Regular follow-up insures that a second primary will be detected while it is still thin and curable. Studies have shown that subsequent melanomas diagnosed in a surveillance program were thinner than the incident melanomas.[35]

Prospective follow-up is especially important in the setting of familial melanoma, and atypical mole syndrome, as well as for those with xeroderma pigmentosa. These individuals have a much greater risk of developing melanoma compared to the general population.

Patients with a history of melanoma should be followed with serial total cutaneous examinations in addition to palpation of the excision site and regional lymph nodes. If cutaneous lesions suspicious for melanoma are noted, they need to be biopsied in a manner similar to that previously described. Total body photographs can be useful in following patients with many atypical nevi.[37] Because the occurrence of distant metastases in patients with thin melanoma is unusual, it is not necessary to perform routine screening for occult visceral lesions unless the patient becomes symptomatic.

Recommendations for the proper follow-up interval vary depending upon the patient. Patients without atypical moles and without a family history for melanoma can be followed up every 6 months. Patients with many risk factors for cutaneous melanoma (that is many atypical moles, family history of melanoma, history of multiple primary melanomas) should be followed up more frequently, from three to four times per year. At 5 years, most patients with thin melanomas can be followed up on an annual basis. Although there appears to be little risk of recurrence in patients with melanoma in situ, it is prudent to follow up these patients given their increased risk of developing a second primary melanoma.

It is important that patients with melanoma be made 'partners' in their own care. Specifically, they should learn what the features of early melanoma are and bring lesions which have the 'ABCD' characteristics to the attention of their physician. They should also perform monthly self-examination of their skin.[38] In addition, patients should be counselled to avoid excessive sun exposure and to use protective clothing and sunscreens.

METHODS TO MAXIMIZE EARLY DETECTION OF CUTANEOUS MELANOMA

The importance of early detection/screening

Since 1985, the American Academy of Dermatology has sponsored free annual skin cancer screening programs as part of the national melanoma/skin cancer prevention campaign (American Academy of Dermatology, unpublished data). To date, more than 400 000 people have been screened (Figure 26.6). Many organizations, including the American Cancer Society and the Skin Cancer Foundation, have supported these programs. Over 40% of dermatologists nationwide volunteer their time for these programs. Almost 1000 melanomas and thousands of non-melanoma skin cancers have been detected through this screening.[39]

In a 1990 study, the sensitivity of cutaneous skin examinations for the detection of melanoma by a dermatologist was 97%.[40] These data support the screening examination of the skin as a useful way to help identify skin cancer in a large population. Clearly, if every American were examined yearly for malignant melanoma, death from this disease would be a rare event.[41] However, the cost–benefit ratio from skin cancer screening as well as the feasibility of screening the entire American population need to be investigated.

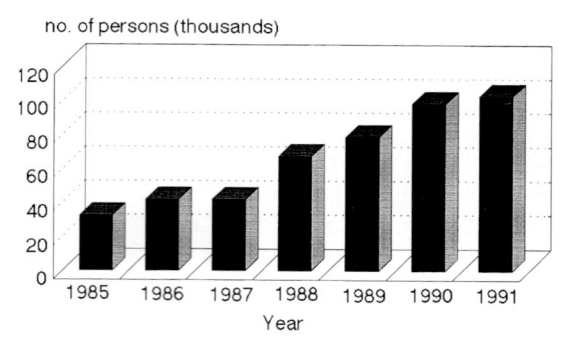

Figure 26.6
Results of the American Academy of Dermatology Skin Cancer Screening Program.

Early melanoma and pregnancy

Melanoma is the most frequent cancer in women between the ages of 25 and 29 years.[42] Since this interval is during the childbearing years, the relationship between pregnancy and melanoma is an important issue. Similarly, the question of oral contraceptives 'causing' malignant melanoma or whether they influence existing 'dormant' melanoma has also been an area of controversy. Although there are reports of patients who have had accelerated metastatic growth from melanoma during pregnancy, there are no specific studies demonstrating that pregnancy influences prognosis in primary melanoma. The only clear conclusion that can be drawn is that the patient with melanoma during pregnancy should be treated promptly, with the status of the fetus as a secondary consideration. However, the prognosis of women who have had a thin melanoma is unchanged if they have subsequent pregnancies.[43] Currently, it is recommended that a 2–3-year waiting period elapse from the time a melanoma is treated until a woman conceives.[44–46]

The use of exogenous estrogens and oral contraceptives is controversial after a melanoma has been treated. The reports in

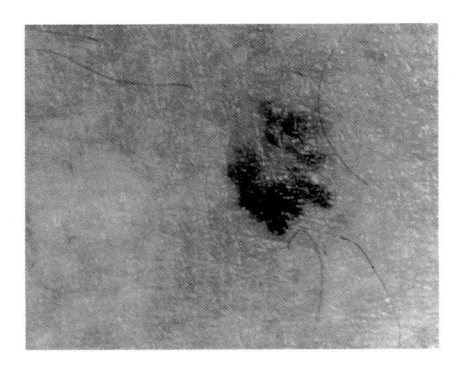

Figure 26.7
Pigmented lesion viewed clinically.

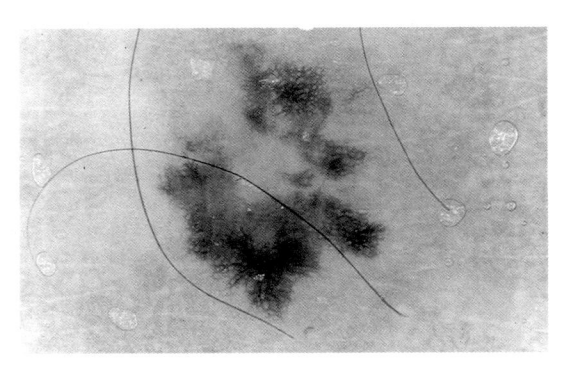

Figure 26.8
Pigmented lesion using dermoscopy. Note the 'network' pattern visible at the periphery and the 'white area' in the center of the lesion.

the literature do not reach a clear consensus.[47–49] Until the issue of potential adverse effects is resolved, it is suggested that women with a history of melanoma, a family history of melanoma, or the classic atypical mole syndrome, should avoid hormonal medications.[50]

Advances in diagnostic techniques

Some advances in technology have the potential to assist in the diagnosis of early cutaneous melanoma. Computer analysis and digital imaging of the skin is being evaluated by several groups to try to detect early malignant changes.[51,52]

Epiluminescence microscopy is another technique that has gained increased use with the development of the hand-held dermatoscope.[53] The dermatoscope, approximately the size of an ophthalmoscope, uses mineral oil placed on the surface of a pigmented lesion to render the stratum corneum translucent. The instrument has a glass plate on one end, which is placed on top of the lesion. It is able to magnify skin lesions by 10-fold. Through epiluminescence microscopy certain features of a pigmented lesion are visible which are not appreciable with routine examination (Figures 26.7 and 26.8). This technique may increase the in vivo diagnostic accuracy for cutaneous melanocytic neoplasms.[54,55] However, further work needs to be done to evaluate this technique.

SUMMARY

Despite continuing research and promising new diagnostic techniques, the current standard of care for thin melanomas remains periodic examination of the skin and surgical excision of the lesion. The combination of routine physician examination augmented by self-examination of the skin provides the best opportunity for the identification of early curable melanomas. Only early diagnosis and treatment can significantly reduce the ever-increasing mortality rate from this serious form of cutaneous cancer.

REFERENCES

1. Kopf AW, Rigel DS, Friedman RJ, The rising incidence and mortality rate of malignant melanoma, *J Dermatol Surg Oncol* (1982) **8**:760–1.

2. Balch CM, Milton GW, Shaw HM et al, eds, *Cutaneous melanoma: clinical management and treatment results*

worldwide (JB Lippincott: Philadelphia 1985) 315–16.

3. Ackerman AB, Clinical diagnosis of malignant melanoma in situ. In: Ackerman AB, ed., *Pathology of malignant melanoma* (Masson Publishing: New York 1981) 57–8.

4. Breslow A, Prognostic factors in the treatment of cutaneous melanoma, *J Cutan Pathol* (1979) **6**:208.

5. Clark WH Jr, From L, Bernardino EA et al, The histogenesis and biologic behavior of primary human malignant melanomas of the skin, *Cancer Res* (1969) **29**:705.

6. Sober AJ, Fitzpatrick TB, Mihm MC et al, Early recognition of cutaneous melanoma, *JAMA* (1979) **242**:2795.

7. Friedman RJ, Heilman ER, Gottlieb GJ et al, Malignant melanoma clinicopathologic correlations. In: Friedman RJ, Rigel DS, Kopf AW et al, eds, *Cancer of the skin* (WB Saunders: Philadelphia 1991) 171.

8. Friedman RJ, Rigel DS, Kopf AW, Early detection of malignant melanoma: the role of physician examination and self-examination of the skin, *CA* (1985) **35**:130–51.

9. Friedman RJ, Heilman ER, Gottlieb GJ et al, Malignant melanoma clinicopathologic correlations. In: Friedman RJ, Rigel DS, Kopf AW et al, eds, *Cancer of the skin* (WB Saunders: Philadelphia 1991) 148–76.

10. Ackerman AB, ed., *Pathology of malignant melanoma* (Masson Publishing: New York 1981) 57–91.

11. Evans RD, Kopf AW, Leu RA et al, Risk factors for the development of malignant melanoma: I. Review of case-control studies, *J Dermatol Surg Oncol* (1988) **14**:393–408.

12. Gellin GA, Kopf AW, Garfinkel L, Malignant melanoma: a controlled study of possibly associated factors, *Arch Dermatol* (1969) **99**:43–8.

13. Pearl DK, Scott EL, The anatomical distribution of skin cancers, *Int J Epidemiol* (1986) **15**:502.

14. Lee JAH, Yongchaiyudha S, Incidence of and mortality from malignant melanoma by anatomical site, *J Natl Cancer Inst* (1971) **47**:253.

15. Rigel DS, Friedman RJ, Kopf AW et al, Importance of complete cutaneous examination for the detection of malignant melanoma, *J Am Acad Dermatol* (1986) **14**:857–60.

16. Balch CM, Milton GW, Shaw HM et al, eds, *Cutaneous melanoma: clinical management and treatment results worldwide* (JB Lippincott: Philadelphia 1985) 73–5.

17. Harris MN, Gumport SL, Biopsy technique for malignant melanoma, *J Dermatol Surg* (1975) **1**:24–7.

18. Lederman JS, Sober AJ, Does biopsy type influence survival in clinical stage I cutaneous melanoma? *J Am Acad Dermatol* (1985) **13**:983–7.

19. Lees VC, Briggs JC, Effect of initial biopsy procedure on prognosis in stage I invasive cutaneous malignant melanoma: review of 1086 patients, *Br J Surg* (1991) **78**:1108–10.

20. Epstein E, Bragg K, Linden G, Biopsy and prognosis of malignant melanoma, *JAMA* (1969) **208**:1369–71.

21. Knutson CO, Hori JM, Spratt JS, Melanoma, *Curr Probl Surg* (1971) December, 1–55.

22. Wagner DE, Cullen RA, Primary melanoma: pitfalls in diagnostic biopsy techniques and interpretations, *Am J Surg* (1984) **148**:99–102.

23. Friedman RJ, Rigel DS, Kopf AW et al, eds, *Cancer of the skin* (WB Saunders: Philadelphia 1991) 171–3.

24. Au FC, Maier WP, Malmud LS et al,

Preoperative nuclear scans in patients with melanoma, *CA* (1984) **53**:2095–7.

25. Veronesi U, Cascinelli N, Narrow excision (1-cm margin) a safe procedure for thin cutaneous melanoma, *Arch Surg* (1991) **126**:438–41.

26. Veronesi U, Cascinelli N, Adamus J et al, Thin stage I primary cutaneous malignant melanoma. Comparison of excision with margins of 1 or 3 cm, *N Engl J Med* (1988) **318**:1159–62.

27. Ackerman AB, Scheiner AM, How wide and deep is wide and deep enough? A critique of surgical practice in excision of primary cutaneous malignant melanoma, *Hum Pathol* (1983) **14**:743–4.

28. Ho VC, Sober AJ, Therapy for cutaneous melanoma: an update, *J Am Acad Dermatol* (1990) **22**:159–76.

29. Day CL, Lew RA, Malignant melanoma prognostic factors 3: surgical margins, *J Dermatol Surg Oncol* (1983) **9**:797–801.

30. Breslow A, Macht SD, Optimal size resection margin for thin cutaneous melanoma, *Surg Gynecol Obstet* (1977) **145**:691–2.

31. Zitelli JA, Moy RL, Abell E, The reliability of frozen sections in the evaluation of surgical margins for melanoma, *J Am Acad Dermatol* (1991) **24**:102–6.

32. de Barker D, Lentigo maligna and Mohs, *Arch Dermatol* (1991) **127**:421.

33. Headington JT, A dermatopathologist looks at Mohs micrographic surgery, *Arch Dermatol* (1990) **126**:950–1.

34. Biess B, Brocker EB, Drepper H et al, Should elective lymph node dissection be used for treatment of primary melanoma? *J Cancer Res Clin Oncol* (1989) **115**:470–3.

35. Titus-Ernstoff L, Erstoff MS, Kirkwood JM et al, Usefulness of frequent skin examination for the early detection of second primary cutaneous melanoma, *Cancer Detect Prev* (1989) **13**:317.

36. Veronesi U, Cascinelli N, Bufalino R, Evaluation of the risk of multiple primaries in malignant cutaneous melanoma, *Tumori* (1976) **62**:127–30.

37. Slue W, Kopf AW, Rivers JK, Total-body photographs of dysplastic nevi, *Arch Dermatol* (1988) **124**:1239–43.

38. Friedman RJ, Rigel DS, Kopf AW, Early detection of malignant melanoma: the role of physician-examination and self-examination of the skin, *CA* (1985) **35**:130–51.

39. Koh HK, Norton LA, Geller AC et al, Confirmed melanomas found in National Skin Cancer Screening, *J Am Acad Dermatol* (in press).

40. Koh HK, Caruso A, Gage I et al, Evaluation of melanoma/skin cancer screening in Massachusetts. Preliminary results, *CA* (1990) **65**:375–9.

41. Devesa SS, Silverman DT, Young JL Jr et al, Cancer incidence and mortality trends among whites in the United States, 1947–84, *J Natl Cancer Inst* (1987) **79**:701–70.

42. Slingluff CL Jr, Reintgen DS, Vollmer RT et al, Malignant melanoma arising during pregnancy. A study of 100 patients, *Ann Surg* (1990) **211**:552–7.

43. MacKie RM, Bufalino R, Morabito A et al, Lack of effect of pregnancy on outcome of melanoma. For the World Health Organisation Melanoma Programme, *Lancet* (1991) **337**:635.

44. Wong DJ, Strassner HT, Melanoma in pregnancy, *Clin Obstet Gynecol* (1990) **33**:782–91.

45. McManamny DS, Moss AL, Pocock PV et al, Melanoma and pregnancy: a long-term follow-up, *Br J Obstet Gynaecol* (1989) **96**:1419–23.

46. Sober AJ, Fitzpatrick TB, Mihm MC Jr, Primary melanoma of the skin: recognition and management, *J Am Acad Dermatol* (1980) **2**:179–97.

47. Franceshi S, Baron AE, La Vecchia C, The influence of female hormones on malignant melanoma, *Tumori* (1990) **76**:439–49.

48. Lederman JS, Lew RA, Koh HK et al, Influence of estrogen administration on tumor characteristics and survival in women with cutaneous melanoma, *J Natl Cancer Inst* (1985) **74**:981–5.

49. Brinton LA, The relationship of exogeneous estrogen to cancer risk, *Cancer Detect Prev* (1984) **7**:159–71.

50. Ellis DL, Pregnancy and sex steroid hormone effects on nevi of patients with the dysplastic nevus syndrome, *J Am Acad Dermatol* (1991) **25**:467–82.

51. Perednia DA, White RG, Schowengerdt RA, Localization of cutaneous lesions in digital images, *Comput Biomed Res* (1989) **22**:374–92.

52. Cascinelli N, Ferrario M, Tonelli T et al, A possible new tool for clinical diagnosis of melanoma: the computer, *J Am Acad Dermatol* (1987) **16**:361–7.

53. Stolz W, Bilek P, Landthaler M et al, Skin surface microscopy, *Lancet* (1989) **Oct:** 864–5.

54. Steiner A, Pehamberger H, Wolff K, In vivo epiluminescence of pigmented skin lesions. II. Diagnosis of small pigmented skin lesions and early detection of malignant melanoma, *J Am Acad Dermatol* (1987) **17**:584–91.

55. MacKie RM, An aid to the preoperative assessment of pigmented lesions of the skin, *Br J Dermatol* (1971) **85**:232–8.

Chapter 27

MOHS MICROGRAPHIC SURGERY FOR MELANOMA

Frederic E. Mohs

Melanoma is the most dangerous common cutaneous neoplasm. It not only tends to have contiguous 'silent' ramifications that are not clinically visible or palpable, but it also may have noncontiguous satellites and in-transit metastases that can result from the tendency for melanoma cells to invade walls of lymphatics and break off as emboli. Moreover, melanoma cells may be transplantable so if an outgrowth or a microsatellite is transected by conventional surgical excision, the melanoma might disseminate during undermining to permit primary closure or concealed by a graft or flap until the melanomatous implant becomes dangerously enlarged.

Mohs micrographic surgery, fixed-tissue technique (MMS-fixed), can largely solve these problems. First, all incisions are through fixed (killed) tissues, avoiding the danger of transecting a viable outgrowth or microsatellite and disseminating melanoma cells in the adjacent tissues. Removal of the melanoma in successive layers and examination of the undersurface of each layer in the microscope makes it possible to detect and selectively follow the outgrowths with the least loss of adjacent normal tissues. This is in contrast to conventional surgery, which requires the sacrifice of a wide 'surgical margin' of the entire periphery because there is no way to know where or how wide the outgrowths might be.

Also MMS-fixed is effective management for clinically invisible satellites or in-transit metastases because these embolic foci are not moved or disturbed. When they become visible they can be removed with MMS-fixed in the safest manner. Finally, after removal of a melanoma by MMS-fixed the wound is left to heal by second intention rather than by primary closure.

THE NAMING OF THE METHOD

The term 'Mohs micrographic surgery' is a relatively new name for a method that was initially called 'chemosurgery' in 1936, when this method was first used at the Wisconsin General Hospital. It was named 'chemosurgery' because the cancerous tissues were subjected to in situ chemical fixation prior to the excision of successive layers of skin for complete microscopic examination of the undersurface of each horizontally cut layer by the systemic use of frozen sections. However, the name became a misnomer when the fresh-tissue technique was initiated in 1953 because the in situ chemical fixation was omitted and the layers were excised in a fresh, unfixed state. At first, the fresh-tissue technique was only partially accepted, but, after a report of a 100% 5-year cure of 66 basal cell carcinomas and 4 squamous cell carcinomas of the eyelids,[1] the acceptance was accelerated. However, the fixed-tissue technique continued to be used in the treatment of melanoma, and at the Mohs Surgery Clinic of the University of Wisconsin Hospital and Clinics at least 95% of melanomas are still removed by the fixed-tissue technique, although at least 95% of the basal and squamous cell carcinomas are now excised with the fresh-tissue technique.

To more clearly indicate the preference for the fresh-tissue technique, the members of the American College of Chemosurgery voted in 1986 to change the name of the organization to the American College of Mohs Micrographic Surgery and Cutaneous Oncology. The names of the two techniques and their abbreviated forms became Mohs micrographic surgery, fixed-tissue technique (MMS-fixed) and Mohs micrographic surgery, fresh-tissue technique (MMS-fresh).

THE FIXED-TISSUE TECHNIQUE

The following case illustrates the MMS-fixed technique. A relatively early nodular melanoma of 6-months duration arose in an area of melanosis of 3 years duration (there was no lentigo maligna, superficial spreading melanoma or nevus) (Figure 27.1A). Dichloroacetic acid was applied to the lesion and slightly beyond (Figure 27.1B). The zinc chloride fixative was applied (Figure 27.1C). The fixative was held in place by a thin layer of cotton. This in turn was covered with a layer of cotton spread with petrolatum for occlusion and taped in place. Treatment was completed after three stages (Figure 27.1D). The final layer of fixed tissue separated at the eleventh day (Figure 27.1E) and the scar was depigmented at 1 year (Figure 27.1F). The patient refused a prophylactic dissection of the regional nodes at the completion of treatment because of family illness. Six months after completion of treatment, a nodule appeared in the preauricular area and a superficial-lobe parotidectomy revealed four nodes with melanoma, but 22 cervical nodes were not involved. The facial nerve was preserved. At 5 years there was no recurrence in the primary or lymph node areas.

IMPORTANT TECHNICAL DETAILS

In preparation for use of MMS-fixed, a number of details for treatment of melanoma should be considered.[3-19] To minimize discomfort from the application of dichloroacetic acid for keratolysis and the fixative for fixation, an analgesic such as acetaminophen 300 mg plus codeine 30 mg may be prescribed and used as needed. If the lesion is large and in a location where a local anesthetic can be injected without getting so near to the melanoma that possible outgrowths or satellites might be disturbed, a local analgesic such as lidocaine 1% with epinephrine 1:100 000 is satisfactory. Often treatment of a small lesion does not hurt enough to require a local anesthetic.

The dichloroacetic acid, full strength, is applied until the skin is white. The melanoma remains black even though the skin overlying it has been penetrated. If the keratin is thick, scraping with a dull knife accelerates the penetration of the keratolytic.

The fixative is applied in a thickness that is calculated to produce fixation of the main mass of melanoma. After a period that may vary from 4 to 24 h the main mass of the melanoma is excised with a sharp scalpel and a gentle touch to avoid trauma to the underlying viable melanoma. Hemostasis is achieved by application of a

MOHS MICROGRAPHIC SURGERY FOR MELANOMA

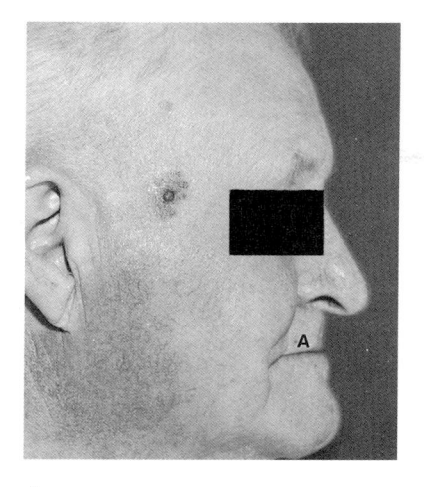

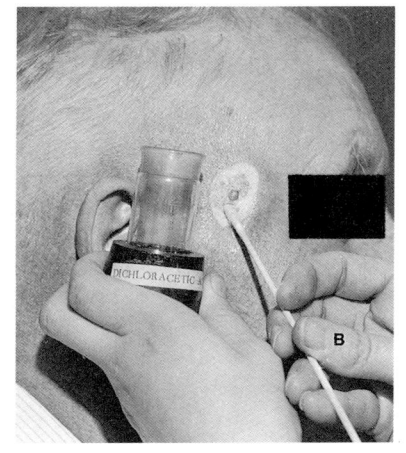

Figure 27.1
(A) Nodular melanoma Clark's level III. (B) Application of dichloroacetic acid. (C) Application of zinc chloride fixative. (D) Lesion when a negative plane was reached. The marks with 20% merbromin show the location of each specimen. (E) Removal of final layer of fixed tissue after 11 days. (F) Lesion after 1 year. After 5 years there was no recurrence in the primary or regional node areas. (Reproduced with permission.[2])

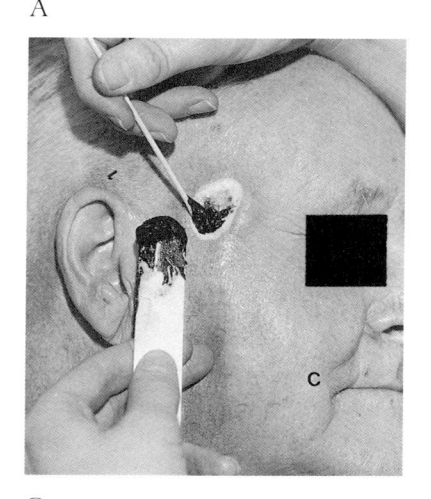

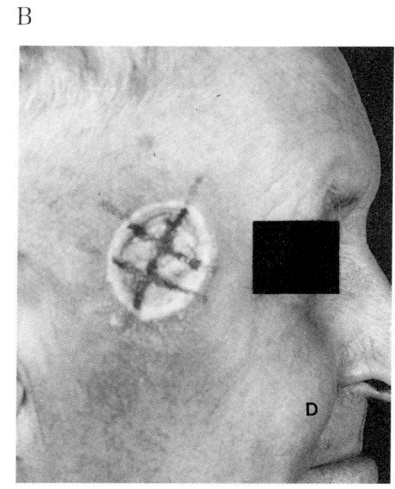

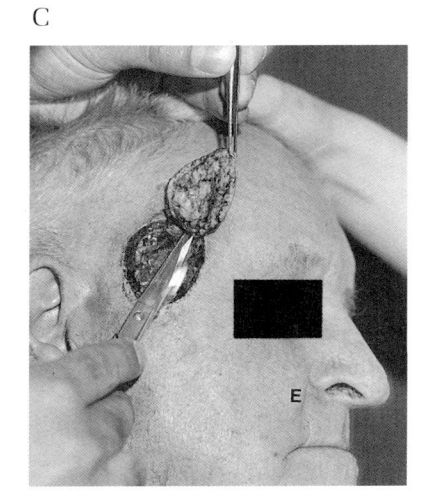

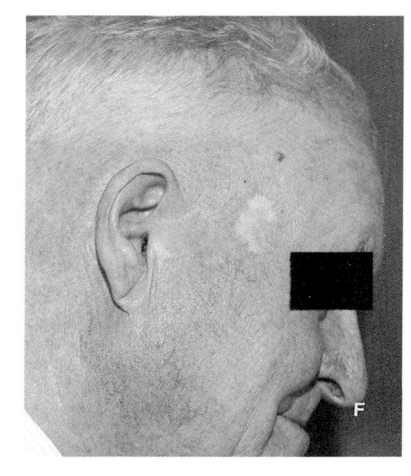

253

small square of gauze impregnated with the fixative under momentary pressure. Fulgeration, or any other source of heat, should be avoided because the tissue steam may impel emboli of melanoma cells into lymphatics according to Amadon.[20]

The first specimen is cut vertically and the frozen section is examined by the surgeon to assess the damage of malignancy as determined by the degree of anaplasia, invasion of vessel walls, extravasation and the number of mitoses. As successive layers are excised, the peripheral edges are incised at a 45° angle so the skin edge of the specimen can be readily assessed. It is important that a saucerized excision is used instead of making incisions with a 90° angle.

As the horizontally excised layers are removed and the melanoma is no longer grossly visible, the specimens are removed for frozen sections of their undersides. The thin sections (6 µm) that are cut with a cryostat, and hematoxylin and eosin staining, make the frozen sections easy to read.

Some clinicians prefer to wait for paraffin sections, but when one gets used to histologically interpreting the ramifications with frozen sections, the 4-h paraffin sections now available are not needed. Recognizing the unique pathology of the particular melanoma one is working with is essential.

Lessons Learned from Some Melanoma Cases

The following cases bring out points about the management of melanoma that are worth consideration. The first melanoma removed with MMS-fixed was a nodular melanoma above the ankle. It invaded the dermis and was 20 mm thick (Figure 27.2A). (Thirty years later, after publication of two classic articles, it would be Clark's level V[21] and Breslow's 20-mm thickness.[22])

The first lesson from this case was that radiation therapy is generally not effective in the treatment of melanoma. The radium plaque that had been used elsewhere had no detectable effect on the melanoma.

A second lesson concerned the question of how wide a surgical margin should be appropriate for this lesion. The melanoma was excised with MMS-fixed to a melanoma-free level (Figure 27.2B), but no extra margin was excised, though the microscopic sections showed moderate anaplasia, invasion of vessel walls, and extravasation. Six weeks later, several tiny satellites appeared and the MMS-fixed was extended for 2 cm beyond the satellites (Figure 27.2C). The lesson was that in view of the danger signs in the sections an extra layer should have been removed to see if there were satellites. The larger defect would have been acceptable since even the larger wound healed satisfactorily (Figure 27.2D).

Another lesson from this case is that satellites (up to 5 cm from the primary melanoma) and in-transit metastases (5 cm or more from the primary lesion, but within the same lymphatic drainage system) should not cause one to give up. Especially on the legs, the lymphatics can provide a filtering system that sometimes can prevent emboli from reaching the inguinal nodes.[11]

The value of a prophylactic groin dissection is unclear. There were no palpable nodes, but, considering the satellites, it was decided that dissection was probably indicated. Microscopic examination revealed no melanoma in the nodes. However, 6 weeks later a node appeared in the pubic area, a considerable distance medial to the groin dissection. This was excised and the patient remained free of melanoma for 30 years. The lesson is that prophylactic regional node dissection may not be indicated because the positive node may be in the backwaters of the lymphatic drainage system where the circulation is more sluggish and more likely to permit implantation of the melanomatous emboli.

Another lesson came from a patient whose lesion was on the preauricular

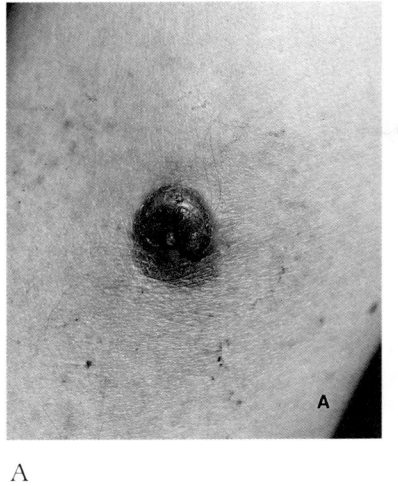

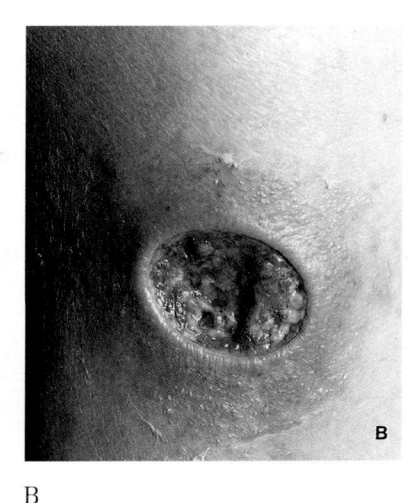

Figure 27.2
(A) A nodular melanoma, Clark's level V, above the ankle had not responded to radium treatment. (B) Granulations after removal to a negative level with MMS-fixed. (C) Six weeks later several tiny satellites appeared. With MMS-fixed the satellites and 2 cm beyond were removed. (D) Healed lesion. No recurrence in 30 years in spite of one metastasis in the pubic area that was surgically excised. (Reproduced with permission.[5])

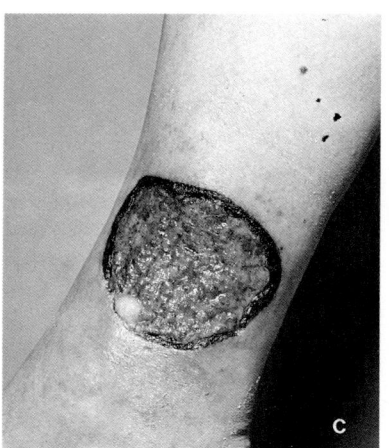

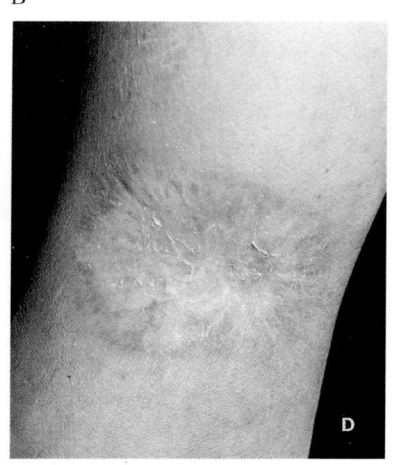

cheek. This was removed with MMS-fixed. Again, the regional nodes were not palpable, but it was deemed advisable to have a prophylactic dissection. Again the nodes were all negative for melanoma, but a few weeks later a palpable node appeared in the postauricular neck area a considerable distance from the usual radical neck dissection. The postauricular node was widely excised, but further positive nodes and systemic metastases led to a fatal outcome.

After these cases, the thought developed that prophylactic dissection often might be contraindicated. Close observation for enlarged nodes could be a preferable alternative although this may be controversial.

THE EFFECT OF THE TYPE OF MELANOMA ON THE WIDTH OF MARGINS

Melanomas of different types need different marginal widths because some have a greater tendency to develop

SURGICAL DERMATOLOGY

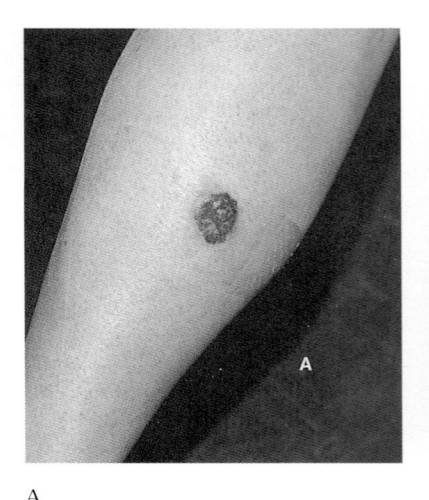

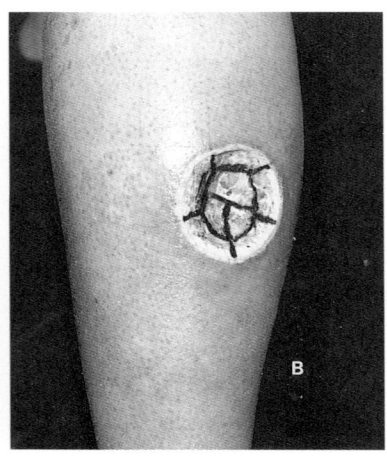

A B C D

Figure 27.3
(A) Nodular melanoma, Clark's level IV on the calf of the leg. (B) Lesion at end of excision of three layers with merbromin markings showing origin of the eight specimens. (C) Granulation tissue after separation of the final layer at 8 days. (D) Healed by second intention. No recurrence in 10 years. (Reproduced with permission.[2])

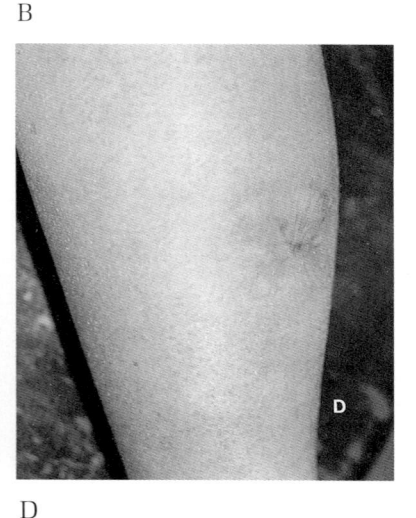

microsatellites than others. Usually, nodular melanomas are more likely to develop microsatellites than are superficial spreading or lentigo maligna melanomas. However, as shown in the melanoma in Figure 27.2, the microscopic appearance of the first excised layer can be important in making a decision. Thus, in the patient with a nodular melanoma on the calf of the leg, the first excised specimen showed anaplasia and some invasion of vessel walls, but no extravasation (Figure 27.3). This was a borderline case, but a third layer was removed to be sure whether or not there were minisatellites. At this level, the lesion was free of tumor and the patient remained free of melanoma for the usual 10-year follow-up.

Another example was a superficial spreading melanoma on the lower leg, Clark's level III, with no adverse microscopic features. This permitted cessation of treatment at a more conservative level (Figure 27.4). Again there was no recurrence in 10 years. The same good result occurred in a patient with a larger superficial spreading melanoma on the triceps area of the upper arm (Figure 27.5).

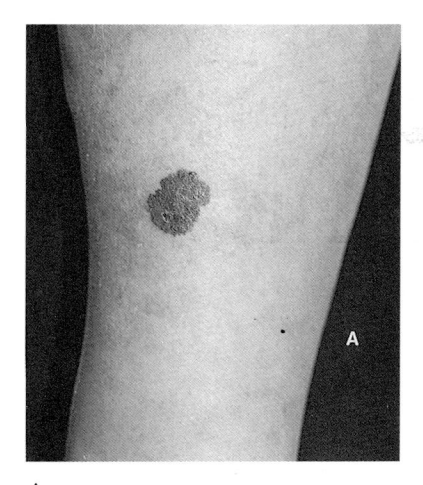

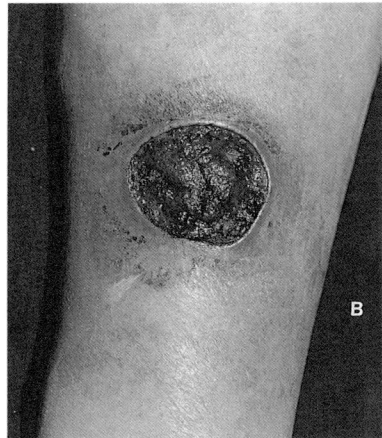

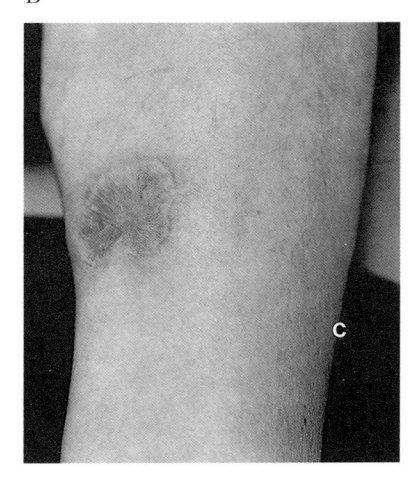

Lentigo maligna melanoma (LMM) is also less likely to develop microsatellites, but it can extend farther than the visible pigmentation. Often, outlying areas of pigmentation may appear to be entirely separate from a lentigo maligna (LM), but with the microscopic visualization is found to be connected.[19] Another example is the patient in Figure 27.6. There are no definite outlying foci of LMM, but the LM did extend considerably farther than the clinically visible border. However, the LM was very superficial so it was possible to save tissue, though the LMM did invade deeply in one area. Conservation of tissue as shown at the completion of treatment (Figure 27.6C), is the reason for the good result by second intention (Figure 27.6E).

FRESH-TISSUE TECHNIQUE FOR MELANOMA

The use of the fresh-tissue technique is limited at the University of Wisconsin Hospital to relatively small melanomas in locations where the local anesthetic can be injected without danger of the needle puncturing a tumor outgrowth or minisatellite. An example of such a case was an 89-year-old man with a small LMM

Figure 27.4
(A) Superficial spreading melanoma, Clark's level III on lower leg. (B) Granulation tissue 7 days later. (C) At 1 year the scar was pink, but this faded 6 months later. No recurrence in 10 years. (Reproduced with permission.[2])

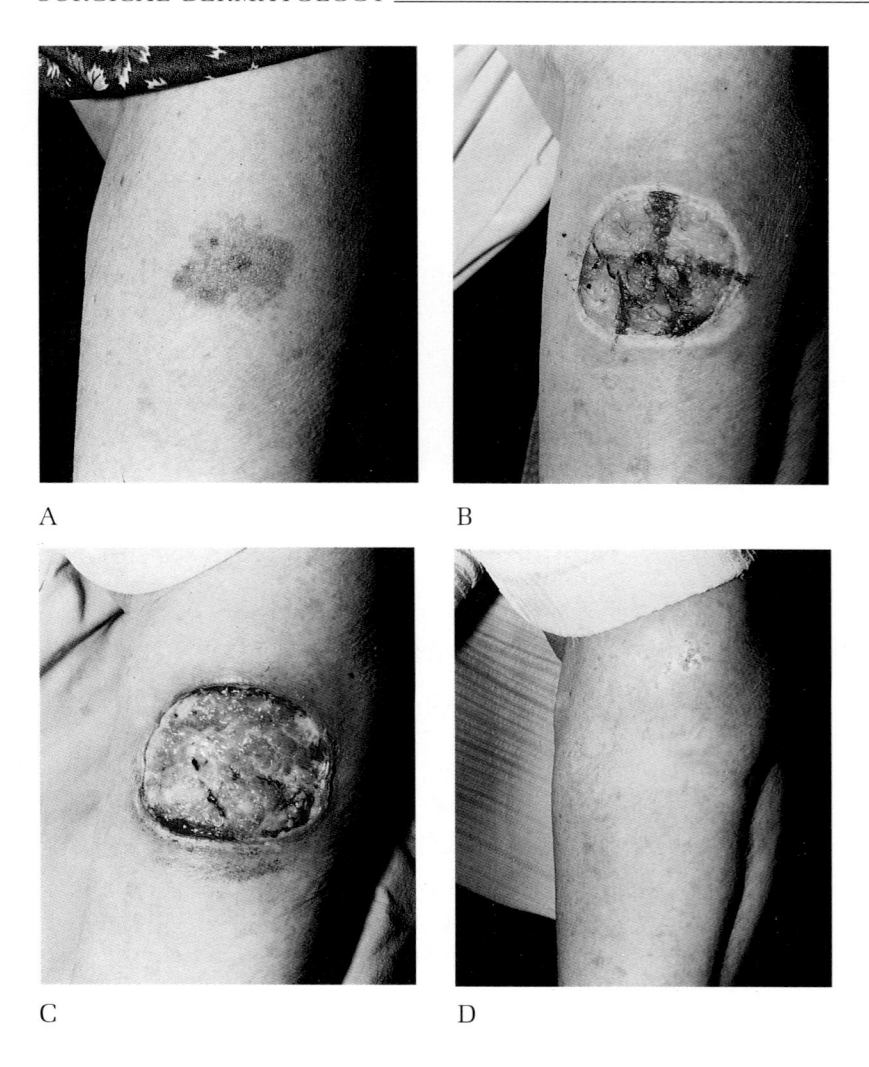

Figure 27.5
(A) Superficial spreading melanoma, triceps area of arm. (B) Lesion at completion in three stages. (C) Granulation tissue 7 days later. (D) Healed lesion after a year. No recurrence in 10 years.

on the lobe of the ear. He and his family were anxious to have the operation done in 1 day. The first layer was excised and the incisional surface was cauterized with dichloroacetic acid, not only to obtain hemostasis, but also to kill any melanoma cells that might be on the incisional surface. Then the second layer was excised and the surface was again cauterized with dichloroacetic acid. The underside of the layer was negative for melanoma. The patient and family drove home, the wound was left to heal by second intention and there was no recurrence when he died of other causes at age 93.

PERIORBITAL MELANOMA

Because melanoma in close contact with the eye cannot be treated with the fixed-tissue technique, the fresh-tissue technique is used as demonstrated by the following cases.[10] One patient had a superficial spreading, Clark's level V melanoma that began a year before in the medial canthus and spread over the cornea, halfway to the

MOHS MICROGRAPHIC SURGERY FOR MELANOMA

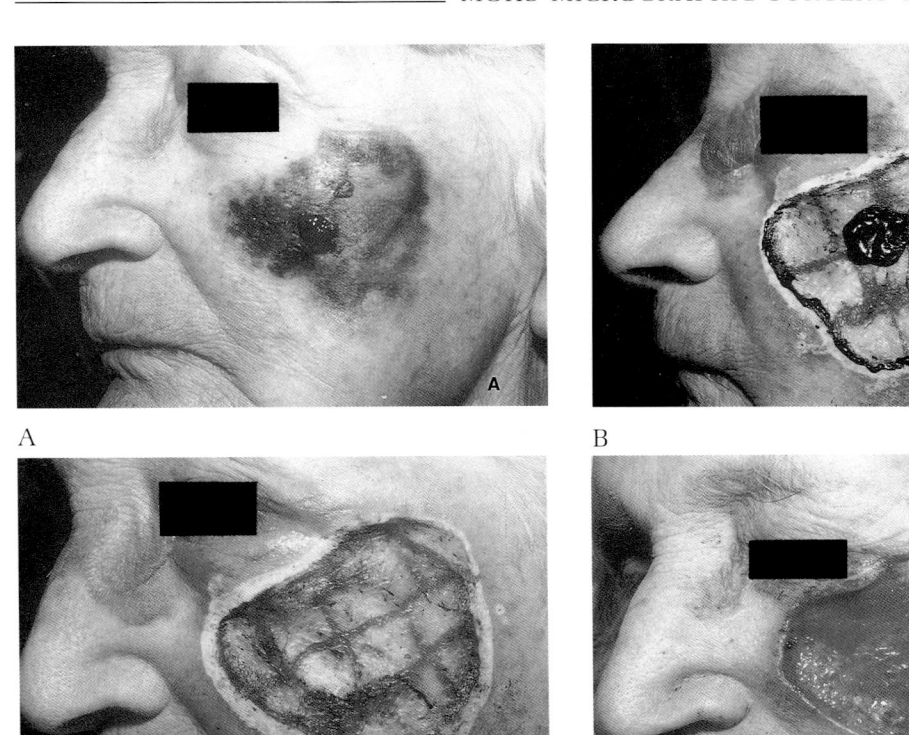

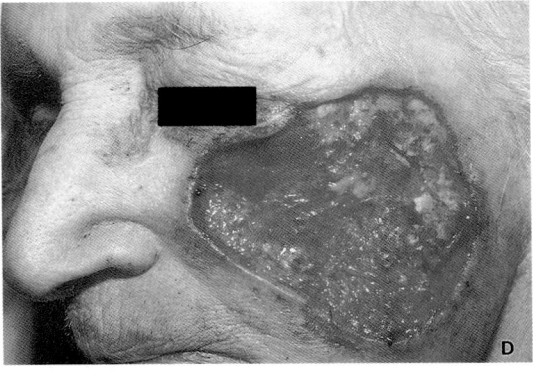

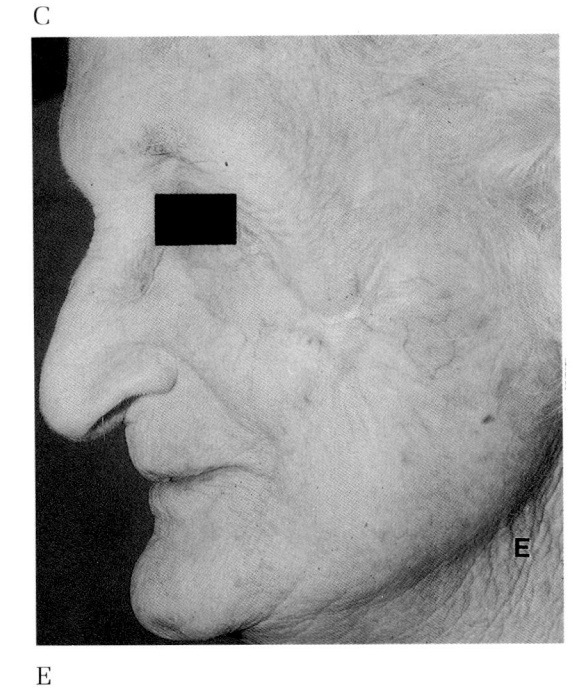

Figure 27.6
(A) Lentigo maligna melanoma, Clark's level V, in a large area of lentigo maligna. (B) The LMM extended deeply in one area, but LM was quite superficial though widespread. (C) At completion of MMS-fixed. (D) Granulation tissue after 8 days. (E) After 1 year. No recurrence in 4 years, when she died of a cardiac ailment. (Reproduced with permission.[2])

iris. Medially, the melanoma invaded the fossa of the lacrimal sac besides invading the medial eyelid margins and the medial canthus. Dichloroacetic acid was momentarily used for hemostasis, but the area was immediately irrigated with 4% boric acid solution. Because the melanoma extended as far as the lacrimal sac, that part was excised with MMS-fixed. The wounds healed by second intention and the eye and lids operated well at the 1-year checkup.

Another patient had an extensive superficial spreading melanoma that started on the medial lower lid and kept on spreading to involve all of both lid margins and canthi, despite various operations by an otolaryngologist and an oculoplastic surgeon. All of the excisions with MMS-fresh were performed under local anesthesia and the canthi were sutured so she could open and close her eye normally. A metastatic node in the right neck led to neck dissection by an oncologic surgeon. The patient continued her schoolteaching with bilateral vision for 3½ years but then developed a lung metastasis that caused her death.

Two other patients, each with nodular melanomas, one near the medial canthus and the other on the junction of the eyelid and cheek, were treated with MMS-fixed and were well for long-term follow-ups of 5 and 30 years. Both of these melanomas were far enough from the lid margins to make it safe to use MMS-fixed.

More use of the fresh-tissue technique may be feasible as the trend to earlier diagnosis of melanoma continues.

Table 27.1
Five-year results for three types of melanoma treated by fixed-tissue micrographic surgery[16]

Type of melanoma	Total number[a]	Indeterminate cases[b]	Determinate cases Total	Successful	Cure rate[c] (%)
Nodular	91[d]	18	73	38	52
Superficial spreading	66	14	52	40	77
Lentigo maligna	43	13	30	23	77
Total (all types)	200	45	155	101	65.2

[a]Series of consecutive patients with stage 1 melanomas.
[b]Patients without evidence of melanoma when they died or who were lost to follow-up before 5 years.
[c]Cure is defined as no evidence of local recurrence or metastases.
[d]Note the unusually high proportion of nodular melanomas.

Table 27.2
Effect of level of invasion on 5-year results of melanoma treated by fixed-tissue micrographic surgery[16]

Level (Clark)	Total number[a]	Indeterminate cases[b]	Determinate cases Total	Successful	Cure rate[c] (%)
II	45	9	36	32	89
III	45	11	34	30	88
IV	42	15	27	17	63
V	68[d]	10	58	22	38
Total	200	45	155	101	65.2

[a]Series of consecutive patients with stage I melanomas.
[b]Patients without evidence of melanoma when they died or who were lost to follow-up before 5 years.
[c]Cure is defined as no evidence of local recurrence or metastases.
[d]Note the unusually high proportion of level V melanomas.

Table 27.3
Results of Mohs surgery for melanomas treated by the fresh-tissue technique by Zitelli[16]

	Total number[a]	Indeterminate cases[b]	Determinate cases Total	Successful	Cure rate[c] (%)
5-year follow-up	36	10	26	23	88
2½-year follow-up	95	18	77	72	94

[a]Patients without evidence of melanoma when they died or who were lost to follow-up before 5 years or before 2½ years.
[b]Cure is defined as no evidence of local recurrence or metastases.
[c]Cure rate; no recurrence at 5-year follow-up or 2½-year follow-up.

However, as pointed out by Zitelli, the technique will differ from that used for other tumors.[16] First, the excision of the first layer is wider and deeper than is usual with basal or squamous cell carcinoma. Then the excisional surface is cauterized with dichloroacetic acid to eradicate melanoma and, with clean instruments, a second layer is excised more deeply than usual—3 mm or more, for microscopic scanning of the undersurface. Hemostasis can be by application of oxycel cotton or if necessary by suture ligation.

RESULTS

Meaningful statistics to compare the results of MMS with the results of conventional surgical excision will probably require a few more years of involvement by a greater number of participants in the melanoma registry that is under way. Our experience at the University of Wisconsin began in 1936 when the 5-year cure rate in the literature varied from 2–38% for conventional surgery.[16] Our series also includes many far-advanced lesions so the cure rate is not indicative of the present rate.

The results of fixed-tissue micrographic surgery for 200 stage I melanomas, with 5-year cure rates, are given for the three main types of melanoma in Table 27.1 and for the four Clark's levels of invasion in Table 27.2. The 5-year cure rate of 65.2% was achieved despite the high proportion of nodular melanomas and of those invading to Clark's level V.

The results of fresh-tissue micrographic surgery for 36 stage I melanomas at the 5-year follow-up and for 95 melanomas at 2½-year follow-up are given in Table 27.3. Innovations are constantly being developed to improve our treatment of one of the most dangerous forms of cancer. Hopefully, the idea of excising melanoma with complete microscopic control will soon be as widely accepted as it has been for the other forms of cutaneous cancer.

REFERENCES

1. Mohs FE, Cancer of eyelids, *Bull Am Coll Chemosurg* (1970) **3**:10–13.
2. Mohs FE, *Chemosurgery. Microscopically controlled surgery for skin cancer* (Charles C Thomas: Springfield, IL 1978) 225–48.
3. Mohs FE, Chemosurgery, a microscopically controlled method of cancer excision, *Arch Surg* (1941) **42**:279–95.
4. Mohs FE, Chemosurgical treatment of melanoma: a microscopically controlled method of excision, *Arch Dermatol Syph* (1950) **62**:269–79.
5. Mohs FE, *Chemosurgery in cancer, gangrene and infections* (Charles C Thomas: Springfield, IL 1956) 168–78.

6. Mohs FE, Chemosurgery for melanoma, *Arch Dermatol* (1977) **113**:285–91.

7. Mohs FE, Bloom RF, Sahl WL, Chemosurgery for familial malignant melanomas, *J Dermatol Surg Oncol* (1979) **5**:127–31.

8. Mohs FE, Chemosurgery, *Clin Plast Surg* (1980) **7**:349–60.

9. Mohs FE, The width and depth of malignant melanoma as observed by a chemosurgeon, *Am J Dermatopathol* (1984) **113**:285–91.

10. Mohs FE, Micrographically controlled surgery for periorbital melanoma. Fixed tissue and fresh tissue techniques, *J Dermatol Surg Oncol* (1985) **11**:284–91.

11. Mohs FE, Micrographic surgery for satellites and in-transit metastases of malignant melanoma, *J Dermatol Surg Oncol* (1986) **12**:471–6.

12. Fewkes J, Mohs FE, Microscopically controlled excision (the Mohs technique). In: Fitzpatrick TB, Eisen AZ, Wolf K et al, eds, *Dermatology in general medicine* (McGraw-Hill: New York 1987) 2557–63.

13. Mohs FE, Microscopically controlled surgery for skin cancer. In: Stark RB, ed, *Plastic surgery of the head and neck* (Churchill Livingstone: New York 1987) 253–60.

14. Mohs FE, Microcontrolled surgery for skin cancer. In: Epstein E, Epstein E Jr, eds, *Skin surgery* (WB Saunders: Philadelphia 1987) 380–95.

15. Mohs FE, Fixed-tissue micrographic surgery for melanoma of the ear, *Arch Otolaryngol Head Neck Surg* (1988) **114**:625–31.

16. Zitelli JA, Mohs FM, Larson PO et al, Micrographic surgery for melanoma. In: Lang PJ, Osguthorpe JD, eds, *Dermatologic clinics. Mohs micrographic surgery of the head and neck: a multidisciplinary approach* (WB Saunders: Philadelphia 1989) 833–43.

17. Mohs FE, Snow SN, Larson PO, Mohs micrographic surgery fixed-tissue technique for melanoma of the nose, *J Dermatol Surg Oncol* (1990) **16**:1111–20.

18. Zitelli JA, Mohs surgery for melanoma. In: Mikhail GR, ed., *Mohs micrographic surgery* (WB Saunders: Philadelphia 1991) 275–88.

19. Mohs FE, Snow SN, Malignant lesions. In: Parish LC, Lask GP, eds, *Aesthetic dermatology* (McGraw-Hill: New York 1991) 65–73.

20. Amadon PD, Electrocoagulation of the melanoma and its dangers, *Surg Gynecol Obstet* (1933) **56**:943–6.

21. Clark WJ, From L, Bernadino EA et al, Histogenesis and biologic behavior of primary human melanoma of the skin, *Cancer Res* (1968) **29**:705–27.

22. Breslow A, Thickness, cross-sectional area and depth of invasion in the prognosis of cutaneous melanoma, *Ann Surg* (1970) **172**:902–8.

Chapter 28

METASTASIS AND DEATH FROM THIN MELANOMA

Edward T. Creagan

There has been virtually universal acceptance of the importance of the thickness of a primary malignant melanoma in prognosis. The initial description of Clark's levels 1 to 5 has been subsequently refined by the Breslow technique, which initially indicated that lesions less than 0.76 mm have an excellent prognosis. A revision of that prognostic discriminant based upon data supplied by New York University and Massachusetts General Hospital clearly indicated at least a 90% 8-year disease-free survival for lesions less than 1.69 mm. Clinical observations at the Mayo Clinic are certainly consistent with those general guidelines. However, these observations have given the impression that there are a minority of patients whose lesions appear to be relatively 'favorable' but who succumb from metastatic disease.

In order to obtain adequate follow-up, 1370 patients seen at the Mayo Clinic were analyzed with a diagnosis of primary malignant melanoma.[1] Of these, 410 individuals were deemed to have 'thin melanomas', defined as lesions less than 0.76 mm. A single pathologist, Dr Edward H Soule, retrospectively reviewed the Breslow's thickness on each lesion. Twenty individuals who experienced metastatic disease from these lesions were then documented. Upon subsequent review, eight patients did not have sufficiently documented thickness or possibly had metastatic disease from some other lesion and hence these patients were not included in the study.

For 12 individuals, 1–10 blocks of tissue were available; six of these 12 were biopsied at Mayo Clinic, and six patients were seen after a biopsy at some other institution. That tissue was reviewed at Mayo. As noted in Table 28.1, there was a prominence of men with an age range of 30–69 years. There did not seem to be a predominant primary site of the primary lesion nor did there appear to be a predominance of metastatic disease in a specific organ.

These findings have led the author to the careful redefinition and reappraisal of the notions of primary malignant melanoma. The situation is remotely comparable to that of stage I breast cancer or stage I bronchogenic carcinoma of the non-small-cell variety. The vast majority of patients may well be cured by a surgical procedure, but there is a minority of perhaps 10–15% who may develop recurrent disease and succumb at 5 years from their lesions. It is certainly true that lesions less than 0.76 mm in thickness are

Table 28.1
Poor survival in patients with thin melanomas

Patient No.	Sex	Age	Tissue source	Type of melanoma	Thickness (mm)	Level	Primary site	Date of Dx of primary	Metastasis site	Date of metastasis	Status of patient
1	M	64	EW	SS	0.43	II	Left subscapular region	19/4/76	Neck Abdomen	4/78	Dead 10/80
2	M	43	EW	SS	0.75	III	Left clavicle	1966[a]	Vertebral	10/74	Dead 6/75
3	M	36	MC	SS	0.3	III	Mid-back	1/73	Pulmonary hepatic	8/75	Dead 6/76
4	M	63	EW	Nodular	0.45	IV	Left scapular	10/72	Pulmonary	5/74	Dead 10/74
5	F	51	EW	Nodular	0.52	III	Left thigh	5/69[a]	Left groin	10/71	NED 1981 (10 year postsurgery)
6	M	64	EW	SS	0.75	IV	Right breast	10/74	Right axilla Chest wall	1/77	Dead 11/77
7	M	59	MC	SS	0.75	IV	Right upper posterior neck	10/74	Brain	10/78	Dead 1/79
8	M	50	MC	SS	0.53	IV	Right forehead	2/75	Brain	9/77	Dead 12/77
9	M	50	MC	SS	0.75	IV	Left lower back	1/73	Lung	?	Dead 7/74
10	F	69	MC	SS	0.48	II	Sacral area	6/70	Inguinal Generalized	1/73 1/75	Dead 9/76
11	F	30	MC	SS	0.63	III	Right arm	4/72	Abdominal	5/72	Dead 1/73
12	M	43	EW	SS	0.75	IV	Scalp	12/70	Neck Brain Liver	7/76 4/77	Dead 10/77

[a]Patient first seen at Mayo Clinic after 1969 but original tissue blocks procured EW, elsewhere; SS, superficial spreading; MC, Mayo Clinic; NED, no evidence of disease.

essentially innocuous, but patients must be aware that there is still the risk of metastatic disease, albeit remote.

Although the series reported here is relatively small and there certainly could be technical factors accounting for the findings, the senior consulting pathologist involved has had extensive experience in the investigation of malignant melanoma, and it seems highly unlikely that there is some type of error in the thickness determinations. On the other hand, it is conceivable that a deeper penetration of the tumor was not detected on the reviewed section. However, it would seem unlikely that this event would apply to the 12 patients in this study. It should be pointed out that if one 'discarded' the six patients whose biopsies were elsewhere and relied only on the initial biopsy from the Mayo Clinic, there are still six individuals who developed metastatic disease from lesions which should have had a more hopeful prognosis.

It is certainly possible that the patients who died from melanoma had a primary lesion which was not detected. Upon careful clinical review of pertinent medical data, it seems highly improbable that all the patients or even a majority of patients in this study had an occult primary lesion. Another possibility is that the patient's initial lesion may have been relatively thick but under the influences of immunologic factors may have regressed. However, there was no histological evidence to suggest that patients initially had 'thick' lesions which subsequently underwent regression.

The caveat from this relatively meager sample is that regardless of the thickness of the malignant melanoma, patients and primary caregivers and certainly dermatologists should be aware that a small percentage of patients, 1 or 2%, may develop metastatic disease, and this typically results in the demise of the patient.

SURVEILLANCE

It is obvious that all malignant melanomas beyond level I have metastatic potential regardless of their thickness and regardless of their levels of invasion. There are relatively few rigid guidelines for every patient with malignant melanoma, but the following generalities might provide a framework for surveillance.[2,3] For individuals with lesions less than 0.85 mm the prognosis is sufficiently hopeful so that patients could be reassessed with a history and physical examination, chest radiograph routine hematologic and chemical indices, including liver function parameters, as well as a careful total skin examination at quarterly intervals for approximately 1 year, then every 6 months during the second and third years, and then on a yearly basis thereafter. For the exceptionally thin lesion, there is probably a greater risk of the patient developing a second primary malignant melanoma than metastasis from the initial lesion.

For lesions of more ominous thickness (0.85–1.69 mm), it would seem reasonable to re-evaluate the patient at quarterly intervals for 2 years and then at 6-month intervals for an indefinite period of time. For lesions greater than 1.69 mm or individuals with nodal involvement, it would seem appropriate to reassess the individual at quarterly intervals for 3 years and then at 6-month intervals for an indefinite period of time. It is acknowledged and recognized here that these guidelines of surveillance are subjective and arbitrary and should be appropriately modified according to clinical circumstances.

The role of routine CT studies of the chest, abdomen and pelvis, bone scan, and an MR study of the brain is controversial and must be recommended in the appropriate clinical context. Generally speaking, the yield of these techniques in the asymptomatic patient is vanishingly low. However, the author has had the experience of patients with melanoma whose complaints seem completely trivial and innocuous and yet who were shown to have metastatic disease by imaging techniques. Therefore, the importance of a history cannot be overestimated. Individuals with frontal lobe metastases may have subtle and transient cognitive dysfunction which ordinarily would not warrant a CT study, but this certainly would be appropriate if there is a history of malignant melanoma. Likewise, patients with symptoms which ordinarily might be thought to be functional should be appropriately investigated.

A detailed discussion of cytotoxic, immunomodulatory, adoptive immunotherapeutic and regional perfusion techniques is beyond the scope of this chapter, but the following guidelines are generally applicable to patients being considered for systemic therapy for malignant melanoma (Figure 28.1).

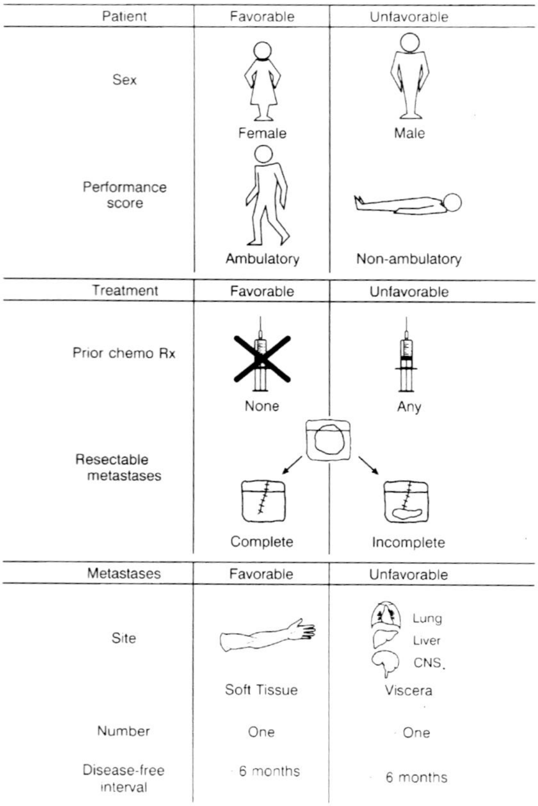

Histological documentation of presumed metastatic disease, especially if there has been a prolonged interval between the initial diagnosis and the current clinical situation

With the advent of CT- and ultrasound-directed biopsies and refinements in fine-needle aspiration technologies, most lesions are accessible to at least cytological documentation.

Progressive symptoms or rapidly accelerating disease

Although the tempo of advanced melanoma is usually that of relentless progression, some patients may have relatively indolent metastatic disease which would not necessarily warrant an aggressive systemic intervention. The individual with a small number of asymptomatic pulmonary lesions or patients with relatively quiescent subcutaneous nodules might be well served by close surveillance rather than a potentially toxic and obviously palliative systemic approach. It would also seem appropriate to 'debulk' extensive subcutaneous disease, especially if it can be performed without general anesthesia. The procedure may obviate the development of painful, necrotic lesions. However, there appears to be little merit in attempting to debulk extensive visceral metastases.

Individuals with more than 10% weight loss within the previous 3 months or those

Figure 28.1
Prognostic factors in disseminated malignant melanoma.

consuming less than 1200 calories per day are high-risk patients for systemic therapy for malignant melanoma. The patient who is bedfast or sedentary for at least 50% of his waking hours (Eastern Cooperative Oncology Group performance score of 3 or 4) and the cachectic, debilitated patient are at high risk for therapy-induced sequelae and there is very little possibility of long-term benefit.

Adequate psychosocial support

Since virtually any therapy for malignant melanoma is potentially toxic, the implications for the patient and the nuclear and extended family are profound. A marginally informed patient, especially without a core nucleus of caregivers, is hardly an ideal candidate for investigational or conventional therapies. Obviously, the patient who is alone would never be excluded from therapy but factors of community support cannot be discarded in considering potentially toxic treatments which are virtually never curative in this setting.

Patients and relevant caregivers should be aware of the obvious risks, benefits, options and alternatives relating to systemic therapies. Patients should be informed that treatment is almost never 'curative' in the usual sense of the word, and even if an objective response is obtained, there is little evidence that this event would meaningfully impact upon survival. As noted in Figure 28.2, the median times of progression and survival from a typical clinical trial are approximately 2 months and 6 months, respectively. Nevertheless, there may be some long-term survivors. Patients should also understand the option of symptomatic and supportive care with palliative interventions. If patients do not elect to participate in an investigational or conventional systemic approach, they should be offered the security of close follow-up to address symptomatic issues as they might arise.

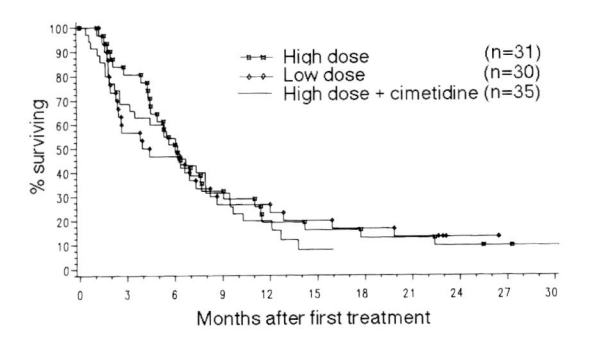

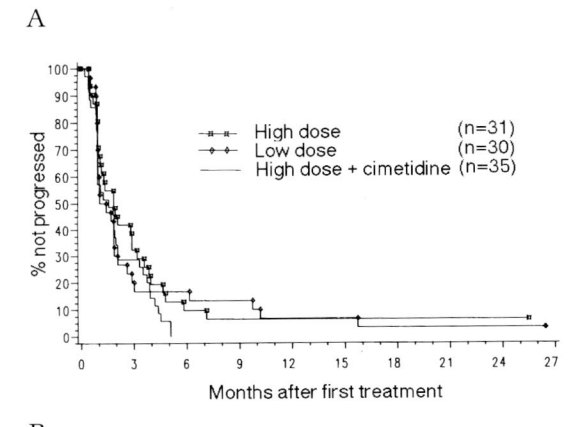

Figure 28.2
Typical survival (A) and progression (B) curves for patients with advanced melanoma receiving high- or low-dose interferon + cimetidine.[2]

For patients participating in investigational phase II studies and also for those receiving conventional therapy, it is important to have an objective measurable or assessable parameter by which to address the efficacy of therapy. This typically would consist of lesions detected on chest radiograph, CT studies, or palpable abnormalities on physical examination. The conscientious and reliable reporting of these parameters is crucial so that patients are not needlessly treated with a therapy which is clearly ineffective.

Although, as with any tumor system, there is an enormous spectrum of response rates from various therapies, it does appear from ongoing evaluations that the objective response rate from interferon, interleukin 2 and various types of chemotherapy is approximately 20%.[4-7] Obviously, there are isolated case reports typically involving a relatively small number of patients with much higher response rates, but a reasonable figure to share with patients and their family members would be the aforementioned number. From most studies the median duration of response is approximately 4-6 months with a median survival of approximately 8-10 months from the onset of therapy. However, it is important to recognize that these numbers are general guidelines for discussion, and there are some individuals who do extraordinarily well from systemic therapies, albeit a minority.

References

1. Woods JE, Soule EH, Creagan ET, Metastasis and death in patients with thin melanomas (less than 0.76 mm), *Ann Surg* (1983) **198**:63–5.
2. Creagan ET, Regional and systemic strategies for metastatic malignant melanoma, *Mayo Clin Proc* (1989) **64**:852–60.
3. Creagan ET, Malignant melanoma. In: Brain MC, Carbone PP, eds, *Current therapy in hematology-oncology 3* (BC Decker: Philadelphia 1988) 305–9.
4. Creagan ET, Schaid DJ, Ahmann DL et al, Disseminated malignant melanoma and recombinant interferon: analysis of seven consecutive Phase II investigations, *J Invest Dermatol* (1990) **95**:188S–92S.
5. Rosenberg SA, Lotze MT, Muul LM et al, A progress report on the treatment of 157 patients with advanced cancer using lymphokine-activated killer cells and interleukin-2 or high-dose interleukin-2 alone, *N Engl J Med* (1987) **316**:889–97.
6. van Haelst-Pisani CM, Pisani RJ, Kovach JS, Cancer immunotherapy: current status of treatment with interleukin-2 and lymphokine-activated killer cells, *Mayo Clin Proc* (1989) **64**:451–65.
7. Quirt IC, Tannock IF, Interleukin-2 for metastatic melanoma: treating polyuria with insulin? *J Clin Oncol* (1990) **8**:1125–7.

Section III

LASERS

29. LOW–FLUENCE CO_2 LASER IRRADIATION
Jeffrey S. Dover, Mitra Mofid

30. THE SUPERPULSED CO_2 LASER
Richard E. Fitzpatrick, Javier Ruiz-Esparza

31. NEWER USES FOR THE CO_2 LASER
Pamela K. Miller, Rokea A. el-Azhary, Randall K. Roenigk

32. HUMAN PAPILLOMAVIRUS
Mark W. Cobb

33. THE LASER PLUME
Neil P.J. Walker

34. SUPERFICIAL VASCULAR LASERS: YELLOW LIGHT AND 532 NM
Timothy J. Rosio

35. PSYCHOLOGICAL DISABILITIES OF HEMANGIOMA
J.A. Cotterill

36. PHOTODYNAMIC THERAPY FOR SKIN CANCER
Scott M. Dinehart, Stephen Flock

37. THE Q–SWITCHED RUBY AND Nd–YAG LASERS
Ronald G. Wheeland

38. NEODYMIUM YAG LASER
Dudley Hill, Diamondis J. Papadopoulos, Hubert T. Greenway

Chapter 29

LOW-FLUENCE CO_2 LASER IRRADIATION

Jeffrey S. Dover
Mitra Mofid

The carbon dioxide (CO_2) laser has been used primarily as a tool to cut, coagulate, char or vaporize tissue using high-energy radiant exposures (fluences) from 20 to over 20 000 J/cm².[1] By the use of lower fluences, however, the CO_2 laser can be used to selectively damage the epidermis, thereby providing the ability to selectively destroy epidermal lesions. The 10.6-µm CO_2 laser wavelength is well absorbed by water-containing cells. All epidermal cells within the first 10–20 µm of skin, except the stratum corneum, nonselectively absorb the laser energy, and subsequent damage to underlying tissue occurs via heat conduction.[2] Kamat et al demonstrated that selective damage limited primarily to the epidermis could be achieved with low-dose CO_2 laser irradiation of skin using fluences limited to 3.8–5.7 J/cm² in human explanted skin,[2] and similar results have been found in guinea pig skin.[1] At these fluences, little or no immediate clinical alteration was seen. Histological evidence of thermal damage began in the basal layer, at the dermal–epidermal (D–E) junction, and extended throughout the entire epidermis.[2] Limiting thermal damage to the papillary dermis was predicted to lead to a decreased chance of scarring, and results suggested that low-dose CO_2 lasers could be used in the treatment of epidermal lesions.[2]

CO_2 IRRADIATION OF LENTIGINES

Clinical studies

To evaluate the therapeutic effectiveness of low-dose CO_2 laser irradiation for epidermal pigmented lesions, Dover et al focused on solar lentigines as examples of benign epidermal lesions in which the response to treatment could be measured by the disappearance of pigment.[3]

Based on the results of a dose–response study in a patient with lentigines caused by treatment with methoxsalen and ultraviolet A light (PUVA), 146 solar lentigines located on the face, trunk and upper extremities in five patients were irradiated with fluences of 3.0, 3.7 or 4.4 J/cm², without anesthesia of any kind. Neighboring lentigines were left untreated to serve as controls. For a period of 6 weeks following therapy, patients were asked to gently clean treated sites with soap and water and to apply Bacitracin ointment daily as well as to avoid sun exposure and to apply sunscreen with a sun protection factor of 15. Patient discomfort, lesion edema, erythema, crusting, atrophic or hypertrophic scarring and pigmentary change were recorded immediately (within 15 min) at 1, 7, 14, 21 and 42 days after irradiation. Lesions were followed with photographs taken under standardized conditions, and color change was assessed by comparing both the treated site and a photograph of the treated site with the photograph taken before treatment. Strict criteria were established regarding lesion lightening, and only when abnormal pigmentation was uniformly and fully removed was the result considered to be 'completely clear'.

Laser irradiation of solar lentigines resulted in degrees of pain, opalescence, erythematous flare, edema and crusting at the fluences of 3.0, 3.7 and 4.4 J/cm². Of the 146 solar lentigines treated, 25 of the 30 lesions that underwent biopsy, which included all lentigines treated at 3.0 J/cm², were clinically unevaluable, leaving 121 solar lentigines that were followed up clinically for 6 weeks. Of these, almost 10% cleared completely, and more than two-thirds lightened substantially (Figure 29.1). Although the results showed a trend for more complete clearing at the higher fluence, chi-squared analysis failed to show a statistically significant difference.

None of the patients had significant complications as a result of therapy. Slight erythema remained at 6 weeks in 10 treatment sites but resolved completely at 10 weeks in all cases. There was no resultant depigmentation, hyperpigmentation or hypertrophic scarring, although slight atrophic textural change was noted in two sites treated with 4.4 J/cm². One of the two patients with psoriasis did, however, develop an isomorphic response at three of the sites treated while the psoriasis was active.

Histological study

A total of thirty 2-mm biopsy specimens of treated solar lentigines from five patients

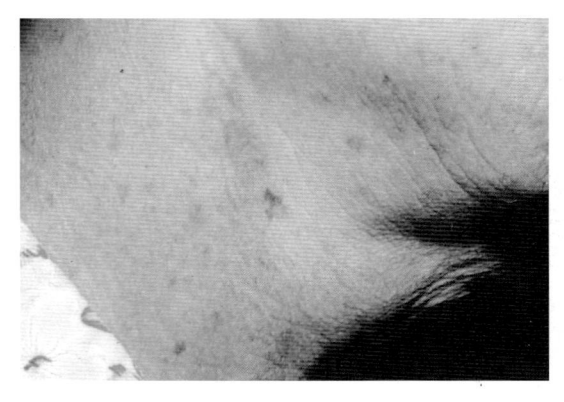

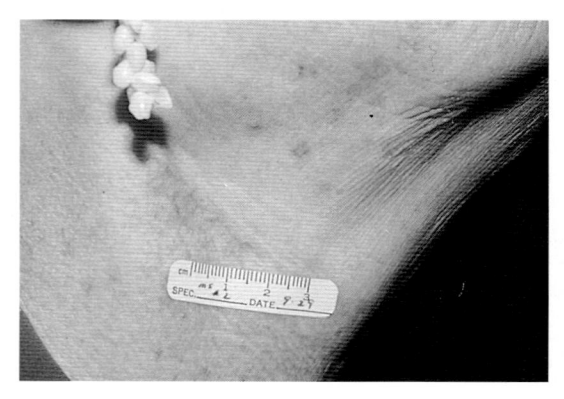

Figure 29.1
(A) Lateral neck of a 60-year-old woman with extensive lentigines. (B) Three weeks after treatment of the dark brown lentigo appearing in the center of (A) with 9 W of low-fluence CO_2 for a 0.1-s exposure.

receiving three different doses of laser radiation at 0, 1, 7 and 42 days were examined.[3] Each patient had biopsies performed on from three to seven treated sites, and specimens were obtained under local anesthesia with 1% lidocaine solution without epinephrine. All of the specimens were fixed in 4% buffered formaldehyde solution and cut at 4–6 μm before being stained with hematoxylin and eosin, Verhoff and van Gieson, and

Masson's trichrome. Each specimen was evaluated independently by two pathologists, who were blinded to treatment specifics, on a four-point scale with regard to parameters of: epidermal pigmentation; dermal and epidermal inflammation; basilar epidermal vacuolization and spindling; necrosis; clefting of the D–E junction; cautery effect; and epidermal regeneration.

The specimens that were obtained immediately after treatment showed extensive basal epidermal pigmentation, consistent with their classification as solar lentigines. Immediate histological injury consisted of marked vacuolization and spindling of the basilar epidermis, with dose-dependent clefting of the D–E junction and cautery effect (stromal condensation and basophilia) extending up to 0.1 mm into the papillary dermis present in the specimens treated with the highest-energy dose. No inflammation or necrosis was present.

Twenty-four hours after laser therapy, extensive epidermal necrosis with focal epidermal regeneration (Figure 29.2) and marked basilar vacuolization could be appreciated. Clefting along the basement membrane, as well as a predominantly lymphocytic infiltrate within the epidermis and perivascular papillary dermis, were present in all '24-h' biopsy specimens. Alterations were, again, dose-dependent.

By 1 week after treatment, epidermal regeneration was complete. Pigment lightening depended on the dose of radiation received, but in all cases new scattered pigment-laden macrophages could be identified. A scant amount of dermal inflammatory infiltrate could still be noted, and a residual cautery effect extending up to 0.1 mm below the D–E junction was seen in lesions other than those treated with the lowest energy levels.

Melanophages persisted at 6 weeks, but there was no evidence of lentiginous elongation of the rete ridges. The inflammatory infiltrate had cleared, and epidermal pigmentation had returned to normal.

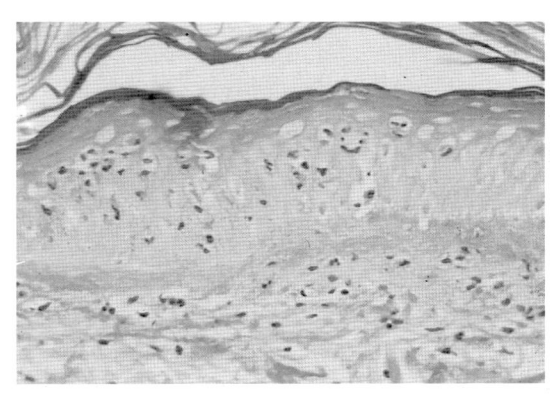

Figure 29.2
Twenty-four hours after treatment with 0.1 s of 6.0-W low-fluence CO_2 exposure. Extensive epidermal necrosis with focal epidermal regeneration may be appreciated above subtle clefting along the basement membrane. Also noted is a predominantly lymphocytic infiltrate within the epidermis and perivascular papillary dermis.

Immunohistochemical study

As epidermal regeneration depends on an intact dermis to act as a foundation, low-fluence CO_2 laser irradiation, by virtually sparing dermal tissue, provides a natural tool for the study of epidermal regeneration. Although immunohistochemical analyses of the structural proteins of mature epidermis and routine histological examinations of the developing epidermis have been previously performed,[4] Smoller et al were the first to use low-dose CO_2-laser-irradiated human epidermis to study expression characteristics of maturational markers to gain a better understanding of the regenerating epidermis following thermal injury.[5]

Cytokeratins, a family of proteins with molecular weights ranging from 40 000 to 70 000, are responsible for the formation of tonofilaments within epidermal keratinocytes. The proteins are found stratified by weight within the epidermis, with lower molecular weight keratins being found throughout the normal epidermis and higher molecular weight keratins usually localized to the higher layers of the epidermis. Monoclonal antibodies to the various classes of keratins have been prepared.[6] AE1 preferentially stains the basal layer of normal human epidermis and AE3 stains all suprabasilar keratinocytes, especially those appearing within the stratum granulosum.

Involucrin is a protein bound to the membranes of keratinocytes that acts as a substrate for keratinocyte-specific transglutaminase. In normal squamous epithelium, involucrin is expressed only in cells within the stratum granulosum and therefore serves as a marker for terminal squamous differentiation.

Skin punch biopsies from the previous study[3] were cut for immunoperoxidase studies. After the tissue was deparaffinized, sections were incubated first with primary and then with secondary antibodies before being localized with avidin–biotin peroxidase complexes, which could be visualized using diaminobenzidine as the chromagen. AE1, AE3 and involucrin expression within the tissues were evaluated by investigators blinded to the interval after treatment. The results of the immunoperoxidase studies were correlated with routine histological findings.

Immediately after treatment, AE1-staining low molecular weight cytokeratins that had been extruded from dying keratinocytes could be seen diffusely throughout the epidermis; by 24 h, they could be found within the dermis. Also at 24 h, the cytoplasm of newly formed keratinocytes could be stained with AE1 with a resultant granular character of variable intensity. By 1 week following laser injury, keratinocytes throughout the epidermis could still be stained by AE1, although a basal predominance to the pattern was beginning to emerge. Six weeks after treatment, the normal pattern of predominantly basilar, AE1 staining returned.

AE3-staining high molecular weight cytokeratins extruded from dying keratinocytes could also be seen immediately following treatment, and they rapidly appeared within dermal macrophages. Nascent keratinocytes stained strongly and diffusely with AE3 and persisted with this pattern until 6 weeks, when staining of the stratum granulosum was found to predominate.

Involucrin expression also changed with laser therapy. After treatment, this protein marker for terminal differentiation could be found throughout the entire epidermis, as well as within dermal macrophages. At 24 h following injury, involucrin expression was virtually absent. By 1 week after treatment, significant involucrin production could be found diffusely throughout 80% of the epidermis, although the most mature keratinocytes stained with greatest intensity. By 6 weeks following initial injury, the normal pattern of intense involucrin staining limited to the stratum granulosum had returned.

The orderly pattern of cellular protein production within mature epidermal tissue is well known.[6,7] The immunohistochemical study by Smoller et al, however, followed rapidly growing epidermis after laser-induced thermal injury to describe a dynamic state of keratinocyte protein expression which undergoes several transitions before attaining the stratified pattern of mature epidermis.[5] Their findings suggest that nascent keratinocytes extend from neighboring unaffected epidermis within a day of thermally-induced injury. The new cells then extend into the defect along the D–E junction, forming a layer that is a few cells thick by 24 h. The initial keratinocytes produce cytokeratins and involucrin without obvious stratification, appearing to be stimulated to express a wider range of proteins than they do under the stable conditions found in fully developed skin.

One week after injury, although routine histological evaluation depicts a relatively normal-appearing full-thickness epidermis, the picture afforded by the added detail of immunohistochemical staining suggests that the new keratinocytes differ from cells found at the steady state by retaining their ability to produce a spectrum of various proteins. By 6 weeks after laser treatment, both the histological picture and the staining profile of epidermis return to the baseline stratified steady state.

The Smoller et al study supported results from previous work[4] in concluding that antigen expression within individual keratinocytes is capable of being modified during maturation or regeneration. Investigations to date support a pattern of keratinocyte protein expression within regenerating epidermis that is independent of the manner of injury.

Although the pattern of epidermal regrowth appears to be constant and without regard to the mode of injury, it has been shown that wounds that are laser-induced heal more slowly than those caused by mechanical forces.[8] It is not known whether the difference can be ascribed to differences in keratinocyte proliferative capacity or to differences in migratory capability, or even a combination of the two. These aspects of keratinocyte biology following laser-induced thermal injury will have to await the results of subsequent studies.

CONTROLLED COMPARATIVE TRIALS OF LOW-DOSE CO_2 WITH OTHER LASER AND NONLASER MODALITIES

In the last 5 years, several new lasers have been developed for the treatment of benign epidermal and dermal pigmented lesions such as solar lentigines. Some of these medical devices have been approved for the treatment of lentigines while others still await FDA sanctioning. Physicians gladly offer and patients often seek laser treatment for cutaneous diseases in the belief that lasers are superior to conventional therapies, with regard to both efficaciousness and scarring. Yet well-controlled comparative studies that assess the relative efficacy and safety of these new technologies are lacking, even for the cutaneous applications in which they are most often used.

Although both the low-fluence CO_2 laser and the argon laser using a shuttered scanning delivery system (Dermascan) are safe and effective in reducing the pigmentation of solar lentigines, the role of these expensive therapies has not been established in the treatment of benign epidermal pigmented lesions through comparative trials that include both competing new technologies and long-established low-technology treatments which are considered the standard of care. Recently, these two laser technologies were compared by Stern et al, in a prospective, controlled fashion, to cryotherapy, the long-established standard therapy of lentigines.[9]

In the trial, Stern et al compared low-fluence CO_2 laser radiation (LFCO$_2$), argon laser light delivered by a Dermascan shuttered delivery system (ADS), and cryosurgery with liquid nitrogen (LN$_2$), for the treatment of solar lentigines. A total of 99 sites were treated in 13 patients who completed the study. For each patient, from five to nine 4-cm^2 areas, each of which contained at least one lentigo, were treated with one of three options.

1. A Coherent CO_2 laser model 450XL (Coherent lasers, Palo Alto, CA) providing fluences ranging from 3 to 5 J/cm^2 was used with an exposure time of 0.1 s on a spot size of 4.5 mm employing irradiances of 3, 4.5 and 6 W.

2. A Coherent Radiation model 1000 argon laser and a Coherent Dermascan Delivery System (Argon Dermascan (ADS)) provided power ranging from 0.5 to 0.9 W and resulted in fluences of less than 1 J/cm². The areas were treated both horizontally and vertically, so that all hyperpigmented areas within the treatment square received two exposures of a beam moving at a rate of 1 cm/s.
3. Cryosurgery (LN$_2$) was performed with liquid nitrogen from an Owens Cryovac-R pressurized thermos canister (Brymill Corp., Vernon, CT) fitted with a 0.3-mm tip that was held 3 cm from the lesion and sprayed continuously for 1–5 s after the entire pigmented area turned white.

Optimal doses for all treatment modalities were based on previous studies. Photographs were taken immediately prior to and after treatments as well as 1 and 8 weeks later using standardized photographic equipment. The treated sites were assessed independently by four dermatologists, who viewed color kodachromes of the same site obtained both before and 8 weeks after treatment. Each rater separately evaluated decrease in pigmentation and textural (for example atrophic) change based on a point scale. An excellent result required a substantial decrease in pigmentation or a return to normal skin color and no textural change. At least moderate lightening corresponding to no more than slight textural change was deemed sufficient to merit a good result. Statistical methods were employed to evaluate the data.

Treatment with LN$_2$ was approximately four times more likely to achieve lightening to the point of normal skin than ADS or LFCO$_2$ therapy ($P < 0.05$). Moderate scarring was rarely appreciated and occurred with the use of all three modalities. The magnitude of lightening related positively to the frequency of textural change ($P < 0.0009$, Mann Whitney Test). A good or excellent result was noted in comparable portions of lesions treated with LFCO$_2$ or ADS, with the result of either of these therapies being only about 60% as great as those obtained with LN$_2$.

As one rater was significantly more likely to give a good or excellent rating than other raters and lesions on the back were more likely to respond to all three types of therapy than lentigines of the upper extremity, multiple logistic regression was performed to adjust for rating physician and anatomical site. The resulting adjusted odds of achieving a good or excellent result were about twice as high with LN$_2$ as with either laser modality. The efficacy of LN$_2$ therapy was also greater than that achieved in a study by Rafal et al using topical tretinoin.[10] Therefore, cryotherapy, the most established of the three methods studied, is superior with respect to the proportion of lesions that responded and is simpler to use, less time-consuming and much less expensive than the newer laser therapies.

All three forms of treatment produced excellent results in at least some lesions, and all appear to have a low frequency of substantial iatrogenic textural change. Had the study been an open trial, the results for any of the three treatment modalities might have been interpreted as supporting claims that the treatment is safe and effective, meeting current FDA regulations for approval.

Stern et al raise the point that a magnitude of biases toward a positive rating is likely to occur in unblinded studies, especially those in which the rater is an advocate of a new treatment. Despite the lack of adequate comparative controlled investigations, new laser systems, some costing more than $100 000, for the treatment of benign epidermal pigmented lesions have been approved on the basis of data from open studies performed by individuals working under company sponsorship.

The data from the Stern et al study demonstrate that preliminary results from open studies of an emerging technology require confirmation under more stringent experimental conditions. Given the rapidly increasing costs of emerging technologies, it would seem appropriate that physicians, patients and regulatory agencies demand that the advocates of any new treatment supply answers to these questions:

1. Does the new technology truly represent an improvement in care?
2. What is the frequency and amount of improvement?

Answers to these questions lay the groundwork for addressing the ethical issue of whether the results of new and expensive therapies are sufficient to justify their higher cost.

In conclusion, Stern et al have shown that cryotherapy, a simple, quick and relatively inexpensive method of treating solar lentigines, has an efficacy approximately twice as great as that achieved by expensive high-technology modalities such as LFCO$_2$ and ADS lasers. None of the laser systems approved, or awaiting approval, by the FDA for the treatment of epidermal benign pigmented lesions, such as the Q-switched ruby, Q-switched Nd:YAG, or pigmented lesions pulsed dye laser, have undergone the scrutiny of a comparative blinded controlled trial with cryotherapy. One wonders what the results might show if such studies were to be performed.

REFERENCES

1. Herbich G, Epidermal changes limited to the epidermis of guinea pig skin by low-power carbon dioxide laser irradiation, *Arch Dermatol* (1986) **122**:132.

2. Kamat BR, Tang SV, Arndt KA et al, Low-fluence CO$_2$ laser irradiation: selective epidermal damage to human skin, *J Invest Dermatol* (1985) **85**:274–8.

3. Dover JS, Smoller BR, Stern RS et al, Low-fluence carbon dioxide laser irradiation of lentigines, *Arch Dermatol* (1988) **124**:1219–24.

4. Mansbridge JN, Knapp AM, Changes in keratinocyte maturation during wound healing, *J Invest Dermatol* (1987) **89**:253–63.

5. Smoller BR, Dover JS, Hsu A, Keratinocyte protein expression in rapidly regenerating epidermis following laser-induced thermal injury, *Lasers Surg Med* (1989) **9**:264–70.

6. Woodcock-Mitchell J, Eichner R, Nelson WG et al, Immunolocalization of keratin polypeptides in human epidermis using monoclonal antibodies, *J Cell Biol* (1982) **95**:580–8.

7. Smoller BR, Kwan TH, Said JW et al, Keratoacanthoma and squamous cell carcinoma of the skin: immunohistochemical localization of involucrin and keratin protein, *J Am Acad Dermatol* (1986) **14**:226–34.

8. Hall RR, The healing of tissues incised by CO$_2$ laser, *Br J Surg* (1971) **58**:222–5.

9. Stern RS, Dover JS, Levin J et al, Safe and effective are not sufficient to justify the adoption of a new medical device: a case study of laser therapy, *JAMA* (in press).

10. Rafal ES, Griffiths CEM, Ditre CM et al, Topical tretinoin (retinoic acid) treatment for liver spots associated with photodamage, *N Engl J Med* (1992) **326**:368–74.

Chapter 30

THE SUPERPULSED CO_2 LASER

Richard E. Fitzpatrick
Javier Ruiz-Esparza

INTRODUCTION

Shortly after the invention of the laser by Maiman in 1960,[1] the exploration of its uses for medical purposes began. Much of the early work was spearheaded by Goldman[2] and involved the use of the laser for the treatment of cutaneous disorders. Today dermatologic applications are among the most common uses of lasers in medicine. The CO_2 laser, developed in 1964, was one of the first medical lasers. As our understanding of light–tissue interactions in the skin has increased, modifications in laser equipment and application techniques have greatly improved results.

The CO_2 laser operates in the invisible far-infrared portion of the light spectrum at 10 600 nm. It is absorbed nonselectively. Its target is tissue water and a beam at this wavelength is entirely absorbed by water. Since skin is approximately 80% water, the CO_2 laser is effective in the treatment of cutaneous disorders and may be used as an incisional or vaporizational device, making it a very versatile surgical instrument.

Though the beam is absorbed within the outer 0.05 mm of tissue[3] with minimal scatter, tissue effects occur as a consequence of rapid heat transfer from the beam to the tissue. Cellular water is rapidly heated past its boiling point, resulting in a cellular explosion that produces steam and cellular debris or the laser plume.[4] This may result in heat conduction and zones of necrosis and damage that extend further than the visualized impact site. This unintended thermal necrosis beyond the target area may interfere with wound healing and increase the risk of scarring.[5]

Treatment techniques will undoubtedly influence this process and will be discussed in detail; however, modifications in the delivery of the laser beam to minimize unwanted thermal damage are equally important. The 'superpulse' feature of the CO_2 laser is the most significant modification in equipment since the original introduction of the CO_2 laser. Prior to a discussion of the specific features of this modification it is necessary to understand basic laser terminology and concepts.

LASER TERMINOLOGY

Misuse of terminology has resulted in confusing and sometimes bewildering situations where communication is difficult or impossible.[6] We will review the basic terms and their significance in laser surgery.

Energy

Energy is the capacity to do work and is expressed as force × length, or mass × velocity.[2] The unit of measurement is a joule. This is also measured as power × time of application, and is a dosage measurement.

Power

Power is the rate of performance of energy. It is energy divided by the time of application. The unit of measurement is the watt. For example, one watt equals one joule per second. This measures the flow of energy.

Power output (the speed of energy emission from the laser tube) is important in limiting the severity of the conduction burn that occurs during use of the laser, but surgical control of the laser is largely a function of the power density and the spot size.

Power density

Power density, or irradiance, is the rate of energy delivery per unit of target tissue area. Power density is expressed in watts per square centimeter and is determined as the power divided by the surface area of the beam or spot size. Because the area of a circle varies with the square of its radius, any reduction in spot size will produce a four-fold increase in energy at the impact site. Increases in power output from the tube, however, result in only a corresponding linear increase in the power density. Power density is the principal determinant of the rate at which tissue is vaporized. High power densities (irradiance) vaporize tissue rapidly.

Spot size

The spot size of the laser may be controllable by use of focusing lenses or by simply moving the handpiece toward or away from the target tissue. It is important to realize that small variations in the handpiece-to-target distance may produce dramatic alterations in the diameter of the beam or spot size and consequently in power density. The irradiance across the beam is distributed in a Gaussian fashion, peaking at the center of the beam and falling off to zero at the edges. A larger spot size allows for smoother, more uniform vaporization of tissue but requires that a much higher power be used in order to compensate for the dilution of power density over the increased area of the larger spot size. The smaller the spot size, the greater the tendency to create uneven ridges, furrows and bleeding. The use of a larger spot size has been shown to result in a decrease in peripheral thermal damage.[7]

The power density, or irradiance, is a static measurement and does not account for time. Laser dosage takes account of time of delivery and is expressed in joules. The number of watts of power multiplied by the delivery time equals the number of joules. Both 1 watt × 1 second and 10 watts × 0.1 second equal 1 joule. This gives a measure of dosage, but does not describe the concentration of the dosage. Fluence combines the concepts of irradiance and dosage.

Fluence

Fluence is the total energy divided by the cross-sectional area of the beam and is expressed as joules per square centimeter. Fluence is the product of irradiance and exposure time. When the power density is greater than about 100 W/cm², the amount of tissue damage that occurs is proportional to the time of application of the beam, not to the irradiance.[4] While irradiance determines the rate at which tissue is vaporized, the volume of tissue removed is entirely a function of the amount of energy applied. A given amount of energy to vaporize a given volume of tissue can be obtained by an infinite combination of powers and times. When heat dispersion in tissue is considered, time of application is the most critical factor.

Laser pulse

Laser energy from the continuous beam of the CO_2 laser can be delivered in short pulses of energy by a variety of techniques. The most common is simply mechanically shuttering the beam so that it is physically blocked for short periods, resulting in an on–off repetitive sequence of pulses. 'Beam chopping' permits very short duration mechanically shuttered pulses by employing a fan-like device. 'Superpulsing' is a process of delivery of very short pulses of very high peak powers by electronically pumping the laser tube. 'Q-switching' employs rotating mirrors and other methods which result in accumulation of laser energy and generation of a giant pulse of very high power and extremely short duration.

Duty cycle

When a laser is used in a repetitive pulsed mode, the duty cycle refers to the time period that the laser is actually 'on'. It is the product of the pulse duration and the repetition rate expressed as a percentage. Duty cycles typically range from 2–50%. It should be noted that the average power of the laser can be increased by increasing the repetition rate. When this is done, the duty cycle is increased, but the irradiance (power density) remains the same. The power has not been 'turned up', but the delivery of that same power per pulse has been accelerated, the faster delivery of power resulting in a higher average power.[5] The same is true of increasing the pulse width. This results in a higher average power but does not alter irradiance.

Thermal relaxation time

The thermal relaxation time of tissue is the time required for the heated tissue to cool by loss of 50% of its heat through diffusion. Significant thermal diffusion will not occur if the pulse duration is short compared to the time it takes the heated layer to cool. Minimal thermal damage is expected if there is insignificant diffusion of heat during the pulse. The thermal relaxation time for pure water has been calculated to be 325 µs for the CO_2 laser.[8] Calculations for human skin have resulted in a value of 695 µs.[8] These are regarded as only 'order of magnitude' estimates but pulse widths of 200 µs[9] and 600 µs[8] have been shown in animal studies to be effective in limiting heat diffusion in treated skin. It is thought that a pulse width of less than 950 µs should be short enough to prevent thermal damage that would be of clinical significance (Coherent Medical Lasers, Palo Alto, CA, unpublished data).

LASER–TISSUE INTERACTION

When laser energy interacts with tissue it does so in accordance with Beer's law. This can be simplified to the statement that tissue damage at the absorption site decreases exponentially with increasing distance from the crater edge. This means that epidermal cells at the wound edge remain viable and can participate in wound healing.[10]

According to Beer's law, laser energy heats a critical tissue volume until the tissue temperature exceeds the vaporization threshold. If fluence is sufficient to deliver adequate energy during a single laser pulse and that pulse is less than the thermal relaxation time of tissue, then one critical volume of tissue will be cleanly vaporized with each laser pulse and without thermal damage occurring beyond the impact site.

If the fluence used results in a pulse energy that is below the minimum necessary to vaporize tissue, then tissues will coagulate and desiccate and carbonize as tissue heat accumulates from the additive effects of multiple pulses or a continuous beam. Continued irradiance of carbonized tissue results in crater temperatures of more than 600°C (the temperature of red-hot coal), rather than the desired temperature of 100°C required for vaporization (the boiling point of water).[10]

When vaporization occurs, the temperature of the crater wall of the impact site is limited to 100°C, because this is the maximum temperature reached during the explosive vaporization process. However, when tissue is heated slowly with low irradiance, burning, desiccation and charring of tissue occur. Gross carbonization is a sign that tissue temperatures exceed 300°C and additional radiation of the black carbon creates a 'heat sink' and tissue temperatures over 600°C.[5] This situation obviously creates extensive peripheral thermal damage secondary to thermal diffusion. Conduction burns similar to those that occur with electrocautery may result. Instead of a narrow zone of thermal damage of 50–100 µm, lateral zones of thermal necrosis measuring 1–5 mm may result with such thermal diffusion.

Though irradiance has been thought to be intimately related to peripheral thermal damage, based on calculations of McKenzie using a one-dimensional model,[11] recent investigations show qualitative agreement but no systematic relationship of peripheral thermal damage to irradiance.[12] McKenzie's calculations show the thickness of the coagulation zone decreasing from about 500 µm at 100 W/cm² to 55 µm at 1000 W/cm² and 20 µm at 10 kW/cm² However, Schomacker et al[12] found almost identical damage zones with irradiances that differ by more than a factor of 40. Damage zones were found to be of the order of 80 µm for irradiances of 1 kW/cm² or greater. Fuller has also shown that above 800 W/cm² the rate of peripheral necrosis decreases and little additional change occurs with further increases in irradiance.[13,14] Thus the influence of irradiance alone on the size of the necrotic zone is minor when compared to the impact that irradiation time has on heat transfer and resulting thermal damage.

However, it is clear that irradiance controls the rate at which tissue is vaporized and therefore the depth of the vaporization crater. Though it is commonly advised that the highest irradiance which can be controlled should be used by the laser surgeon, this requires a rapid sweep speed with a continuous beam or a very short pulse of application. In order to control the depth of incision or vaporization, low power densities have been attempted. This is particularly dangerous in the 'airbrush' vaporization technique using a continuous beam. As can be seen from the previous discussion, this maneuver requires an increased time of application and creates the ideal set of parameters for increasing peripheral thermal diffusion.[5,10,15]

The ideal CO_2 laser for cutaneous surgery must incise or vaporize tissue effectively and rapidly, coagulate blood vessels, and allow rapid and normal healing from adnexal structures as well as from nontreated adjacent epidermis, and should not interfere with graft survival. The continuous-wave and mechanically shuttered CO_2 lasers have been shown to provide hemostasis[9] and surgical speed as their only advantages over the use of conventional instrumentation. The 300–1000-µm layer of thermal damage reported with these lasers is adequate to automatically seal blood vessels of 0.5 mm diameter or smaller and may provide hemostasis of vessels as large as 2 mm in diameter.[4] However, this layer of thermal necrosis also impedes wound healing, tensile strength and skin graft survival.

The use of pulsed lasers with irradiances of 4–19 J/cm² has been shown to produce precise tissue ablation (20–40 μm of tissue removed per pulse impact), while limiting peripheral thermal damage to a zone measuring less than 100 μm in thickness.[9,16] In summary, the CO_2 laser can be used most effectively to vaporize cutaneous lesions if used in a pulsed mode with a pulse less than the thermal relaxation time of skin (approximately 695 μs) and irradiance of 1000 W/cm² or higher. Such short exposure times and high irradiances can be achieved only with a superpulsed CO_2 laser.

SUPERPULSED CO_2 LASER

Superpulsed CO_2 lasers emit a controlled train of short-duration, high-power pulses. Typically, peak powers are generated which are as much as 10 times the power the laser is capable of producing in the continuous-wave mode. The laser tube is pumped electronically to produce high-power pulses in repetitive short pulses. The repetition rate varies from laser to laser, but may be a critical parameter as well. In some lasers the repetition rate is fixed by the choice of the other parameters; in others, it may be chosen by the surgeon. Repetition rates vary from 1 to 5000 per second (hertz).

For most superpulsed CO_2 lasers, each individual short pulse does not contain adequate energy per pulse to ablate tissue with a single pulse. In this situation the repetition rate needs to be rapid enough to avoid interpulse cooling, so that a series of four to five pulses accumulates enough heat to reach the tissue vaporization threshold. This creates a situation that may allow thermal diffusion beyond the intended site of treatment. This is particularly true for rapid repetition rates (>1000 Hz). In this situation the superpulsed CO_2 laser behaves essentially as a continuous-wave laser. Repetition rates as low as 10–100 Hz are estimated to allow slight accumulation of thermal energy.[7] However, recent calculations have suggested an ideal repetition rate to avoid unwanted thermal damage with the CO_2 laser to be 93 Hz[17] or less. Additionally, the use of repetition rates of 1–50 Hz has been suggested to allow better manual control of the superpulsed CO_2 laser.[18]

The cumulative effects of multiple-pulse exposures versus a single-pulse exposure were studied by Schomacker et al.[12] A single 100-ms pulse of 830 W/cm² resulted in a crater depth of approximately 125 μm and a layer of thermal necrosis at the base of the crater measuring 100 μm. Five repetitive pulses at 0.1 Hz (500 times the estimated tissue relaxation time) resulted in a crater depth of approximately 400 μm and a residual layer of thermal necrosis measuring 160 μm. Clearly, multiple pulses lead to increased damage. This multiple-pulse effect explains the difference between the 100-μm damage zones typical of single 50–100-ms pulse exposures[12] and the 750-μm damage zones reported by Walsh et al[8] using 100 or more 50-ms pulses at 510 W/cm².

This multiple-pulse effect with a high repetition rate also explains the relative lack of clinically significant improved wound healing that we found in the clinical use of the Coherent Ambulase Superpulsed CO_2 laser.[19] The superpulse parameters of this particular laser allow only the choice of a repetition rate of 250 or 500 Hz. The most significant improvement in clinical results occurred only with shuttering this superpulsed beam with a secondary pulse of 50 ms. This shuttering cuts the stream of pulses into short bursts of 10–12 pulses that accumulate adequate energy to vaporize tissue. The 'off' period protects the peripheral tissue from excessive thermal damage.

The threshold fluence for ablation of skin has been reported as 4.75 J/cm² based on measurements by Walsh et al[8] and 2.6

J/cm^2 (95% confidence interval: 1.9–3.2) based on studies by Green et al.[9] From these measurements it is estimated that the effective fluence required to ablate skin is 5 J/cm^2 or higher. The requirement to reach this threshold necessitates the use of a cumulative effect of multiple pulses for most superpulsed lasers. To modulate the unwanted thermal effects, as well as to add a further increment of control over the beam, a second duty cycle is superimposed on the superpulsed cycle by use of a mechanically pulsed shutter. This adds additional on–off periods and cuts the train of continuous superpulse impacts into smaller groups of several pulses, separated by a longer cooling time. Typical increments of 50 ms to 0.5 s are provided and these repeat in cycles of 2–10 per second. This is an excellent means of controlling the high-irradiance superpulsed laser. There have been experimental data using CO_2 laser ablation of guinea pig skin suggesting that less thermal damage occurs with a 50-ms pulse than with longer shuttered pulses.[12,20] We have confirmed this on human skin, both with continuous CO_2 laser ablation and with superpulsed CO_2 laser ablation, using only single impacts,[21] as well as in clinical use in treatment of patients[19] (Figures 30.1 and 30.2).

Experimental data suggest a thermal relaxation time of 19 ms for a liquid phase which forms during laser–tissue interaction.[12] This liquid tissue phase is thought to act as a conduit of heat from the impact crater to the surrounding tissue. The shuttered pulse may be significant in controlling heat conduction through this phase. The tissue effects of shuttered pulses shorter than 50 ms have not been reported.

A recent study has demonstrated normal healing of skin ablated with a mechanical scanning device using a spot size of 400 μm, pulse energy of 23 mJ and radiant exposure of 18 J/cm^2 per pulse. The mechanical scanner produced a grid of

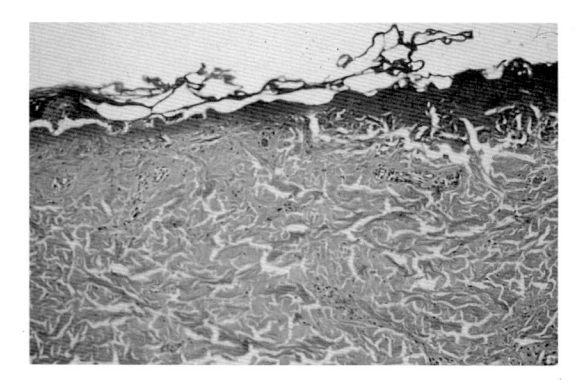

Figure 30.1
Thermal necrosis of the epidermis and papillary dermis resulting from a single impact of continuous-wave CO_2 laser, 4 W, 0.05 s pulse.

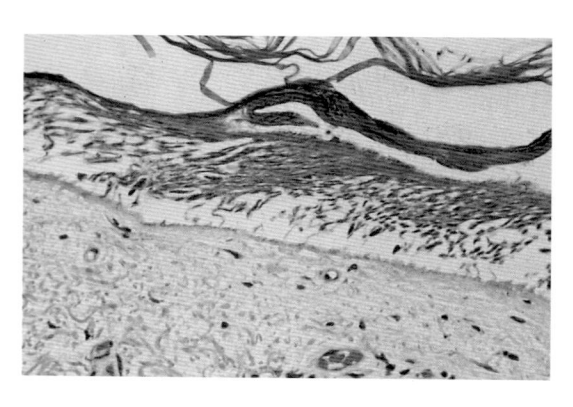

Figure 30.2
Thermal damage of epidermis only, resulting from a single impact of 0.05 s of superpulsed CO_2 laser with average power of 4 W (pulse width 200 μs, pulse rate 250 Hz). There is much more control of thermal damage even with this high superpulse repetition rate.

overlapping pulses while moving at a speed of 25.4 mm per second. The epidermis and dermis were removed to a depth of 856 ± 230 μm and thermal necrosis measured only 85 ± 15 μm. The healing of these wounds was compared to that caused by a dermatome and measuring 871 ± 200 μm. There were no differences in the healed wounds or in healing time of the wounds. The authors recognized the difficulty in reproducing these parameters clinically and suggested modification of existing laser systems to allow a larger spot size with radiant energies of 4–19 J/cm^2 and a slow repetition rate of 1–50 Hz.[18] It must be realized that the extent of tissue damage that occurs is technique and user dependent as well and that these factors will affect the ultimate clinical result. However, by use of the most ideal laser parameters, the variance from operator to operator will be minimized and results will not be so technique dependent.

Recently, Coherent Medical Lasers has introduced a new type of superpulsed CO_2 laser having pulse energies five to seven times higher than the conventional superpulsed lasers. This laser has a peak pulse power of >450 W, an average power of up to 100 W, and an energy per pulse of up to 250 mJ. This is delivered with a pulse width no greater than 950 µs and may be used with a pulse spot size as large as 2.5 mm and still deliver 5 J/cm^2 per pulse. This laser is called the Ultrapulse laser. These delivery parameters are ideal for tissue vaporization without unwanted thermal damage and in early trials on cutaneous lesions this laser has proven to be exceptional.

Clinical Applications

Vaporization

The extreme precision that is achievable with the use of the proper pulse parameters of a superpulsed CO_2 laser makes this laser a unique instrument for the treatment of various dermatologic conditions. When it is used as a vaporization instrument, a large beam diameter is appropriate, preferably 2 mm or larger. The fact that unwanted thermal diffusion is controllable by the choice of the appropriate pulse parameters allows for precise clinical control of vaporization of epidermal as well as dermal lesions without risk of significant scarring or prolonged healing time.

The clinical use of the laser must be guided by close attention to detailed observation of certain parameters during the procedure. These clinical parameters and their significance with regard to depth of tissue ablation have been well characterized in an article by Reid.[10] He characterized opalescent bubbling of the skin surface accompanied by audible cracking sounds as an indication that only the epidermis had been ablated. This surface can be wiped clean with saline to reveal an intact, smooth, pink plane representing the surface of the papillary dermis. When this layer is vaporized, there is visible contraction of the tissue and the development of a yellowish, roughened appearance similar to chamois cloth. When the reticular dermis is reached, coarse collagen bundles are seen, having an appearance resembling waterlogged cotton threads. Healing of the skin down to this point will occur without scarring. To proceed deeper may increase the risk of scarring. It is important to note that close attention must be paid to tissue charring. If charring occurs, there will be thermal diffusion and unwanted tissue necrosis beyond the depth of vaporization. When charring is noted, this can often be remedied by decreasing the spot size of the beam, resulting in an increased fluence.

Use of the superpulsed CO_2 laser for vaporization of actinic cheilitis of the lower lip offers the best example of the unique clinical usefulness of this laser. Our patients having actinic cheilitis who were treated with a continuous-wave CO_2 laser required an average of 5.5 weeks to heal and 44% healed with visible scarring (Figure 30.3). Those patients treated with a continuous rapidly pulsed low-fluence superpulsed laser required 4.5 weeks to heal and had a 33% incidence of visible scarring. Patients who were treated with

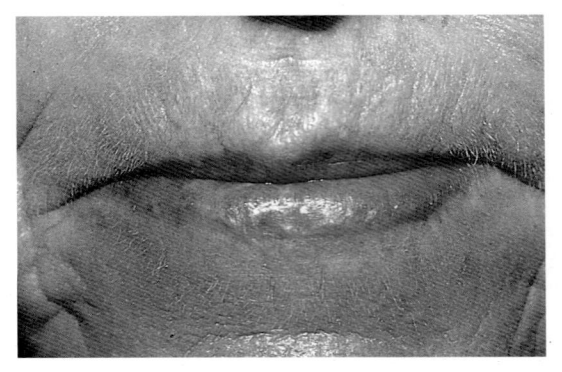

SURGICAL DERMATOLOGY

Figure 30.3
Scarring of lower lip following vaporization of actinic cheilitis, using continuous-wave CO_2 laser.

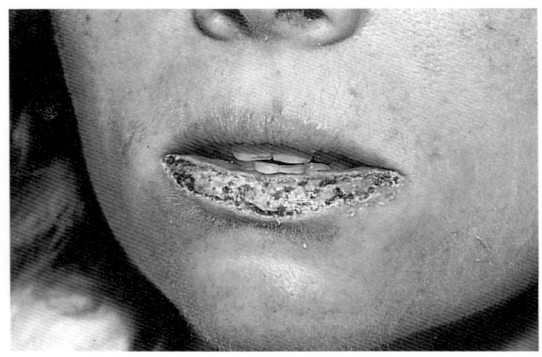

Figure 30.4
Patient with actinic cheilitis immediately following treatment with continuous-wave CO_2 laser. Tissue charring of this type indicates temperatures in excess of 300°C and is a high-risk situation for unwanted thermal necrosis that may cause prolonged wound healing and scarring.

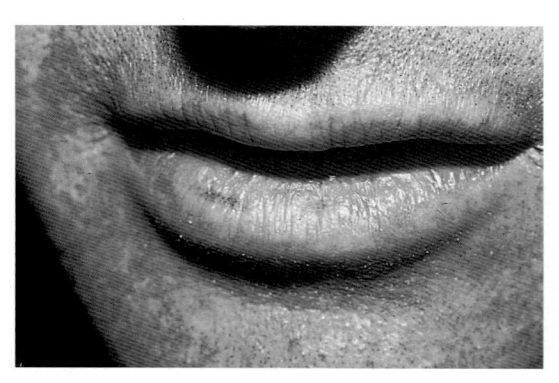

A

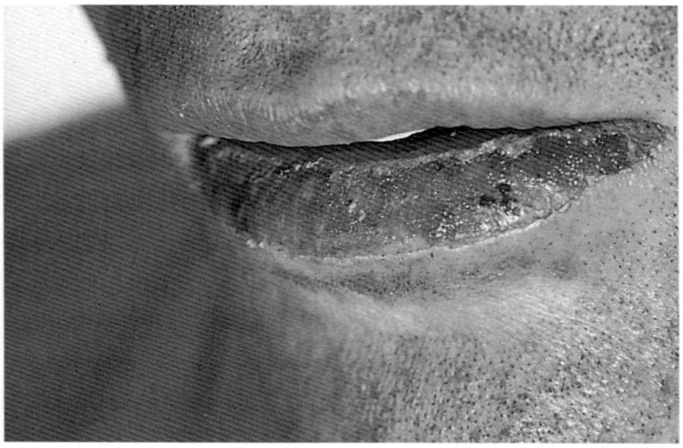

B

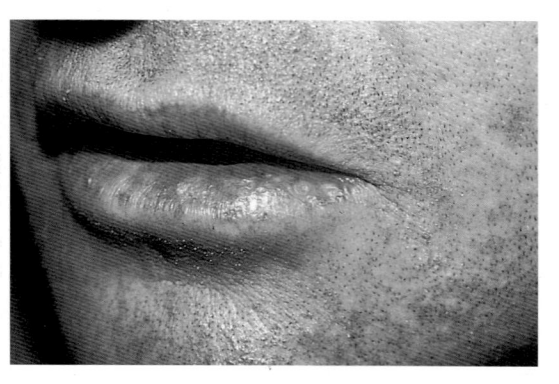

Figure 30.5
(A) Lesions typical of actinic cheilitis across the lower lip. (B) Lower lip immediately following vaporization with the ultrapulse CO_2 laser (pulse width 547 μs, repetition rate 40 Hz, average power 8 W, 250 mJ per pulse). Note absence of charring of treated tissue. (C) Clinical healing 3 weeks after treatment. The surface had completely re-epithelialized 12 days after treatment.

C

the same superpulsed laser, but with the addition of a 50-ms shuttered pulse, required 2.5 weeks to heal and had no scarring.[19] The final group was treated with the ultrapulse laser having ideal pulse parameters. This group of patients required an average of 12 days to heal and none had scarring. It should be mentioned that those patients treated with the continuous-wave CO_2 laser and the continuous superpulsed CO_2 laser were treated without attention being focused on the avoidance of tissue charring (Figure 30.4). The comparison of these four groups of patients offers a valuable demonstration of the dramatic improvement in results that can be achieved by attention to the selection of proper pulse characteristics as well as attention to details of clinical technique (Figures 30.5A,B,C).

The treatment of verrucae vulgaris can be achieved very successfully with the use of the superpulsed CO_2 laser. Cure rates of 71–95% have been reported with the CO_2 laser[22,23] and with precision enough to avoid onychodystrophy in patients having periungual verrucae.[22] All commonly used destructive treatment modalities, including the use of various acids, electrocautery, liquid nitrogen cryosurgery, intralesional bleomycin and continuous-wave CO_2 laser ablation, result in imprecise tissue destruction and a clinically unknown layer of tissue necrosis beyond the application site. This may result in a high incidence of scarring or inadequate treatment and lesion recurrence. The precise vaporization achievable with the superpulsed CO_2 laser allows destruction of lesional tissue with much greater accuracy and improved clinical results. Because wart virus has been demonstrated in normal perilesional epidermis as far away as 1 cm, consideration can be given to selectively ablating the adjacent epidermis without risk of dermal necrosis in this area by carefully controlled use of the superpulsed CO_2 laser. This cannot be achieved with the use of the other modalities commonly used for the treatment of warts without adding significant risk of scarring and prolonged healing.

The CO_2 laser has a long history of use in the removal of decorative amateur as well as professional tattoos. Scarring is inevitable if the complete removal of all tattoo pigment in one treatment session is attempted because of the fact that tissue containing tattoo pigment is vaporized during the treatment process. Because tattoo pigment may be present in the deep reticular dermis, vaporization to this level will invariably be followed by significant scarring. An alternative treatment is the ablation of only 30–50% of the tattoo pigment followed by application of 50% urea.[24] This treatment technique has proven to be very successful in limiting the extent of scarring while providing pigment removal in one treatment session. Because of the extremely precise vaporization that can be performed with the CO_2 laser, we have been very successful in the removal of cosmetic eyeliner tattoo without visible scarring or loss of eyelashes.[25] This is achieved by tissue vaporization without the use of urea (Figure 30.6A,B,C).

Many tumors of the skin have been shown to be responsive to vaporization with the CO_2 laser. These include rhinophyma,[26,27] adenoma sebaceum,[28] xanthelasma,[29,30] syringomas,[31,32] trichoepitheliomas,[33,34] superficial basal cell carcinoma,[35] hydrocystomas,[34] lymphangiomas,[36] actinic keratoses,[34] lentigos,[37,38] ephelides,[19] seborrheic keratoses,[20,34] neurofibromas,[39] Cowden's disease,[40] bowenoid papulosis,[41] and epidermal nevi[42] (Figures 30.7A,B).

Incision

When the laser is used as an incisional instrument, a small focal point of 0.1–0.2 mm is used.[43] Such a small spot size results in tremendously high fluences

SURGICAL DERMATOLOGY

A

B

C

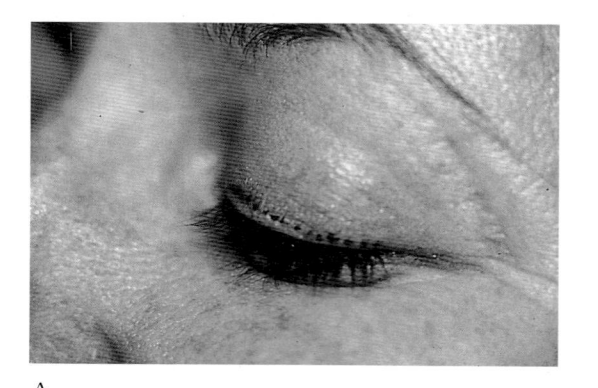

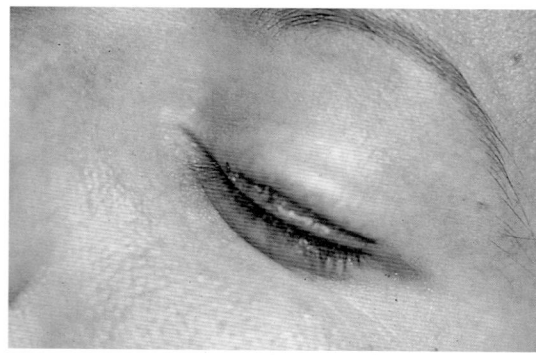

Figure 30.6
(A) A cosmetic 'eyeliner' tattoo was misapplied, causing the patient to request removal. (B) The CO_2 laser offers precise vaporization, preserving the eyelash hair follicles and avoiding scarring that could cause ectropion and lid distortion. (C) Clinical results are excellent in this case.

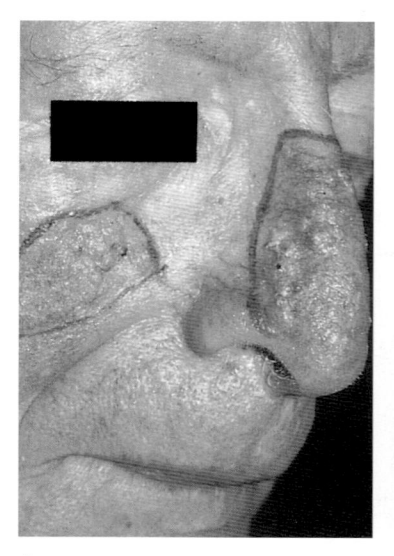

A

B

Figure 30.7
(A) Multiple lesions of hyperkeratotic nodules and erythema which on biopsy proved to be superficial squamous cell carcinoma. Because of the widespread nature and variable thickness of the lesions, they had been unresponsive to liquid nitrogen cryosurgery. (B) One month following ablation with the superpulsed CO_2 laser (average power 8 W, 400-μs pulse, 250 Hz). Lesions of this nature are ideal candidates for selective ablation with the superpulsed CO_2 laser. Close visualization of the lesion during the procedure is necessary to assure complete lesion removal, and postoperative biopsy follow-up may be necessary.

which can make the depth of incision difficult to control unless a slow repetition rate (around 50 Hz) can be chosen or a shuttered pulse of 50 ms can be superimposed. The primary advantage of the laser scalpel is the speed achieved because of the relatively bloodless field resulting from coagulation of dermal vessels smaller than 0.5 mm. When larger vessels are encountered, the handpiece may be moved away from tissue to produce a larger spot size and lower fluence, and the vessel may then be selectively cauterized. The use of the superpulsed mode results in avoidance of unwanted thermal necrosis at the cut edge that may interfere with wound healing or with histological interpretation of wound borders. The use of the laser scalpel has been most apparent in the excision of skin cancers in patients with various coagulation disorders from medicinal or medical etiologies and in the excision of highly vascular tissue.[41,44] Bailin et al have described the advantages of the CO_2 laser for selected cases in Mohs micrographic surgery.[44] There has also been considerable experience with the use of the CO_2 laser in the performance of blepharoplasty and demonstration of lowered operative time with decreased ecchymosis, bleeding, swelling, pain and healing time.[45]

REFERENCES

1. Maiman TH, Stimulated optical radiation in ruby, *Nature* (1960) **187**:493–4.
2. Goldman L. *Biomedical aspects of the laser* (Springer-Verlag: New York 1967).
3. Kamat BR, Tang SV, Arndt KA et al, Low fluence CO_2 laser irradiation: selective epidermal damage to human skin, *J Invest Derm* (1985) **85**:274–8.
4. Absten GT, Laser biophysics for the physician. In: Ratz JL, ed., *Lasers in cutaneous medicine and surgery* (Yearbook Medical Publishers: Chicago 1986) 1–28.
5. Hobbs ER, Bailin PL, Wheeland RG et al, Superpulsed lasers: minimizing thermal damage with short duration high irradiance pulses, *J Dermatol Surg Oncol* (1987) **13**:955–64.
6. Fisher JC, A short glossary of laser terminology for physicians and surgeons, *J Clin Laser Med Surg* (1991) **10**:345–8.
7. Zweig AD, Meierhofer B, Muller OM et al, Lateral thermal damage along pulsed laser incisions, *Lasers Surg Med* (1990) **10**:262–74.
8. Walsh JT, Flotte TJ, Anderson RR et al, Pulsed CO_2 laser tissue ablation: effect of tissue type and pulse duration on thermal damage, *Lasers Surg Med* (1988) **8**:108–18.
9. Green HA, Domankevitz Y, Nishioka NS, Pulsed carbon dioxide laser ablation of burned skin: in vitro and in vivo analysis, *Lasers Surg Med* (1990) **10**:476–84.
10. Reid R, Physical and surgical principles governing carbon dioxide laser surgery on the skin, *Dermatol Clin* (1991) **9**:297–316.
11. McKenzie AL, A three-zone model of soft-tissue damage by a CO_2 laser, *Phys Med Biol* (1986) **31**:967–83.
12. Schomacker KT, Walsh JT, Flotte TJ et al, Thermal damage produced by high-irradiance continuous wave CO_2 laser cutting of tissue, *Lasers Surg Med* (1990) **10**:74–84.
13. Fuller TA, Laser tissue interaction: the influence of power density. In: Baggish MS, ed., *Basic and advanced laser surgery in gynecology* (Appleton-Century-Crofts: Norwalk 1985).
14. Mage G, Pouly JL, Bruhat MA, Laser microsurgery of the oviducts. In:

Baggish MS, ed., *Basic and advanced laser surgery in gynecology* (Appleton-Century-Crofts: Norwalk 1985).

15. McKenzie AL, How far does thermal damage extend beneath the surface of CO_2 laser incisions? *Phys Med Biol* (1983) **28**:905–12.

16. Walsh JT, Deutsch TF, Pulsed CO_2 laser ablation: measurement of the ablation rate, *Lasers Surg Med* (1988) **8**:264–75.

17. Van Gemert MJC, Welch AJ, Time constants in thermal laser medicine, *Lasers Surg Med* (1989) **9**:405–21.

18. Green HA, Burd E, Nishioka NS et al, Mid dermal wound healing, *Arch Dermatol* (1992) **128**:639–45.

19. Fitzpatrick RE, Ruiz-Esparza J, Goldman MP, Clinical advantage of the superpulse carbon dioxide laser, *Lasers Surg Med* (1990) **2**(Supplement):52 (abst 218).

20. Lanzafame RJ, Naim JO, Rogers DW et al, Comparison of continuous-wave, chop-wave, and super-pulse laser wounds, *Lasers Surg Med* (1988) **8**:119–24.

21. Fitzpatrick RE, Ruiz-Esparza J, Goldman MP, The depth of thermal necrosis using the CO_2 laser: a comparison of the superpulsed mode and conventional mode, *J Dermatol Surg Oncol* (1991) **17**:340–4.

22. Street ML, Roenigk RK, Recalcitrant periungual verrucae: the role of carbon dioxide laser vaporization, *J Am Acad Dermatol* (1990) **23**:115–20.

23. McBurney EI, Rosen DA, Carbon dioxide laser treatment of verruca vulgares, *J Dermatol Surg Oncol* (1984) **10**:45–8.

24. Ruiz-Esparza J, Goldman MP, Fitzpatrick RE, Tattoo removal with minimal scarring: the chemo-laser technique, *J Dermatol Surg Oncol* (1988) **14**:1372–6.

25. Fitzpatrick RE, Ruiz-Esparza J, Goldman MP, CO_2 laser removal of 'permanent eyeliner', *Lasers Surg Med* (1990) (Supplement 2):51 (abst 212).

26. Haas A, Wheeland RG, Treatment of massive rhinophyma with the carbon dioxide laser, *J Dermatol Surg Oncol* (1990) **16**:645–9.

27. Bohigegian RK, Shapshy SR, Hybey RL, Management of rhinophyma with carbon dioxide laser: Lahey Clinic experience, *Lasers Surg Med* (1988) **8**:397–401.

28. Wheeland RG, Bailin PL, Kantor G et al, Treatment of adenoma sebaceum with carbon dioxide laser vaporization, *J Am Acad Dermatol* (1986) **14**:257–62.

29. Apfelberg DB, Maser MR, Lash H et al, Treatment of xanthelasma palpebrum with the carbon dioxide laser, *J Dermatol Surg Oncol* (1987) **13**:149–51.

30. Apfelberg DB, Maser MR, Lash H et al, Treatment of xanthelasma palpebrarum with the carbon dioxide laser, *J Dermatol Surg Oncol* (1987) **13**:149–51.

31. Apfelberg DB, Maser MR, Lash H et al, Superpulse CO_2 laser treatment of facial syringomata, *Lasers Surg Med* (1987) **7**:533–7.

32. Wheeland RG, Bailin PL, Reynolds O et al, Carbon dioxide (CO_2) laser vaporization of multiple facial syringomas, *J Dermatol Surg Oncol* (1986) **12**:223–8.

33. Wheeland RG, Bailin PL, Kronberg E, Carbon dioxide (CO_2) laser vaporization for the treatment of trichoepitheliomata, *J Dermatol Surg Oncol* (1984) **10**:470–4.

34. Dover J, Arndt K, Geronemus R et al (eds), *Illustrated cutaneous laser surgery: a practitioner's atlas* (Appleton & Lange: Norwalk, CT 1990).

35. Wheeland RG, Bailin PL, Ratz JL et al, Carbon dioxide laser vaporization and curettage in the treatment of large or multiple superficial basal cell carcinomas, *J Dermatol Surg Oncol* (1987) **13:**119–24.

36. Bailin PL, Kantor GR, Wheeland RG, Carbon dioxide laser vaporization of lymphangioma circumscriptum, *J Am Acad Dermatol* (1986) **14:**257–62.

37. Benedict LM, Cohen B, Treatment of Peutz-Jeghers lentigines with the carbon dioxide laser, *J Dermatol Surg Oncol* (1991) **17:**954–5.

38. Dover JS, Smoller B, Stern RS et al, Low fluence CO_2 laser irradiation of lentigines, *Arch Dermatol* (1988) **124:**1219–24.

39. Roenigk RK, Ratz JL, CO_2 laser treatment of cutaneous neurofibromas, *J Dermatol Surg Oncol* (1987) **13:**187–90.

40. Wheeland RG, McGillis ST, Cowden's disease—treatment of cutaneous lesions using carbon dioxide laser vaporization: a comparison of conventional and superpulsed techniques, *J Dermatol Surg Oncol* (1989) **15:**1055–9.

41. Polnikorn N, Bowenoid papulosis: treatment with carbon dioxide laser vaporization, *J Clin Laser Med Surg* (1992) **10:** 27–30.

42. Ratz JL, Bailin PL, Lakeland RF, Carbon dioxide laser treatment of epidermal nevi, *J Dermatol Surg Oncol* (1986) **12:**567–70.

43. Garden JM, Geronemus RG, Dermatologic laser surgery, *J Dermatol Surg Oncol* (1990) **16:**156–68.

44. Bailin PL, Ratz JL, Lutz-Nagey L, CO_2 laser modification of Mohs' surgery, *J Dermatol Surg Oncol* (1981) **7:**621–3.

45. David LM, Laser blepharoplasty—1991, *Lasers Surg Med* (1991) (Supplement 3): 71 (abst 288).

Chapter 31

NEWER USES FOR THE CO$_2$ LASER

Pamela K. Miller
Rokea A. el-Azhary
Randall K. Roenigk

INTRODUCTION

The carbon dioxide (CO$_2$) laser is a versatile surgical tool that has been used to treat various skin disorders with unique precision. This laser emits an invisible beam of light energy with a wavelength in the far-infrared range (10 600 nm) which is absorbed by tissue water and leads to instantaneous heating and conversion of the water to steam. The cells then rapidly expand and explode or vaporize.

The CO$_2$ laser can be used in two ways. The beam can be focused to a very small spot and function as a scalpel to cut. Alternatively, the beam can be defocused to a larger spot size and allow superficial destruction of successive layers of tissue. When the laser is used properly at low fluences or 'superpulsed', heat conduction to surrounding tissues is minimal and its effects are well localized.

One major advantage of using the CO$_2$ laser is that a bloodless surgical field is produced due to the sealing of small-diameter dermal blood vessels. The surgeon can clearly visualize vaporizing tissue and precisely control its destruction.

Due to the focal and superficial way in which the CO$_2$ laser can destroy tissue, this tool is ideally suited to treat some epidermal and superficial dermal lesions. Conditions commonly treated with the CO$_2$ laser include actinic cheilitis, condyloma acuminata, epidermal nevi, verrucae vulgaris and rhinophyma. Less common uses for CO$_2$ laser therapy include adnexal tumors, acne scarring, infectious processes, pigmentation disorders, vascular tumors, disorders of keratinization, genodermatoses, metabolic diseases and inflammatory diseases (see Table 31.1). In this chapter these less common uses of the CO$_2$ laser will be listed and the authors' experience or opinion given as to whether this is a reasonable therapy in each case.

TUMORS

Apocrine hidrocystoma

Apocrine hidrocystomas are benign appendeal tumors which commonly occur on the face. Bickley et al[1] reported their experience treating four facial lesions with the CO$_2$ laser at 5 W in a defocused fashion. The lesions reportedly healed well with excellent cosmetic results. Electrosurgery or shave excision are the authors' preference.

Cylindroma

Cylindromas are benign adnexal tumors which commonly involve the face, scalp and neck. Reported treatments such as excision and local irradiation commonly result in recurrence, or may be impractical, especially when multiple tumors are present.

Stoner and Hobbs[2] reported the first case in which the CO_2 laser was used to successfully treat these lesions. They treated 70 cylindromas in one patient with the CO_2 laser in the continuous-mode, focused fashion, with the 400-mm handpiece at 8 W to vaporize the overlying epidermis. Many tumors spontaneously extruded, leaving a shell of normal dermis. The patient experienced minimal postoperative discomfort, the wounds healed by second intention, and cosmesis was excellent. The authors have combined CO_2 laser with dermabrasion, but still expect recurrences long term.

Syringoma

Syringoma is a benign tumor of eccrine gland origin. It commonly appears in women as multiple, 1–5 mm, yellow or flesh-colored papules on the face, predominantly around the eyes.

Other treatment for this tumor includes dermabrasion, excision, topical trichloroacetic acid, or argon laser photocoagulation. As with other adnexal tumors, use of the CO_2 laser allows precise destruction of multiple lesions and very acceptable cosmetic results.[3]

Several reports describe use of the CO_2 laser for eyelid syringomas. Nerad and Anderson[4] treated three patients using 2–5 W of power, 1–2 mm spot size, and the intermittent mode for isolated lesions and continuous mode for confluent lesions. Six-month follow-up showed no evidence of recurrence and no tendency for ectropion or lower lid retraction.

In a report by Apfelberg et al,[5] eight patients were treated with a CO_2 laser with superpulse capability. Moderate defocusing was utilized to vaporize sufficiently to remove the epidermis and expose the underlying cyst. The cyst was then removed with a fine-tooth forceps or 25-gauge needle. Healing and re-epithelialization occurred within 7–10 days. The patients were followed for up to 3 years, with satisfactory results in five out of the eight patients. In the authors' experience, the laser is helpful in more extensive cases, especially when ectropion is a concern. Otherwise, electrosurgery or punch excision are used. Dermabrasion is another technique used successfully for multiple syringomas.

Myxoid cyst

In the treatment of myxoid cysts, the CO_2 laser provides the clinician with a bloodless operative field and precise tissue destruction. Huerter et al[6] treated 10 lesions in 10 patients by using the laser in the defocused fashion at 5 W to vaporize lesions until clinically tumor-free margins were achieved. Follow-up (average 35.2 months) revealed no recurrences. Patients experienced minimal discomfort, complete wound healing in 3 weeks, and excellent cosmesis. Laser is promising, but these tumors can extend to the synovial space, so a deeper excision must still be considered standard therapy.

Pearly penile papules

Pearly penile papules are characterized histologically by fibrous and angiomatous proliferation in the dermis. Magid and Garden[7] successfully treated lesions in two patients with the superpulsed CO_2 laser in the defocused fashion at 5 W. Healing occurred within 2 weeks of the procedure and cosmetic and functional results were excellent.

ACNE SCARRING

Pitted acne scarring

Various modalities have been used to help correct acne scarring. The CO_2 laser may be utilized as an alternative to other standard scar revision methods to correct 'icepick' or deeply pitted, well-demarcated scars. Garrett et al[8] treated a total of eight patients; four with the superpulsed CO_2 laser, three with the continuous-wave laser, and one with both laser types during separate treatment sessions. The centers and margins of scars were treated in a defocused fashion at 4–25 W in one or two passes to achieve a uniform depth over the base of the scar and contouring of the wound edges. The treated scars were softer and more shallow. Patients were quite satisfied with the cosmetic result (Figure 31.1). Treating individual, pitted scars with the CO_2 laser allows one to accurately control the depth of tissue destruction and contour the wound edges. The superpulsed mode adds even more control as the short-duration, high-energy pulses result in less heat transfer peripheral to tissue and minimal thermal damage. This method helps smooth the sharp contours of some acne scars, but often results in hypopigmentation. This is minimized when laser is followed by a full-face dermabrasion in the authors' experience.

Acne keloidalis nuchae

Acne keloidalis nuchae is characterized by pustules and firm, skin-colored papules on the occipital scalp and posterior neck that later coalesce to form keloidal plaques. Treatment of the early stages of the disease includes topical cleansers, intralesional steroids, epilation and local or systemic antibiotics. The later and chronic stages of the disease usually require surgical excision with primary closure or split-thickness skin grafts, electrodesiccation or

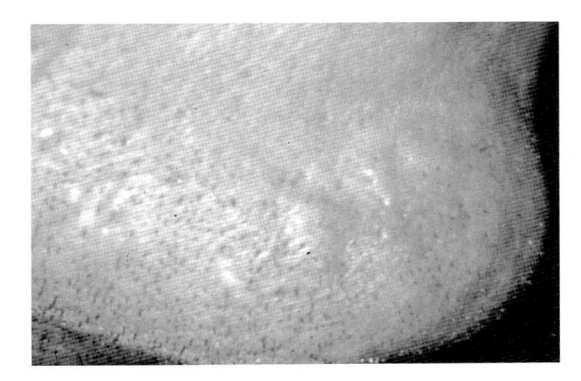

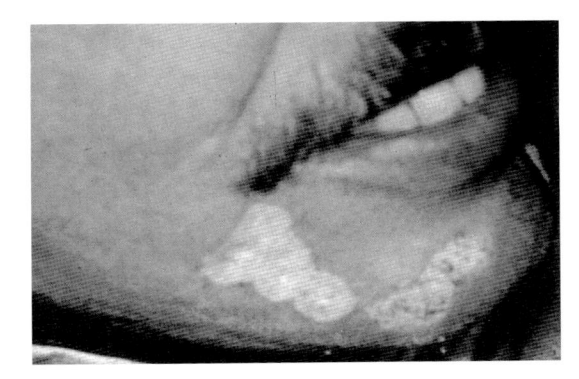

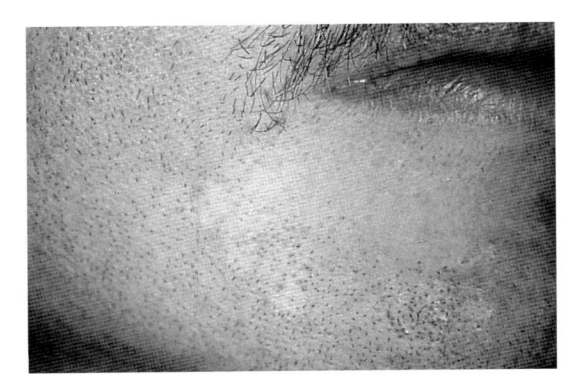

Figure 31.1
Acne scars. (A) Preoperatively, focal, well-demarcated scars. (B) Immediately postoperative. (C) Three months postoperatively. (Case of Dr PL Bailin, Cleveland Clinic Foundation, reproduced with permission.)

radiation therapy. Eight patients who were refractory to other forms of treatment underwent CO_2 laser excision by Kantor et al.[9] Their lesions had been present for a mean duration of 10.1 years, and ranged in size from 3 to 15 cm. The CO_2 laser was used in a focused mode at an irradiance of 64 000 W/cm^2 to excise through the fibrotic tissue to the subfollicular level of the deep dermis or subcutaneous fat. Hemostasis was accomplished by using the laser in the defocused mode. Healing was generally complete within 6 weeks postoperatively. Slight hypertrophic scars developed in two patients 3 months postoperatively. The hypertrophic scarring responded to intralesional triamcinolone at a concentration of 20–40 mg/ml. There were no recurrences in six of the eight patients at 1 year follow-up. The authors recommend the excision mode over vaporization since the two patients treated by vaporization developed recurrences. In their experience this method is excellent, but the key is excision down to subcutaneous fat and the removal of all the hair follicles. Scalpel excision with or without grafting may be equally effective.

INFECTIOUS PROCESSES

Blastomycosis

Blastomycosis, caused by the fungus *Blastomyces dermatitidis*, usually presents as a primary pulmonary infection which occasionally may disseminate to the skin, bone and central nervous system; primary cutaneous inoculation is rare. Therapy usually involves prolonged courses of systemic antibiotics. The CO_2 laser may be used as an alternative or adjunct to medical therapy to ablate cutaneous lesions, particularly primary cutaneous inoculation as reported by Kantor et al.[9] As with all infectious lesions listed below, extra precautions may be necessary to avoid the CO_2 laser plume which is contaminated with the etiologic agent.

Botryomycosis

Cutaneous botryomycosis is a chronic skin infection caused by *Staphylococcus aureus* mimicking a deep fungal infection. The disease responds variably to oral and intravenous antibiotic therapy and, in some cases, surgical excision may be necessary. When conservative medical management fails and excision is not practical, the CO_2 laser can be used to successfully ablate these cutaneous lesions. Leffell et al[11] demonstrated complete resolution of an infection at 6-month follow-up after vaporization of a large plaque on the dorsum of the right foot.

Chromomycosis

Chromomycosis is a chronic and slowly progressive infection of the skin and subcutaneous tissue caused by several species of saprophytic, dematiaceous fungi. As in botryomycosis, response to a number of medical regimens is variable. Thus, scalpel excision with wide margins has become a preferred treatment for localized, small lesions. Excision with the CO_2 laser offers the advantage of immediate hemostasis during surgery and theoretically reduces the risk of disseminated infection due to sterilization of the surgical field and sealing off of blood vessels and lymphatics as described by Kuttner and Siegle.[12]

Leishmaniasis

In a recent report by Babajev et al,[13] 108 patients with cutaneous leishmaniasis were treated with the CO_2 laser. Of 108 patients, 101 were young or middle-aged and 82% were men. The duration of their disease was 3 months or more. The skin manifestations ranged from a single ulcer to one or more lesions, located mainly on the extremities, trunk, or head and neck. The CO_2 laser was used in a continuous mode with powers from 40 to 100 W, and power densities of 2.3–3.0 kW/cm². Single tuberculi of leishmaniasis lesions were vaporized using a defocused laser beam. With multiple lesions, the largest and most infected ulcers were removed in one session, and the remainder were treated as soon as the first ones re-epithelialized. Epithelialization of the wound began by day 5–7 and was complete by day 10–30. Cultures showed that the wound produced by the laser was 96% sterile. Cosmetic results were reported to be satisfactory, especially on the face and neck. Since medical therapy for cutaneous leishmaniasis is not readily available or routinely effective, destructive therapy seems to hold promise. This problem has increased in the USA since the soldiers returned from the Gulf War. Cryosurgery has always been effective, but CO_2 laser vaporization would be more precise.

Atypical mycobacteria

There have been no reports regarding CO_2 laser treatment for localized atypical mycobacterial infections, for example *Mycobacterium marinum* or sporotrichoid-like lesions. One might consider laser vaporization as an option for the treatment of these indolent cutaneous lesions.

Perifolliculitis capitis abscedens et suffodiens

Perifolliculitis capitis abscedens et suffodiens is a chronic disease of the scalp characterized by multiple firm nodules or fluctuant abscesses scattered over the occiput and vertex which are connected through sinus tracts. The end-result of this process is usually a severe, scarring alopecia. The cause is unknown.

Perifolliculitis capitis abscedens et suffodiens tends to be resistant to medical treatments which include antiseptic wet dressings, hot compresses, topical or intralesional corticosteroids or systemic retinoids. Aggressive therapy with local irradiation or total scalp excision with grafting leads to permanent alopecia. Glass et al[14] reported one case in which the CO_2 laser was utilized in the focused fashion to excise a large fluctuant nodule. Second intention wound healing was complete after 6 weeks, and there was no evidence of recurrence after 4 months of follow-up.

Pigmentation disorders

Lentigines

Carbon dioxide laser vaporization of the skin with fluences of 3.8–5.7 J/cm² induces primarily epidermal damage with little or no involvement of the underlying dermis. Dover et al[15] have demonstrated that this mode of therapy is an effective way to lighten actinic lentigines with little scarring or postinflammatory hypo- or hyperpigmentation. The authors still feel that cryotherapy is the best option because of its simplicity and low cost. The pigmented lesion lasers are newer and theoretically more precise because of selective chromophore (melanin) destruction. However, the cost of these lasers makes this therapy more expensive than necessary and several treatments are required. Clearly these lasers are being used as advertising to attract patients intrigued by laser therapy.

Ochronosis

Endogenous ochronosis is a rare inborn error of metabolism in which homogentisic acid oxidase is absent. This results in yellow, brown or ochre pigment deposition within connective tissues. Exogenous ochronosis can result from the repeated topical use of several chemically related compounds such as phenol, resorcinol, quinine and hydroquinone.

Treatment of exogenous ochronosis is difficult. Most cases show little resolution over time while topical retinoids and corticosteroids lack efficacy. The CO_2 laser was useful in removing this dermal pigmentation in one study by Diven et al.[16] The CO_2 laser was used in a defocused fashion at 3–6-W settings to remove pigment from the skin around the eyes, nose and forehead. After healing, the cosmetic result was very acceptable.

Vascular tumors

Lymphangioma circumscriptum

Carbon dioxide laser vaporization of lymphangioma circumscriptum has been reported in adult patients by Bailin et al[17] and in infants by Kaplan.[18] The rationale for using the CO_2 laser for this type of lesion stems from the use of the CO_2 laser for the treatment of portwine stains, whereby a decrease in the number of ectatic blood vessels and erythrocytes has been described. Furthermore, it is known that the CO_2 laser seals small lymphatic and blood vessel channels. Successful treatment depends upon vaporization of the entire lesion, including the deep communicating cistern. The authors have had very good results in both primary and secondary lymphangioma when limited to the skin. If there are significant deeper soft tissue communications, some cases heal slowly and are subject to infection.

Angiofibromas

Janniger and Goldberg[19] compared treatment results of the CO_2 and argon lasers in one patient with tuberous sclerosis and multiple facial angiofibromas. The CO_2 laser was used in a defocused mode at 5 W power with a continuous wave and a 2-mm spot size, resulting in an irradiance of 160 W/cm², to vaporize each lesion in two passes. Healing occurred within 3 weeks without postinflammatory pigmentary changes.

Cosmetic results were excellent. In general, both lasers work, but scarring and abnormal hypopigmentation are more common with the CO_2 laser.[20–22] If the angiofibromas have a significant vascular (red) component, argon, tunable dye or other yellow light lasers might be more effective. Dermabrasion may also be considered. Recurrences should be expected.

Disorders of keratinization

Porokeratosis of Mibelli

Porokeratosis of Mibelli consists of one or more keratotic plaques surrounded by a distinct, raised border of epidermal proliferation. When extensive areas are involved, treatment has been generally unsuccessful. Groot and Johnston[23] reported CO_2 laser treatment of porokeratosis of Mibelli in a patient with lesions over the entire foot and leg. By the use of the CO_2 laser at 10 W with a 10-mm spot size, the lesions were vaporized in staged procedures every 3 months. Follow-up 2 years later showed no clinical evidence of recurrence. It appears that the CO_2 laser may be very helpful in these cases, but dermabrasion might also be considered.

Linear porokeratosis

Linear porokeratosis was also reported to be successfully treated by the CO_2 laser. Barnett[24] reported successful treatment in a patient with a lifelong history of linear porokeratosis, as well as of the hyperkeratotic type on the fingers and the zosteriform type on the right side of the neck and shoulder. The CO_2 laser was used at 4–6 W in a pulsed mode with a spot size of 0.3 mm and a power density of 5700–8600 W/cm². Healing was within 3 weeks with minimal pain and slight scar formation and hypopigmentation. No recurrences were noted 1 year later. The specific advantages of CO_2 laser vaporization are in the controlled epidermal and dermal destruction (when needed), and that difficult anatomic locations not traditionally accessible by dermabrasion can be vaporized (laserabrasion).

Genodermatoses

Hailey–Hailey and Darier's disease

McElroy et al[25] used the CO_2 laser for the treatment of symptomatic plaques of Hailey–Hailey and Darier's disease (Figures 31.2 and 31.3). Two patients with recalcitrant Darier's disease and two other patients with recalcitrant Hailey–Hailey disease were treated. Vaporization was carried to the reticular dermis. The epidermal appendages were not completely destroyed. Only one patient with Darier's disease experienced a recurrence in one of eight treated plaques. Since this report Kartamaa and Reitamo[26] and others[27] have treated more patients with similar success. In the authors' opinion this therapy holds great promise. Many other surgical modalities may be effective if used properly, such as cryosurgery, dermabrasion, dermatomal planing, and excision with or without grafting. Rather than remissions with medical therapy in 4–6 months, surgical

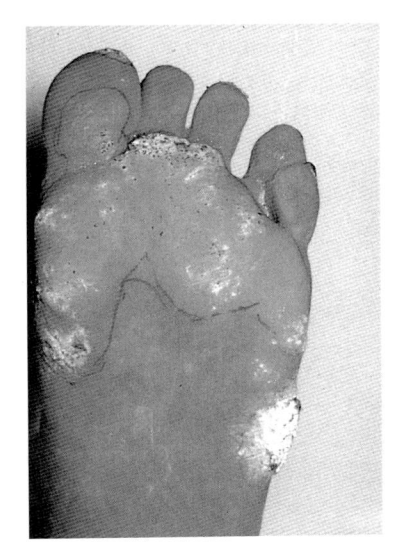

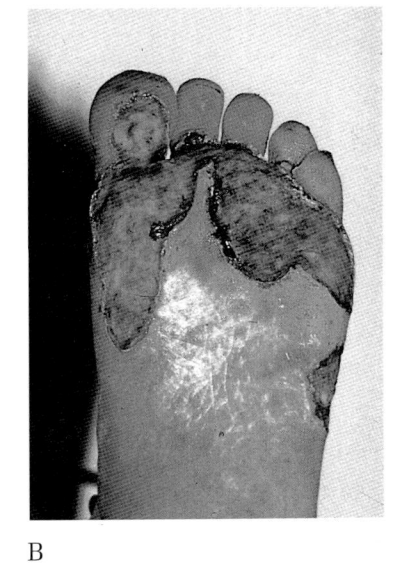

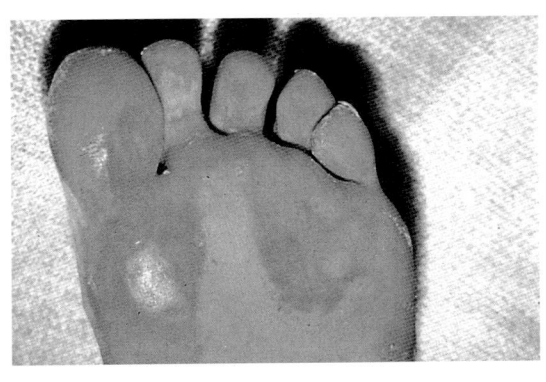

Figure 31.2
Darier's disease. (A) Preoperatively involving the foot. Patient unable to walk. (B) Immediately after CO_2 vaporization. (C) Three months postoperatively. Symptoms gone and patient able to walk normally.

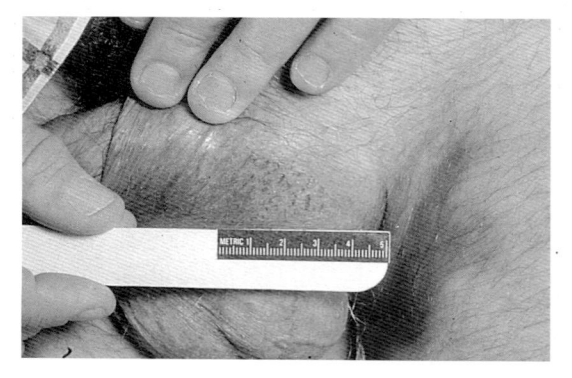

SURGICAL DERMATOLOGY

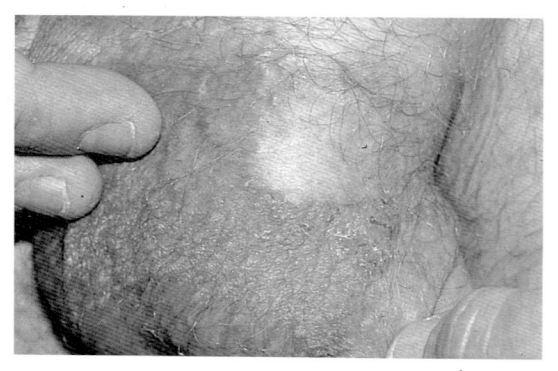

Figure 31.3
Hailey–Hailey disease. (A) Preoperatively. (B) One year postoperatively. Treated site has healed well and is asymptomatic. Recurrence at periphery, previously not treated.

Figure 31.4
Neurofibromas. (A) Preoperatively. (B) One month after CO_2 laser vaporization. Tumors do not rub on clothing and are less symptomatic.

treatment may be effective for 5–10 years at the treated site. The reason for lack of recurrence is unclear but probably has to do with the dermal–epidermal interface and its role in the pathogenesis of Hailey–Hailey disease or Darier's disease.

Neurofibromatosis

Cutaneous benign neurofibromas are the most common skin manifestation of neurofibromatosis. Patients may develop several to hundreds of cutaneous tumors in a lifetime. The majority of these tumors are small (less than 2 cm) and treatment usually involves simple or punch excision. Roenigk and Ratz[28] have shown that many (over 100) neurofibromas can easily, quickly and efficiently be treated using the CO_2 laser in one session with results equal to or better than excision (Figure 31.4).

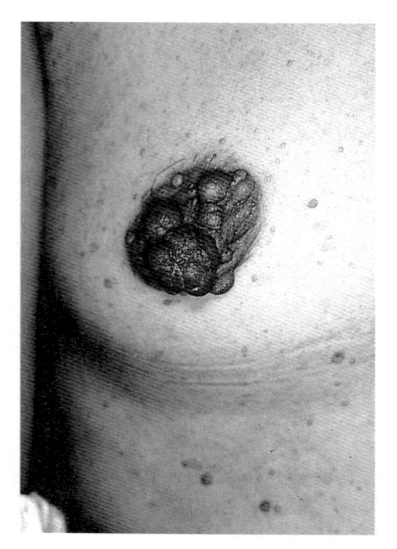

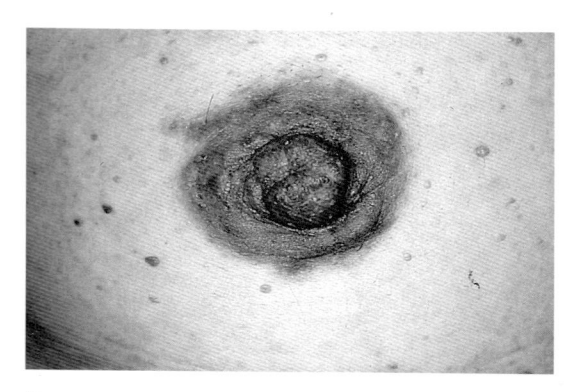

When the resultant wounds are small, second intention wound healing leads to excellent cosmesis. Larger or deeper defects may be sutured with absorbable sutures for more rapid healing. If completely removed, lesions seldom recur, but this treatment does not prevent the development of new neurofibromas.

METABOLIC DISEASES

Amyloidosis

Nodular primary localized cutaneous amyloidosis is an uncommon disorder which is difficult to treat. In one case report by Truhan et al,[29] a 3.7 × 4.6 cm scalp lesion was treated with the CO_2 laser on two occasions, 3 months apart. Re-epithelialization was complete within 3–4 weeks. A repeat biopsy showed persistent amyloid in the reticular dermis and subcutaneous tissue; however, the clinical appearance was cosmetically acceptable with complete regrowth of the terminal hairs. Nine-month follow-up revealed an area adjacent to the treated site which developed a nodular appearance and was positive for amyloid. The authors elected to observe that area.

INFLAMMATORY DISEASES

Balanitis xerotica obliterans and vaginal lichen sclerosis et atrophicus

Balanitis xerotica obliterans is a chronic, painful condition of the glans penis characterized by longstanding inflammation leading to atrophic, friable, eroded skin. Medical treatments are not always successful. In one case report by Ratz,[30] treatment with the CO_2 laser set at 20 W in the defocused mode yielded complete resolution of disease after 12 weeks healing time with no evidence of recurrence at 21 months. The authors have used the low-fluence CO_2 laser to treat painful vaginal lichen sclerosis et atrophicus with similar benefit (Figure 31.5). Gynecologists have used the flashlamp dye laser to treat vulvodynia. Precise de-epithelialization, superficial dermal vaporization, and wound healing with a soft supple scar (analogous to the procedure commonly followed for actinic cheilitis) may be improving this problem, but we do not know why.

Granuloma faciale

Granuloma faciale is characterized histologically by a dense, band-like collection of acute and chronic inflammatory cells involving the upper reticular dermis but sparing a narrow zone of papillary dermis. Wheeland et al[31] treated a patient with a single lesion on the nose with the CO_2 laser in the continuous, defocused mode at 5 W and 638 W/cm² power density. They found that the nonselective vaporization by the CO_2 laser is an alternative to traditional therapies with more rapid healing, with lack of significant scarring, and without recurrence. The authors have also tried the argon laser with variable results.

Hidradenitis suppurativa

Hidradenitis suppurativa is manifested by painful dermal and subcutaneous cystic nodules that are interconnected by draining sinus tracts. The most effective treatment has been exteriorization or wide excision of the entire apocrine gland-bearing tissue. This can lead to extensive wounds and functionally difficult scars. Sherman and Reid[32] treated 11 patients with chronic hidradenitis of the anogenital region using the CO_2 laser to vaporize the fibrotic tissue, abscessed areas and sinus tracts only. The adjacent, uninvolved skin was left untreated. Wounds were closed primarily or allowed to heal by second

SURGICAL DERMATOLOGY

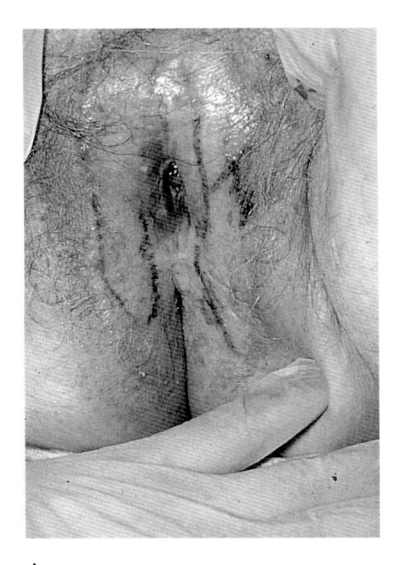

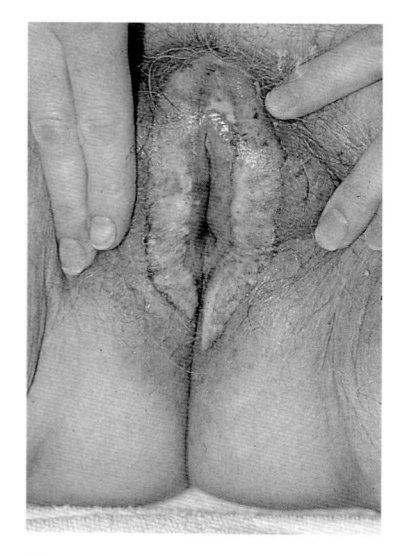

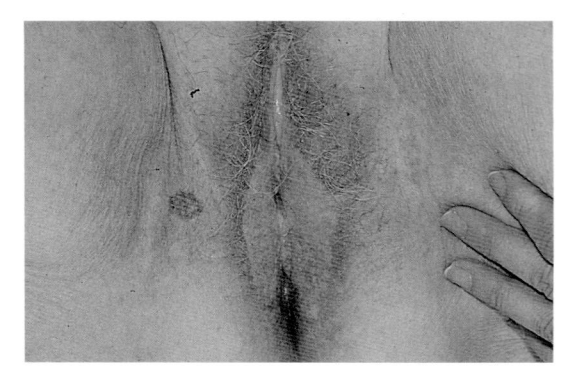

Figure 31.5
Lichen sclerosis et atrophicus: painful. (A) Preoperatively, area to be treated marked with gentian violet. (B) Immediately after CO_2 laser vaporization, removing mucosal epithelium only. (C) Five months postoperatively; healed with pigment alteration but symptoms gone.

intention. Patients reported little postoperative morbidity, satisfactory cosmetic appearance, and no disease recurrence to date. Others have also reported their experiences using the CO_2 laser.[33]

SUMMARY (TABLE 31.1)

The principal advantage of using the CO_2 laser is the precise destruction of tissue. This is important for two reasons. First, difficult anatomic locations such as the eyelids, lips, fingers, genital areas, etc. are not as easy to treat precisely with other destructive methods (cryosurgery, electrosurgery, dermabrasion). The CO_2 laser allows this option. If the subsequent wound does not include the entire dermis, second intention healing often results in a soft, supple, functionally and cosmetically acceptable scar.

Second, it is important to consider the pathology of the lesion being treated. Epidermal and superficial dermal

Table 31.1
Cutaneous lesions treated with the carbon dioxide (CO_2) laser

Common indications for CO_2 laser
    Actinic cheilitis
    Condyloma acuminatum (recalcitrant)
    Epidermal nevi
    Hand and digital verrucae (recalcitrant)
    Periungual verrucae
    Plantar verrucae (recalcitrant)
    Rhinophyma

CO_2 laser used as one of several alternative therapies
    Adenoma sebaceum
    Basal cell carcinoma (superficial)
    Bowenoid papulosis
    Bowen's disease
    Keloids
    Neurofibromas
    Organoid nevi
    Plantar keratoderma
    Sebaceous adenoma
    Squamous cell carcinoma (in situ)
    Tattoos (professional)
    Trichoepithelioma
    Xanthelasma

CO_2 laser occasionally used
    Angiokeratoma (Fordyce)
    Balanitis xerotica obliterans
    Blastomycosis (primary inoculation)
    Chromomycosis
    Cutaneous amyloid
    Cylindroma
    Darier's disease
    Digital mucous cyst
    Erythroplasia of Queyrat
    Hailey-Hailey disease (benign familial pemphigus)
    Lichen myxedematosus
    Lichen planus
    Pearly penile papules
    Zoon's balanitis

Reproduced with permission from Fairhurst et al, Carbon dioxide laser surgery for skin disease, *Mayo Clinic Proceedings* (1992) **67**:49–58.

processes may be effectively managed by the CO_2 laser, including some traditionally treated medically (that is Hailey–Hailey disease, Darier's disease, balanitis xerotica obliterans, lichen sclerosis et atrophicus). More deeply invasive tumors need deeper vaporization, excision or a combination of surgical therapies.

While new lasers are available for more specific chromophore destruction (yellow light lasers, pigmented lesion laser, Q-switched ruby laser), there is still a need in dermatology for the CO_2 laser. Besides the most common indications listed earlier, its ability to precisely destroy some less common skin lesions still makes the CO_2 laser a useful clinical tool.

References

1. Bickley LK, Goldberg DJ, Imaeda S et al, Treatment of multiple apocine hydrocystomas with the carbon dioxide (CO_2) laser, *J Dermatol Surg Oncol* (1989) **15**:599–602.

2. Stoner MF, Hobbs ER, Treatment of multiple dermal cylindromas with the carbon dioxide laser, *J Dermatol Surg Oncol* (1988) **14**:1263–67.

3. Wheeland RG, Bailin PL, Reynolds OD et al, Carbon dioxide (CO_2) laser vaporization of multiple facial syringomas, *J Dermatol Surg Oncol* (1986) **12**:225–8.

4. Nerad JA, Anderson RL, CO_2 laser treatment of eyelid syringomas, *Ophthal Plast Reconstr Surg* (1988) **4**:91–4.

5. Apfelberg DB, Maser MR, Lash H et al, Superpulse CO_2 laser treatment of facial syringomata, *Lasers Surg Med* (1987) **7**:533–7.

6. Huerter CJ, Wheeland RG, Bailin PL et al, Treatment of digital myxoid cysts with carbon dioxide laser vaporization, *J Dermatol Surg Oncol* (1987) **13**:723–7.

7. Magid M, Garden JM, Pearly penile papules: treatment with the carbon dioxide laser, *J Dermatol Surg Oncol* (1989) **15**:552–4.

8. Garrett AB, DuFresne RG, Ratz JL et al, Carbon dioxide laser treatment of pitted acne scarring, *J Dermatol Surg Oncol* (1990) **16**:737–40.

9. Kantor GR, Ratz JL, Wheeland RG, Treatment of acne keloidalis nuchae with carbon dioxide laser, *J Am Acad Dermatol* (1986) **14**:263–7.

10. Kantor GR, Roenigk RK, Bailin PL et al, Cutaneous blastomycosis: report of a case presumably acquired by direct inoculation and treated with carbon dioxide laser vaporization, *Cleve Clin J Med* (1987) **54**:121–4.

11. Leffell DJ, Brown MD, Swanson NA, Laser vaporization: a novel treatment of botryomycosis, *J Dermatol Surg Oncol* (1989) **15**:703–5.

12. Kuttner BJ, Siegle RJ, Treatment of chromomycosis with a CO_2 laser, *J Dermatol Surg Oncol* (1986) **12**:965–8.

13. Babajev KB, Babajev OG, Korepanov VI, Treatment of cutaneous leishmaniasis using a carbon dioxide laser, *Bull WHO* (1991) **69**:103–6.

14. Glass LF, Berman B, Laub D, Treatment of perifolliculitis capitis abscedens et suffodiens with the carbon dioxide laser, *J Dermatol Surg Oncol* (1989) **15**:673–6.

15. Dover JS, Smoller BR, Stern RS et al, Low-fluence carbon dioxide laser irradiation of lentigines, *Arch Dermatol* (1988) **124**:1219–24.

16. Diven DG, Smith EB, Pupo RA et al, Hydroquinone-induced localized exogenous ochronosis treated with dermabrasion and CO_2 laser, *J Dermatol Surg Oncol* (1990) **16**:1018–22.

17. Bailin PL, Kantor GR, Wheeland RG, Carbon dioxide laser vaporization of lymphangioma circumscriptum, *J Am Acad Dermatol* (1986) **14**:257–62.

18. Kaplan I, The Sharplan CO_2 laser in neonatal surgery, *Ann Plast Surg* (1982) **8**:426–8.

19. Janniger CK, Goldberg DJ, Angiofibromas in tuberous sclerosis: comparison of treatment by carbon dioxide and argon laser, *J Dermatol Surg Oncol* (1990) **16**:317–20.

20. Spenier CW, Achauer BM, Vanderkam VM, Treatment of extensive adenoma sebaceum with a carbon dioxide laser, *Ann Plast Surg* (1988) **20**:586–9.

21. Weston J, Apfelberg DB, Maser MR et al, Carbon dioxide laserbrasion of treatment of adenoma sebaceum in tuberous sclerosis, *Ann Plast Surg* (1985) **15**:132–7.

22. Wheeland RG, Bailin PL, Kantor GR et al, Treatment of adenoma sebaceum with carbon dioxide laser vaporization, *J Dermatol Surg Oncol* (1985) **11**:861–4.

23. Groot DW, Johnston PA, Carbon dioxide laser treatment of porokeratosis of Mibelli, *Lasers Surg Med* (1985) **5**:603–6.

24. Barnett JH, Linear porokeratosis: treatment with the carbon dioxide laser, *J Am Acad Dermatol* (1986) **14**:902–4.

25. McElroy JA, Mehregan DA, Roenigk RK, Carbon dioxide laser vaporization of recalcitrant asymptomatic plaques of Hailey–Hailey disease and Darier's disease, *J Am Acad Dermatol* (1990) **23**:893–7.

26. Kartamaa IM, Reitamo S, Gamilial benign chronic pemphigus (Hailey-Hailey disease): treatment with carbon dioxide laser vaporization, *Arch Dermatol* (1992) **128**:646–8.

27. Don PC, Camey PS, Lynch WS et al, Carbon dioxide laserbrasion: a new approach to management of familial benign chronic pemphigus (Hailey–Hailey disease), *J Dermatol Surg Oncol* (1987) **12**:1187–94.

28. Roenigk RK, Ratz JL, CO_2 laser treatment of cutaneous neurofibromas, *J Dermatol Surg Oncol* (1987) **13**:187–90.

29. Truhan AP, Garden JM, Roenigk HH, Nodular primary localized cutaneous amyloidosis: immunohistochemical evaluation and treatment with the carbon dioxide laser, *J Am Acad Dermatol* (1986) **14**:1058–62.

30. Ratz JL, Carbon dioxide laser treatment of balanitis xerotica obliterans, *J Am Acad Dermatol* (1984) **10:**925–8.

31. Wheeland RG, Ashley JR, Smith DA et al, Carbon dioxide laser treatment of granuloma faciale, *J Dermatol Surg Oncol* (1984) **10:**730–3.

32. Sherman AI, Reid R, CO_2 laser for suppurative hidradenitis of the vulva, *J Reprod Med* (1991) **36:**113–17.

33. Dalrymple JC, Monaghan JM, Treatment of hidradenitis suppurative with the carbon dioxide laser, *Br J Surg* (1987) **74:**420.

Chapter 32

HUMAN PAPILLOMAVIRUS

Mark W. Cobb

INTRODUCTION

Throughout history, medical science has recognized and studied the most common manifestation of the human papillomavirus (HPV) infection: the wart. The ancient Greeks and Romans knew that anogenital warts were transmitted sexually[1] and as early as the first century AD, Celsus[2] described three types of warts: 'ficus' (fig), referring to genital warts; 'thymion' (thyme plant), indicating the common wart; and 'myrmecia' (anthill), meaning the deep plantar wart. Work by Ciuffo[3] in 1907 and Strauss et al[4] in 1949 strongly suggested the viral etiology of warts. Subsequently, the etiologic agent has been identified as a double-stranded DNA virus, belonging to the Papovaviridae family. The human papillomavirus has recently been implicated in a variety of benign cutaneous and mucosal lesions as well as the development of some forms of human cancer, most notably anogenital cancer and squamous cell carcinoma of the skin. The dermatologic surgeon should be well versed in this important viral infection; he or she may be called upon to treat a benign or malignant lesion resulting from HPV infection. Of recent concern is evidence that several therapeutic modalities employed in the treatment of warts have the potential of transmitting the infection to members of the surgical team.

VIROLOGY

The human papillomavirus contains double-stranded, circular, supercoiled DNA enclosed in an icosahedral capsid made up of 72 capsomeres and measuring 55 nm in diameter. The virus has no envelope and is resistant to ether inactivation, freezing, desiccation and prolonged storage at −20°C. It has never been successfully propagated in tissue culture. Different HPV types have been identified by means of DNA hybridization. By convention, a virus is classified as a new type if it hybridizes by less than 50% with other known types.[5] It is important to realize that 50% hybridization implies approximately 90% identity at the DNA sequence level.[1] To date there have been approximately 60 HPV types identified and new types are continuing to be isolated.[6,7] For many of these HPV types, a significant clinicopathological correlation exists (Table 32.1).

Table 32.1
HPV types and their clinical associations

HPV-1	Deep plantar warts, common warts
HPV-2	Common warts, flat warts
HPV-3, -10, -41	Flat warts
HPV-4	Common warts, plantar warts
HPV-5, -8, -9, -12, -14, -15, -17, -19 to -25, -36, -37 -38, -46, -47, -49, -50	Epidermodysplasia verruciformis (EV)
HPV-6, -11, -43, -44, -55	Genital warts, laryngeal papillomas
HPV-7	Common warts in meat handlers
HPV-13	Focal epithelial hyperplasia
HPV-16, -18, -31, -32, -42, -51 to -54	Genital warts, bowenoid papulosis, cervical dysplasia, cervical carcinoma
HPV-26 to -29	Common warts, flat warts
HPV-30	Laryngeal carcinoma, genital warts
HPV-33	Cervical carcinoma
HPV-34, -48	Bowenoid papulosis, Bowen's disease
HPV-35	Cervical dysplasia, cervical carcinoma
HPV-39	Bowenoid papulosis, cervical carcinoma

Adapted from ref. 8.

Epidemiology and Natural History of HPV Infection

A number of surveys involving both pediatric and adult populations have documented warts in 3.5–5% of patients.[9] In Great Britain, 10–25% of new patients presenting to dermatologic clinics do so for warts.[10] The incidence of warts peaks between the ages of 12 and 16, where 70% are common warts, 24% are plantar warts, and 3.5% are plane warts. Anogenital warts are one of the most common viral sexually transmitted diseases and have recently increased in incidence as documented by a 28-year epidemiologic survey at Mayo Clinic of patients from Rochester, Minnesota.[11] Between 1950 and 1978, a general rise in the average annual incidence rate of condylomas was noted, with an average annual rate of 106.5 per 100 000 in the period 1975–78. A report from the MMWR documents a five-fold increase in office visits for condylomas from 1966 to 1981.[12] Young adults in the third decade of life are most likely to have anogenital warts. The incidence of HPV infection is increased in immunocompromised patients; up to 43% of kidney transplant patients have warts.[13] These patients may also progress more rapidly from wart to malignancy.

Transmission of HPV usually occurs by close contact with an infected individual, although desquamated keratinocytes may also transmit the virus.[1] Small breaks in the skin may be necessary to inoculate HPV, explaining the frequent localization of warts to traumatized areas (hands, feet, knees) and the Koebner phenomenon seen with flat warts. Autoinoculation may cause warts to spread locally and appear on adjacent digits. The infectivity of HPV depends on many factors, including the number of viral particles in the lesion(s) contacted (determined in part by lesion type and location), the degree of exposure to the lesion(s), local factors such as skin moisture, and the host's defenses against HPV infection. Experimental inoculation studies have shown that verrucae take 1–6 months to become clinically apparent.[14]

The study of anogenital warts has taught us much about the infectivity and subsequent incubation period of HPV infection. One large, single-center study found that 64% of sexual partners of individuals with known genital warts developed genital warts themselves after 9 months.[15] The average incubation time for the development of genital warts in this study was 2.8 months, with a range of 3 weeks to 8 months. Others have found the incubation period to range from 1 to 20 months.[16] Although the majority of genital warts contain HPV-6, -11 or -16 and most common and plantar warts contain HPV-1, -2 and -4, there have been isolated reports of the detection of HPV-1 and HPV-2 in genital warts, supporting occasional nonvenereal transmission.[17,18]

Anogenital warts are being reported more frequently in children.[16,19] Because of concern about potential child abuse, the route of transmission becomes of paramount importance. Pediatric patients may acquire genital HPV infection during delivery or from close nonsexual contact.[16] Recent literature, however, implicates sexual transmission in at least some and possibly the majority of cases. An American Academy of Dermatology Task Force examining genital warts and sexual abuse in children concluded that at least 50% of pediatric cases of genital warts can be documented by investigators as sexual abuse and that when anal or genital warts are found in children under the age of 12 years, sexual abuse should be considered.[20] Nonvenereal transmission is more likely when there is no physical evidence of child abuse, when the lesions are located some distance from the anus or introitus, and when the child is less than 9 months old when the lesions first appear.[21]

Spontaneous regression of warts is a well-documented phenomenon, occurring in about two-thirds of warts on children when followed for 2 years.[22] Several studies have provided evidence that the cell-mediated immune response to HPV infection as measured by lymphocyte transformation and leukocyte migration inhibition may play a role in wart regression.[23,24]

Clinical Manifestations of HPV

Clinical lesions resulting from HPV infection may be divided into two broad categories: cutaneous and extracutaneous. Cutaneous lesions include common warts (verruca vulgaris), filiform warts, flat warts (verruca plana), plantar warts (including myrmecia and mosaic types), anogenital warts, and bowenoid papulosis. Extracutaneous lesions occur on mucous membranes and include oral common warts, oral condyloma acuminata, focal epithelial hyperplasia, oral florid papillomatosis, nasal papillomas, conjunctival papillomas, laryngeal papillomatosis, and cervical warts.

Common warts are rough, keratotic papules that may appear singly or grouped on any cutaneous surface, most commonly on the dorsal hands and extremities. Butcher's warts, caused by HPV-7 as well as types 1–4, are common warts that are found on the hands and fingers of meat cutters.[25] Warts may occasionally have an overlying cutaneous horn or appear as long, slender, filiform lesions. Flat warts are slightly elevated, smooth, flesh-colored-to-tan papules that are generally less than 5 mm in size. They usually occur as multiple lesions on the face, hands and legs of children, often in a linear array. Plantar warts usually have a rough, keratotic surface studded with punctate black dots, representing thrombosed capillaries, and a peripheral rim of thickened skin. They may coalesce to form a mosaic wart or may present as a deep, endophytic lesion called a myrmecia wart. When hyperhidrosis is present, plantar warts are frequently widespread and refractory to therapy.

Anogenital warts have three basic morphologies: hyperplastic, cauliflower-like lesions (condylomata acuminata), sessile papules, and keratotic, verruca vulgaris-like lesions. The hyperplastic type are typically found on moist areas like the glans penis, inner surface of the prepuce, urethral meatus, anal mucosa, perianal area and labia. The sessile papules and keratotic lesions are seen on the penile shaft. Recently, small macular and slightly elevated lesions have been detected on apparently normal penile skin after the application of 5% acetic acid (aceto white test) and with the aid of magnification (colposcopy for example).[26-28] These show histological changes consistent with condylomata acuminata or intraepithelial neoplasia. This has become an important adjunctive diagnostic technique for the detection of HPV infection of the male genitalia. A disorder termed *bowenoid papulosis* has been described, consisting of multiple small, verrucous or velvety, often pigmented papules involving the anogenital region of young adults.[29-31] Histological examination reveals changes of carcinoma in situ suggestive of Bowen's disease. These lesions may behave in a manner similar to condylomata acuminata, responding to conservative surgical removal and topical 5-fluorouracil, and even undergoing spontaneous regression.[30-32] In the majority of cases, HPV-16 has been demonstrated.[33,34] The benign nature of this condition has been questioned, for it may be associated with cervical dysplasia and has been reported to progress to Bowen's disease.[35] Vulvar papillomatosis is another newly described condition, presenting as a velvety, granular or cobblestone-like surface on the vulvar vestibule and at times causing vulvodynia.[36,37]

A variety of extracutaneous HPV infections involve orificial mucous membranes. Common warts and condylomata acuminata may be seen in the oral cavity. Similarly, nasal and conjunctival papillomas are manifestations of HPV infection. Focal epithelial hyperplasia, consisting of multiple, discrete and confluent papules on the oral mucosa, is a condition described primarily in children of American Indian descent.[38] These lesions contain HPV-13, a type unique to this condition.[39] Laryngeal papillomas, a potentially life-threatening manifestation of HPV infection, not only involve the larynx, but may also extend into the tracheal, bronchial and pulmonary epithelia.[40] They may become sufficiently large to cause airway obstruction and death. Although the papillomas tend to regress, recurrences and treatment failures are common. Since HPV-6 and HPV-11 have been frequently found in this condition and are commonly isolated from anogenital warts, it is postulated that infants may acquire the disease during birth from mothers with condylomata acuminata. Cervical condylomas may present as exophytic papillomatous lesions or more commonly as white patches visualized with the aid of acetic acid whitening and colposcopic examination.[41,42]

Finally, latent HPV infection may involve clinically normal skin adjacent to genital condylomas, as evidenced by the presence of HPV DNA.[43] When present, latent infection is associated with a higher rate of recurrent clinical disease after laser ablasion of condylomata acuminata.

HPV INFECTION IN IMMUNOSUPPRESSED PATIENTS

Epidermodysplasia verruciformis (EV) is a rare, genetic disorder characterized by persistent, refractory HPV infection that is believed to result from a specific defect in cell-mediated immunity. These patients have disseminated flat wart-like lesions and erythematous, hyperpigmented or hypopigmented macules.[44–47] About one-third of patients will develop malignant degeneration of their cutaneous lesions, almost always in sun-exposed areas. The cancers are usually multiple and tend to be in situ or invasive squamous cell carcinoma. At least 23 different HPV types occur in EV patients and most are found almost exclusively in this disorder. HPV-5 is the most common type isolated.

A variety of other patients with immune deficiency states may present with extensive or unusual manifestations of HPV infection. Renal transplant patients, on chronic immunosuppressive therapy, have a high frequency of warts and may develop plaque lesions similar to those seen in EV.[48] Interestingly, these lesions may contain HPV-5/8 DNA, originally thought to be exclusively associated with EV.[48–50] Renal transplant recipients, like EV patients, have a markedly increased incidence of sun-induced squamous cell carcinoma.[51,52] These patients are also at increased risk for genital tract HPV infection and neoplasia.[53,54] Warts have been found to occur with increased frequency in patients with lymphoma, chronic lymphocytic leukemia and Hodgkin's disease.[55,56] Patients with AIDS appear not only to be more readily infected with HPV, but once infected may have persistent, atypical or unique lesions and may be at greater risk for malignant transformation.[57–61]

Detection of HPV

With the use of transmission electron microscopy, HPV has been visualized as 55-nm particles within the nuclei of infected cells.[62] Their presence varies among the different HPV-induced lesions. Antisera have been generated to HPV capsid antigens and may be either type specific or group specific depending on laboratory methods. These antisera, in combination with immunohistochemical or immunofluorescence techniques, can demonstrate productive HPV infection (one in which intact virions are produced) in lesional tissue. Tissue infected with HPV but not actively producing viral particles, such as dysplastic or carcinomatous lesions, will be negative. Several new methods for detecting HPV take advantage of recent advances in molecular biology such as nucleic acid hybridization, site-specific cleavage of DNA by restriction endonucleases, and DNA cloning.[63] Southern blotting[64] and dot-blotting[65] involve extracting DNA from lesional tissue and allowing it to hybridize with a specific labeled DNA probe, in this case cloned HPV DNA. In situ hybridization uses labeled DNA probes to detect HPV DNA within formalin-fixed, paraffin-embedded or frozen-tissue biopsy specimens, preserving lesional architecture.[66] A newly described technique, the polymerase chain reaction, allows targeted DNA sequences to be enzymatically amplified prior to Southern blotting so that a single molecule of HPV DNA can be detected in 10^5 cells.[67,68]

Relationship between HPV infection and cancer

Over 50 years ago a certain animal papillomavirus infecting the cottontail rabbit was shown to induce papillomas that would often progress to carcinoma.[69] More recently, a number of human carcinomas have been associated with HPV infection, including cervical carcinoma, squamous cell carcinoma associated with lesions of epidermodysplasia verruciformis and warts in immunocompromised patients, carcinomas arising in the aerodigestive tract, verrucous carcinoma, and Bowen's disease.

Of those carcinomas listed, cancer of the uterine cervix has received the most attention. HPV DNA has been demonstrated in a variety of cervical lesions using the DNA hybridization techniques described above. HPV-6 has been found in CIN and HPV-11 in a few cervical carcinomas, although these two types are usually associated with benign condylomas. More importantly, HPV-16 and HPV-18 have been repeatedly demonstrated in a majority (60–80%) of invasive cervical carcinomas.[70–72] HPV-33 and HPV-35 have also been isolated from cervical carcinomas. The HPV DNA found in cervical carcinomas is integrated into the host genome and no longer produces virions. This integration of HPV DNA results in deregulated expression of two viral genes involved with transformation, E6 and E7, providing further evidence for the role of HPV in cervical cancer.[73]

Although less studied, other human cancers have been associated with HPV infection. Epidermodysplasia verruciformis patients and renal transplant recipients with warts have an increase in sun-induced squamous cell carcinoma. HPV has also been implicated in cases of carcinoma of the nasal cavity and paranasal sinuses, laryngeal carcinoma, bronchogenic carcinoma, and esophageal carcinoma.[74] Periungual squamous cell carcinoma has been associated with HPV-16,[75] while HPV-34 DNA has been isolated from a lesion of Bowen's disease on the periungual region.[76] HPV-6 and HPV-11 are the most common types found in anogenital verrucous carcinoma.[77] Keratoacanthoma has also been associated with HPV infection.[78,79]

THERAPY FOR HPV INFECTION

A brief overview of wart therapy, including physical and chemical destructive methods, chemotherapeutic agents and immune modulators, will be given. Among the physical modalities, cryosurgery with liquid nitrogen is one of the most commonly used techniques. It is simple to perform, inexpensive and efficacious in the majority of warts. Electrosurgery, usually reserved for recalcitrant warts, may result in more scarring. Warts removed by blunt surgical dissection tend to recur more frequently than those treated by cryosurgery or electrosurgery. A more recent physical modality is the carbon dioxide laser. This has the advantages of control of surgical destruction, a bloodless surgical field, and possibly less postoperative pain.[80] Disadvantages include expense and the risk of spreading HPV in the laser plume.[81]

Chemical destructive methods include the use of salicylic acid, trichloroacetic acid, cantharidin, formalin and glutaraldehyde. Salicylic acid is available in a variety of vehicles, including solutions, plasters and adhesive patches, at concentrations ranging from 15 to 40%. Its keratolytic action destroys HPV-infected epidermis. It is an inexpensive, relatively effective therapy that may be applied at home. Trichloroacetic acid has the potential for causing more local destruction and subsequent scarring and should only be applied by a physician. Cantharidin, a mitochondrial poison produced by the blister beetle, destroys warts by inducing a blister at the site of application. Infrequently the wart recurs as a ring at the periphery of the blister. Formalin and glutaraldehyde are both topical solutions that destroy warts by dehydration. Both may cause an irritant or allergic contact dermatitis.

Regarding the chemotherapeutic agents employed in the therapy of warts (podophyllin, 5-fluorouracil and bleomycin), two recent advances will be discussed. First is the use of podophyllotoxin (Condylox Oclassen Pharmaceuticals Inc., San Rafael, CA) in the treatment of condylomata accuminata. Podophyllotoxin is the purified active ingredient in podophyllin, a plant extract derived from *Podophyllum peltatum* or *Podophyllum emodi*. Podophyllotoxin appears to be significantly less toxic than podophyllin with as yet no systemic reactions reported.[82] Unlike podophyllin, it may be applied at home by the patient. Several studies have documented its efficacy when applied twice daily for 3 consecutive days per week for 1–6 weeks.[82–84] Side-effects of this therapy are generally mild but may include erythema, swelling, burning and erosions.

The second recent advance has been a newly described technique for using bleomycin sulfate in the treatment of warts.[85] A small volume of bleomycin solution (1 U/ml) is placed over the wart. It is then introduced into the wart via multiple punctures with a small bifurcated needle (designed initially for smallpox vaccination) using approximately 40 punctures per 5 mm^2 wart tissue. These authors report a cure rate of 92%. Advantages of this technique vis-à-vis intralesional injection of bleomycin sulfate with a tuberculin syringe include a much smaller dose of bleomycin (each puncture introduces only 0.001 U) and much less chance of sublesional injection, for the bifurcated needle does not penetrate the dermis easily. Vasospastic complications were not encountered in this study of 258 warts.

Methods involving modulation of the host immune response to HPV infection include induction of a local allergic contact dermatitis with dinitrochlorobenzene (DNCB) or squaric acid dibutyl ester and the use of agents such as interferon or retinoids. Dinitrochlorobenzene is a potent topical sensitizer that may stimulate an immunologic or at least inflammatory reaction to eliminate warts.

Interferon (IF) is theoretically attractive in the treatment of HPV infection for a number of reasons.[86] The antiviral activity of IF should limit HPV replication in lesional as well as clinically normal infected skin. Its antiproliferative effect should slow the rapidly dividing keratinocytes seen in some warts and dysplastic genital lesions. Finally, IF may modulate the host's immune response to HPV infections.

Several clinical trials have demonstrated the efficacy of IF-α in the treatment of condylomata acuminata.[86–90] When it is used intralesionally two to three times weekly for up to 8 weeks, clearing rates of 36–62% are reported, varying with the type of IF-α used. Systemic IF, delivered either subcutaneously or intramuscularly, has also been shown to be beneficial in the treatment of genital warts in several uncontrolled studies. Interferon beta has been used intralesionally[91] and intramuscularly[92] with some success for condylomata acuminata. Finally, IF-α has been shown to be beneficial in two other HPV-related conditions, laryngeal papillomas[93] and epidermodysplasia verruciformis.[94] Side-effects of IF therapy include fatigue, fever, chills, myalgias, headache, malaise and a transient leukopenia.

Retinoids are another theoretically promising modality for the treatment of HPV disease. These agents have been demonstrated to enhance both humeral and cell-mediated immunity[95] and are well-known regulators of cellular differentiation. HPV replication, which appears to be linked to the state of keratinocyte differentiation, may be inhibited by retinoids. Finally, malignant transformation of HPV-induced lesions may be prevented. In several case reports systemic retinoids have caused partial regression of HPV lesions in immunosuppressed patients.[96–98] However, discontinuation of therapy generally results in relapse. Topical retinoic acid (Retin-A) may be used to treat flat warts.

References

1. Lowy DR, Androphy EJ, Warts. In: Fitzpatrick TB, Elsen AZ, Wolff K, eds, *Dermatology in general medicine* (McGraw-Hill: New York 1987) 2355–64.

2. Lutzner MA, The human papillomaviruses, a review, *Arch Dermatol* (1983) **119**:631–5.

3. Ciuffo G, Innesto positivo con filtrato di verrucae volgare, *Giorn Ital Mal Venereol* (1907) **48**:12–17.

4. Strauss MJ, Shaw EW, Bunting H et al, 'Crystalline' virus-like particles from skin papillomas characterized by intranuclear inclusion bodies, *Proc Soc Exp Biol Med* (1949) **72**:46–50.

5. Coggin J Jr, Zur Hausen H Workshop in papillomaviruses and cancer, *Cancer Res* (1979) **39**:545–6.

6. Beutner KR, Human papillomavirus infection, *J Am Acad Dermatol* (1989) **20**:114–23.

7. DeVilliers EM, Heterogeneity of the human papillomavirus group, *J Virol* (1989) **63**:4898–903.

8. Cobb MW, Human papillomavirus infection, *J Am Acad Dermatol* (1990) **22**:547–66.

9. Beutner KR, Becker TM, Stone KM, Epidemiology of human papillomavirus infection, *Dermatol Clin* (1991) **9**:211–18.

10. Nagington J, Rook A, Highet AS, Virus and related infections. In: Rook A, Wilkinson DS, Ebling FJG, eds, *Textbook of dermatology* (Blackwell Scientific: Oxford 1986) 668–79.

11. Chuang T, Perry HO, Kurland LT et al, Condyloma acuminatum in Rochester, Minn., 1950–1978. I. Epidemiology and clinical features, *Arch Dermatol* (1984) **120**:469–75.

12. Condyloma acuminatum—United States, 1966–1981. *MMWR* (1983) **32**:306–8.

13. Briggaman RA, Wheeler CE, Immunology of human warts, *J Am Acad Dermatol* (1979) **1**:279–304.

14. Rowson KEK, Mahy BWJ, Human papova (wart) virus, *Bacteriol Rev* (1967) **31**:110–3.

15. Oriel JD, Natural history of genital warts, *Br J Vener Dis* (1971) **47**:1–13.

16. DeJong AR, Weiss JC, Brent RL, Condyloma acuminata in children, *Am J Dis Child* (1982) **136**:704–6.

17. Fleming KA, Venning V, Evans M, DNA typing of genital warts and diagnosis of sexual abuse of children, *Lancet* (1987) **2**:489.

18. Krzyzek RA, Watts SL, Anderson DL et al, Anogenital warts contain several distinct species of human papillomavirus, *J Virol* (1980) **36**:236–44.

19. Shelton TB, Jerkins GR, Noe HN, Condylomata acuminata in the pediatric patient, *J Urol* (1986) **135**:548–9.

20. Norins AL, Caputo RV, Lucky AW et al, Genital warts and sexual abuse in children, *J Am Acad Dermatol* (1984) **11**:529–30.

21. Rock B, Naghashfar Z, Barnett N et al, Genital tract papillomavirus infection in children, *Arch Dermatol* (1986) **122**:1129–32.

22. Massing AM, Epstein WL, Natural history of warts, *Arch Dermatol* (1963) **87**:74–8.

23. Ivanyi L, Morison WL, In vitro lymphocyte stimulation by wart antigen in man, *Br J Dermatol* (1976) **94**:523–7.

24. Lee AKY, Eisenger M, Cell-mediated immunity to human wart virus and wart-associated tissue antigens, *Clin Exp Immunol* (1976) **26**:419–24.

25. Orth G, Jablonska S, Favre M et al, Identification of papillomaviruses in butcher's warts, *J Invest Dermatol* (1981) **76**:97–102.

26. Barrasso R, De Brux J, Croissant O et al, High prevalence of papillomavirus-associated penile intraepithelial neoplasia in sexual partners of women

with cervical intraepithelial neoplasia, *N Engl J Med* (1987) **317**:916–23.

27. Sedlacek TV, Cunnane M, Carpiniello V, Colposcopy in the diagnosis of penile condyloma, *Am J Obstet Gynecol* (1986) **154**:494–6.

28. Berman A, Berman JE, New concepts in viral wart infection, *Compr Ther* (1988) **14**:19–24.

29. Patterson JW, Kao GF, Graham JH et al, Bowenoid papulosis. A clinicopathologic study with ultrastructural observations, *Cancer* (1986) **57**:823–36.

30. Wade TR, Kopf AW, Ackerman AB, Bowenoid papulosis of the genitalia, *Arch Dermatol* (1979) **115**:306–8.

31. Wade TR, Kopf AW, Ackerman AB, Bowenoid papulosis of the penis, *Cancer* (1978) **42**:1890–903.

32. Berger BW, Hori Y, Multicentric Bowen's disease of the genitalia, *Arch Dermatol* (1978) **114**:1698–9.

33. Ikenberg H, Gissmann L, Gross G et al, Human papillomavirus type 16-related DNA in genital Bowen's disease and bowenoid papulosis, *Int J Cancer* (1983) **32**:563–5.

34. Obalek S, Jablonska S, Beaudenon S et al, Bowenoid papulosis of the male and female genitalia: risk of cervical neoplasia, *J Am Acad Dermatol* (1986) **14**:433–44.

35. De Villez RL, Stevens CS, Bowenoid papules of the genitalia: a case progressing to Bowen's disease, *J Am Acad Dermatol* (1980) **3**:149–52.

36. Growdon WA, Fu YS, Lebherz TB et al, Pruritic vulvar squamous papillomatosis: evidence for human papillomavirus etiology, *Obstet Gynecol* (1985) **66**:564–8.

37. di Paola GR, Rueda NG, Deceptive vulvar papillomavirus infection. A possible explanation for certain cases of vulvodynia, *J Reprod Med* (1986) **31**:966–70.

38. Archard HO, Heck JW, Stanley HR, Focal epithelial hyperplasia: an unusual oral mucosal lesion found in Indian children, *Oral Surg* (1965) **20**:201–12.

39. Pfister H, Hettich I, Runne U et al, Characterization of human papillomavirus type 13 from focal epithelial hyperplasia Heck lesions, *J Virol* (1983) **47**:363–6.

40. Steinberg BM, Laryngeal papillomas. Clinical aspects and in vitro studies. In: Salzman NP, Howley PM eds, *The papovaviridae. 2. The papillomaviruses* (Plenum: New York 1987) 265–92.

41. Meisels A, Fortin R, Roy M, Condylomatous lesions of the cervix and vagina. II. Cytologic, colposcopic and histopathologic study, *Acta Cytol* (1977) **21**:379–90.

42. Meisels A, Roy M, Fortier M et al, Human papillomavirus infection of the cervix. The atypical condyloma, *Acta Cytol* (1981) **25**:7–16.

43. Gissmann L, de Villiers E-M, zur Hausen H, Analysis of human genital warts (condylomata acuminata) and other genital tumors for human papillomavirus type 6 DNA, *Int J Cancer* (1982) **29**:143–6.

44. Lewandowsky F, Lutz W, Ein fall einer bisher nicht beschriebenen hauterkrankung (epidermodysplasia verruciformis), *Arch Dermatol Syphilol* (1922) **141**:193–203.

45. Howley PM, Broker TR, eds, *Papillomaviruses. Molecular and clinical aspects* (Alan R. Liss: New York 1985).

46. Orth G, Epidermodysplasia verruciformis. In: Salzman NP, Howley PM, eds, *The papovaviridae. 2. The papillomaviruses* (Plenum: New York 1987) 199–243.

47. Lutzner MA, Blanchet-Bardon C, Epidermodysplasia verruciformis (Lewandowsky–Lutz syndrome). In: Fitzpatrick TB, Eisen AZ, Wolff K, eds, *Dermatology in general medicine* (McGraw-Hill: New York 1987) 2364–72.
48. Barr BBB, Benton EC, McLaren K et al, Human papilloma virus infection and skin cancer in renal allograft recipients, *Lancet* (1989) **1**:124–8.
49. Lutzner M, Croissant O, Ducasse MF et al, A potentially oncogenic human papillomavirus (HPV 5) found in two renal allograft recipients, *J Invest Dermatol* (1980) **75**:353–6.
50. Van der Leest RJ, Zachow KR, Ostrow RS et al, Human papillomavirus heterogeneity in 36 renal transplant recipients, *Arch Dermatol* (1987) **123**:354–7.
51. Hoxell EO, Mandel JS, Murray SS et al, Incidence of skin carcinoma after renal transplantation, *Arch Dermatol* (1977) **113**:436–8.
52. Boyle J, Mackie RM, Briggs JD et al, Cancer, warts and sunshine in renal transplant recipients, *Lancet* (1984) **1**:702–5.
53. Halpert R, Fruchter RG, Sedlis A et al, Human papillomavirus and lower genital neoplasms in renal transplant patients, *Obstet Gynecol* (1986) **68**:251–8.
54. Rudlinger R, Smith IW, Lunney MH et al, Human papillomavirus infections in a group of renal transplant recipients, *Br J Dermatol* (1986) **115**:681–92.
55. Savin JA, Noble WC, Immunosuppression and skin infection, *Br J Dermatol* (1975) **93**:115–20.
56. Morison WL, Viral warts, herpes simplex and herpes zoster in patients with secondary immune deficiencies and neoplasms, *Br J Dermatol* (1975) **92**:625–30.
57. Valle S-L, Dermatologic findings related to human immunodeficiency virus infection in high-risk individuals, *J Am Acad Dermatol* (1987) **17**:951–61.
58. Goodman DS, Teplitz ED, Wishner A et al, Prevalence of cutaneous disease in patients with acquired immunodeficiency syndrome (AIDS) or AIDS-related complex, *J Am Acad Dermatol* (1987) **17**:210–20.
59. Kaplan MH, Sadick N, McNutt NS et al, Dermatologic findings and manifestations of acquired immunodeficiency syndrome (AIDS), *J Am Acad Dermatol* (1987) **16**:485–506.
60. Milburn PB, Brandsma JL, Goldsman CI et al, Disseminated warts and evolving squamous cell carcinoma in a patient with acquired immunodeficiency syndrome, *J Am Acad Dermatol* (1988) **19**:401–5.
61. Fisher BK, Warner LC, Cutaneous manifestations of the acquired immunodeficiency syndrome, Update 1987, *Int J Dermatol* (1987) **26**:615–30.
62. Almeida JD, Howatson AF, Williams MG, Electron microscope study of human warts: sites of virus production and nature of the inclusion bodies, *J Invest Dermatol* (1962) **38**:337–45.
63. Wickenden C, Malcolm ADB, Coleman DV, DNA hybridization of cervical tissues, *CRC Crit Rev Clin Lab Sci* (1987) **25**:1–18.
64. Southern EM, Detection of specific sequences among DNA fragments separated by gel electrophoresis, *J Mol Biol* (1975) **98**:503–17.
65. Merz B, DNA probes for papillomavirus strains readied for cervical cancer screening, *JAMA* (1988) **260**:2777.
66. Todd J, Jou L, Yang HL, Use of biotinylated DNA probes for *in situ* detection of HPV in biopsy specimens.

In: *Proc. Sixth Internal Papillomavirus Workshop*, Washington, DC, June 1987.

67. Young LS, Bevan IS, Johnson MA et al, The polymerase chain reaction: a new epidemiological tool for investigating cervical human papillomavirus infection, *Br Med J* (1989) **298**:14–18.

68. Morris BJ, Flanagan JL, McKinnon KJ et al, Papillomavirus screening of cervical lavages by polymerase chain reaction, *Lancet* (1988) **2**:1368.

69. Rous P, Beard JW, The progression to carcinoma of virus-induced rabbit papilloma (Shope), *J Exp Med* (1935) **62**:523–48.

70. Gissman L, Boshart M, Durst M et al, Presence of human papillomavirus in genital tumors, *J Invest Dermatol* (1984) **83**:26s–8s.

71. Gissmann L, Schwarz E, Persistence and expression of human papillomavirus DNA in genital cancer. In: Evered D, Clark S, eds, *Papillomaviruses*, Ciba Foundation Symposium 120 (John Wiley & Sons: Chichester 1986) 190–7.

72. Macnab JCM, Walkinshaw SA, Cordiner JW et al, Human papillomavirus in clinically and histologically normal tissue of patients with genital cancer, *N Engl J Med* (1986) **315**:1052–8.

73. Howley PM, Schlegel R, The human papillomaviruses, an overview, *Am J Med* (1988) **85**(supplement 2A): 155–8.

74. Kashima H, Mounts P, Tumors of the head and neck, larynx, lung and esophagus and their possible relationship to HPV. In: Syrjanen K, Gissmann L, Koss LG, eds, *Papillomaviruses and human disease* (Springer-Verlag: Berlin 1987) 138–57.

75. Moy RL, Eliezri YD, Nuovo GJ et al, Human papillomavirus type 16 DNA in periungual squamous cell carcinomas, *JAMA* (1989) **261**:2669–73.

76. Kawashima M, Jablonska S, Favre M et al, Characterization of a new type of human papillomavirus found in a lesion of Bowen's disease of the skin, *J Virol* (1986) **57**:688–92.

77. Yeager JK, Findley RF, McAleer IM, Penile verrucous carcinoma, *Arch Dermatol* (1990) **126**:1208–10.

78. Pfister H, Iftner T, Fuchs PG, Papillomaviruses from epidermodysplasia verruciformis patients and renal allograft recipients. In: Howley PM, Broker TR, eds, *Papillomaviruses: molecular and clinical aspects* (Alan R. Liss: New York 1985) 85–100.

79. Scheurlen W, Gissmann L, Gross G et al, Molecular cloning of two new HPV types (HPV 37 and HPV 38) from a keratoacanthoma and a malignant melanoma, *Int J Cancer* (1986) **37**:505–10.

80. Goldfarb MT, Gupta AK, Gupta MA et al, Office therapy for human papillomavirus infection in nongenital sites, *Dermatol Clin* (1991) **9**:287–96.

81. Sawchuk WS, Weber PJ, Lowy DR et al, Infectious papillomavirus in the vapor of warts treated with carbon dioxide laser or electrocoagulation: detection and protection, *J Am Acad Dermatol* (1989) **21**:41–9.

82. Beutner KR, Friedman-Kien AE, Conant MA et al, Patient-applied podofilox for treatment of genital warts, *Lancet* (1989) **1**:831–4.

83. Von Krogh G, Penile condylomata acuminata: an experimental model for evaluation of topical self-treatment with 0.5–1.0% ethanolic preparations of podophyllotoxin for three days, *Sex Transm Dis* (1981) **8**:179–86.

84. Edwards A, Atma-Ram A, Nicol Thin R, Podophyllotoxin 0.5% v podophyllin 20% to treat penile warts, *Genitourin Med* (1988) **64**:263–5.

85. Shelley WB, Shelley ED, Intralesional bleomycin sulfate therapy for warts. A novel bifurcated needle puncture technique, *Arch Dermatol* (1991) **127**:234–6.

86. Weck PK, Buddin DA, Whisnant JK, Interferons in the treatment of genital human papillomavirus infections, *Am J Med* (1988) **85**(supplement 2A):159–64.

87. Eron LJ, Judson F, Tucker S et al, Interferon therapy for condylomata acuminata, *N Engl J Med* (1986) **315**:1059–64.

88. Friedman-Kien AE, Eron LJ, Conant M et al, Natural interferon alfa for treatment of condylomata acuminata, *JAMA* (1988) **259**:533–8.

89. Vance JC, Bart BJ, Hansen RC et al, Intralesional recombinant alpha-2 interferon for the treatment of patients with condyloma acuminatum or verruca plantaris, *Arch Dermatol* (1986) **122**:272–7.

90. Gross G, Roussaki A, Schopf E et al, Successful treatment of condylomata acuminata and bowenoid papulosis with subcutaneous injections of low-dose recombinant interferon-alpha, *Arch Dermatol* (1986) **122**:749–50.

91. Reichman RC, Oakes D, Bonnez W et al, Treatment of condyloma acuminatum with three different interferons administered intralesionally, *Ann Intern Med* (1988) **108**:675–9.

92. Schonfeld A, Nitke S, Schattner A et al, Intramuscular human interferon-beta injections in treatment of condylomata acuminata, *Lancet* (1984) **1**:1038–42.

93. Haglund S, Lundquist P-G, Cantell K et al, Interferon therapy in juvenile laryngeal papillomatosis, *Arch Otolaryngol* (1981) **107**:327–32.

94. Androphy EJ, Dvoretzky I, Maluish AE et al, Response of warts in epidermodysplasia verruciformis to treatment with systemic and intralesional alpha interferon, *J Am Acad Dermatol* (1984) **11**:197–202.

95. Weiner SA, Meyskens FL, Surwit EA et al, Response of human papilloma-associated diseases to retinoids (vitamin A derivatives). In: Howley PM, Broker TR, eds, *Papillomaviruses. Molecular and clinical aspects* (Alan R. Liss: New York 1985) 249–55.

96. Lutzner MA, Inserm GR, Blanchet-Bardon C, Oral retinoid treatment of human papillomavirus type 5-induced epidermodysplasia verruciformis, *N Engl J Med* (1980) **302**:1091.

97. Boyle J, Dick DC, Mackie RM, Treatment of extensive virus warts with etretinate (Tigason) in a patient with sarcoidosis, *Clin Exp Dermatol* (1983) **8**:33–6.

98. Gross G, Pfister H, Hagedorn M et al, Effect of oral aromatic retinoid (Ro 10-9359) on human papilloma virus-2-induced common warts, *Dermatologica* (1983) **166**:48–53.

Chapter 33

THE LASER PLUME

Neil P.J. Walker

In many instances the clinical application of lasers results in vaporization of human tissue. Use of the carbon dioxide laser for superficial abrasion produces large amounts of plume but other lasers can similarly produce quantities of smoke emissions. It has been known since 1967 that the very short pulses of Q-switched lasers can disseminate quite large particles of viable material.

In 1967 Hoye et al[1] were able to demonstrate the presence of viable tumor cells in the tissue fragments produced during neodymium-YAG laser treatment of S91 mouse melanoma. In contrast, the early attempts to isolate viable material following carbon dioxide laser treatments were unsuccessful.[2-4] Following exposure of tongue tissue, Mihashi et al[2] demonstrated intact cells which did not grow in culture, and Oosterhuis et al[3], working with a mouse melanoma model, had similar results. In 1982 when Bellina et al[4] treated condylomas the few intact cells they collected showed no metabolic activity. In 1981 Tomita et al[5] demonstrated the mutagenicity of smoke condensates induced by carbon dioxide laser irradiation and electrocauterization. The first firm evidence of viable material came in 1985.[6,7] Mullarkey et al[6] demonstrated in vitro that during carbon dioxide laser treatment infected tissue was not sterilized and that the plume contained viable material. Walker et al[7] demonstrated the presence of viable bacterial spores in the plume and splatter produced by low-irradiance (<750 W/cm^2) vaporization of freshly inoculated post-mortem skin and in similar subsequent work demonstrated the dissemination of viable poliovirus.[8] In our discussion we emphasized that the virus used is relatively heat labile and that more heat-resistant viruses such as hepatitis B, human papillomaviruses (HPV) and possibly human immunodeficiency virus (HIV) may survive more readily.

Studies in clinical situations by other workers soon confirmed these conclusions by the demonstration of intact HPV DNA[9] and viable viruses.[10] Many clinicians have sought consolation in the absence of any clinical case reports of operation-acquired infection, but the recent development of laryngeal papillomatosis in a laser surgeon who had been treating anogenital condylomas[11] should persuade everyone concerned of the potential risks. Similarly, doubts have been cast by some studies[12] that have failed, like the earliest reported studies, to demonstrate viable material, but many other studies have confirmed the presence of HPV DNA.

Of more practical importance has been the demonstration of the in vitro production of viable bacteriophage in both carbon dioxide and argon laser plumes.[13] Previous experience would suggest that such in vitro results can be justifiably extrapolated to the clinic and this work emphasizes that the smoke emissions produced by any physical procedure on the skin should be regarded as potentially infectious. No solace should be drawn from the recent failure of Starr et al[14] to demonstrate the presence of simian immunodeficiency virus in an in vitro study analysing carbon dioxide laser plumes. When carbon dioxide laser light strikes body tissue the intracellular water boils almost instantaneously and the rapid expansion disrupts the cells, producing the particulate matter and debris which is disseminated. This is a very different scenario from the cell-free virus-containing fluid used in these studies. If we consider that, although there has been no recorded transmission of HIV infection by split body fluids, the virus can survive for about 6 days when dried onto glass coverslips, adequate measures need to be taken to control and evacuate tissue plumes.

Practically, the laser surgeon must either take a decision to regard every procedure as being potentially hazardous or make a clinical evaluation of each case. Most prudently, all personnel will now be immunized against hepatitis B and no laser procedure which might involve the production of a plume should be conducted without adequate smoke evacuation and personal protection with operating gown, gloves, wrap-around goggles and small-pore facemasks. Whether to carry out a procedure on an HIV-positive patient must be a decision for the individual but no reliance should be placed on antibody tests alone and a careful history and elucidation of at-risk behavior is probably of greatest importance. In such cases double gloving will afford extra protection[15] and procedures and techniques must be strictly followed. Remember, for instance, that for most smoke evacuators the distal end must be no more than 2 cm from the irradiated site or significant escape occurs. Many such smoke evacuators are available and the relative efficacy of some has recently been evaluated.[16]

Improvements in many evacuators may be made by the introduction at the distal end of the suction tubing of a Pall Laser Smoke Filter (Pall Biomedical Ltd, Portsmouth, UK) which will protect the tubing and equipment from contamination. The Smog-Rova System (United Air Specialists, Leamington Spa, UK) which has an orifice flow of 20 000 l/min has sufficient flow (850 l/min) at a distance of 300 mm to collect emissions and may provide a useful system in purpose-built laser suites.

References

1. Hoye RC, Ketcham AS, Riggle GC, The air-borne dissemination of viable tumour by high-energy neodymium laser, *Life Sci* (1967) **6**:119–25.

2. Mihashi S, Jako GJ, Ineze J et al, Laser surgery in otolaryngology: interaction of carbon dioxide laser and soft tissue, *Ann NY Acad Sci* (1975) **267**:263–94.

3. Oosterhuis JW, Verschueren RCJ, Eibergen R et al, The viability of cells in the waste products of carbon dioxide laser evaporation of Cloudman mouse melanomas, *Cancer* (1982) **49**:61–7.

4. Bellina JH, Stjernholm RL, Kurpel JE, Analysis of plume emissions after papovavirus irradiation with the carbon dioxide laser, *J Reprod Med* (1982) **27**:268–70.

5. Tomita Y, Mihashi S, Nagata K et al, Mutagenicity of smoke condensates

induced by carbon dioxide laser irradiation and electrocauterisation, *Mutat Res* (1981) **89**:145.

6. Mullarkey MB, Norris CW, Goldberg IV, The efficacy of the carbon dioxide laser in the sterilization of skin seeded with bacteria: survival at the skin surface and in the plume emissions, *Laryngoscope* (1985) **95**:186–7.

7. Walker NPJ, Matthews J, Newsom SWB, Possible hazards from irradiation with the carbon dioxide laser, *Lasers Surg Med* (1986) **6**:84–6.

8. Walker NPJ, Matthews J, Newsom SWB, Viral dissemination during carbon dioxide laser vaporisation. Presented at the *7th International Congress of Dermatologic Surgey* (1986) September, London, UK.

9. Garden JM, O'Bavian MK, Shelnitz LS et al, Papillomavirus in the vapor of carbon dioxide laser treatment for verrucae, *JAMA* (1988) **259**:1199–202.

10. Sawchuk WS, Weber PJ, Lowy DR et al, Infectious papillomavirus in the vapor of warts treated with the carbon dioxide laser or electrocoagulation: detection and protection, *J Am Acad Dermatol* (1989) **21**:41–9.

11. Hallomo P, Naess O, Laryngeal papillomatosis with human papillomavirus DNA contracted by a laser surgeon, *Eur Arch Otorhinolaryngol* (1991) **248**(7):425–7.

12. Abramson AL, DiLorenzo TP, Steinberg BM, Is papillomavirus detectable in the plume of laser-treated laryngeal papilloma? *Arch Otolaryngol Head Neck Surg* (1990) **116**(5):604–7.

13. Matchette LS, Faaland RW, Royston DD et al, In vitro production of viable bacteriophage in carbon dioxide and argon laser plumes, *Lasers Surg Med* (1991) **11**(4):380–4.

14. Starr JC, Kilmer SL, Wheeland RG, Analysis of carbon dioxide laser plume for simian immunodeficiency virus, *J Dermatol Surg Oncol* (1991) **18**(4):297–300.

15. Cohen MS, Do JT, Tahery DP et al, Efficacy of double gloving as a protection against blood exposure in dermatologic surgery, *J Dermatol Surg Oncol* (1992) **18**(10):873–4.

16. Smith JP, Topmiller JL, Shulman S, Factors affecting emission collection by surgical smoke evacuators, *Lasers Surg Med* (1990) **10**(3):224–33.

Chapter 34

SUPERFICIAL VASCULAR LASERS: YELLOW LIGHT AND 532 NM

Timothy J. Rosio

INTRODUCTION

'What I tell you three times is true.'
The Hunting of the Snark

'The question, said Alice, is whether you can make words mean so many things.'
Through the Looking Glass

Lewis Carroll

Laser hardware choices abound, and expectations of patients and physicians for the successful treatment of cutaneous vascular lesions have never been higher. The last decade has witnessed our continuing progress with a proliferation of lasers, laser settings, and techniques for the treatment of malformations and hemangiomas. Our choices comprise a disparate array of treatment recipes, each claiming optimal treatment. Individual laser operators characteristically developed skill and judgment, for example with the argon laser, and mastered one of several techniques (for example 'point by point technique', 'air-brush' or 'painting', 'tracing' or 'Scheibner' technique). But often omission of a key ingredient or experience in the expert's technique or patient selection hindered reproducibility and wider adoption.

Side-by-side vascular lesion treatment comparisons are few due to long 'treatment time-lines', the lack of simultaneous availability of different types of costly technology and scarce expertise with various techniques. This is also complicated by biological variability between patients (Figure 34.1). Confusion and disagreement has reigned in the marketplace, exacerbated by inadequate terminology ('what shade of yellow, how fast is your pulse; is your 'pulse' really a pulse?') and marketing enthusiasm. Laser marketing materials promise 'clearing' within a number of treatments, but does clearing mean truly 'clear' or partially lightened?

What things have we learned? A single ideal laser for all superficial vascular lesions does not yet exist. Limited financial and laser hardware resources are a practical reality in most settings, so some choices will have to be made about vessel size, type, depth and anatomic locations to be treated. The features of current vascular lasers overlap along a continuum. Good to excellent clinical results are achievable with a variety of old and newer lasers employing various settings and new accessories, despite some departures from the theoretical ideal wavelength, power, spot size and exposure duration. Two

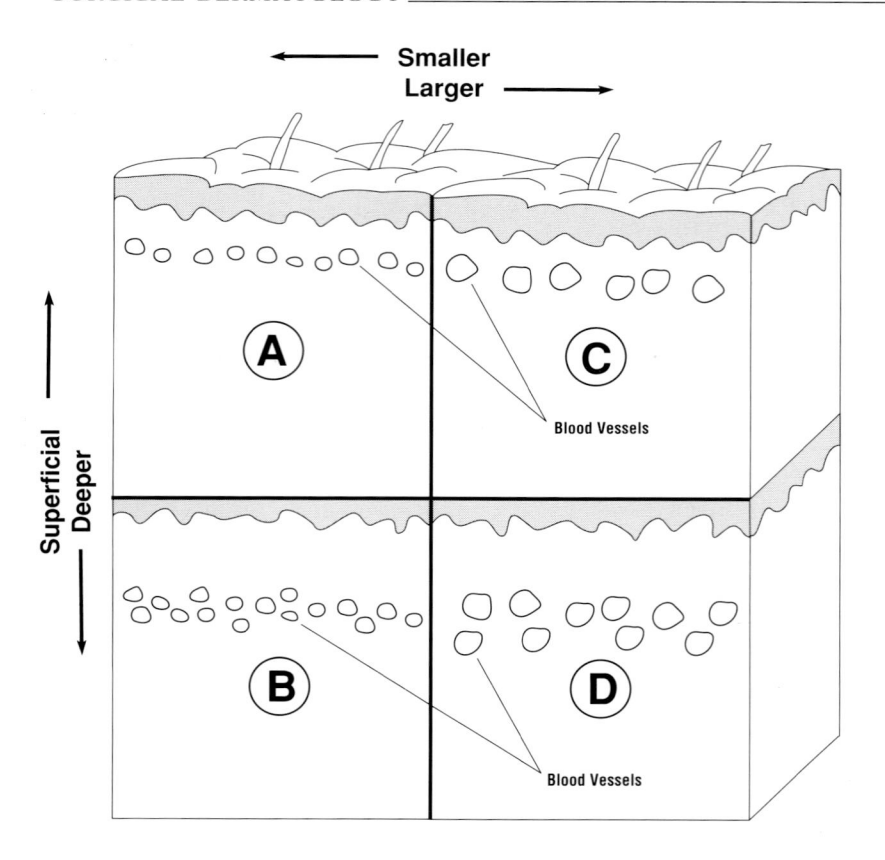

Figure 34.1
Vascular size and distribution variations affect clinical appearance and response to different laser therapies. The volume of blood in abnormal vessels B > A, and D > C. Clinical impressions between the pairs may be comparable due to greater depth in B and D. Number of treatments may be greater and final results less complete in B, and even less in D.

types of vascular lasers will be required for optimal treatment of some patients. Regardless of approach, many portwine stain (PWS) patients lighten but do not completely clear, and end points of treatment in these patients are ill-defined. Some approaches appear to offer improvement with fewer treatments and lower cost; but is this at some increased scarring risk? These realities challenge us to ask, what are the relative effectiveness and economies of vascular laser treatment technologies and approaches? This requires more precise clinical subsets (age, location, sex, ethnic group, skin type, etc.), and the consideration of patient risk, cost, number of treatments, morbidity, and side-effects from treatments (for example pain, swelling, textural alterations, and temporary or permanent coloration changes).

Clinicians (often with a very basic laser physics background) need to understand this dynamic topic and related questions to treat or refer patients appropriately, and also to make informed decisions on expensive capital equipment. This chapter summarizes and compares current laser approaches for superficial vascular lesions, emphasizing yellow light and 532-nm lasers and treatment trends. The reader is assumed to be familiar with basic laser physics. A brief discussion of pertinent laser terms and key principles to hardware and technique comparisons is provided.

Key Principles and Terms

Nomenclature, selective photothermolysis and vascular classification

Our understanding and selection of cutaneous vascular laser therapies has made large gains in the last decade due to three components: first, the use of standard nomenclature for specifying laser techniques and parameters;[1] second, development of selective photothermolysis concepts;[2-4] and third, formulation and application of a more precise classification of vascular lesions.[5,6] We are increasingly able to select a therapeutic course, then estimate and prescribe idealized ranges of wavelengths, pulse durations, peak powers, etc. for vessel size ranges or tissues with calculated thermal relaxation times ($T_r = G(D^2C)/K$). Though equipped with increasingly 'menu-driven' technology the laser surgeon must operate mindful of variation and unpredictability of real-world clinical responses with attendant risks such as scarring, pigmentary alterations, etc.

Laser–skin interaction

The key to understanding differences between vascular lasers is their wavelength, and distribution of the laser energy in time and space. Comparison of vascular lasers and their effectiveness uses this physical specification of the beam produced (wavelength, power density, fluence, temporal and spatial beam profile), its delivery (temporal and spatial distribution of beam at tissue), and finally its optical-thermal interaction with tissue (four possible fates) with subsequent biological responses (damage and healing).

Laser energy encountering a skin target predominantly results in photothermal transformation, subject to four main fates: absorption, transmission, reflection and scattering. The relative proportions of these depend on the relative transmission and absorption efficiencies of the chosen wavelength, target tissue and competing chromophores. Despite a wealth of such laboratory-measured values and clinical research, the skin remains optically complex and sometimes defies prediction of its properties.[7,8] Examples include 'tissue lensing', and the nonpeak absorption wavelength of oxyhemoglobin being superior to the peak absorption wavelength for clinical therapy (585 versus 577 nm).

General thermal principles

Photothermal effects range in a linear fashion from protein denaturation and coagulation (>50°C) to vaporization (>100°C), depending on the amount of energy, the delivery rate and target size. However, very high power (MW) and rapid (≤ ns) pulsed energy delivery induces nonlinear photomechanical target disruption typified by Q-switched lasers. Cutaneous tissue may recover from brief exposures in excess of 50°C temperatures, thereby decreasing the likelihood or quantity of fibrosis (Figure 34.2). Absolute temperature and duration are both important in determining marginally recoverable laser thermal injuries. It is the goal of selective photothermolysis to spatially confine irreversible thermal injury to the target tissue (for example vessels), while limiting heat diffusion injury to the surrounding stromal tissue (for example collagen, fibroblasts, adnexal structures). Inadequate energy delivery or insufficient depth leads to treatment failure while excessive energy delivery may result in scarring, pigmentary and textural changes.

Undesirable or abnormal superficial vascular structures are preferably treated by visible laser wavelengths which act selectively upon the intravascular oxyhemoglobin chromophore. While oxyhemoglobin absorbs a considerable range of wavelengths, optimal treatment depends on wavelengths which

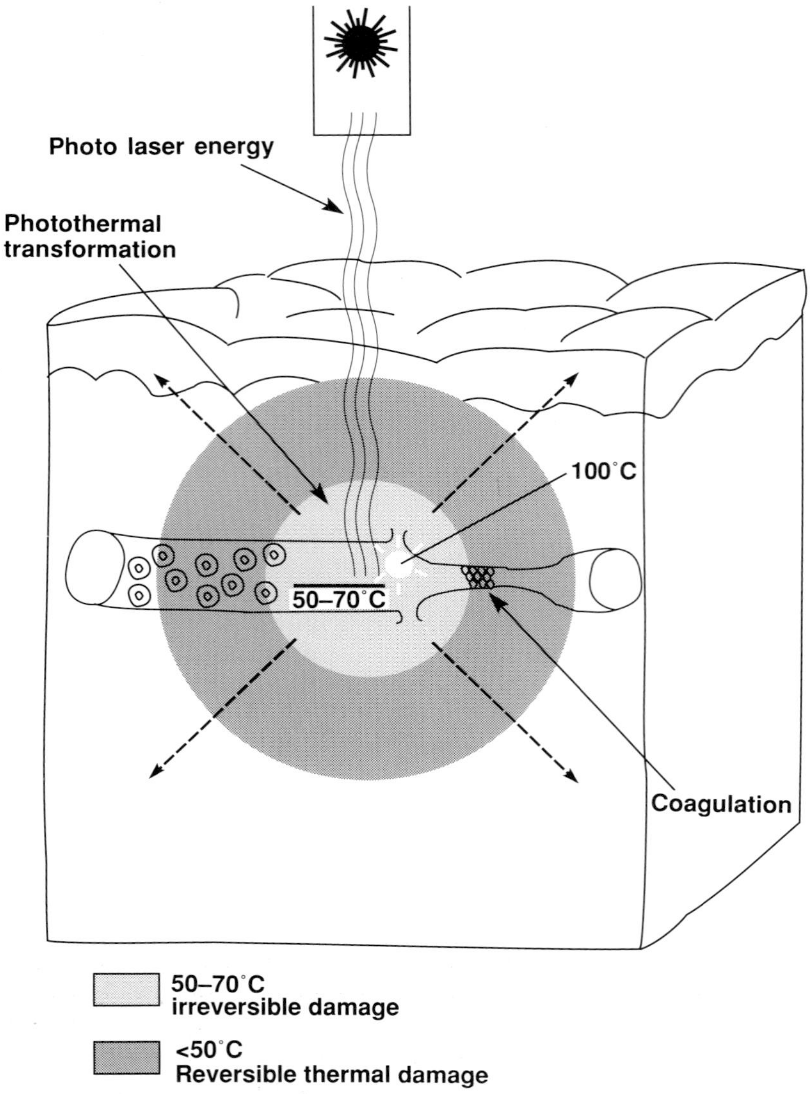

Figure 34.2
Photothermal damage gradient.

- 50–70°C irreversible damage
- <50°C Reversible thermal damage

are relatively poorly absorbed by competing chromophores (for example melanin) and can penetrate to sufficient depth with enough energy to eliminate target vessels. It is important to realize that the advantages of particular wavelengths are reduced or lost completely with longer exposure times. So one must consider simultaneously all major variables—exposure time, spot size, energy density, and wavelength—in the context of the chromophores and thermal relaxation times.

Wavelength and depth

Long visible wavelengths of light travel further than shorter ones in tissue. Therefore at the longer (yellow) wavelength end of oxyhemoglobin's absorption curve, cutaneous penetration is deeper and

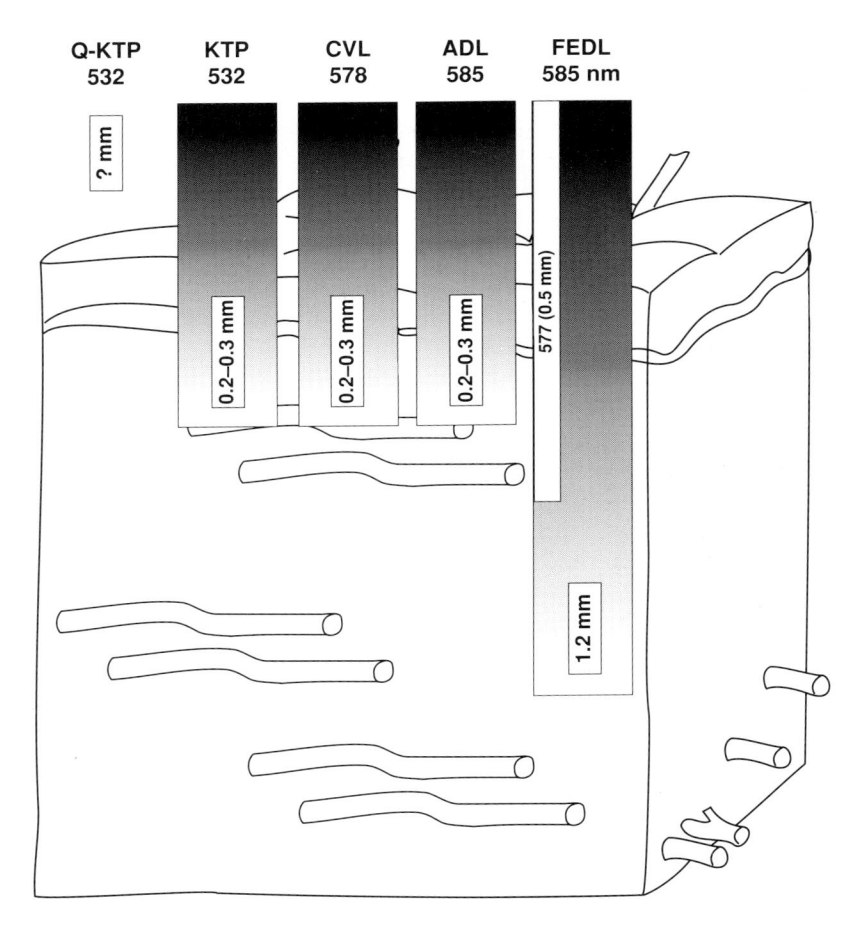

Figure 34.3
Wavelength relative penetration depth with selectivity. CVL, copper vapor laser; ADL, argon-dye laser; FEDL, flashlamp excited dye laser.

scatters less, while melanin absorption is relatively low. This is in contrast to the 418-nm (Soret band) oxyhemoglobin peak where absolute absorption efficiency is greatest but tissue penetration by blue light is minimal due to greater scatter, and superficial melanin, epidermis and dermal tissue absorbs substantial amounts of energy before it can reach the dermal vessels. Oxyhemoglobin's secondary absorption peaks in the green–yellow light range at approximately 542 and 577 nm come closer to satisfying both requirements.[9]

Where on the spectrum of green–yellow wavelengths is the trade-off between absorption efficiency and tissue penetration actually optimized? Research with a 540-nm wavelength 3-W continuous-wave laser demonstrated selective photothermolysis to 0.3 mm effective dermal depth with a very narrow safety-efficacy window of 5–6.5 J/cm^2, using 100–200 ms exposures and 2 mm spot size.[9] Lesser energy densities were ineffective clinically, while greater densities caused nonselective coagulation. Flashlamp excited dye laser (FEDL) experiments showed that 577 nm (coinciding with the ß-oxyhemoglobin absorption peak) achieved selective vessel coagulation to 0.8 mm in pig skin, whereas 585 nm reached 1.2 mm.[8] A still longer wavelength of 590 nm was tried, but reached a depth of only 0.8 mm (Figure 34.3).

Selectivity, tissue exposure time and energy density (when is a 'pulse' a 'pulse'?)

Selective photothermolysis also relies upon delivering the requisite energy within a sufficiently short time window (thermal relaxation time) to both coagulate the vascular target and spare other tissues, resulting in spatial confinement of irreversible injury to the targeted structure. Thermal relaxation time is the calculated period required for a structure's original temperature to decline by 50%. Microvessels are characterized by thermal relaxation times approximating to 100–1000 µs (Figure 34.4). Much shorter (nanosecond) high-energy exposures completely destroy the vessel with abrupt vaporization; a vaporization phase change induces vessel disruption and pressure wave effects on the surrounding tissue. Lower fluences with much longer exposures (milliseconds) minimize vaporization, increase vessel coagulation severity but also allow sufficient heat to diffuse to the surrounding tissue to cause nonspecific epidermal and dermal damage (and possible visible scarring).

Very brief (nanosecond) low-power pulses closely spaced, for example 2–5 kHz (2000–5000 pulses per second), may be referred to as 'quasi-continuous-wave' lasers. Examples are the copper vapor and KTP lasers. The total energy contained in an individual pulse is low despite a moderate peak power, due to brief duration. The rapid repetition rate allows minimal thermal relaxation between pulses, and therefore the tissue responds to the average power similarly to a continuous wave. If some thermal relaxation occurs between continuous-wave copper vapor laser or KTP pulses then more pulses of energy will have to be delivered over a longer period to raise tissue temperature in a 'stair-step' fashion to coagulation.

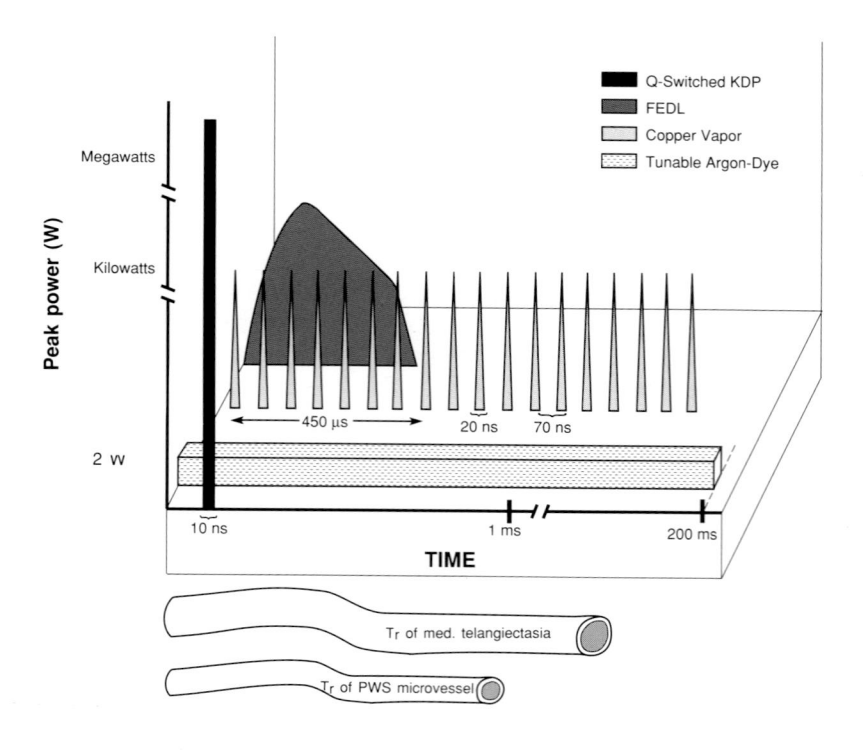

Figure 34.4
Thermal relaxation time related to lasers' power and exposure times. FEDL, flashlamp excited dye laser.

The Q-switched YAG-KDP laser is distinctly different in its energy profile. Q-switching provides for it several orders of magnitude greater peak energy delivery. Therefore photovaporization and photodisruption occur with the Q-switched YAG-KDP laser (1064/532 nm), resulting in tearing of vessels rather than coagulation. Its primary application is for treatment of pigmented lesions at 1064 nm. It is undergoing research testing at present for applicability in treatment of vascular disorders.

Thermal relaxation time varies depending on the size of the vessel and may be an order of magnitude longer for larger vessels, telangiectasias, and vascular blebs. Flashlamp excited dye laser systems have a fixed exposure time of 450 µs, which is too brief for larger vessels. Continuous-wave systems have longer adjustable exposure times sufficient for larger vessels, but effective minimum shuttered exposure times (100 ms) which still exceed the smallest microvessel thermal relaxation times by several to many times.

Energy density

Energy density and spot size are the remaining components of selective photothermolysis to address (fluence = J/cm² = W × T/cm² where W = watts and T = time). A high fluence rate (joules/exposure time) per pulse is a distinguishing difference between FEDL (pulsed, high peak power) lasers and continuous-wave (shuttered, low power continuous or quasi-continuous) lasers. Continuous-wave laser systems using 3–5-mm spot sizes (equivalent to FEDL systems) must deliver four to five times the total energy delivered by a FEDL to achieve purpura in normal-sized experimental animal vessels.[10] This increases the risk of clinical scarring. The alternative is to reduce the spot-size component of the energy density equation to compensate for the lower peak power, and come closer to calculated ideal microvessel thermal relaxation times. Some focusing handpieces on recent continuous-wave lasers can achieve beam sizes of 0.1 mm. Such small spot sizes allow current continuous-wave sources to more closely approach FEDL energy densities, but continuous-wave sources still require minima of 150–250% greater total energy, partly because the lower peak energy is distributed over a 100–10 000 times longer period than FEDL, and partly because of shallower penetration of small spot sizes.

Oversimplified, the objective in the continuous-wave systems is to obtain the highest power possible that allows a corresponding reduction in tissue exposure time. Remember that the product (power × time) = joules is the basis for the 'energy' delivered to tissue. Tunable dye systems are now available that provide nearly 3 W or more at 585 nm. Some KTP systems could provide 20 W at 532 nm. Higher powers such as these allow sufficient energy (for example 18–30 J) to be delivered along with selection of the shortest available exposure time for continuous-wave lasers when used in conjunction with robotized scanning devices (that is 30 ms).

Spot size

Research has demonstrated that laser spot sizes of 3 mm or more have superior penetration compared to smaller ones due to tissue scattering effects. They point to experimental evidence that deeper effective laser light doses derive from wider beam profiles.[11] Wider beams provide more numerous coincident scattered rays, resulting in higher effective total energy absorption at targets. This phenomenon has been dubbed 'tissue lensing'. Despite this depth advantage of 3 mm and larger FEDL beam sizes, 1.0-mm or even smaller continuous-wave beams do achieve therapeutic clinical success. However, it comes at the expense of longer exposure times. The smaller the beam at diameters less than 3 mm, the shallower the penetration at a given power and time exposure. Increased power or time exposure can only partially restore some of the reduced penetration depth due to smaller spot sizes, while sacrificing some selectivity. The trade-off in continuous wave may be, then, a narrower treatment safety margin (especially in scar-prone areas or patients) or poorer response in patients with deeper small vessel constituents, in a PWS for example.

The advantage of continuous wave will certainly remain providing longer exposure times and greater total energy required in the treatment of large telangiectasias, hypertrophic nodules, blebs and venous lakes,[12] for which FEDL systems are ineffective. Also, in more moderately sized telangiectasias continuous-wave systems may be capable of achieving cosmetic acceptable vessel destruction in fewer treatments than FEDL.[13] Finally, more deeply located, resistant and high-flow vascular malformations, 'spider angiomas', may be effectively and aesthetically treated in a single continuous-wave session; very small spot sizes (150–500 µm) vaporize a narrow shaft to the 'central source vessel' with superimposed 100–200-ms pulses.[14]

LASER SYSTEMS COMPARISON

Tunable-dye (argon-dye) laser

Tunable-dye lasers or argon-dye lasers comprise an argon laser used as an optical energy pumping source to excite organic rhodamine dye molecules (Figure 34.5). The rhodamine dye in turn emits a secondary laser light in the yellow–red range. The yellow-range beam (577–585 nm) matches the β-absorption peak of oxyhemoglobin. The specific mixture of rhodamine has been designed to emit a range of laser wavelengths (577–630 nm) when stimulated by the blue–green laser light. The precise wavelength is selected in the optical resonator by adjusting the refraction angle of an optical crystal in the laser light path. The laser surgeon may 'tune' or select any wavelength within the range of the rhodamine dye at any time, or revert to 488, 514 nm argon wavelengths; hence the designation 'tunable-dye'. This is in contrast with 'fixed' wavelength and pulse duration dye lasers of the FEDL type, which are changeable only with major factory servicing modifications to the dye mixture, software, and possibly hardware.

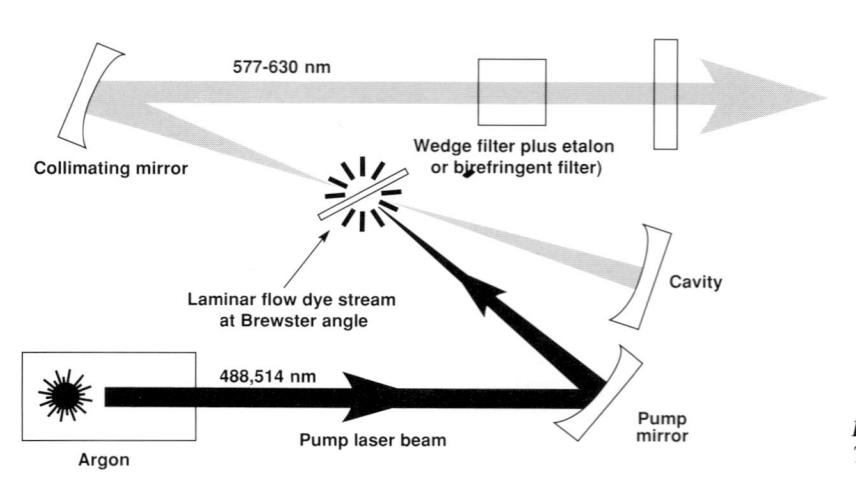

Figure 34.5 Tunable argon-dye laser.

Table 34.1
Superficial vascular laser hardware comparison

Laser	Wavelength (nm)	Time exposure (effective)[a]	Peak power (effective)[b]	Spot size[c]	Depth of penetration (selectivity maintained)	Efficacy small vessels	Efficacy large vessels	Safety (normal color, texture)	Price + scanner ($)	Consumable	Service (annual) + scanner service
Argon	488, 514	200 ms	2.5 W	0.5–2+ mm	Not selective	+	++	+	39k+25k		$5500+1000
Tunable-dye (Argon-dye)	488, 514, 577–630	200 ms	1–2 W	0.5–2+ mm	0.2–0.3 mm	++	++	++	90k+25k	1–2 dye changes/year in service contract	$9500+1000
Copper vapor(CV)	578, 511	200 ms	1–2 W	0.5–2+ mm	0.2–0.3 mm	++	++	++	129k+0k (included with CVL) scanner alone 21.5k	Tube replaced every 1000 h operation in service contract	$7800 (laser and scanner)
KTP	532	100–200 ms	12–20 W	0.15, 1,2 mm	0.2–0.3 mm	+++	+++	++	105–130k +25k		$12 000 +1000
FEDL (Flashlamp excited dye)	585	450 μs	4–8 kW	5 mm, 2 mm	1.2 mm	+++	0	+++	160k	$1000/dye fixed pulse kit = 5000 shots	$20 000
Q-switched KTP/YAG	532, 1064	10 ns fixed pulse	MW	2 mm	?	+	0 (under study)	+++	78k		$6000

Note: Hardware and service costs in round figures from recent contracts or telephone survey; may vary by manufacturer, or vendor.
[a] Electronically shuttered average exposure time required for common applications (unless fixed pulse noted).
[b] Quasi-continuous-wave lasers transient energy peaks require summation (average power) for clinical significance.
[c] May require special handpiece or add-on lenses at extra cost up to $1000–3000.

The argon-dye laser produces laser light at modest power (1–3 W) as a continuous wave. Electromechanical timed shuttering (comparable to a camera) allows user-selectable exposure times ranging from 2.0 to 0.02 s. In laser terminology, low-power brief exposures are most correctly referred to as 'shuttered' or 'gated' exposures. 'Pulsed' should be reserved for extremely short laser emissions, with very high peak energies orders of magnitude higher than those of standard lasers. However, even expert users will occasionally lapse into applying the term 'pulsed' to describe low-power, shuttered, brief exposures. This is not surprising, since manufacturers often print this descriptor on the timed exposure controls of many nonpulsed lasers.

The yellow–red laser light is delivered through an optical fiber or cable. Most commonly this is coupled to a focusing handpiece that can produce spot sizes from 0.05 to 6 mm; occasionally a set of fixed focal length lens attachments is employed. The optical cavity alignment is crucial to obtain normal power output. Significant movement of the laser may require a service call for mirror alignment or to

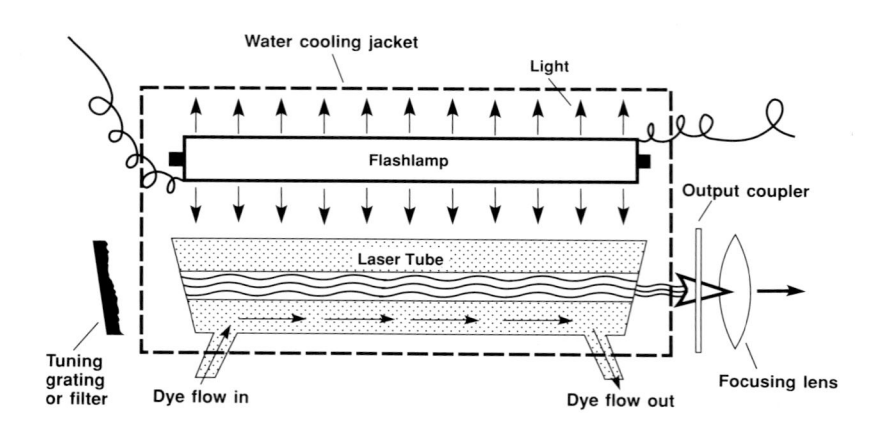

Figure 34.6
Flashlamp excited dye laser linear flashlamp design.

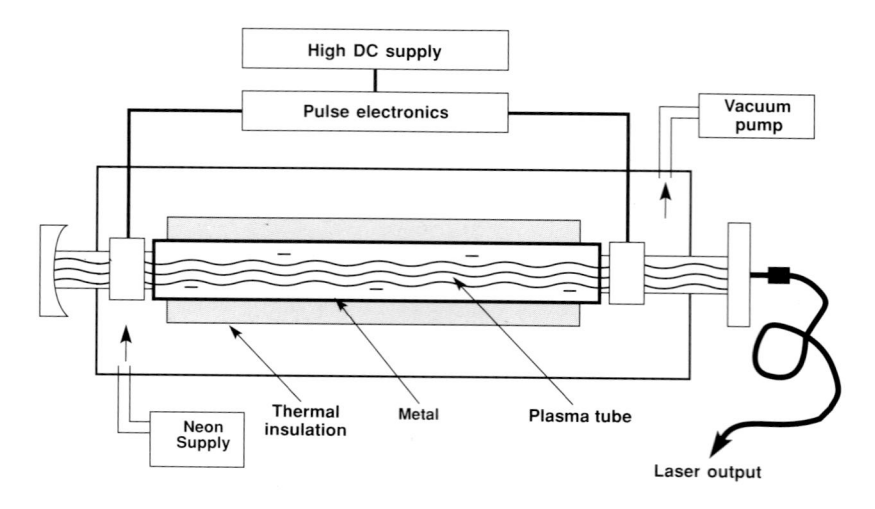

Figure 34.7
Copper vapor laser.

replace very expensive light conduction cables that may break when bumped or stretched. Dye is replaced on average once between 6 and 12 months. This much less frequent rate (compared to FEDL systems) is due to the lower dye photodegradation at relatively low-power argon laser pumping. The longevity, stability, relative simplicity and large installed base of argon lasers make the cost of purchase, operation and maintenance moderate compared to other lasers (Table 34.1). Tunability allows use in photodynamic therapy but may require a different dye mixture for optimization of power and prolonged 630-nm output. Robotized scanners may also be attached.

Flashlamp excited dye laser (FEDL)

FEDLs operate by storing high quantities of energy in a capacitor; sudden energy release powers a very brief intense flashlamp burst to excite laser production in rhodamine dye (Figure 34.6). Related chemical structures in the rhodamine group allow selection of specific compounds with different wavelength outputs. Filters and resonators may be adjusted in series with the optical cavity to restrict wavelength and duration of output to the currently desired 585 nm, 450 µs. Neither setting is user adjustable. Approximately 4–8 kW peak output is produced. Two main flashlamp designs (linear versus coaxial) are available in clinical systems. Linear flashlamps excite the dye mainly from one direction, possibly aided by reflecting surfaces. A patented design that is claimed to be more efficient utilizes a coaxial flashlamp which surrounds the dye medium with more uniform light.

The treatment beam is delivered by an optical fiber coupled to a fixed focal length handpiece with a 5-mm spot size, at a rate of 1 pulse every 3 s. A 2-mm handpiece, and a finger-activated control (alternative to the standard foot pedal), are available at extra cost. A recent more expensive unit (+15%) supplies energy more rapidly and delivers 1 pulse per second.

Software systems and electronic controls are used to assure safe and accurate energy densities. Software, hardware or simultaneous problems can cause prolonged treatment interruptions and downtime ranging from 30 min up to several days. Therefore, the more expensive service contracts with these lasers are indispensable. Long downtimes were far too common in early models (occasionally several per month). This is very disruptive to patient and physician scheduling. Current models are much more reliable, and scheduled preventative maintenance visits reduce to a manageable level the frequency and severity of downtime.

The much higher peak energies used in FEDLs to excite the dye medium cause rapid photodegradation, requiring fresh dye to maintain output levels. Replacement of dye containers (~$1000) after some thousands of pulses should be considered in the operating cost projections prior to purchase. A busy unit treating patients with extensive portwine stains could easily use one or two dye changes per week in treating as few as 5–10 patients. Also, in our experience, flashlamp replacement may be required four times yearly or more along with an equal number of preventative maintenance visits.

Copper vapor lasers

The copper vapor laser emits two harmonic wavelengths, 510.6 nm (green) and 578.2 nm (yellow) (Figure 34.7). The yellow beam matches the β-absorption peak of oxyhemoglobin. The copper vapor laser uses vaporized copper as its laser medium, generated from metal beads in a vaporization chamber. Electrical energy pumping leads to stimulated emission of extremely brief, very rapidly repeating, moderately high peak power, but low average power pulses. Power output is 2–3 W. Typical pulses have a duration of 15–20 ns, a frequency of 15 kHz (15 000/s), an interval of 70 ns, a peak energy of 90 μJ and a peak power of 5 kW. The minimal energy contained in any one brief pulse, together with the very rapid repetition rate, result in the classification of this as a 'quasi-continuous' beam. Shuttered operation allows exposures from 0.05 to 2.0 s. Variable spot size handpieces allow beam diameters from less than 0.5 mm to greater than 5 mm. Fiber optic delivery is standard. Raising the temperature of copper to achieve vaporization requires long warm-up times, commonly 45 min. Interruption of the vaporization during treatment may necessitate noticeable delays to resume treatment. The copper vapor laser system has been used in a variety of scientific and industrial applications, where it has proven very reliable. Copper tube replacement is required every 600 h of operation. The system is not tunable but allows switching from yellow to green wavelength for treatment of epidermal melanocytic lesions. Another possibility is substitution of the vaporization chamber (at significant cost) to use a gold tube and produce 628-nm red light suitable for photodynamic therapy. The purchase price is slightly higher than for argon-dye lasers but maintenance costs are competitive with other lasers. Robotized scanners may be attached. At present a scanner and its service is included with the laser, which makes the combined purchase and service price more competitive with argon-dye lasers.

KTP-YAG lasers (KTP)

The KTP laser begins with a 1060-nm Nd:YAG crystal-produced beam which is generated by a high-intensity optical pumping source such as a xenon flashlamp (Figure 34.8). The wavelength is halved (by either a frequency-doubling potassium titanyl phosphate crystal or photoacoustic method), resulting in 532 nm beam output. The green 532-nm beam comes close to the α-absorption peak of oxyhemoglobin. The KTP beam is quasi-continuous, similar to the copper vapor laser. Average power peak outputs may be from 5 to 20 W, and minor variations on the following beam specifications occur

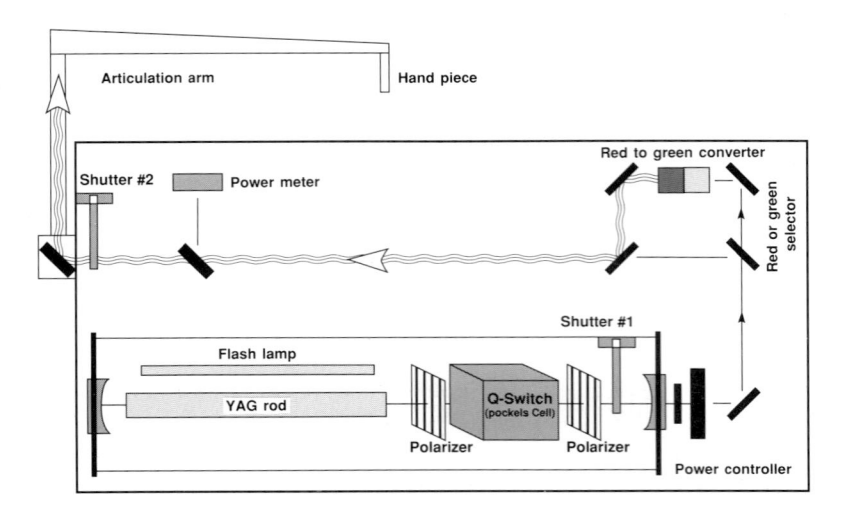

Figure 34.8
Frequency-doubled Q-switched KTP-YAG. The standard KTP-YAG lacks the Pockels cell and polarizing filters depicted here. A 1 060-nm Nd:YAG crystal-produced beam is generated by a xenon flashlamp. The wavelength is halved (by either a frequency-doubling crystal or photoacoustic method), resulting in a 532-nm quasi-continuous beam.

depending on the make and model. Typical beams have continuous-appearing power peaks with duration of 150 ns, frequency of 5 kHz (5000/s), and interval of 200 ns. While the intervals between pulses are three times longer than those of the copper vapor laser, thereby allowing some thermal relaxation, the total energy per pulse is insufficient to accomplish coagulation. Therefore, as with the copper vapor laser, the energy from a train of pulses must be summated to achieve sufficient temperature for coagulation. Shuttered exposure times include 0.05–2.0 s. Interchangeable lenses are available with spot sizes of 0.15, 0.2, 1.0 and 2.0 mm at extra charge; some vendors have offered a variable spot size handpiece with a minimum of 1.0–5.0 mm.

Nd:YAG lasers are touted as 'solid-state' lasers with few moving parts and minimal consumables. No dyes are used. Only the flashlamp pumping source will need replacement based on use. Many systems are now primarily air cooled, which is advantageous where plumbing difficulties or mobility are concerned. However, heat generation could be undesirable in smaller rooms or ones with less generous air exchange and cooling rates. Stability and performance are felt to be strong due to infrequent alignment problems and service requirements. Robotized scanners may be attached for treating large areas with a point-by-point technique.

Q-switched KTP-YAG lasers (Q-KTP)

The Q-KTP laser is fundamentally a frequency-doubled KTP-YAG laser; the addition of a 'Q-switch' mechanism provides thousands of times greater peak energy delivery over much shorter time intervals (millions of watts equivalence, 10 ns), providing selective photothermolysis capabilities at 1064 nm or 532 nm. The Q-switch Pockels cell mechanism interrupts the optical path by rotating the polarity of the laser light as long as power is supplied to the switch. A polarizing filter oriented 90° out of phase with the powered Pockels cell prevents release of the optical laser beam. Deactivating the Pockels cell suddenly allows transmission of all the now parallel phase laser energy through the polarizing filter in nanoseconds.

Delivery is through an articulated arm system, with a 2-mm spot size and repetition rate of 1–10 Hz. The Nd:YAG laser foundation makes this a 'solid-state' laser with few moving parts and without consumables. The flashlamp pumping source will need replacement based on use, and, due to the very high intensity of the beam, optics (chiefly lenses and their coatings) life may be limited. Further field use will clarify this. This system is air cooled. Stability and performance are felt to be strong due to infrequent alignment problems, a stable crystal, and claimed low service requirements. The current commercial unit is also referred to as Q-switched KDP.

Although it was designed to be a tattoo and other pigment removal laser (not a vascular laser), studies are nevertheless underway to further investigate its suitability for treating very small anomalous vessels. The very short pulse duration physically disrupts (explodes) small vessels due to intense phase change, rather than there being photocoagulation effects induced by more gradual heating as in previously discussed vascular lasers. Studies in progress show small vessel disappearance with purpura, and no scarring noted (Weiner P, Waner M, personal communications).

Continuous-wave scanners

Can continuous-wave lasers routinely achieve effective, uniform and safe treatment of microvessel lesions (for example PWS)? Scanners are hardware attachments to continuous-wave lasers designed for treatment of superficial vascular or benign pigmented lesions. Precise delivery of countless measured microbeam laser exposures from continuous-wave lasers was impractical until development of these automatic scanning devices.[15–17] Equipped with their own software and electro-mechanical controls, current scanners provide for more predictable and precise spatial and temporal distribution of continuous-wave or quasi-continuous-wave beams for treating larger surface areas. They also provide more readily available information (such as conversion to energy density in joules), and can deliver shorter exposure times than most currently available continuous-wave shuttered systems. They succeed in making treatment of larger areas safer, more predictable, more uniform, and less fatiguing for doctor and patient than traditional continuous-wave freehand methods. Holding the bulkier handpiece exactly in place for each 30-s cycle can be quite fatiguing in large cases, however.

The main vendors' products (Hexascan (available from Lihtan Technologies, San Rafael, CA, and other licensed dealers), Autolase (Metalaser Technologies, Pleasanton, CA)) are similar in most practical respects. The Autolase offers adjustability of spot size, number, and interspot distances, and claims more uniform center-to-edge spot shape (and therefore power density). The Autolase is being promoted primarily for the copper vapor laser, but connection to other continuous-wave lasers is feasible. A connecting fiber to the laser runs to the control-monitoring box, and another leads from the control box to the user handpiece. Similarities include a preprogrammed hexagonal grid with up to approximately 127 (Hexascan) or 397 (Autoscan) potential 1-mm spots (when filled). The laser spots are delivered in a discontiguous sequence during the average 30 s required for one cycle, allow-

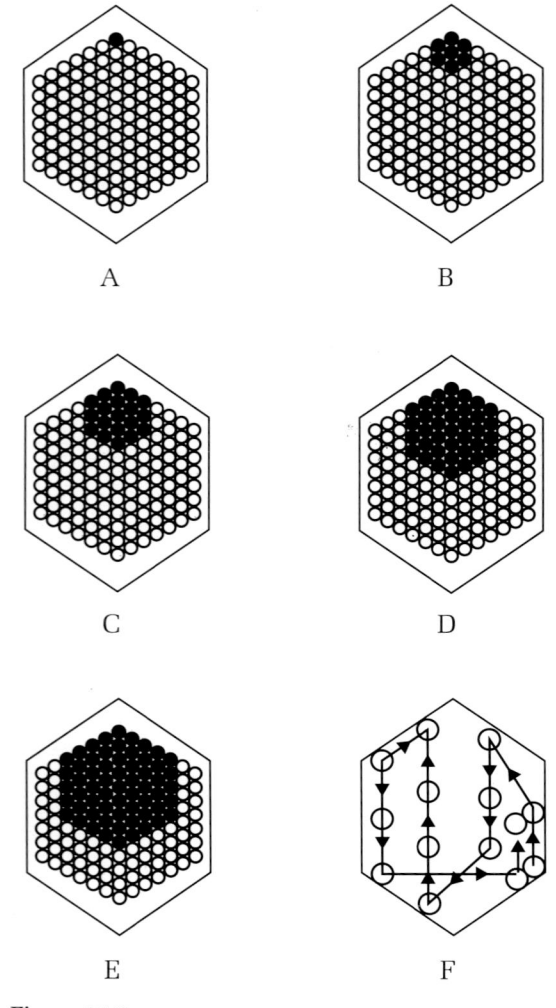

Figure 34.9
Continuous-wave scanner spot array and discontiguous sequence. Selectable hexagonal grouped laser impulse patterns from scanner. (A) Single spot in potential 13-mm grid. (B–E) 3-, 5-, 7- or 9-mm preprogrammed scanner target patterns; each requires approximately 30 s. (F) Sequence of discontiguous laser impulses to allow cooling.

ing local cooling between adjacent impulses (Figure 34.9). The basic hexagonal grid measures 13 mm, but smaller hexagonal grids of 11, 9, 5 and 3 mm may be delivered as well as a 1-mm single spot. An alternating 'skipped' rows option is available at each size, purportedly offering 'faster healing' in patients who blister and form more pronounced eschars. This investigator finds skipped lines of dubious benefit since future alignment with these skip patterns is very difficult, and will leave untreated spots. A feature of the hexagonal shape is tesselation, the ability of certain regular polygons to fit together like blocks or a mosaic, completely covering their combined surface area. This ideally is accomplished without overlapping impulses (as circles require), or missing areas resulting in residual undertreated vascular lesion. Exact matching is more difficult than it looks. Returning to small areas to treat with smaller spot arrays is common.

The shortest time exposure available is 30 ms. The longest is 990 ms. The power requirement is at least 0.5 W up to 9.9 W, but for most uses more than 1.0 W should be considered an effective minimum to reduce thermal injury to perivascular tissues. Even more desirable to achieve desired energy densities for the treatment of PWS while keeping near the 30-ms equipment minimum exposure time would be 3.0–5.0 W (30 ms already considerably exceeds the thermal relaxation times of microvessels). Minimizing tissue exposure time in some circumstances takes precedence even over wavelength. Equivalent joules of green laser light delivered as shorter exposures (2.5–3.0 W of argon 488, 514 nm) appear to produce less acute and subacute eschar (tissue injury) than slightly longer yellow laser light exposures (≤1 W of 585 nm) from the same argon-dye laser.

The author's experience with several of the Hexascan scanners has been in combination with two different tunable argon-dye lasers and with two KTP lasers. The scanners have performed smoothly and reliably in all instances where laser power is at least 1 W. The Autolase was not provided for review.

CLINICAL CRITERIA FOR SELECTION OF SUPERFICIAL VASCULAR LASERS: VISUAL CONCEPTUAL BLUEPRINT

The vascular lasers discussed in this chapter address very similar problems, despite the numerous differences in hardware. The author offers a conceptual blueprint to visually summarize clinical criteria he finds most helpful in deciding which of the functionally overlapping laser groups are to be preferred for a particular lesion (Figure 34.10). The goal is the safest and most effective treatment with the fewest sessions and least overhead cost. Assuming both categories of lasers (FEDL and continuous wave) are available, vessel size and pattern are assessed. The smallest vessels are not individually distinguishable by the naked eye, for example macular portwine stains less than 60 μm (Figure 34.1A). Such lesions found on infant skin more prone to scarring or texture change (especially in anatomic areas like the eyelid and neck) may be better treated with the more selective FEDL.

Children or adults with flat vascular lesions may be treated with either the FEDL or a continuous-wave laser; if CW is chosen, preferably with a scanner attachment to the continuous-wave laser to allow safer, more predictable and precise spatial and temporal distribution of the numerous beam exposures. Continuous-wave laser selection should emphasize adequate power to insure that the necessary joules are attainable at close to the shortest exposure time on current scanners (30 ms). Powers of 2.0–3.0 W are preferable, and slightly higher available power is desirable.

Small to large individual telangiectatic vessels, particularly if elevated, are more suitably treated with continuous-wave lasers freehand (without scanner) utilizing small (1.0–0.1 mm) spot sizes, and shuttered tracing to the point of vessel

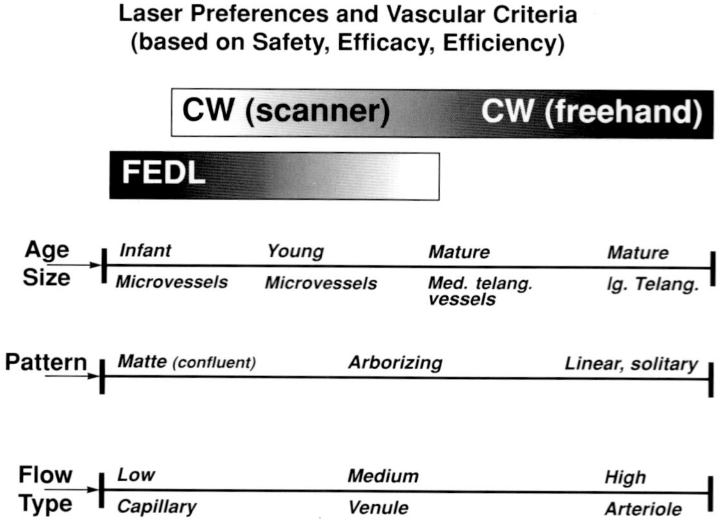

Laser Preferences and Vascular Criteria
(based on Safety, Efficacy, Efficiency)

Age	Infant	Young	Mature	Mature
Size	Microvessels	Microvessels	Med. telang. vessels	lg. Telang.
Pattern	Matte (confluent)	Arborizing		Linear, solitary
Flow	Low	Medium		High
Type	Capillary	Venule		Arteriole

Figure 34.10
Laser preferences and vascular criteria. CW, continuous wave; FEDL, flashlamp excited dye laser.

disappearance or minimum blanching; this provides the necessary energy and control needed for vessels with longer thermal relaxation times and avoids the temporary purpura of the FEDL. More confluent lesions with larger vessels may be treated with same approach with or without a scanner (Figure 34.10).

Patients with ruddy complexions require special feathering techniques when treating telangiectasias with the FEDL to avoid leaving a circular hypopigmentation pattern. Recently, 2-mm handpieces have become available for FEDL which decrease the diameter of the purpura, but it is still present. Patients conscious of being 'in the public eye' may prefer the less conspicuous continuous-wave technique. The smaller and more densely arborized the vessels are, the better candidates they are for FEDL, where all branches are easily removed in each 5-mm shot diameter.

Blood flow rate and vessel type/wall thickness may affect treatment efficacy. Low flow rate capillary/venules may be treated with either system. A nearly flat proliferating hemangioma in an infant would be better treated with FEDL. Higher flow rates and thicker walls associated with arteriolar lesions respond poorly if at all to FEDL and are best approached with freehand continuous wave.

A functional gap exists in our ideal laser approach to superficial vascular lesions beyond a certain depth and size. One must then choose whether to risk a scar potentially worse than the vascular lesion it would replace. The author has studied patients repeatedly treated with 9–10 J FEDL settings and residual vessel sizes of 100 µm are seen with thickened walls near 1 mm depth. Increasing the output of current FEDL vascular systems (especially beyond 10 J, which is feasible) results in loss of vascular specificity. Large vascular lesions ≥3 mm increasingly yield visible scars even when treated with the finest techniques.

Investigators have tried to selectively damage larger vessels with two different modalities (for example sclerotherapy and FEDL) but side-effects are increased over sclerotherapy alone.[18] Physical compression of enlarged vascular lesions prior to or during treatment (diascopy) may increase success and decrease complications with continuous-wave systems set at high power, 0.5–1.0-mm spot sizes.[12] Also, shuttered drilling methods with minimal spot sizes may augment cosmesis and effectiveness for spider angiomas that are larger or deeper, or have thicker walls or high flow rates.[14]

There is a final note of caution. The observed phenomenon of lightening can occur from either one or both of 'selective vascular removal' and vascular compression and optical interference caused by fibrosis. All current laser systems are capable of causing scarring, on a continuum from the microscopic subclinical and focal to the grossly evident. Not that scar tissue is intrinsically 'bad'. Fibrosis in small amounts and properly distributed may even be necessary, or unavoidable for certain lesions with current technology. Remember that surgical excision is still a reasonable option for selected deeper vascular malformations.

However, adoption of different vascular treatment regimens should be implemented, scrutinized and reported with due care. Cicatricial injury to dermal tissue may be focal and subtle, and recognition delayed for many months. Even then photographs from different angles, flat lighting and overexposure may hide or reduce the perceivable degree of such changes. A high complication rate in specific clinical groups (for example children), or in anatomic areas (nasolabial, mandible, maxillary lip) may occur regardless of the type of laser system used and despite normal test patches. Dosimetry and margin of safety may vary significantly between different yellow light or 532-nm laser systems, so a simultaneous analysis of all major variables must be performed. A given patient may require more than one type of vascular laser for optimal response. In the final analysis we must continue to exercise the 'art' of medicine along with the increasingly technical 'science' of lasers.

REFERENCES

1. Arndt KA, Noe JM, Noutham DB et al, Laser therapy. Basic concepts and nomenclature, *J Am Acad Dermatol* (1981) **5:**649–54.

2. Anderson RR, Parrish JA. Microvasculature can be selectively damaged using dye lasers: a basic theory and experimental evidence in human skin, *Lasers Surg Med* (1981) **1:**263–76.

3. Morelli JG, Tan OT, Garden J et al, Tunable dye laser (577 nm) treatment of port wine stains, *Lasers Surg Med* (1986) **6:**94–9.

4. Tan OT, Carney JM, Margolis R et al, Histologic responses of port-wine stains treated by argon, carbon dioxide, and tunable dye lasers. A preliminary report, *Arch Dermatol* (1986) **122:**1016–22.

5. Burrows PE, Mulliken JB, Fellows KE et al, Childhood hemangiomas and vascular malformations: angiographic differentiation, *AJR* (1983) **141:**483–8.

6. Finn MC, Glowacki J, Mulliken JB et al, Congenital vascular lesions: clinical application of a new classification, *J Pediatr Surg* (1983) **18:**894–900.

7. Wan S, Parrish J, Anderson RR et al, Transmittance of nonionizing radiation in human tissues, *Photochem Photobiol* (1982) **34:**679–81.

8. Tan OT, Morelli MD, Whitaker D et al, Ultrastructural changes in red blood cells following pulsed irradiation in

vitro, *J Invest Dermatol* (1989) **92**:100–104.

9. Hulsbergen HJ, van Gemert MJ, Port wine stain coagulation experiments with a 540-nm continuous wave dye-laser, *Lasers Surg Med* (1983) **2**:205–10.

10. Tan OT, Stafford TJ, Murray S et al, Histologic comparison of the pulsed dye laser and copper vapor laser effects on pig skin, *Lasers Surg Med* (1990) **10**:551–8.

11. Keijzer M, Light distributions in artery tissue: Monte Carlo simulations for finite-diameter laser beams, *Lasers Surg Med* (1989) **9**:148–54.

12. Rosio TJ, Tunable dye laser plus diascopy for venous lake. In: Apfelberg DB, ed. *Atlas of cutaneous laser surgery* (Raven Press: New York 1992) 398–9.

13. Rosio TJ, Tunable dye laser treatment of large telangiectasias. In: Apfelberg DB, ed. *Atlas of cutaneous laser surgery* (Raven Press: New York 1992) 351–3.

14. Rosio TJ, Tunable dye laser treatment of spider angiomas. In: Apfelberg DB, ed. *Atlas of cutaneous laser surgery* (Raven Press: New York 1992) 378–9.

15. Rotteleur G, Mordon S, Buys B et al, Robotized scanning laser handpiece for the treatment of port wine stains and other angiodysplasias, *Lasers Surg Med* (1988) **8**:283–7.

16. McDaniel DH, Mordon S, Hexascan: a new robotized scanning laser handpiece, *Cutis* (1990) **45**:300–5.

17. Smithies DJ, Butler PH, Pickering JW et al, A computer controlled scanner for the laser treatment of vascular lesions and hyperpigmentation, *Clin Phys Physiol Meas* (1991) **12**:261–7.

18. Goldman MP, Fitzpatrick RE, Pulsed-dye laser treatment of leg telangiectasia: with and without simultaneous sclerotherapy, *J Dermatol Surg Oncol* (1990) **16**:338–44.

Chapter 35

PSYCHOLOGICAL DISABILITIES OF HEMANGIOMA

J. A. Cotterill

'And the blots of Nature's hand
Shall not in their issue stand:
Never mole, hare-lip, nor scar,
Nor mark prodigious, such as are
Despised in nativity,
Shall upon their children be.'

A Midsummer Night's Dream, IV, i

INTRODUCTION

These Shakespearean lines, the silent thoughts of an Elizabethan bride, become all the more poignant with the realization that people with unusual birthmarks in medieval England were likely to be suspected of being witches and therefore tormented and often executed in the most horrific way.[1] Things have changed in this respect, but the stigma of a birthmark remains, especially if visible.

All dermatologists are aware of the stigma associated with skin diseases.[2] Skin disease in readily visible areas, such as the face and hands, can be expected to produce a lowering of self-esteem and body image perception, loss of confidence and reactive depression.[3] The teenager with facial acne, facial psoriasis or facial eczema comes readily to mind in this regard. It must also be remembered that even the smallest lesion can produce disparate anxiety and depression if it is present in an important cutaneous body image area. Thus a tiny spider nevus on the end of the nose can produce as much cosmetic distress as severe and extensive facial acne. Moreover, some individuals have very vulnerable personalities. An example of this group of individuals are those patients who present to dermatologists with virtually no clinical acne but demanding treatment with 13-*cis*-retinoic acid and threatening suicide if they do not get it.[4] These patients seem quite unable to tolerate even a hint of acne on the face, possibly because of their obsessional, compulsive type of personality. It is against this type of background that we have to see our patients with vascular birthmarks.

BODY IMAGE

The face is one of the most important body image areas and, sadly, is an area often affected by a portwine stain. We all have a mental impression, a body image, of what we look like, and we all tacitly assume that this is how others see us. This personal psychological body image is a curious mixed abstraction, partly perceptual, partly conceptual and partly intellectual. Corporeal awareness in man is very largely cutaneous, with nose, face and hair all featuring prominently. It is ironic that although we all think we know how we look, we have never personally seen our own face, but only images of it in a mirror.

The simplest and most useful definition of body image is that of Macdonald Critchley,[5] who defined corporeal awareness as 'the idea which an individual possesses as to the physical properties of his own anatomy which he carries over into the imagery of himself'.

Factors which may modify body image

Age

It is no accident that body image is often inappropriately young in a given individual. Thus, most artists painting their self-portraits represent themselves as being much younger than they actually are. This aspect of art was highlighted by Macdonald Critchley[6] when he described the portraits of Beatrice Turner, who at 58 was still painting herself to look like a woman years younger than she actually was. Moreover, this artist painted a nude self-portrait showing a young woman of ample proportions shortly before she died, thin and emaciated from starvation.

At times of adversity and strife, body image may conform more to actuality. It is probably true that the only escape from corporeal awareness, apart from death, may occur during moments of ecstasy, for instance as part of orgasmic experience.[5]

Cosmetic changes

It is known that an individual may try to modify his or her body image. For instance, it is not uncommon for young men to grow a moustache to try and appear older, or for older men to grow a beard, perhaps to try and appear more virile. It could also be argued that the use of cosmetics and tattoos in Western society also fulfils a desire to modify body image, while those more enthusiastic for more radical change seek cosmetic surgery, particularly on the nose, but also on the face, scalp or breasts. Cosmetic camouflage is also utilized, mainly by female patients with portwine stains, to alter the reality of their perceived facial disfigurement.

Social norms

The average Western female is encouraged by women's magazines, the media and advertisements in general to be infantile in her cutaneous desires.[7] It is no accident that in many advertisements for soap, lotions and potions, particularly those stressing skin care and youth, the incredibly young-looking mother is usually standing alongside a pre-adolescent daughter; the message is clear that a caring, mature woman of the Western world should strive for perfection and thus for a childlike skin.

It is not surprising, therefore, that there can be a large gap between an adult female's expectations and reality in terms of body image and actual appearance. Moreover, it is not surprising that the obsessional woman who has a powerful magnifying lens and a mirror soon makes herself miserable by regarding the lunar landscape of her face in between the howls of her children, the demands of her husband and the mortgage repayments. The unfortunate woman with a facial portwine stain can never aspire to the ideals of conventional physical beauty set by, for instance, women's magazines and the media at large.

A positive body image leads to positive feelings about self-esteem and confidence. Negative ideas about body image lead to significant loss of self-esteem and confidence, and, ultimately, to depression, which may become quite profound.

Body image in dermatology

Until recent times there has been little systematic investigation into the relationship of body image to dermatological problems. However, it would be surprising if dermatological pathology on the face did not produce some changes in body image.

Such a prediction was made by Shuster et al,[3] who found that, in acne, with increasing severity there was a progressive, dramatic and highly significant decrease both in the quality of self-image and in the perception of what others thought. Control subjects with eczema and psoriasis showed less severe damage to body image, which was thought to be related to the non-facial involvement of disease in these patients. The changes were also more marked in females than in males.

Clinical experiences of patients with portwine stains

Those dermatologists working with patients with portwine stains cannot fail but be impressed by the cheerful courage with which most of these patients, even with very visible portwine stains, go about their everyday life. From time to time some patients are referred for laser treatment after they have tried to commit suicide on account of their portwine stain, but this is most unusual.

That portwine stains do have a significant effect on the quality of life of affected individuals can be readily ascertained by talking to the patients. Many men with portwine stains fail to marry. Many affected women have never allowed their husbands to see them as they really are, choosing to cover up the portwine stain with cosmetic camouflage rather than face the possibility of rejection by their partner. In addition, many women with portwine stains will not open the front door unless they are wearing cosmetic camouflage. One of my patients nearly died of thyrotoxicosis which failed to come under medical control. She refused surgery because she was afraid that the surgeon or anaesthetist might disturb her cosmetic camouflage while she was having surgery. Another of my patients wrote me an angry three-page letter because I had sent her an appointment to come for treatment of her portwine stain. The appointment envelope had been automatically franked by the hospital and the patient was concerned that her husband would see this and learn for the first time that she had a portwine stain on her arm. She was adamant that all appointments for people with portwine stains should be sent in plain envelopes. A rude remark to a little girl with a portwine stain led many years later to the creation of the largest charity in the UK devoted to disfigurement and led ultimately to the provision of several pulsed tunable dye lasers to treat children and adults with portwine stains.

Additional stigmas which some children with portwine stains have to face include seizures, because of cerebral involvement and inequality of growth of limbs, hands and feet caused by an arterial element in the vascular naevus. Fortunately, only a rare minority face blindness because of glaucoma.

Interestingly, I was referred my first totally blind patient with a portwine stain seeking treatment of her birthmark as I was preparing this chapter. The referring doctor commented that the patient did not like the lumps and bumps which she had developed on her portwine stain with increasing age, and, as the patient was totally blind, could we phone with an appointment rather than send one through the post.

The horror, disbelief and feeling of failure that initially overwhelm a young couple when their child is born with a portwine stain can be very moving for the involved empathic practitioner. Acceptance of the portwine stain proves difficult, or frankly impossible, for some families and they may be driven into a restless pursuit of treatment, whatever the associated risks.

The problems can be compounded by interfering bystanders who may accuse the mother of assaulting her child. Bleeding and pain from an ulcerated strawberry nevus may induce understandable anxiety in both parents and other family members.

This clinical experience of the psychological disabilities experienced by patients and their relatives as a result of portwine stains has led to several studies of objective psychological disabilities in such patients.

Two previous studies concerning psychological effects of laser therapy in patients with portwine stains using standard psychological and psychiatric tests showed no differences from normal controls,[8,9] but patients were found to be perfectionist and many had unrealistic expectations of the outcome of laser treatment.[10] However, it was felt that such studies were ignoring considerable psychological burdens in these patients, so we undertook a further study in 1989 in Leeds of patients with portwine stains using a questionnaire designed to elicit feelings of stigmatization and poor self-image, and difficulties in interpersonal relationships.[11]

PSYCHOLOGICAL DISABILITY IN PATIENTS WITH PORTWINE STAINS

To facilitate this study a questionnaire was devised containing 16 general questions, including an assessment by the patient of the severity of the birthmark in terms of the extent of involvement, colour change and surface features. In addition, 26 direct questions requiring a 'yes' or 'no' answer were also given to each patient. These included questions such as 'I feel an outcast because of my birthmark', and 'I am resentful of people with normal skin'. The questions with a high positive response rate are shown in Table 35.1. This questionnaire was administered to 90 patients over the age of 15 years with portwine stains. In addition, they were given a General Health Questionnaire and a Hospital Anxiety and Depression Inventory. Finally, 71 patients completed this study, 46 females and 25 males. The study showed that cosmetic camouflage was used successfully by 22 of the 39 females, but hardly ever by the males. Fifty per cent of the patients felt embarrassed, anxious or depressed because of their portwine stain. Forty-one per cent felt envious of people with normal skin and a similar number felt that people avoided looking at them. Twenty-

Table 35.1
Questions with a high positive response rate

Question	Positive response (%)
I feel people stare at me because of my birthmark	75
I have been hurt by what other people say to me because of my birthmark	73
I feel the need to hide my birthmark	72
If my birthmark is improved by treatment I will feel more comfortable with people of the same sex	71
My birthmark has affected my self-confidence	71
Having a birthmark makes me feel different from other people	67
If my child were to have a birthmark I would feel guilty	67
I feel physically unattractive and sexually undesirable because of my birthmark	54

three per cent said they avoided sexual activity because of their portwine stain.

This latest study from Leeds in 71 patients has shown that there is a significant degree of psychological morbidity which will not be detected in standard psychiatric screening tests, such as the Hospital Anxiety and Depression Inventory or the General Health Questionnaire.

There seems no doubt that patients with portwine stains experience feelings of stigmatization, difficulties in relationships, particularly with members of the opposite sex, embarrassment, guilt feelings, anxiety and depression. Older patients in our study were still often embarrassed because of their birthmarks and avoided social situations because of them, suggesting that with increasing age there is little adaptation to the portwine stain. Nearly three-quarters of the patients felt the need to hide their birthmark and this need was reflected in the common use of cosmetic camouflage in females. Patients also felt that the treatment of their portwine stain would result in an improvement in the quality of their lives.

Treatment of portwine stains in the newborn

When a baby is born with a portwine stain it is the parents who feel stigmatized. The child is unlikely to be at all concerned about the portwine stain for many years, but the parents are anxious to get treatment under way as soon as possible. In a way, the parents are the index patients and it is they who are asking for treatment. It can be argued that the surface area of the portwine stain is probably smaller just after birth than at any other time in life and so there may be economic reasons for treating a patient at this age. There are those therapists who carry out a test patch very early on in life without any sedation. Thus, young babies have been treated with the pulsed tunable dye laser using physical restraint. Child psychologists are not happy about this approach and there could be some risk of damage to the retina if great care is not taken to protect the eyes. On the other hand, a general anaesthetic is not without risks in a young baby.

The writer feels that some sort of compromise is necessary here. It is often possible to perform an initial trial area in a child with a portwine stain under cover of EMLA cream at about the age of 3 or 4 years and in many children it is possible to initiate therapy before they begin primary school at the age of 4 or 5 years. Most children do not experience any psychological problems at this time in their life. Teasing on account of portwine stains begins to become a more marked feature of life by the age of 8 or 9 years, becoming more common with increasing years as the child moves into the early teens.

Conclusions

Patient expectations of laser therapy, and of the laser therapist in particular, are high, often unrealistically so. A careful pretreatment consultation must set out to explain the procedure and its chances of success, and also to establish the fact that the involved area may need to be treated on several occasions. In short, excellent communication is necessary to dispel future unrealistic expectations. During the consultation it is important to try and empathize with the patient and the family, realizing that in most individuals the portwine stain is producing significant psychological morbidity and in a minority of adults these feelings can be profound enough to induce thoughts of suicide.

It is heartening to see how a good result, even in a tiny test area, can lead to a new self-confidence and bolster self-esteem in the treated patient. A determined effort should be made to get treatment under way before affected children begin school so that the child is not set apart from classmates.

REFERENCES

1. Cotterill JA, Shakespeare on the skin, *Br J Dermatol* (1972) **86**:533–42.
2. Ginsberg IH, Link BG, Feelings of stigmatization in patients with psoriasis, *J Am Acad Dermatol* (1989) **20**:53–63.
3. Shuster S, Fisher GH, Harris E et al, The effect of skin disease on self-image, *Br J Dermatol* (1978) **99**(supplement 16):18–19.
4. MacDonald-Hull S, Cunliffe WJ, Hughes BR, Treatment of the depressed and dysmorphophobic acne patient, *Clin Exp Dermatol* (1991) **16**:210–11.
5. Macdonald Critchley, *The divine banquet of the brain and other essays* (Raven Press: New York 1979) 93.
6. Macdonald Critchley, *The divine banquet of the brain and other essays* (Raven Press: New York 1979) 121–9.
7. Cotterill JA, What is really true about cosmetics, *Int J Dermatol* (1988) **10**:682.
8. Kalick SM, Goldwin RM, Noe JM, Social issues and body concerns of port wine stain patients undergoing laser therapy, *Lasers Surg Med* (1981) **1**:205–313.
9. Kalick SM, Laser treatment of port wine stains: observations concerning psychological outcome. In: Arndt KA, Noe JM, Rosen S, eds, *Cutaneous laser therapy: principles and methods* (John Wiley & Sons: 1983) 215–29.
10. Dixon JA, Rotering RH, Huether SE, Patients' valuation of argon laser therapy of port wine stains, decorative tattoos and essential telangiectasia, *Lasers Surg Med* (1984) **4**:181–90.
11. Lanigan SW, Cotterill JA, Psychological disabilities amongst patients with port wine stains, *Br J Dermatol* (1989) **121**:209–15.

Chapter 36

PHOTODYNAMIC THERAPY FOR SKIN CANCER

Scott M. Dinehart
Stephen Flock

Photodynamic therapy (PDT), previously known as photochemotherapy and photoradiation therapy, involves the use of a photosensitizer and nonionizing radiation to produce a beneficial therapeutic effect. Photodynamic therapy is not a new concept to dermatologists, who for decades have used the Goeckerman regimen of topically applied crude coal tar and ultraviolet light to treat psoriasis. More recently, 8-methoxypsoralen as a photosensitizer combined with an ultraviolet A light source (PUVA) has enjoyed widespread use for psoriasis and other cutaneous diseases. Although the Goeckerman regimen and PUVA are common examples of PDT, it is the use of PDT for the treatment of malignant disorders, most often using porphyrin as a sensitizer and a laser producing red light as the light source, that has recently generated increasing interest. This chapter discusses the history, mechanism of action, clinical applications and future of PDT for the treatment of cutaneous malignancies.

History

Photodynamic therapy had its beginnings in 1900 when Raab observed that exposure of paramecia to an acridine dye and light could be lethal.[1] The combination of the dye and light was shown to be effective in a dose-dependent fashion while neither dye nor light alone was effective. In 1903 Tappenier and Jesionek attempted treatment of cutaneous malignancies with sunlight exposure after first painting them with eosin.[2] Meyer-Betz, in 1913, personally observed the photosensitizing effects of porphyrins in man by intravenously injecting himself with these compounds.[3] The concept that porphyrins could be taken up in significant amounts by tumors was first envisioned by Policard, who reported in 1924 that porphyrins were the probable cause of reddish fluorescence seen in experimental rat sarcomas illuminated by a Wood's lamp.[4] Policard postulated that this fluorescence was due to excitation of endogenous porphyrins present in the sarcomas because of secondary infection by hemolytic bacteria.

The uptake of hematoporphyrin in neoplastic tissue was first described by Auler and Banzer in 1942.[5] Figge et al confirmed this uptake in 1948 using the intrinsic fluorescence of hematoporphyrins.[6] A significant advance in the development of PDT use for malignancy came when Lipson et al reported in 1961 on the use of hematoporphyrin derivative, the acid-washed derivative of hematoporphyrin which remains the major clinical photosensitizer for fluorescence detection of tumor tissue.[7] This group followed their work concerning detection of tumors by treating a patient with recurrent breast cancer using sensitization with hematoporphyrin derivative followed by light exposure.[7]

Whereas previous studies had concentrated on using porphyrins in detection of cancer, a series of articles began to be published concerning therapeutic use of porphyrin sensitization followed by exposure to light. Diamond et al reported in 1972 that hematoporphyrin, activated by white light, caused regression of experimental gliomas in rats.[8] In 1976, Dougherty et al successfully treated transplanted mammary tumors in mice using intraperitoneally administered hematoporphyrin derivative and tumor-directed red light from a filtered xenon arc lamp.[9] At about the same time Tomson et al utilized lasers as a light source for PDT.[10] They reported that acridine orange, activated by an argon laser, could destroy a mouse epithelial tumor. In 1978 Dougherty et al reported their favorable experience with treatment of cutaneous malignancies, including human basal and squamous cell carcinomas, using hematoporphyrin derivative and red light.[11]

THE PHOTODYNAMIC EFFECT

The use of PDT for treatment of cutaneous malignancy is dependent on the ability of photosensitizing agents to undergo various photochemical reactions upon absorbing light. Excitation of the sensitizer by light that falls within its absorption band initiates the photodynamic effect. Light absorption by porphyrin sensitizers in the presence of oxygen has been shown to produce singlet oxygen in vitro.[12] Singlet oxygen is a short-lived excited form of oxygen which can cause irreversible oxidation of some essential cellular molecules. Purportedly, this is the mechanism which causes death of the neoplasm.[13]

The primary sites of photodynamic activity are thought to be cellular and mitochondrial membranes, although a large number of other intracellular structures, including nucleic acids and proteins, are also damaged by photo-oxidation.[14-18] It is not entirely clear how this process takes place, but it is felt that singlet oxygen is responsible for much of the damage. This species can produce organoperoxides which are able to disrupt cellular membranes.[16] Other highly reactive oxygen species are produced by PDT but appear to play a minor role in producing cell death.[19-21] Photodynamic therapy has been seen to have a marked effect on the vasculature although the precise mechanism by and extent to which the microcirculation of tumors is destroyed during PDT is a current subject of investigation.[22] It may be that nonporphyrin photosensitizers will be proven to act by entirely different mechanisms.

PHOTOSENSITIZERS

The ideal photosensitizer for use in PDT is one which can be specifically concentrated in neoplastic tissue, is nontoxic, and is photoactivated by a wavelength of light that penetrates deeply into tissues. Of course the photosensitizer should also have a potent photosensitizing potential. While no photosensitizer currently approaches this ideal, porphyrins are the most widely used and studied. Hematoporphyrin is obtained from hemoglobin present in cow's blood.[7] Hematoporphyrin derivative (HPD) is a mixture of porphyrins derived from hematoporphyrin after successive alkalinization and acetylation.[7] A variety of porphyrin compounds can be identified when HPD is subjected to high-performance liquid chromatographic analysis. The acid-washed product of HPD is dihematoporphyrin ester/ether (DHE) and is currently marketed as photofrin. Dihematoporphyrin ester/ether is currently the only FDA-approved cancer photosensitizing agent available for human studies.

One of the difficulties with porphyrin sensitizers has been that these are biologically extracted materials which have been difficult to characterize or artificially synthesize. Nuclear magnetic resonance (NMR) studies suggest that DHE is probably a mixture of both ethers and esters.[23] It is clear that DHE is a more effective photosensitizer than HPD.[24] Estimates from studies conducted on animals suggest that twice as much HPD as DHE is required to achieve a given photosensitizing level.[24]

Following intravenous administration HPD is rapidly cleared from most tissues but is retained in neoplastic tissue as well as in certain organs, including the skin.[25] The liver is the primary metabolic and excretory organ for porphyrins and is the site of highest accumulation.[26] Other organs such as the spleen, adrenal cortex, kidney and those tissues rich in reticuloendothelial cells also readily retain porphyrins.[27,28] It is not known why porphyrins are retained longer by some tumors but it is postulated that perhaps the tumor microvasculature delivers increased amounts of intravenously injected porphyrins and poorly developed lymphatics in tumors hinder clearance.[29] It is also speculated that some photosensitizers may bind to a plasma lipoprotein.[30] Neoplastic tissues contain high levels of low-density lipoprotein (LDL) receptors[31] and therefore these receptors may participate in the selective retention of porphyrins by neoplasms.

Investigators are realizing some of the limitations and disadvantages of porphyrins as sensitizers. Thus, there is a great desire to find sensitizers that are more pure, less toxic and more compatible with longer wavelength light sources. Phthalocyanines are an entirely separate class of sensitizers that have received much attention because of their effectiveness at selectively killing tumor cells in tissue culture after exposure to longer wavelength light sources of 680–720 nm.[32] They have the added advantage of being water soluble, which expedites clearance from tissues. While the photosensitizing effects of lipid-soluble HPD can last as long as 6 months, estimates are that phthalocyanine photosensitivity will last little more than a week. Results are promising in tissue cultures;[32] however, little experience with use in animals or humans is available. Additionally, photosensitizing efficiency of the phthalocyanines has been questioned and may be a drawback to the use of these compounds. Other sensitizers such as the rhodamines, benzophenoxonines, triphenylmethanes, chlorins, purpurins, verdins, bacteriochlorophyll a and naphthalocynanne along with many other compounds are all being studied in the hope of finding a photosensitizer superior to Photofrin.

The wavelength specificity of photosensitizers is directly related to their molecular structure. It appears that increasing the number of alternating single and double bonds in a molecule can lead to increased absorption at longer wavelengths.[33–36] Once the mechanism and mechanics of the photodynamic process are more fully understood it may be possible to chemically manipulate photosensitizers in this manner to bring them closer to the ideal.

LIGHT

The optimal light wavelength for PDT is entirely determined by the absorption spectrum of the sensitizer and the characteristics of light penetration through the tissue being treated. Tissue optical properties, pigmentation, bloodflow and irradiation geometry all affect light penetration and efficacy of treatment.[37,38] Red light has been chosen for PDT in cancer patients because this wavelength offers a greater depth (approximately 5–10 mm) of tissue penetration and does not correspond to a minor porphyrin absorbency peak.[39] Unfortunately DHE absorbance is 35 times greater at lower, less penetrating blue light wavelengths (363 nm) than at red light wavelengths of 626 nm.[40]

Although optically filtered xenon arc lamps were used in earlier times it has become more standard to use lasers to obtain the red light needed for PDT. Lasers have the advantage of providing pure, reproducible, intense, easily measured monochromatic light. Currently the argon-dye laser and the pulsed gold vapor laser emit light within the red region of the electromagnetic spectrum and are suitable for PDT.[41] The argon-dye laser can be configured to emit light at 630 nm and the gold vapor emits light at 627 nm. While these two lasers dominate the field of PDT, it is inevitable that as more emphasis is placed on longer wavelength photosensitizers, new or different lasers will become more prevalent.

Clinical applications in treating cutaneous malignancy

Most current treatment modalities for nonmelanoma skin cancer provide greater than 90% cure for primary (nonrecurrent) tumors.[42] Mohs micrographic surgery routinely provides 95% cure rates for some recurrent or difficult to treat skin tumors.[42] Despite these successes, there is still a small group of patients with tumors that are difficult to treat or situations in which a treatment modality such as PDT would be in the patient's interest. Currently, photodynamic therapy is considered for skin cancer patients who are not good surgical candidates or those patients with multiple tumors or widespread disease. Patients with basal cell nevus syndrome often have hundreds of tumors over widespread areas and are frequently a therapeutic problem. These patients may benefit greatly from routine use of PDT.[43] Ill-defined tumors may be ideal for PDT as less emphasis is placed on defining margins with the photodynamic technique. There are also a group of patients with tumors that are located in critical functional or cosmetic areas who would benefit from the selective tumor cell death produced by PDT.[44] As therapeutic trials continue, the indications for PDT will inevitably be expanded.

Several types of cancer that commonly develop within skin have been treated with PDT. Since basal cell carcinoma (BCC) is the most common cancer in man, it is appropriate that this tumor was one of the first to be treated by Dougherty and his colleagues.[11] They treated two lesions and noted complete response in both. One treatment site was observed at 7 months to be clinically free of tumor. After a 12–14-month follow-up, Tse et al found that only 10.8% of 40 BCCs that they had treated in two patients with nevoid BCC had recurred.[43] Tumor recurrences tended to be at peripheral margins and they recommended wider light irradiation to correct this. A topical porphyrin derivative utilized as a photosensitizer in 14 cases of BCC was found to give complete remission in lesions less than 2 mm in thickness, but only partial remission in thicker lesions.[45] Gregory and Goldman reported several cases of BCC treated with PDT, including a recurrent lesion which remained clinically clear after 9 months of follow-up.[46]

In situ and invasive squamous cell carcinoma (SCC) have both been treated with PDT. Dougherty treated a single lesion of SCC and noted a complete response in that patient.[11] Gross similarly reported a single patient with a large invasive SCC who remained clinically and histologically free of tumor at 6 months.[44] Over 500 lesions in two patients with widespread Bowen's disease completely cleared at 6 months after treatment with PDT.[47] Another single report of treatment of a small patch of Bowen's noted no recurrence.[46]

Not all reports treating SCC and BCC with PDT have been so favorable. In seven patients McCaughan et al treated 36 areas and could document a complete response in only 16.[48] They treated five areas of SCC, and noted a complete response in only three. One of these patients, however, was documented to have a 5-year cure after treatment of a SCC on the eyelid. Poor results 6 months after treatment of 21 BCCs and 32 SCCs led Pennington et al to abandon a trial of PDT on skin cancer patients.[49] Retrospectively, the energy density of the light source they were using may have been too low.

Photodynamic therapy has received mostly poor reviews when used to treat malignant melanoma. All investigators have treated metastases to the skin and not primary lesions. Although results concerning a series of seven intraocular melanomas treated with PDT were reported as encouraging, it should be noted that histological evidence of residual neoplasm was noted in all treated tumors.[50] Out of 27 treatment areas another study could document only five complete responses.[48] Dougherty reported six out of seven complete responses in his initial study but later reviewed other cases and concluded that only lightly pigmented lesions should be expected to respond in a satisfactory manner.[51] When data for PDT treatment of melanoma are examined collectively it appears that malignant melanoma is one of the primary skin tumors least responsive to PDT as it is currently practiced.

Another skin tumor where PDT may find use is Kaposi's sarcoma, where three patients with classical disease have been reported to obtain complete control following treatment.[51] Follow-up was available in two of these cases for over 1 year. A complete response in four of six lesions of cutaneous T cell lymphoma has been reported.[11] A partial response to PDT in a metastatic angiosarcoma has also been reported.[11] Numerous cases of other tumors metastatic to the skin treated with PDT have been reported with impressive response rates.

One of the most exciting applications of PDT is its combination with other therapeutic modalities. Several studies have shown that PDT and ionizing radiation affect cell survival independently and that their effects are additive.[52,53] It has been shown that the effects of ionizing radiation in an animal model can be potentiated by very high doses of HPD.[54] Potentiation is also seen when hyperthermia and PDT are given simultaneously.[55] Even so, PDT seems to be most effective when it precedes hyperthermia.[56] Combination studies involving chemotherapeutic agents and PDT have shown little potential advantage and are less applicable to treatment of tumors which originate in the skin.[57,58] Gregory and Goldman used adjuvant PDT following surgical debulking of a BCC located on the nose.[46] The patient remained free of tumor at 1 year.

Our current protocol for treating BCC or SCC of the skin begins 72 h prior to light activation with the intravenous infusion of 2 mg/kg photofrin. At this time the necessity for photoprotection is reinforced and the patient is given written instructions concerning protective measures to be taken. Seventy-two hours after infusion of photofrin the sensitizer is activated using an argon-pumped dye laser. Exposure is generally for 20–30 min using an energy density of 100 J/cm^2. Depending upon the circumstances, a 0.5–1.0-cm margin of clinically normal skin is irradiated and surrounding skin is protected using black felt. No anesthesia is needed during the laser session and analgesia is given as needed over the next 24–36 h. Within 24 h swelling of the treated area and clinical necrosis of the tumor is seen. The resulting wound is allowed to heal by second intention. Swelling generally diminishes by 1 week and healing is generally complete by 6–8 weeks. All patients are required to have pretreatment histological confirmation of tumor.

Advantages

PDT offers a tumor-specific cancer treatment in which any lesion accessible to light is potentially treatable. Local or general anesthetic agents are not generally needed for skin cancer treatments. Treatments can be repeated and the effects of repeated treatments are cumulative. Unlike treatment with ionizing radiation, no mutagenesis is expected, possibly because the intracellular target site is most likely the cell membrane rather than the DNA.[41] Photodynamic therapy has additional advantages in that it can be easily combined with other treatments. In the case of cutaneous cancers its greatest promise may be in 'mop up' therapy where it is combined with another modality such as surgical excision[46] or ionizing radiation.[53]

Disadvantages

A significant disadvantage of PDT when using porphyrin sensitizers and red light is the generalized sensitivity of normal skin to visible and UV light seen for an average of 6 weeks after intravenous administration of the photosensitizer.[59] A prospective study in which detailed written and verbal photoprotection instructions as well as sunscreens were given to patients undergoing PDT procedures found that three out of every four patients reported cutaneous photosensitivity.[59] Of these patients, 17% experienced blister formation. Other HPD-related complications include skin hyperpigmentation, ocular discomfort, pruritus, urticaria, nausea, pain at the injection site, and a metallic taste sensation.[59] The need to administer photosensitizers intravenously rather than by intralesional injection or topically is also a considerable drawback.

The development and use of PDT has been somewhat hindered by the need for lasers as light sources. Lasers provide an optimal light source because they provide high enough light intensities to make treatments possible in a reasonable amount of time but they are expensive and somewhat cumbersome to use. Additionally, the optimal time to begin light exposure after sensitization has not been determined although most investigators use 72 h. Optimal dosage of sensitizer and energy density of light used are determined by a similar empirical method. Care must also be taken to direct light only to the tumor volume to avoid damage to surrounding normal skin. Therefore it is still necessary to determine clinical margins, although this is less important than in other types of standard treatment.

Future

There is a strong need for new pure sensitizers and light sources that function at longer, more penetrating wavelengths. Local administration of these sensitizers, by either topical or intralesional delivery, would be more optimal than the current intravenous administration. If intravenous delivery is continued, sensitizers should be less dermophilic to avoid cutaneous photosensitivity. A novel method for increasing the specificity of the sensitizers is to conjugate them with tumor-seeking monoclonal antibodies.[60] Recent topical formulations using laurocapram azone to enhance dermal penetration have shown considerable promise in animal trials.[61]

Summary

The ideal cancer treatment provides selective destruction of tumor without significant disruption of normal cell and tissue function. Photodynamic therapy for treatment of cutaneous malignancies has the potential to provide this type of selective tumor cell death. Advances have been significant since Raab's initial experiments with single cell organisms in 1900 and it is estimated that by 1986 between 3000 and 5000 human patients had been treated by PDT. Although this type of treatment remains investigational, it is clear that as the technique improves and more data accumulate as to the potential cure rates, photodynamic therapy will surely find its therapeutic niche in the treatment of skin cancer.

References

1. Raab C, Uber die wirkung fluoreszierender stoffe auf infusoria, *Z Biol* (1900) **39**:524–6.
2. Tappenier H, Jesionek A, Therapeutische reosuche mit fluoreszirenden stoff, *MMW* (1903) **1**:2042.
3. Meyer-Betz F, Untersuchungen uber die biologische (photodynamische) wirkung des hamatoporphyrins und anderer derivate des blut-und gallenfarbstoffs, *Dtsch Arch Klin Med* (1913) **112**:476–503.
4. Policard A, Etude sur les aspects offerts par des tumeurs experimentales examinees a la lumiere de Wood, *C R Soc Biol (Paris)* (1924) **91**:1423–4.
5. Auler H, Banzer G, Unter suchungen uber die rolle der porphyrine BEI geschwul stkranken menschen und tieren, *Z Krebsforsch* (1942) **53**:65–8.
6. Figge FHJ, Weiland GS, Manganiello LOJ, Cancer detection and therapy. Affinity of neoplastic embryonic, and traumatized tissues for porphyrins and metalloporphyrins, *Proc Soc Exp Biol Med* (1948) **68**:640–1.
7. Lipson RL, Baldes EJ, Olsen EM, The use of a derivative of hematoporphyrin in tumor detection, *JNCI* (1961) **26**:1–12.
8. Diamond I, Granelli SG, McDonough AF et al, Photodynamic therapy of malignant tumours, *Lancet* (1972) **2**:1175–7.
9. Dougherty TJ, Gomer CJ, Weishaupt KR, Energetics and efficiency of photoinactivation of murine tumor cells containing hematoporphyrin, *Cancer Res* (1976) **36**:2330–3.
10. Tomson SH, Emmet EA, Fox SH, Photodestruction of mouse epithelial tumors after oral acridine orange and argon laser, *Cancer Res* (1974) **34**:3124–7.
11. Dougherty TJ, Kaufman JE, Goldfarb A et al, Photoradiation therapy for the treatment of malignant tumors, *Cancer Res* (1978) **38**:2628–35.
12. Henderson BW, Miller AC, Effects of scavengers of reactive oxygen and radical species on cell survival following photodynamic treatment in vitro: comparison to ionizing radiation, *Radiat Res* (1986) **108**:196–205.
13. Weishaupt K, Gomer CJ, Dougherty T, Identification of singlet oxygen as the cytotoxic agent in photo-inactivation of a murine tumor, *Cancer Res* (1976) **36**:2326–9.
14. Gibson SL, Hilf R, Photosensitization of mitochondrial cytochrome c oxidase by hematoporphyrin derivative and related porphyrins in vitro and in vivo, *Cancer Res* (1983) **43**:4191–7.
15. Hilf R, Warne NW, Smail DB et al, Photodynamic inactivation of selected intracellular enzymes by hematoporphyrin derivative and their relationship to tumor cell viability in vitro, *Cancer Lett* (1984) **24**:165–72.

16. Foote CS, Mechanisms of photooxygenation. In: Doiron DR, Comer CJ, eds, *Porphyrin localization and treatment of tumors* (Liss: New York 1984) 3–18.
17. Fiel RJ, Datta-Gupta N, Mark EH et al, Induction of DNA damage by porphyrin photosensitizers, *Cancer Res* (1981) **41**:3543–5.
18. Moan J, Waksvik H, Christensen T, DNA single-strand breaks and sister chromatid exchanges induced by treatment with hematoporphyrin and light or by x-rays in human NHIK 3025 cells, *Cancer Res* (1980) **40**:2915–18.
19. Buettner GR, Oberley LW, Apparent production of superoxide and hydroxyl radicals by hematoporphyrin and light as seen by spin-trapping, *FEBS Lett* (1980) **121**:161–4.
20. Buettner GR, Need MJ, Hydrogen peroxide and hydroxyl free radical production by hematoporphyrin derivative, ascorbate and light, *Cancer Lett* (1985) **25**:297–304.
21. Hariharan PV, Courtney J, Eleczko S, Production of hydroxyl radicals in cell systems exposed to haematoporphyrin and red light, *Int J Radiat Biol* (1980) **37**:691–4.
22. Henderson BW, Dougherty TJ, Malone PB, Studies on the mechanism of tumor destruction by photoradiation therapy, *Prog Clin Biol Res* (1984) **170**:601–12.
23. Pandey RK, Dougherty TJ, Syntheses and photosensitizing activity of porphyrins joined with ester linkages, *Cancer Res* (1989) **49**: 2042–7.
24. Dougherty TJ, Potter WR, Weishaupt KR, The structure of the active component of hematoporphyrin derivative. In: Doiron DR, Gomer CJ, eds, *Porphyrin localization and treatment of tumors* (Liss: New York 1984) 301–14.
25. Kessel D, Cheng M, On the preparation and properties of dihematoporphyrin ether, the tumor localizing component of HPD, *Photochem Photobiol* (1985) **41**:277–82.
26. Delaney TF, Glatstein E, Photodynamic therapy of cancer, *Compr Ther* (1988) **14**:43–55.
27. Gomer CJ, Dougherty TJ, Determination of ^{3}H and ^{14}C hematoporphyrin derivative distribution in malignant and normal tissue, *Cancer Res* (1979) **39**:146–51.
28. Ho Y-K, Pandey RK, Misert JR et al, Carbon-14 labeling and biological activity of the tumor-localizing derivative of hematoporphyrin, *Photochem Photobiol* (1988) **48**:445–9.
29. Bugelski PJ, Porter CW, Dougherty TJ, Autoradiographic distribution of HPD in normal and tumor tissue of the mouse, *Cancer Res* (1981) **41**:4606–12.
30. Kessel K, Thompson P, Saatio K, Tumor localization and photosensitization by sulfonated derivatives of tetraphenylporphine, *Photochem Photobiol* (1987) **45**:787–90.
31. Jori G, Reddi E, Salvato B et al, Evidence for a major role of plasma lipoproteins as hematoporphyrin carriers in vivo, *Cancer Lett* (1984) **24**:291–7.
32. Glassberg E, Lewandowski L, Lask GL et al, Laser-induced photodynamic therapy with aluminum phthalocyanine tetrasulfonate as the photosensitizer: differential phototoxicity in normal and malignant human cells in vitro, *J Invest Dermatol* (1990) **94**:604–10.
33. Spikes JD, Photobiology of porphyrins. In: Doiron DR, Gomer CJ, eds, *Porphyrin localization and treatment of tumors* (Liss: New York 1984) 19–39.

34. Woodward RB, Structure and the absorption spectra of a,b-unsaturated ketones, *J Am Chem Soc* (1941) **63**:1123–6.

35. Woodward RB, Structure and absorption spectra. III. Normal conjugated dienes, *J Am Chem Soc* (1942) **64**:72–5.

36. Woodward RB, Structure and absorption spectra. IV. Further observations on a,b-unsaturated ketones, *J Am Chem Soc* (1942) **64**:76–7.

37. Svaasand LO, Optical dosimetry for direct and interstitial photoradiation therapy of malignant tumors. In: Doiron DR, Gomer CJ, eds, *Porphyrin localization and treatment of tumors* (Liss: New York 1984) 91–114.

38. Wan S, Parrish JA, Anderson RR et al, Transmittance of nonionizing radiation in human tissues. *Photochem Photobiol* (1981) **34**:679–81.

39. Doiron DR, Photophysics of and instrumentation for porphyrin detection and activation. In: Doiron DR, Comer CJ, eds, *Porphyrin localization and treatment of tumors* (Liss: New York 1984) 41–73.

40. Manyak MJ, Russo A, Smith PD et al, Photodynamic therapy, *J Clin Oncol* (1988) **6**:380–91.

41. Berns MW, McCullough JL, Porphyrin sensitized phototherapy, *Arch Dermatol* (1986) **122**:871–4.

42. Dinehart SM, Pollack SV, Mohs micrographic surgery for skin cancer, *Cancer Treat Rev* (1989) **16**:257–65.

43. Tse DT, Kersten RC, Anderson RL, Hematoporphyrin derivative photoradiation therapy in managing nevoid basal-cell carcinoma syndrome. A preliminary report, *Arch Opthalmol* (1984) **102**:990–4.

44. Gross DJ, Waner M, Schosser RH et al, Squamous cell carcinoma of the lower lip involving a large cutaneous surface. Photodynamic therapy as an alternative therapy, *Arch Dermatol* (1990) **126**:1148–50.

45. Sacchini V, Melloni E, Marchesini R, Preliminary clinical studies with PDT by topical TPPS administration in neoplastic skin lesions, *Lasers Surg Med* (1987) **7**:6–11.

46. Gregory R, Goldman L, Application of photodynamic therapy in plastic surgery, *Lasers Surg Med* (1986) **6**:62–6.

47. Robinson PJ, Carruth JAS, Fairris GM, Photodynamic therapy: a better treatment for widespread Bowen's disease, *Br J Dermatol* (1988) **119**:59–61.

48. McCaughan JS, Guy JT, Hicks W et al, Photodynamic therapy for cutaneous and subcutaneous malignant neoplasms, *Arch Surg* (1989) **124**:211–16.

49. Pennington DG, Waner M, Knox A, Photodynamic therapy for multiple skin cancers, *Plast Reconstr Surg* (1988) **82**:1067–71.

50. Tse DT, Dutton JJ, Weingeist TA et al, Hematoporphyrin photoradiation therapy for intraocular and orbital malignant melanoma, *Arch Ophthalmol* (1984) **102**:833–8.

51. Dougherty TJ, Photoradiation therapy for cutaneous and subcutaneous malignancies, *J Invest Dermatol* (1981) **77**:122–4.

52. Bellnier DA, Dougherty TJ, Haematoporphyrin derivative photosensitization and gamma damage interaction in Chinese hamster ovary fibroblasts, *Int J Radiat Biol* (1986) **50**:659–664.

53. Winther J, Overgaard J, Ehlers N, The effect of photodynamic therapy alone and in combination with misonidazole or x-rays for management of a retinoblastoma-like tumour, *Photochem Photobiol* (1988) **47**:419–23.

54. Kostron H, Swartz MR, Miller DC et al, The interaction of hematoporphyrin derivative, light, and ionizing radiation in a rat glioma model, *Cancer* (1986) **57**:964–70.

55. Henderson BW, Waldow SM, Mang TS et al, Photodynamic therapy and hyperthermia. In: Jori G, Peria C, eds, *Photodynamic therapy of tumors and other diseases* (Libreria Progetto Editore: Padua 1985) 183–93.

56. Mang TS, Combination studies on hyperthermia induced by the neodymium yttrium aluminum garnet (Nd:YAG) laser as an adjuvant to photodynamic therapy, *Proc SPIE Conf New Directions in Photodynamic Therapy* (1987) **847**:158–62.

57. Cowled PA, Mackenzie L, Forbes IJ, Pharmacological modulation of photodynamic therapy with hematoporphyrin derivative and light, *Cancer Res* (1987) **47**:971–4.

58. Nahabedian MY, Cohen RA, Contino MF et al, Combination cytotoxic chemotherapy with cisplatin or doxorubicin and photodynamic therapy in murine tumors, *JNCI* (1988) **810**:739–43.

59. Wooten RS, Smith KC, Ahlquist DA et al, Prospective study of cutaneous phototoxicity after systemic hematoporphyrin derivative, *Lasers Surg Med* (1988) **8**:294–300.

60. Mew D, Wat C, Towers N et al, Photoimmunotherapy: treatment of animal tumors with tumor specific monoclonal-antibody-hematoporphyrin conjugates, *J Immunol* (1983) **130**:1473–7.

61. McCullough JL, Weinstein GD, Lemus LL et al, Development of a topical hematoporphyrin derivative formulation: characterization of photosensitizing effects in vivo, *J Invest Dermatol* (1983) **81**:528–32.

Chapter 37

THE Q-SWITCHED RUBY AND Nd:YAG LASERS

Ronald G. Wheeland

Introduction

The ruby laser was the first functional system, developed in 1960 by Maiman.[1] Goldman, a dermatologist, began using the ruby laser in the treatment of a variety of different cutaneous conditions soon after its original development.[2,3] Nearly 30 years passed before this laser system received formal United States Food and Drug Administration (FDA) approval for the treatment of decorative tattoos. Dermatologic surgeons have long had a number of techniques available for removing decorative tattoos, including: salabrasion,[4] dermabrasion,[5] split-thickness tangential excision,[6] chemical scarification,[7] cryosurgery,[8] excisional surgery,[9] infrared coagulation,[10] and ablation using the argon[11] or carbon dioxide lasers.[12,13]

None of these techniques was considered to be ideal because they could not ensure complete pigment removal in one step without also producing permanent scars, textural changes, and irregularities in pigmentation. Additionally, with many of the older techniques there was also a need for significant postoperative wound care. Commonly, an extended period of time, up to 18 months in some cases, was required before the final cosmetic result was achieved. As a result, new techniques were constantly being sought for the more effective removal of tattoos. A rekindled interest in the Q-switched ruby laser was stimulated by a 1983 British publication,[14] which convincingly showed that this form of therapy offered significant advantages over the existing treatments for managing patients with tattoos. Since then, the Q-switched ruby laser treatment has become an established and accepted form of therapy for many tattoos.[15,16,17]

The increased availability of the ruby laser for the treatment of tattoos has also resulted in numerous studies being performed to determine the suitability of this laser system as a primary form of treatment for pigmentary conditions.[18–21] In addition, another laser system which employs the same Q-switching mechanism as the ruby laser, the neodymium:yttrium-aluminum-garnet (Nd:YAG) laser, has also recently received FDA approval for the treatment of tattoos after both basic and clinical studies demonstrated significant usefulness.[22,23] This new laser system is also under current investigation as a possible form of treatment for benign pigmented lesions.

The Ruby Laser

Treatment of tattoos

The most important benefit offered by the ruby laser in the treatment of tattoos is its ability to treat the exogenous pigments without causing scarring or permanent changes in texture. This appears to be possible because the high-intensity red light, with a wavelength of 694 nm, which is produced by the ruby laser is selectively absorbed by the blue and black colored carbon particles found in amateur and professional tattoos. In addition, the energy from this laser system is emitted in extremely short pulses of only 20–40 ns, which limits the injury to only the pigmented tissues without damaging the surrounding normal skin. This concept, known as selective photothermolysis,[24] was originally used to develop effective instrumentation for the treatment of portwine stains in infants and young children without scarring using another laser system, the pulsed dye laser.[25,26] Thermal damage is so restricted with the ruby laser treatment of tattoos that only limited injury occurs at the skin surface, resulting in minimal postoperative wound care and rapid healing.

Unfortunately, this technique does have some limitations. Presumably because of differences in the size of the pigment particles and variable energy absorption by the many metals and organic compounds that are used to produce different colors of tattoos, all patients do not respond uniformly to ruby laser therapy. In general, blue and black tattoo pigments have been found to respond best to treatment with the ruby laser. Yellow, green and red pigments will also fade with multiple treatments, which are usually performed at 5–6-week intervals. In addition, more treatments are typically required to remove professional (Figure 37.1) than amateur tattoos. However, even given these generalizations an accurate prediction cannot be made as to the ultimate response or the actual number of treatments that will be required for any given patient. While this procedure is performed in an outpatient setting, local anesthesia is required in approximately 50% of patients, especially if the tattoos are located on sensitive areas like the breast, face or fingers. Despite these limitations, the benefits resulting from rediscovery of this technique are substantial and make it a viable consideration for patients with large tattoos, those with tattoos located in anatomical locations that normally heal poorly, and those individuals who are seeking the ultimate cosmetic result, removal without scarring (Figure 37.2).

Mechanism of action

The 694-nm red light produced by the ruby laser can penetrate further into soft tissue than the shorter wavelengths.[27] Furthermore, there is little absorptive interference caused either by oxyhemoglobin or melanin since neither of these chromophores absorb this wavelength of light very well. Another effect that is seen with the ruby laser pulse is attributed to its thermoacoustic properties.[28–30] It has been shown that mechanical forces are generated in soft tissue by the high-energy pulses produced by the ruby laser. These photoacoustic waves act to fragment the pigment granules[31–33] by a process known as cavitation.

Prior to treatment, the average size of the tattoo pigment clusters range from 147 to 180 μm, but after treatment with the 40-ns pulse, these clusters become superheated to 300°C, causing fragmentation into much smaller particles. Multiple effects result from this action. Some of the smaller pigment clusters are taken up by phagocytic cells and removed from the skin via the lymphatics. Some of the pigment is lost through the epidermis in a process of transepidermal elimination. Finally, some of the pigment is redistributed within the dermis where it is no longer clinically identifiable.

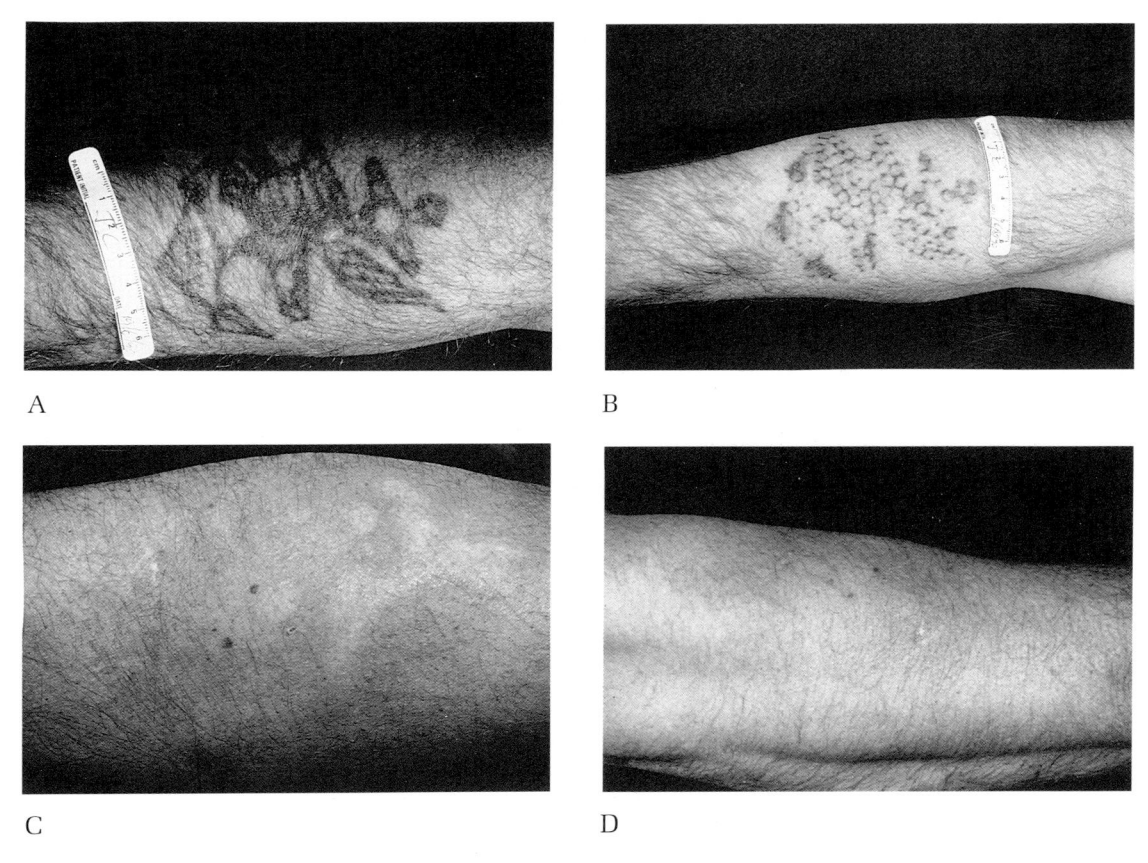

Figure 37.1
(A) Preoperative appearance of a professional tattoo on the forearm. (B) Four months after initiating treatment with the ruby laser, the tattoo pigment has begun to break up. (C) Slight hypopigmentation remains after complete removal of the tattoo pigment. (D) Normal skin color has returned by 12 months after initiating ruby laser treatment. (Courtesy of Dr Adrianna Scheibner.)

Treatment techniques

Initial testing of representative portions and colors of the tattoo at different energy fluences (EF) is recommended in order to determine the most ideal laser parameters. The initial test dose is typically performed without local anesthesia, if possible, beginning at 2 or 3 J/cm² and increasing by a dose of 0.5 J/cm² until an immediate uniform whitening of the skin surface develops.[17] Although initially a source of some debate, the white color that forms on the skin surface, always greater in the tattooed areas than in the surrounding normal skin, appears to be the result of steam generated within the dermis by the photoacoustic wave. It is evanescent in nature, lasting only 20 min in most cases, and is replaced by redness and swelling at higher EFs. Different authors have reported effective EFs for tattoo treatment using the ruby laser ranging from 2 to 10 J/cm², with the optimal fluences most often being between 4 and 8 J/cm².[16]

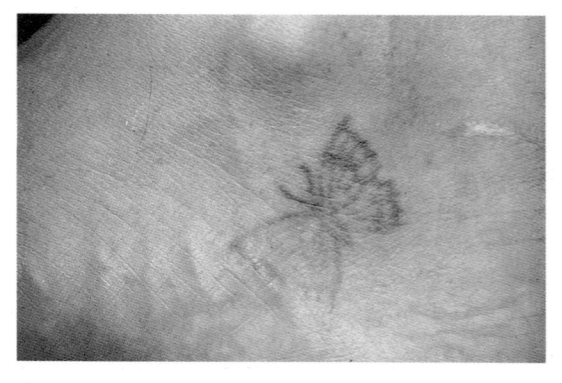

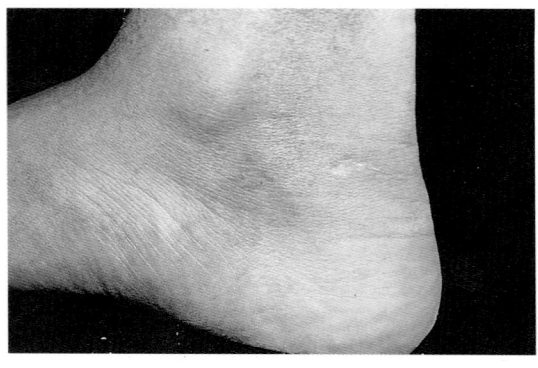

Figure 37.2
(A) Preoperative appearance of a blue–black tattoo. (B) Complete removal of the pigment has been accomplished with the ruby laser without scarring or textural changes 18 months later.

overlapping pulses of approximately 10–20% are delivered to the tattoo so that a uniform whitening response is obtained over the entire surface of the tattoo. When tattoos in hair-bearing areas are treated, a strong malodor will result on impact of the ruby laser pulse unless the hair is removed. If the immediate response causes significant discomfort, topical application of 100% aloe vera gel and ice will help to lessen the postoperative pain, which normally feels like a sunburn for 30–60 min. While bleeding and exudation do not occur, petechiae are commonly seen at higher EFs, and minor vesiculation is typically replaced by superficial crusting within several days following treatment. Usually only minimal postoperative wound care is required and the treated areas are often healed completely within 10–14 days. Residual erythema and transient postinflammatory hypopigmentation may persist for varying periods of time. Tattoo fading typically requires 4–6 weeks in most cases. For that reason, most laser surgeons will delay retreatment for several months.

Results

Even though it is impossible to accurately anticipate the response of tattoos to ruby laser treatment, several rough generalizations can be made. First, amateur tattoos respond better to treatment than professional tattoos and require lower EFs and fewer retreatments to obtain similar degrees of lightening. The average number of treatments for amateur tattoos is typically four to six, while six or more treatments may be required for professional tattoos. Second, professional tattoos with green, yellow and red pigments respond less well than either professional or amateur tattoos composed only of blue or black pigments. While this is generally true, multiple treatments can provide satisfactory lightening of even these colors of tattoos. Third, professional tattoos

Unfortunately, the optimal laser parameters for each patient cannot be determined immediately following testing, since it may take several weeks for the tattoo to fade. However, treatment can begin as soon as lightening has been noted, as long as textural and pigmentary changes or scarring have not resulted from treatment. Treatment is most commonly performed under local anesthesia consisting of intradermal injection of 1% lidocaine with epinephrine. Slightly present for more than 10 years can be expected to respond more favorably than tattoos which have only recently been applied. Fourth, the natural color of the patient's skin influences the outcome of ruby laser treatment of tattoos. Immediate whitening following laser impacts occurs at lower EFs in individuals with dark complexions and results in less fading of the tattoos. Fifth, temporary hypopigmentation can be expected to last 2–6 months in most cases, but permanent textural changes or scarring does not occur with treatment at lower EFs.

The biggest advantage of the ruby laser technique for the treatment of tattoos relates to its ability to remove many tattoos without producing a visible scar. In addition, wound healing is rapid since only minimal postoperative care is required. However, the main disadvantage of this technique is that multiple treatments are virtually always necessary to obtain a satisfactory degree of lightening and the number cannot be accurately determined in advance. Also, the yellow, green and red pigments found in some professional tattoos are exceedingly resistant to treatment and in some cases may not fade completely. However, despite these facts, the ruby laser does appear to be an acceptable method to treat many tattoos.

Treatment of benign pigmented lesions

Shortly after the ruby laser was developed it was used to treat a variety of pigmented lesions of the skin,[2,3] and this clinical research has continued today.[18,21]

Mechanism of action

The ruby laser technique is successful for the treatment of benign pigmentation because the endogenous chromophore, melanin, has a rather broad absorption spectrum from the ultraviolet through visible wavelengths out to the near-infrared regions of the electromagnetic spectrum (EMS). This spectrum is so broad that it overlaps the red emission of the ruby laser.[20] In addition, since light emitted in the 400–600-nm portion of the EMS is strongly absorbed by hemoglobin, vascular damage may predominate. However, at the ruby output of 694 nm, oxyhemoglobin has minimal absorption so the effects will be largely confined to melanin-containing cells of the epidermis and upper dermis.[20]

Melanin is found in relatively large amounts in the melanosomes of many pigmented lesions. This pigment could be effectively targeted for selective photothermolysis[19,34,35] by choosing the ruby laser, whose pulse characteristic of 20–40 ns closely matches the thermal relaxation times for melanosomes (50–100 ns) and is shorter than that for melanocytes (1000 ns). When heavily melanized melanosomes have been exposed to these short pulses, photodisruption has been identified microscopically in both pigmented lesions[36] and normal skin.[37]

Treatment techniques

The ruby laser has been reported to be an effective form of treatment in the management of lentigines, ephelides, cafe au lait spots, Becker's nevus, melasma, nevus of Ota and Peutz–Jegher's spots.[36] The treatment technique is very similar to that used in the treatment of tattoos except that the test pulses are usually delivered over a wider range of EFs, beginning at 4.0 J/cm², with tests also performed at 6.5 J/cm² and 9.0 J/cm². In addition, the small size of many pigmented lesions does not require an overlapping pulse technique in order to effectively treat the entire lesion (Figure 37.3). However, when larger areas of uniform pigmentation are being treated, like a cafe au lait spot, 10–20% overlapping pulses should be used to ensure a uniform response.

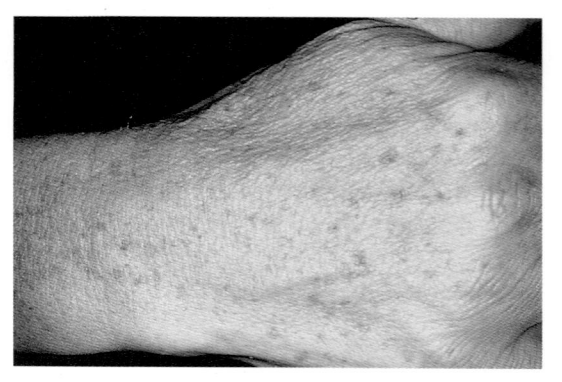

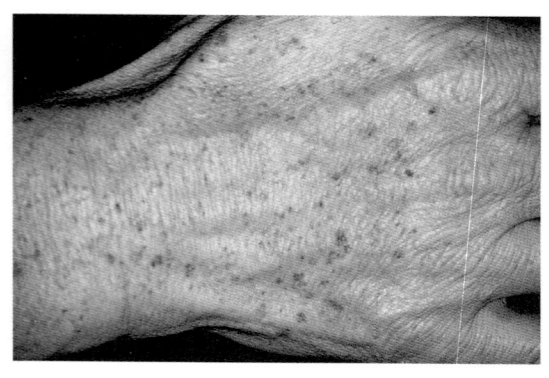

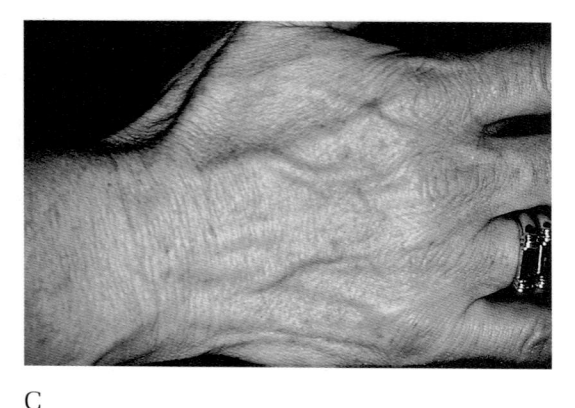

SURGICAL DERMATOLOGY

Figure 37.3
(A) Preoperative appearance of lentigines on the hands. (B) Following treatment with the ruby laser the treated areas darken in color. (C) Complete pigment removal without scarring has been achieved with the ruby laser.

Results

Although very little has been published on the effectiveness of ruby laser treatment of benign pigmentation, it appears from abstracts of presentations made at various scientific meetings that many of these conditions can be effectively managed with this form of treatment. The same quality of results (excellent lightening without scarring, textural or permanent pigmentary changes) described in the treatment of tattoos appears to be true in preliminary reports of treatment for pigmented lesions. Obviously, additional controlled clinical investigation and peer-reviewed publications are necessary before endorsement of this treatment can be given.

THE NEODYMIUM:YTTRIUM-ALUMINUM-GARNET (Nd:YAG) LASER

The Nd:YAG laser is an invisible, near-infrared light source with a wavelength of 1064 nm. Because this wavelength of light is not selectively absorbed by either of the two cutaneous chromophores, melanin or hemoglobin, or by intracellular or extracellular water, like the carbon dioxide laser, it has a deeper penetration of 4–6 mm. This property has limited the usefulness of this laser system in dermatologic conditions largely to the photocoagulation of boggy or proliferative strawberry hemangiomas[38] or nodular portwine stains in older patients[39] using a noncontact delivery technique. Although capable of reducing the volume of these lesions, and sometimes speeding their resolution, this laser system always causes unwanted thermal damage which results in scarring. For that reason, the noncontact mode of operation has only limited usefulness in most cutaneous surgical practices.

A recent development, the synthetic sapphire tip, has greatly expanded the potential dermatologic applications of the Nd:YAG laser. The sapphire tip concentrates the infrared energy to permit incision of the soft tissues with which it is in contact, without signficant thermal damage or bleeding. Hemostasis is provided by the precise delivery of laser energy.[40–42]

The Nd:YAG laser has traditionally been used to photocoagulate blood vessels with relatively low power in either a continuous-discharge mode or as 'long' pulses. However, this laser system can also be Q-switched, like the ruby laser, to produce extremely short pulses (10 ns) of high output power. In this mode of operation, the laser has been investigated for its potential usefulness in treating tattoos in a manner similar to the ruby laser, and pigmented lesions using a frequency-doubled beam of green light at a wavelength of 532 nm.

Treatment of tattoos

Mechanism of action

The same mechanism proposed for the ruby laser is probably operative for the Nd:YAG laser as well. However, because the 1064-nm light produced by this laser system is poorly absorbed by melanin, in contrast to the ruby laser at 694 nm, there is less absorptive interference. Also, this longer wavelength of infrared light can penetrate more deeply into tissue, which may allow it to be more effective in the treatment of some tattoos.

Treatment techniques

The Nd:YAG laser has only recently been approved by the FDA for the treatment of tattoos and only limited published information is currently available.[22,23] From these limited reports, it appears that 10-ns pulses of 1064-nm light at 6–12 J/cm^2 could effectively fade blue, black, red and yellow tattoo pigments, even after previous ruby laser treatments had failed.[23] Treatments are performed at 3–4-week intervals for a total of four treatments.

Results

The best results reported so far occurred at higher EFs and most patients obtained greater than 50% lightening after the first treatment. There was less vesiculation and pain following Nd:YAG laser treatment compared to ruby laser treatment, and no significant side-effects, including pigmentary changes or scarring reported. Treatment with the Nd:YAG laser was better tolerated than the ruby laser and the incidence of hypopigmentation was also reduced over that with the ruby laser.

Treatment of benign pigmentation

If the near-infrared Nd:YAG light with a wavelength of 1064 nm is passed through a special optical crystal, the frequency doubles and the wavelength is halved to 532 nm. The effects on tissue of this Q-switched green light from the frequency-doubled laser are substantially different than the effects produced by the Q-switched infrared light, so the indications for this instrument are different as well.

Mechanism of action

The absorption spectrum of melanin overlaps the green emission from the frequency-doubled Nd:YAG laser. Therefore, this new laser system is an appropriate instrument for the treatment of benign pigmented lesions. Because the pulse duration (10 ns) of this instrument is below

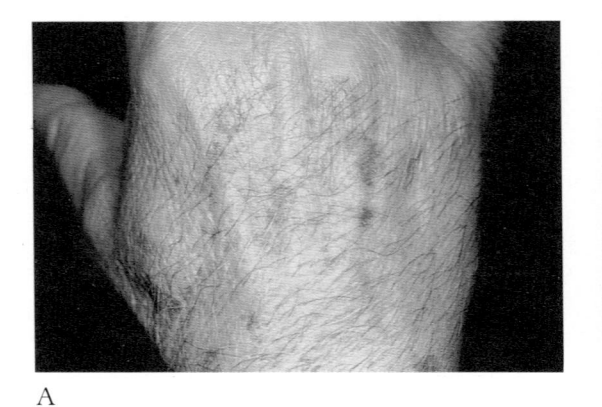

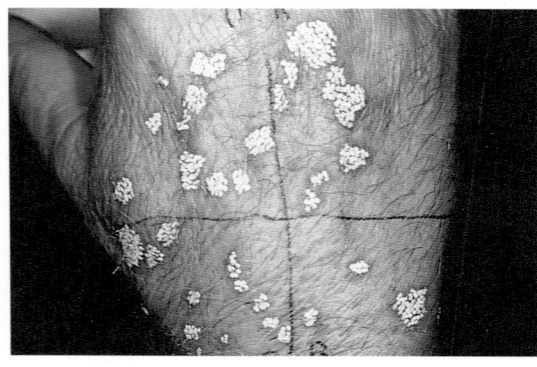

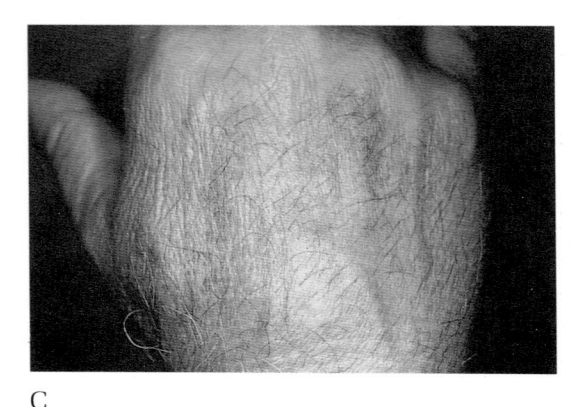

Figure 37.4
(A) Preoperative appearance of lentigines on the hands. (B) Immediate whitening occurs after treatment with the Nd:YAG laser. (C) Three months after a single treatment the pigmentation has cleared completely without scarring or textural change.

the established thermal relaxation times for both melanosomes and melanocytes, selective photothermolysis can be expected to occur.[43]

Treatment techniques

Using no anesthesia, test doses are typically delivered at EFs of 2–5 J/cm^2 using a wavelength of 532 nm, a pulse duration of 10 ns, and a spot size of 1.6 mm to representative pigmented lesions, like lentigines, ephelides and cafe au lait spots. Minimal overlapping is required to produce uniform whitening of the skin and the mild discomfort is well tolerated in most cases (Figure 37.4).

Results

Immediately after treatment the skin turns white, presumably due to the same mechanism as with the ruby laser. This discoloration disappears spontaneously in 15–20 min and the treated areas develop small petechiae or purpura. The petechiae gradually fade in 3–4 days, after which the treated lesions often appear darker, even black in some cases, before the superficial crust separates in 1 week. There is no postoperative pain associated with this procedure. After the crusts disappear, the treated sites remain slightly erythematous for 4–6 weeks but then gradually fade. Persistent hypopigmentation has not been a problem and no scars or textural changes have been reported. Using this new system, lentigines, cafe au lait spots, ephelides and other benign pigmented lesions have responded satisfactorily.

REFERENCES

1. Maiman TH, Stimulated optical radiation in ruby, *Nature* (1960) **187**:493–4.
2. Goldman L, Blaney DJ, Kindel DJ et al, Effect of the laser beam on the skin: preliminary report, *J Invest Dermatol* (1963) **40**:121–2.
3. Goldman L, Wilson RG, Hornby P et al, Radiation from a Q-switched ruby laser. Effect of repeated impacts of power output of 10 megawatts on a tattoo of man, *J Invest Dermatol* (1965) **44**:69–71.
4. Koerber WA Jr, Price NM, Salabrasion of tattoos. A correlation of the clinical and histological results, *Arch Dermatol* (1978) **114**:884–8.
5. Clabaugh W, Removal of tattoos by superficial dermabrasion, *Arch Dermatol* (1968) **98**:515–21.
6. Wheeland RG, Norwood OT, Roundtree JM, Tattoo removal using serial tangential excision and polyurethane membrane dressing, *J Dermatol Surg Oncol* (1983) **9**:822–6.
7. Scutt RWB, The chemical removal of tattoos, *Br J Plast Surg* (1972) **25**:189–94.
8. Dvir E, Hirshowitz B, Tattoo removal by cryosurgery, *Plast Reconstr Surg* (1980) **66**:373–8.
9. Bailey BN, Treatment of tattoos, *Plast Reconstr Surg* (1967) **40**:361–71.
10. Groot DW, Arlette JP, Johnston PA, Comparison of the infrared coagulator and the carbon dioxide laser in the removal of decorative tattoos, *J Am Acad Dermatol* (1986) **15**:518–22.
11. Apfelberg DB, Maser MR, Lash H et al, The argon laser for cutaneous lesions, *JAMA* (1981) **245**:2073–5.
12. Bailin PL, Ratz JL, Levine HL, Removal of tattoos by CO_2 laser, *J Dermatol Surg Oncol* (1980) **6**:997–1001.
13. Apfelberg DB, Maser MR, Lash H et al, Comparison of argon and carbon dioxide laser treatment of decorative tattoos: a preliminary report, *Ann Plast Surg* (1985) **14**:6–15.
14. Reid WH, McLeod PJ, Ritchie A et al, Q-switched ruby laser treatment of black tattoos, *Br J Plast Surg* (1983) **36**:455–9.
15. Vance CA, McLeod PJ, Reid WH et al, Q-switched ruby laser treatment of tattoos: a further study, *Lasers Surg Med* (1985) **5**:179.
16. Taylor CR, Gange RW, Dover JS et al, Treatment of tattoos by Q-switched ruby laser, *Arch Dermatol* (1990) **126**:893–9.
17. Scheibner A, Kenny G, White W et al, A superior method of tattoo removal using the Q-switched ruby laser, *J Dermatol Surg Oncol* (1990) **16**:1091–88.
18. Ohshiro T, Maruyama Y, The ruby and argon lasers in the treatment of naevi, *Ann Acad Med Singapore* (1983) **12**:388–95.
19. Polla LL, Margolis RJ, Dover JS et al, Melanosomes are the primary target of Q-switched ruby laser irradiation in guinea pig skin, *J Invest Dermatol* (1986) **89**:281–6.
20. Dover JS, Margolis RJ, Polla LL et al, Pigmented guinea pig skin irradiated with Q-switched ruby laser pulses, *Arch Dermatol* (1989) **125**:43–9.

21. Scheibner A, Removal of tattoos and benign pigmented lesions using the ruby laser, *Lasers Surg Med* (1990) **2S**:51.

22. Anderson RR, Margolis RJ, Watanabe S et al, Selective photothermolysis of cutaneous pigmentation by Q-switched Nd:YAG laser pulses at 1064, 532, and 355 nm, *J Invest Dermatol* (1989) **93**:38–42.

23. Kilmer SL, Lee M, Farinelli W et al, Q-switched Nd:YAG laser (1064 nm) effectively treats Q-switched ruby laser resistant tattoos, *Lasers Surg Med* (1992) **4S**:72.

24. Anderson RR, Parrish JA, Selective photothermolysis: precise microsurgery by selective absorption of pulsed radiation, *Science* (1983) **220**:524–7.

25. Garden JM, Tan OT, Kerschmann R et al, Effect of dye laser pulse duration on selective cutaneous vascular injury, *J Invest Dermatol* (1986) **87**:653–7.

26. Garden JM, Polla LL, Tan OT, The treatment of port-wine stains by the pulsed dye laser, *Arch Dermatol* (1988) **124**:889–96.

27. Anderson RR, Parrish JA, The optics of human skin, *J Invest Dermatol* (1981) **77**:13–19.

28. Carome SF, Hamrick PE, Laser-induced acoustic transients in the mammalian eye, *J Acoust Soc Am* (1969) **46**:1037–44.

29. Sigrist MW, Kneubuhl FK, Laser generated stress waves in liquids, *J Acoust Soc Am* (1978) **64**:1652–63.

30. Mainster MA, Sliney DH, Belcher D et al, Laser photodisruptors. Damage mechanism, instrument design, and safety, *Ophthalmology* (1983) **99**:973–91.

31. Goldman AI, Ham WT Jr, Mueller HA, Mechanisms of retinal damage resulting from the exposure of rhesus monkeys to ultrashort laser pulses, *Exp Eye Res* (1975) **21**:457–69.

32. Boulnois JL, Photophysical processes in recent medical laser developments: a review, *Lasers Med Sci* (1986) **1**:47–66.

33. Watanabe S, Flotte TJ, McAuliffe DJ et al, Putative photoacoustic damage in skin induced by pulsed ArF excimer laser, *J Invest Dermatol* (1988) **90**:761–6.

34. Murphy GF, Shepard RS, Paul BS et al, Organelle-specific injury to melanin-containing cells in human skin by pulsed laser irradiation, *Lab Invest* (1983) **49**:680–5.

35. Goldman L, Igelman JM, Richfield DF, Impact of the laser on nevi and melanomas, *Arch Dermatol* (1964) **90**:71–5.

36. Ohshiro T, Maruyama Y, Makajima H et al, Treatment of pigmentation of the lips and oral mucosa in Peutz–Jeghers syndrome using ruby and argon lasers, *Br J Plast Surg* (1980) **33**:346–9.

37. Hruza GJ, Dover JS, Flotta TJ et al, Q-switched ruby laser irradiation of normal human skin, *Arch Dermatol* (1991) **127**:1799–1805.

38. Achauer B, VanderKam V, Capillary hemangioma (strawberry mark) of infancy: comparison of argon and Nd:YAG laser treatment, *Plast Reconstr Surg* (1989) **84**:60–69.

39. Dixon JA, Gilbertson JJ, Argon and neodymium:YAG laser therapy of dark nodular port-wine stains in older patients, *Lasers Surg Med* (1986) **6**:5–11.

40. Daikuzono N, Joffe SN, Artificial sapphire probe for contact photocoagulation and tissue vaporization with the Nd:YAG laser, *Med Instrument* (1988) **19**:173.

41. Hukki J, Krogerus I, Castran M et al, Effects of different contact laser scalpels on skin and subcutaneous fat, *Lasers Surg Med* (1988) **8**:276.

42. Apfelberg DB, Smith T, Lash H et al, Preliminary report on use of the neodymium:YAG laser in plastic surgery, *Lasers Surg Med* (1987) **7**:189–98.

43. Lanzafame RJ, Naim JO, Blackman JR et al, Initial assessment of the Con-Bio Laser in-vivo, *Lasers Surg Med* (1992) **4S**:69.

Chapter 38

NEODYMIUM YAG LASER

Dudley Hill
Diamondis J. Papadopoulos
Hubert T. Greenway

In 1961 Johnson[1] developed an Yttrium Aluminum Garnet (YAG) crystal, on which he embedded dopant neodymium (Nd) ions and excited this crystal rod-like structure with a high-powered krypton-arc lamp to emit light energy in the near infrared portion of the spectrum. This first Nd:YAG laser was large, heavy and had an average power output of less than 10 W.[2] Over the past 30 years the delivery capabilities of this laser have become more compact and powerful.

Nd:YAG laser light is invisible, however, a visible aiming beam, commonly of helium-neon red light, is used coaxially with the laser beam. The Nd:YAG laser requires water cooling. Protective eyewear must be worn by every person in the laser suite during the instrument's use. The 1064 nm wavelength emitted by the Nd:YAG laser results in much deeper penetration, up to 5–7 mm in the skin, which is nonspecific and is accompanied by considerable scatter resulting in a large volume of coagulated tissue around the treated area. Nd:YAG laser light has the ability to coagulate blood vessels much larger than those vessels coagulated by the CO_2 or Argon lasers.

Most Nd:YAG lasers operate in a continuous mode and typically produce power outputs of approximately 100 W. Maximum power of the continuous wave can be significantly enhanced if the laser is pulsed. Thus, through super-pulsing or Q-switching, power level increases of 5–100 times can be achieved by means of the induction of very high intensity pulses through a shutter in the optical cavity of the laser.

Currently this laser can be transmitted by fiberoptic technology, enabling the operator to use a thin, flexible and comparatively cheap delivery system. The development of synthetic sapphire tips has enabled the Nd:YAG laser to be used as a direct-contact, bloodless cutting device. Small conical tips concentrate the beam for cutting and vaporization while larger round or flat tips diffuse the laser beam's distribution for greater hemostatic effect.[3]

INDICATIONS AND USES OF THE Nd:YAG LASER IN DERMATOLOGY

The Nd:YAG laser has been used to stop intestinal bleeding, for palliative treatment of obstructive gastrointestinal[4] and endobronchial[5] carcinoma, in gynecologic laparoscopic procedures,[6] as well as in ophthalmology, urology and neurosurgery. Its use in dermatology and plastic surgery has lagged behind the use of the argon, CO_2, tunable dye, and more recently, the copper-vapor and Q-switched ruby lasers. However, there are circumstances when the use of the Nd:YAG has been advantageous.

Capillary and Cavernous Hemangiomas and AV Malformations

The use of Nd:YAG lasers to treat deeper angiomatous lesions in the skin has received the most attention. A number of reports indicate its advantages in treating thickened or deeper lesions both in the skin and on mucous membranes. Due to the delayed tissue coagulation around the treated areas a polka-dot approach is used, requiring some experience. Pre-freezing the treated area with ice helps to reduce coagulation of the overlying epidermis. Treatment with the beam directed through a glass slide to compress the treated area enhances penetration of the laser beam.

Smaller thick lesions such as cherry angiomas and venous lakes have responded well to Nd:YAG laser treatment. Higher flow AV malformations are also particularly suited to Nd:YAG laser treatment because of its excellent hemostatic properties.

Strawberry hemangiomas of infancy may require treatment if they are rapidly growing, ulcerated, recurrently bleeding or interfere with the development of normal function (for example, eyesight, hearing, eating and drinking). Treatment with the Nd:YAG laser may be particularly useful in conjunction with intralesional or systemic steroids with subsequent appropriate cosmetic surgery to remove redundant skin.[7]

Because the Nd:YAG laser coagulates more deeply there is a significant risk of permanent postoperative scarring. Following Nd:YAG laser treatment of deeper cavernous angiomas of mucous membranes, however, the mucous membranes heal with minimal or no scarring even when deep lesions are treated. Combination therapy for deeper hemangiomas using the cutting mode to excise and the coagulating mode to treat residual areas may be a significant advantage.[8]

Keloid scars

In 1984, Abergel et al,[9] reported that the Nd:YAG laser could selectively inhibit collagen deposition in experimental situations, both in vivo and in vitro. They hypothesized that the Nd:YAG laser might therefore provide a new modality for the treatment of keloids. They subsequently treated eight patients with extensive treatment-resistant keloids using skin blanching as an end-point on 1-cm squared, non-overlapping areas with 70 W power. Their report included details of one patient, but they suggested that considerable flattening, softening and reduction in size was progressively noted during twelve treatments at 1–2 week intervals, with similar results in the other seven patients. No recurrence of the keloid was observed over 3 years in the treated area.[10]

Another report by Sherman and Rosenfeld[11] detailed treatment with a Nd:YAG laser of 17 keloids, using 1–4 treatments with between 20 and 70 W. They reported significant resolution in eight patients, but concluded that further study was required before such treatment was of proven value.[11]

Apfelberg et al,[8] reported a series of 12 patients with keloids treated with a Nd:YAG laser. They noted initial shrinkage, prolonged healing time (average 43 days) and recurrence within 3–4 months.

In this report, adjunctive use of intralesional and topical steroids improved the long-term response, although only five of 22 treated keloids were said to have had good results from the treatment.

Condyloma

Although the CO_2 laser has been at the forefront of laser treatment of condylomata there have been reports that the Nd:YAG laser is effective as well. In 1980, Hofstetter and Frank[12] reported the treatment of 30 patients with the Nd:YAG laser with only two exhibiting recurrences in the near term. In 1985, Stein[13] reported 40 patients treated by Nd:YAG laser with only one showing recurrence in a laser-treated area, although several showed recurrences in non-laser treated areas at approximately one year. More recently, Graversen et al[14] reported treating 56 consecutive men with recurrent condylomata either with a CO_2 laser or a Nd:YAG laser or both. Half their patients responded completely to a single treatment and 86% to a maximum of three treatments with no important side-effects encountered and with excellent cosmetic results.

It can be concluded, therefore, that condyloma is the main indication for the Nd:YAG laser. There are two major advantages: first, the use of sapphire tips allow better control; second, less vaporization occurs and thus there is less risk of viral dispersion in the operating suite. One problem encountered is the necessity to keep the Nd:YAG laser in a single operating area as otherwise mechanical problems with alignment of the laser beam may occur.

Clearly, greater investigation is required to better understand the effects of treatment of condylomata by the Nd:YAG laser and, in particular, the coupling of this laser system with other therapeutic modalities (i.e., interferon, the CO_2 laser, etc.) for the eradication of larger bulkier lesions.

Malignant and Premalignant Skin Tumors

The Nd:YAG laser may be used to vaporize or coagulate skin tumors or as a cutting instrument to excise tumors. When used as a scalpel, the Nd:YAG laser has the advantage of excellent hemostasis with smaller diameter, finer, sapphire tips producing less tissue thermal injury.[15]

Brunner et al,[16] reported a series of cutaneous tumors in 90 patients treated by Nd:YAG laser. Lesions treated included basal cell carcinoma, squamous cell carcinoma, Bowen's disease, breast and melanoma skin metastases, genital leukoplakia and bowenoid papulosis. Apfelberg et al advised that treatment of such tumors with the Nd:YAG laser should be approached cautiously in areas of thin skin.[17] They also felt that Nd:YAG laser therapy was particularly indicated in the treatment of multiple tumors (for example, in basal cell nevus syndrome), in older patients presenting operative risks, and those with a hemorrhagic tendency. They stressed the advantages of precise and non-contact surgery, performance under local anesthesia on an outpatient basis, and low risk of bleeding and infection.

References

1. Johnson LF, Optical laser characteristics of rare earth ions in crystals, *J Appl Physiol* (1961) **34**:897–909.
2. Fuller TA, *Surgical lasers, a clinic guide* (MacMillan Publishing Co: New York 1987) 10–11.
3. Apfelberg DB, *Evaluation and installation of surgical laser systems* (Springer-Verlag: New York 1987) 223–4.
4. Krasner N, Palliative laser therapy for

tumours of the gastrointestinal tract, *Boilliers Clinical Gastroenterology* (1991) **5**:37–59.
5. Hetzel MR, Smith SG, Endoscopic palliation of tracheobronchial malignancies, *Thorax* (1991) **46**:325–33.
6. Corson SL, Use of the YAG laser in laparoscopic gynecologic procedures, *Obstet Gynecol Clin North Am* (1991) **18**:619–36.
7. Apfelberg DB, *Atlas of cutaneous laser surgery* (Raven Press: New York 1992) 291–341.
8. Apfelberg DB, Smith T, Study of the benefites of the Nd:YAG laser in plastic surgery. In: Ogura Y, Joffee S, eds, *Advances in Nd:YAG laser surgery* (Springer-Verlag: New York 1988) 213–26.
9. Abergel RP, Meeker CA, Lam TS et al, Control of connective tissue metabolism by lasers: recent developments and future prospects, *J Am Acad Dermatol* (1984) **11**:1142–50.
10. Abergel RP, Lam TS, Lask G et al, Biological effects of lasers, *Invest Clin Laser* (1986) **3**:7–14.
11. Sherman R, Rosenfeld H, Experience with the Nd:YAG laser in the treatment of keloid scars, *Ann Plast Surg* (1988) **21**:231–6.
12. Hofstetter A, Frank F, *The neodymium: YAG laser in urology* (Editiones 'Roche': F Hoffman-LaRoche and Co., Ltd, Basel, Switzerland 1980).
13. Stein BS, Laser treatment of condylomata acuminata. Presented at the *Sixth Congress of the International Society of Laser Surgery and Medicine*, Jerusalem (1985).
14. Graversen PH, Bagi P, Rosenkilde P, Laser treatment of recurrent urethral condylomata in men, *Scand J Urol Nephrol* (1990) **224**:163–6.
15. Hukki T, Krogerus L, Castren M et al, Effects of different contact laser scalpels on skin and subcutaneous fat, *Lasers Surg Med* (1988) **8**:276–82.
16. Brunner R, Landthaler M, Haina D et al, Treatment of benign, semimalignant and malignant skin tumors with the Nd:YAG laser, *Laser Surg Med* (1985) **15**:105–111.
17. Apfelberg DB, Smith T, Lash H et al, Preliminary report on use of the neodymium-YAG laser in plastic surgery, *Laser Surg Med* (1987) **7**:189–98.

Section IV

RECONSTRUCTIVE SURGERY

39. RETINOIDS, DERMABRASION, CHEMICAL PEEL AND KELOIDS
    Kevin S. Pinski, Henry H. Roenigk Jr

40. DERMABRASION FOR SCAR REVISION
    Bruce E. Katz

41. CULTURED EPIDERMAL GRAFTS
    Youn H. Kim, David T. Woodley

42. ADVANCES IN FLAPS AND GRAFTS IN DERMATOLOGIC SURGERY
    Eckart Haneke

Chapter 39

RETINOIDS, DERMABRASION, CHEMICAL PEEL AND KELOIDS

Kevin S. Pinski
Henry H. Roenigk Jr

INTRODUCTION

The therapeutic use of retinoids, especially isotretinoin, is becoming more frequent in dermatology. The effectiveness of isotretinoin has been documented in treating cystic acne, acne rosacea, psoriasis and a variety of disorders of keratinization, such as Darier's disease and pityriasis rubra pilaris.

The side-effects observed with retinoids are well tolerated, are not life-threatening and are dose dependent in incidence and severity. The major symptoms are those of mucocutaneous drying and chapping. Systemic toxicities which have been observed include: transient minor elevations in liver function tests, hyperlipidemia, arthralgias/ myalgias, photosensitivity, and teratogenicity. In addition, patients treated with retinoids may develop calcification of bones and ligaments. Lastly, postoperative wound healing has been reported to be impaired by retinoids.

KELOIDS

The actual cause of keloid formation is uncertain. They may form as a result of breakdown in the synthetic or degradation phase of collagen metabolism. Keloids are more cellular than normal dermis with increased DNA content, increased synthesis of glycoproteins and increased proteoglycan content.[1] Collagen synthesis has also been found to be increased in keloidal tissues; however, it differs from normal collagen. On electron microscopy the organization of the collagen bundles was less discrete in keloids and the fibers were randomly oriented rather than closely packed parallel rows of normal collagen.[2]

The fibrous tissue accumulation in keloids may also result from altered degradation. Although collagenase, the enzyme which initiates collagen degradation in tissue, has been found to have either normal or increased activity in keloid tissue cultures.[3] Collagenase is inhibited by naturally occurring antagonists in serum, including alpha-2-macroglobulin and alpha-1-antitrypsin. Immunofluorescence studies have revealed accumulation of these substances in keloids.[4] It has also been postulated that keloidal tissue may be protected from collagenase degradation by proteoglycans, which are found in excess in such tissues.[5]

Retinoids affect the metabolism of connective tissue in a variety of ways. Although in vitro studies have demonstrated that isotretinoin is a selective inhibitor of procollagen production in fibroblast cultures,[6] it also has been found to inhibit the expression of collagenase.[7] The retinoids have been shown to increase mucopolysaccharides and collagen synthesis[8-10] and to decrease collagenase production.[11,12] Fibronectin synthesis, important in early granulation tissue formation and epidermal migration, can be increased up to three-fold by retinoids.[13] In addition, retinoids may stimulate fibroblasts by increasing the number of available receptor sites for epidermal growth factor.[14] Retinoids may also stimulate epidermal migration,[15] possibly by decreasing the number of tonofilaments and epidermal desmosomal attachments, events known to precede epidermal migration.[16] Tretinoin has also been shown to increase epidermal mitotic activity.[17,18]

There have been numerous reports showing that topical retinoids, particularly topical tretinoin, can enhance wound healing.[19-24] Hung et al[22] studied the effects of topical tretinoin on epithelial wound healing using a porcine model. They applied tretinoin cream, 0.05% daily for 10 days, prior to partial-thickness skin wounding. Daily tretinoin treatment was continued after wounding on two of eight animals. Pretreatment with topical tretinoin accelerated epithelial wound healing, whereas continued tretinoin applications retarded epithelialization. In an open study in humans, Mandy[24] found that pretreatment with tretinoin cream 0.05% for 2 weeks prior to dermabrasion enhanced healing and reduced milia formation. Similarly, Hevia et al[25] concluded that tretinoin cream 0.05% pretreatment for 2 weeks prior to trichloroacetic acid peeling significantly accelerated healing. It has been hypothesized that these beneficial effects of topical tretinoin pretreatment may be due to its ability to stimulate epithelial proliferation and decrease cell transit time.[26] In addition, pretreatment with tretinoin cream involves inflammatory changes and vascular dilatation, both of which are components of normal early wound healing.[22]

There have also been case reports failing to disclose any problems in wound healing or keloid formation among patients taking isotretinoin at the time of and within 6 months of surgery.[27-29] Moy et al[29] examined the effects of systemic isotretinoin on dermal wound healing in a rabbit ear model. They determined that there was no effect on collagen synthesis, as determined by mRNA level measurements between control rabbits and those treated with 4 mg/kg per day of isotretinoin.

In contrast, in a review of the adverse effects of isotretinoin therapy, Bruno et al[30] noted delayed wound healing in two patients being treated with isotretinoin for cystic acne. Various dermatologic surgeons have also reported impaired wound healing and keloid formation in surgical patients attributed to treatment with systemic isotretinoin (Alt TH, Hanke CW, Annual Meeting of the American Academy of Dermatology 1989; Katz B, Annual Meeting of the American Society for Dermatologic Surgery 1990; Pinski JB, personal communication; Boughton RS, personal communication).[31-34]

Dermabrasion and Isotretinoin

With the increase in reliable methods for controlling severe acne, including isotretinoin, one might predict a decline in the need for dermabrasion for acne scars. Nevertheless, dermabrasion is as popular as it was before these developments. However, the increased use of isotretinoin has led to new problems for dermatologic surgeons.

In 1985, Roenigk et al[27] reported on nine patients who underwent dermabrasion while they were on or shortly after discontinuing isotretinoin therapy for acne. No abnormalities in wound healing were noted. In an addendum to that paper Roenigk indicated that he had seen two cases of keloids following dermabrasion while the patients were taking isotretinoin. One year later, members from the same group published a paper describing six patients who developed keloids in atypical sites 1–4 months postdermabrasion.[31] Three of these patients were on isotretinoin at the time of surgery and the remaining three had discontinued isotretinoin 2–6 months prior to dermabrasion (see Table 39.1). All of these patients had normal postoperative healing until 2–6 months later, at which time they spontaneously began to develop hypertrophic and keloidal scarring (Figures 39.1, 39.2 and 39.3). These were not preceded by persistent erythema, which is often the first sign of evolving hypertrophic scars. This change often becomes apparent 3–4 weeks after dermabrasion, when the remaining treated areas are beginning to lighten in color. In addition, many of these atypical keloids developed on the central face, an area rarely subject to scarring after dermabrasion. The authors then suggested that dermabrasion be delayed for at least 6

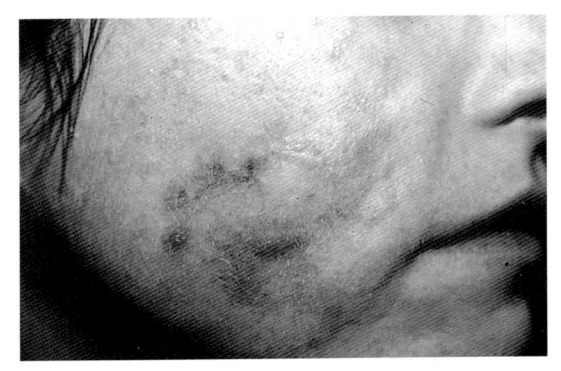

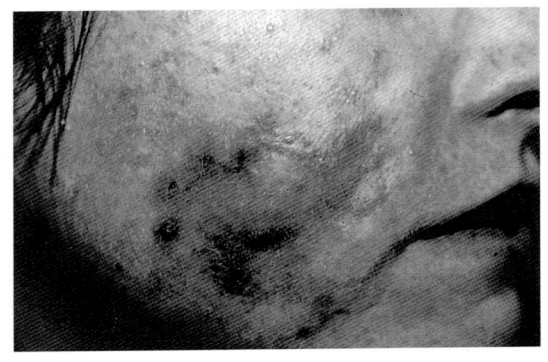

Figure 39.1
(A) Atypical early erythema and keloids 2 months after dermabrasion in patient recently on accutane. (B) Four and a half months after dermabrasion and atyical keloids worse.

Table 39.1
Development of keloidal scarring in patients treated with isotretinoin

Case	Age	Sex	Isotretinoin dose (mg/kg per day)	Total duration isotretinoin therapy (months)	Isotretinoin during dermabrasion (prior)	Time to keloid formation postdermabrasion (months)	Site of keloid	Status
1	32	F	1.0	8	Yes	3	Forehead Cheek	Resolution
2	32	M	0.5	14	Yes	2	Chin Cheek	Resolution
3	30	M	0.5	4	Yes	1	Cheeks	Partial resolution
4	48	F	0.5	4	No (2½ months)	2	Central cheeks	Partial resolution
5	28	M	1.0	5	No (3 months)	2½	Lower cheeks	Partial resolution
6	27	F	1.0	8	No (6 months)	4	Cheeks	Partial resolution

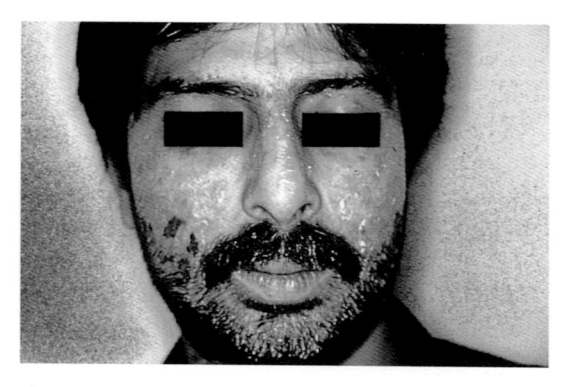

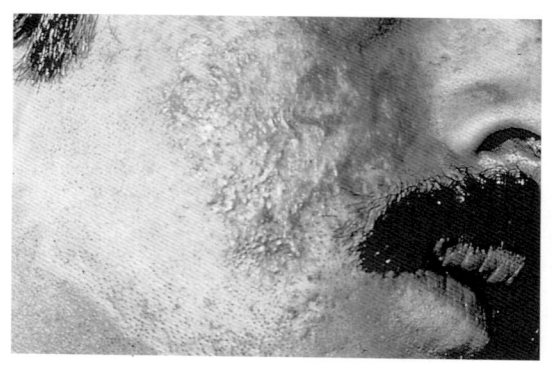

Figure 39.2
(A) Atypical and persistent erythema of cheeks in a patient 2½ months after dermabrasion. (B) Same patient 1 month later with keloidal scarring on cheeks.

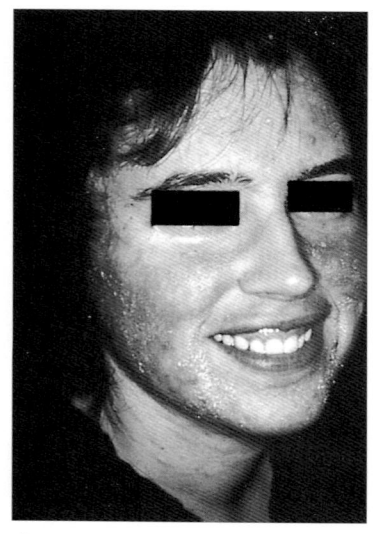

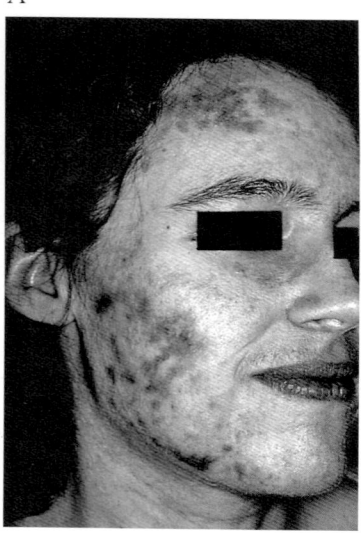

Figure 39.3
(A) Postoperative 2 weeks from dermabrasion in patient who had just completed a 6-month course of accutane. Skin healing normal with erythema. (B) Same patient 6 months later with atypical keloids on cheeks and forehead.

months after retinoid therapy has been discontinued.

In 1988, Zachariae reported on the observation of delayed wound healing and keloid formation in three patients, following dermabrasion or argon laser treatment which was administered while they were receiving isotretinoin for severe acne.[32] It is interesting that two of the patients in this report had similar previous procedures performed while not on isotretinoin without any wound-healing abnormalities. However, while on isotrenitoin repeat procedures resulted in keloid formation. These patients to a certain extent acted as their own controls. Zachariae also recommended that skin surgery in retinoid-treated patients be postponed until after discontinuation of isotretinoin therapy and after the activity of retinoids has had time to subside.

Over the past 3–4 years several other reports have surfaced of atypical scarring in patients dermabraded as long as 38 months after stopping isotretinoin.[35] Unexpected central cheek scars have been reported in a patient who underwent dermabrasion 23 months after discontinuation of isotretinoin. This patient is of particular interest because he had a normal skin biopsy and a normal spot dermabrasion 2 months before the full-face procedure.[33] Several cases of scarring have also been reported on patients who have begun isotretinoin therapy within several months after dermabrasion.[33]

Most recently, Pinski et al[36] published a retrospective analysis of 70 dermabrasion cases. Thirteen of these procedures involved patients who had previously been treated with isotretinoin for cystic acne (see Table 39.2). However, dermabrasion was delayed in all at least 5–6 months (average 12 months) after the cessation of isotretinoin. Of the 13 cases, all exhibited normal postoperative wound healing and were without keloid formation. Three of the remaining 57 patients who had not been treated with isotretinoin did form keloidal scars. However, two of these cases involved deep dermabrasion of the upper extremities for tattoo removal, which often results in keloids. The third procedure was for acne scars overlying the angle of the jaw where hypertrophic scarring also occurs more frequently. This study therefore seems to lend further credence to the previous recommendations of Rubenstein et al[31] and Zachariae[32] to delay dermabrasion for 6 months to 1 year after isotretinoin therapy.

The authors currently wait at least 1 year after discontinuation of isotretinoin therapy before performing dermabrasion.

Table 39.2
Results of dermabrasion in patients previously treated with isotretinoin for cystic acne

Patient	Age	Sex	Isotretinoin dose (mg/kg per day)	Total duration of therapy (months)	Isotretinoin during dermabrasion (prior)	Site of dermabrasion	Lesion dermabraded
1	20 21 21 22	F	0.75	2	No (12 months) No (21 months) No (29 months) No (35 months)	Cheeks Cheeks Cheeks Cheeks	Cystic acne scars
2	17	F	1.0	4	No (13 months)	Full face	Acne vulgaris scars
3	34 34 36	F	1.0	6	No (12 months) No (15 months) No (40 months)	Full face Right cheek, chin Cheeks, chin	Cystic acne scars
4	37	F	1.0	5	No (5 months)	Full face	Acne scarring
5	19	M	1.0	4½	No (5 months)	Full face	Acne scarring
6	31	F	1.0	5	No (12 months)	Full face	acne scarring
7	27	F	1.0	5	No (8 months)	Full face	Acne scarring
8	45	F	0.8	4	No (33 months)	Full face	Acne scarring

Over the past 2–3 years, since using this as a cutoff, we have not seen any new cases of atypical scarring. We also wait at least 6 months after a dermabrasion before initiating isotretinoin therapy. Even longer intervals are preferred if possible. It is important to discuss the potential for scarring with each patient who is a candidate for both dermabrasion and isotretinoin therapy. Some dermatologists now recommend a 2-year delay and a biopsy.[37]

CHEMICAL PEELS AND ISOTRETINOIN

In addition to retinoids causing scarring problems with dermabrasion, there are six cases of hypertrophic scarring associated with isotretinoin and chemical peels that have been reported to date (Pinski K, Annual Meeting of the American Academy of Dermatology 1991). The first two patients each received 50% trichloroacetic acid peels for acne scarring (Boughton RS, personal communication). These procedures were performed 4 months and 7 months, respectively, after completion of a course of isotretinoin 40 mg daily. Both were very slow to re-epithelialize, taking approximately 1 month. Persistent erythema then developed, which later evolved into hypertrophic scarring. Both improved with topical corticosteroids. The third patient underwent a phenol peel approximately 3 years after completing the course of isotretinoin (Pinski JB, personal communication). She developed some hypertrophic scarring of her upper lip at a site of persistent erythema. However, 8 months later she spontaneously developed keloidal scarring of her left cheek without preceding erythema or lesions in this area. This has subsequently improved with intralesional injections of cortisone.

The next two patients had chemical peels performed while they were still on isotretinoin. Both resulted in spontaneous

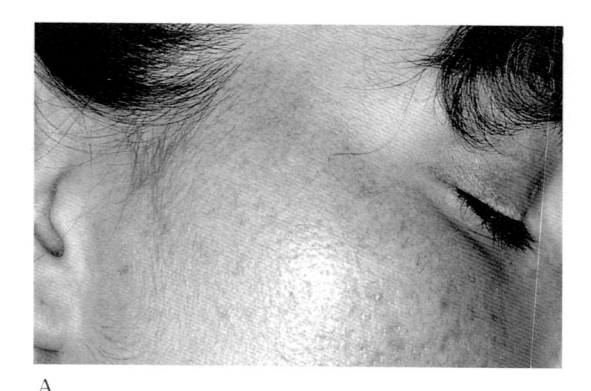

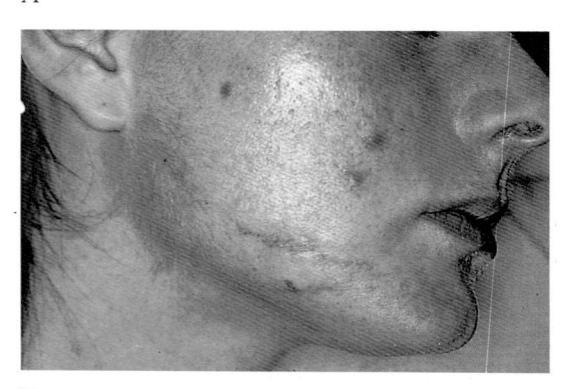

Figure 39.4
(A) Normal healing after spot dermabrasion of left temple, performed 6 months after stopping accutane. (B) Same patient after 25% TCA peel performed while on accutane 10 mg daily.

scarring after uncomplicated healing. Case 4 was a 50% trichloroacetic acid peel while on isotretinoin 40 mg daily for 2 months (Boughton RS, personal communication). Case 5 was initially on isotretinoin for severe cystic acne (Roenigk HH, personal communication). Six months after stopping treatment she received a spot dermabrasion without any problems in postoperative wound healing. Her acne began to flare again 4 months later and she was restarted on isotretinoin 10 mg daily. While on this regimen she had a 25% trichloroacetic acid peel which resulted in atypical scarring (Figure 39.4). One year

dioxide immediately followed by 35% trichloroacetic acid.[34] She healed without complication, but spontaneously scarred when begun on a 4-month course of isotretinoin 3 months after re-epithelialization (Figure 39.5).

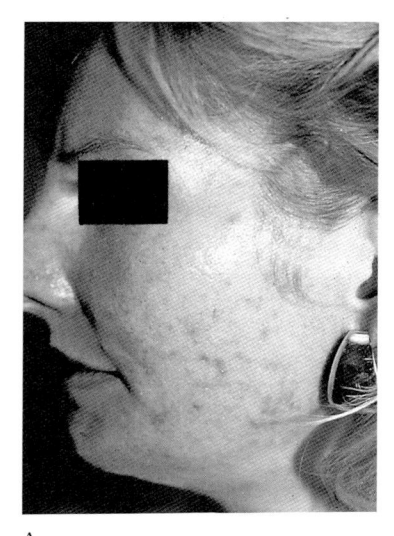

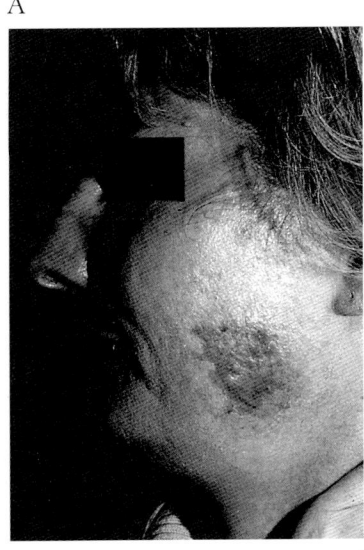

These cases suggest that the use of isotretinoin before, during or even after a chemical peel may be a factor in hypertrophic scar formation. This abnormal scarring may occur because isotretinoin shrinks the adnexal structures from which the epidermis is reconstructed. If they are not ready to produce a normal epidermis, or if the balance of collagen and collagenase is disturbed, then atypical keloid scar formation may result.

CONCLUSION

Scarring after peeling or dermabrasion occurs as a result of many factors such as hereditary predisposition, the time interval between multiple surgical procedures, the depth of wounding, the surgical site, and the possibility of poor postoperative care or resulting infection, and probably exposure to isotretinoin.[38] These procedures are very technique dependent and imprecise. Thus, it is difficult to consistently quantitate the amount of tissue destruction. In addition, since many factors contribute to the final cosmetic outcome it is difficult to directly implicate one single variable such as isotretinoin. At the present time isotretinoin therapy is regarded as a relative contraindication in dermabrasion and chemical peels. However, in time we may find that it is an absolute contraindication.

Figure 39.5
(A) Three months after full-face peel with carbon dioxide and 35% TCA healing normally. (B) Same patient 3 months later while on accutane with the development of spontaneous scarring.

after isotretinoin was stopped she underwent a full-face dermabrasion without problems.

The sixth patient received a medium-depth chemical peel with solid carbon

REFERENCES

1. Kiscuer CW, Shetlar MR, Collagen and mucopolysaccharides in the hypertrophic scar, *Connect Tissue Res* (1974) **2**:205–13.

2. Knapp JR, Damels JR, Kaplan EN, Pathological scar formation, *Am J Pathol* (1970) **56**:47–63.

3. Cohn IK, Diegelmann RF, Keiser HR, Collagen metabolism in keloid and hypertrophic scar. In: Longacre JJ, ed., *The ultrastructure of collagen* (Charles C. Thomas: Springfield, Il 1973) 199–212.

4. Diegelmann RF, Cohan K, Kaplan AM, The role of macrophages in wound repair: a review, *Plast Reconstr Surg* (1981) **59**:107–10.

5. Linares HA, Larson DL, Proteoglycans and collagenase in hypertrophic scar formation, *Plast Reconstr Surg* (1978) **62**:589–93.

6. Oikarinen H, Oikarinen AI, Tan EMI et al, Modulation of procollagen gene expression by retinoids, *J Clin Invest* (1985) **75**:1545–57.

7. Bauer EA, Seltzer JL, Eisen AZ, Inhibition of collagen degradative enzymes by retinoic acid in vitro, *J Am Acad Dermatol* (1982) **88**:603–7.

8. Beach RS, Kenney MC, Vitamin A augments collagen production by corneal endothelial cells, *Biochem Biophys Res Commun* (1983) **14**:395–402.

9. Forest N, Boy-Leteure ML, Duprey P et al, Collagen synthesis in mouse embryonal carcinomas cells: effect of retinoic acid, *Differentiation* (1982) **23**:153–63.

10. Lee KH, Studies on the mechanism of salicylate, III: effect of vitamin A on the wound healing retardation action of aspirin, *J Pharm Sci* (1968) **57**:1238–40.

11. Abergel RP, Meeker CA, Oikarinen H et al, Retinoid modulation of connective tissue metabolism in keloid fibroblast cultures, *Arch Dermatol* (1985) **121**:632–5.

12. Kenney MC, Shin LM, Labermeier U et al, Modulation of rabbit keratinocyte production of collagen, sulfated glycosaminoglycans and fibronectin by retinal acid and retinoic acid, *Biochem Biophys Acta* (1986) **889**:156–62.

13. Elias P, Epidermal effects of retinoids: supramolecular observations and clinical implications, *J Am Acad Dermatol* (1986) **15**:797–809.

14. Jetten AM, Retinoids specifically enhance the number of epidermal growth factor receptors, *Nature* (1980) **2884**:626–9.

15. Williams ML, Elias PM, Nature of skin fragility in patients receiving retinoids for systemic effect, *Arch Dermatol* (1981) **117**:611–19.

16. Clark RAF, Cutaneousd tissue repair: basic biologic considerations I, *J Am Acad Dermatol* (1985) **13**:701–25.

17. Lee KH, Cherny-Chyi Fu, Spencer MR et al, Mechanism of action of retinyl compounds on wound healing. III: effect of retinoic acid homologs on granuloma formation, *J Pharm Sci* (1973) **62**:896–99.

18. Zil JS, Vitamin A acid effects on epidermal mitotic activity, thickness and cellularity on the hairless mouse, *J Invest Dermatol* (1972) **59**:228–32.

19. Herman JB, Woodward SC, An experimental study of wound healing accelerators, *Am Surg* (1972) **38**:26–34.

20. Prutkin L, Wound healing and vitamin A acid, *Acta Derm Venereol* (1972) **52**(supplement):489–92.

21. Lee KH, Tong TG, Mechanism of action of retinyl compounds on wound healing: I structural relationship of retinyl compounds and wound healing, *J Pharm Sci* (1970) **59**:851–4.

22. Hung VC, Lee JY, Zitelli JA et al, Topical tretinoin and epithelial wound healing, *Arch Dermatol* (1989) **125**:65–9.

23. Dlein P, Vitamin A acid and wound healing, *Acta Derm Venereol* (1975) **74**(supplement):171–3.
24. Mandy S, Tretinoin in the preoperative and postoperative management of dermabrasion, *J Am Acad Dermatol* (1986) **15**(supplement):878–9.
25. Hevia O, Nemeth AJ, Taylor JR, Tretinoin accelerates healing after trichloroacetic acid chemical peel, *Arch Dermatol* (1991) **127**:678–82.
26. Plewig G, Braun-Falco O, Kinetics of epidermis and adnexa following vitamin A acid in the human, *Acta Derm Venereol* (1975) **74**(supplement):86–98.
27. Roenigk HH, Pinski JB, Robinson JK et al, Acne, retinoids and dermabrasion, *J Dermatol Surg Oncol* (1985) **11**:396–8.
28. Lask G, David L, No scarring from dermabrasion from Accutane, *Schoch Lett* (1985) **35**:21.
29. Moy RL, Moy LS, Bennett RG et al, Systemic isotretinoin effects on dermal wound healing in a rabbit ear model in vivo, *J Dermatol Surg Oncol* (1990) **16**:1142–6.
30. Bruno NP, Beacham BE, Burnett JW, Adverse effects of isotretinoin therapy, *Cutis* (1984) **33**:484–9.
31. Rubenstein R, Roenigk HH, Stegman SJ et al, Atypical keloids after dermabrasion of patients taking isotretinoin, *J Am Acad Dermatol* (1986) **15**:280–5.
32. Zachariae H, Delayed wound healing and keloid formation following argon laser treatment or dermabrasion during isotretinoin treatment, *Br J Dermatol* (1988) **118**:703–6.
33. Alt TH, Coleman WP III, Hanke CW et al, Dermabrasion. In: Coleman WP III, Hanke CW, Alt TH et al, eds, *Cosmetic surgery of the skin* (BC Decker: Philadelphia 1991) 147–95.
34. Brody HJ, Hailey CW, Medium depth peeling of the skin: a variation of superficial chemosurgery, *J Dermatol Surg Oncol* (1986) **12**:1268–74.
35. Alt TH, Avoiding complications in dermabrasions and chemical peel, *Skin and Allergy News* (April 1990) 2.
36. Pinski KS, Roenigk HH, Pinski JB, Dermabrasion and retinoid therapy, *Dermatology Today and Tomorrow* (1989) **16**:30–3.
37. Coleman WP III, Dermabrasion and hypertrophic scars, *Int J Dermatol* (1991) **30**:629–31.
38. Brody HJ, Complications of chemical peeling, *J Dermatol Surg Oncol* (1989) **15**:1010–19.

Chapter 40

DERMABRASION FOR SCAR REVISION

Bruce E. Katz

History

The first attempts to improve scars and surface irregularities of the human skin date back to antiquity. In the Egyptian Papyrus Ebers, which was published circa 1500 BC, descriptions of abrasive pastes of pumice and alabaster particles in honey and milk used to smooth skin defects are found. Variations of this formulation endured over many centuries. In fact, the great European dermatologist Unna, in the late nineteenth century, applied compounds of pumice to facial skin to improve its cosmetic appearance.

In 1905, Kromayer described rudimentary motor-powered dermabrasion instrumentation which he used to plane down facial scars and defects.[1] Considered the father of modern dermabrasion, he first applied cylindrical knives and then later dental burrs and rasps to treat tattoos, nevi, warts, freckles, pigmentation and scars. His contributions also included freezing with carbon dioxide snow and ether spray to provide the rigidity and anesthesia that are suitable for dermabrasion. In his book *Cosmetic Treatment of Skin Complaints*, Kromayer detailed the evolution of his technique and its applications. However, there was little interest in this new area of surgery until the 1930s.

In 1935, Janson described the use of a stiff-bristled brush to remove a tattoo with good cosmetic results.[2] Iverson, in 1947, drew more attention to skin abrasion by successfully removing traumatic tattoos with common carpenters' sandpaper.[3] McEvitt then applied sandpaper abrasion to the treatment of acne pits with a satisfactory outcome.[4] However, this method of abrasion had several significant limitations: general anesthesia was necessary; selective abrasion of anatomical sites was obscured by the bloody field; and the development of foreign body silica granulomas was a frequent complication.

Abner Kurtin, in the early 1950s, is credited with refining much of Kromayer's original work and for reawakening the interest of dermatologists in this field.[5] He developed motor-driven wire brushes and used ethyl chloride as a skin refrigerant, which permitted controlled abrasion in a relatively bloodless field. His technique was applied successfully to such conditions as acne pits, traumatic scars, tattoos, fine wrinkles, keratoses, keloids and freckles.

Traditional approach to scar revision

The traditional approach for the revision of scars with dermabrasion has been to perform abrasion 6 months or longer after the original surgery or injury.

Vukas, in 1974, reflected this consensus by stating that the aesthetic results were better when the scar was older.[6] It was found subsequently that when dermabrasion was performed after this interval of time, there was only marginal improvement. Thus, enthusiasm for dermabrasion as a useful tool for scar revision waned. Other techniques—such as Z-plasty, W-plasty and geometric broken line closures, which were also postponed until scar maturation—increased in popularity. These procedures did not erase the scar tissue, although they did change a straight line into a broken line (thus making the scar less apparent to the eye). It was only 13 years ago that earlier intervention was first suggested. In his book, Burks stated that 'pox scars, like other scars, may be dermabraded 6–8 weeks after their appearance'.[1] No references to studies were given.

Collins and Farber reported that in selective cases, diamond fraise dermabrasion effectively enhanced the cosmetic outcome of nasal scars when they were treated 2–6 weeks after suture removal.[7] Yarborough found that facial scars, when planed with a wire brush 4–8 weeks after injury, healed without evidence of residual scarring, compared to mature scars abraded 3 months to 13 years after injury, which were not eradicated.[8] Since the author's surgical experience seemed to support these latter observations, it was decided to critically evaluate the effects of spot dermabrasion, or, as it came to be known, 'scarabrasion' (SA), on the appearance and healing of surgical scars.

A CONTROLLED STUDY OF SCARABRASION

In the first controlled investigation of its type, four parameters were studied:

1. Does scarabrasion significantly improve the appearance of scars?
2. What is the optimal length of time after injury to perform SA?
3. As only facial scars had been studied in the past, the efficacy of SA was assessed on various regions of the body.
4. The effects of SA were tested with a diamond fraise.

A controlled study with a split-scar paradigm was designed.[9] Linear scars that were produced by full-thickness surgical excisions on the face, trunk and extremities were chosen randomly for abrasion 4, 6 or 8 weeks after surgery. The results of spot dermabrasion of the left (top) half of each scar were compared to the untreated right (bottom) half of each scar. Ratings were performed by physicians, lay persons and the patients themselves after viewing color photographs of the scars taken at 1, 3 and 6 months postabrasion.

Dichlorotetrafluoroethane (Frigiderm, Dermatologic Laboratory and Supply, Council Bluffs, Iowa) spray was applied for 15 s and then the upper (left) half of the scar was abraded to the mid-reticular dermis using a 12×3 mm extra-coarse diamond fraise driven by a Bell Hand Engine, rotating at 20 000 rev/min. One operator performed all of the abrasions.

Forty-eight scars in patients ranging in age from 25 to 86 years were included in the study. The judges' mean scores on the scarabrasion rating scale in percentage of patients are illustrated in Table 40.1. According to the data, none of the abraded halves of the scars appeared worse than the nonabraded halves and between 6% and 23% showed no change. Although a majority of abraded scars were improved at 4 and 6 weeks, a significantly greater percentage were improved when treated at 8 weeks ($P < 0.05\%$). A trend was seen at 8 weeks where 50% of the abraded scars were undetectable. No statistically significant differences were noted between the scars abraded in various regions of the body.

In summary, the findings of this study were:

1. SA significantly improved the appearance of surgical scars.
2. The appearance of the scars was not worsened by SA.
3. Scars improved with SA at all time intervals, but the result was significantly improved ($P < 0.05$) at 8 weeks after surgery, when 50% of the scars disappeared.
4. The face, trunk and extremities showed comparable improvement with SA.
5. The diamond fraise was found to be an effective instrument for SA.

Table 40.1
Scarabrasion rating scale: distribution by time

Weeks after surgery	N	-1	0	+1	+2	+1 & +2	Overall mean
4	13	0	23	54	23	77	1.06
6	19	0	21	63	16	79	1.01
8	16	0	6	44	50	94	1.39

[a]
-1 The half of the scar marked '0' is worse than the other half.
+1 The half of the scar marked '0' is noticeably improved compared to the other half.
0 There is no difference between each half of the scar.
+2 The half marked '0' is not detectable, i.e. there is no evidence of any scar.

Mechanism of action

In order to determine the mechanism by which SA improves the appearance of surgical scars, the histological differences between abraded and nonabraded halves of scars were explored in four cases. In routine hematoxylin and eosin (H & E) and orcein stained specimens, no gross microscopic differences were noted.

How SA improves the healing of surgical scars is therefore not readily apparent. It may work merely by creating a more diffused, less perceptible scar. Alternatively, SA may affect collagen matrix formation and the remodeling phase of wound healing.

Hyaluronic acid is a glycosaminoglycan, a major component of the wound matrix during the process of granulation tissue formation in early wound repair. It stimulates cellular migration and proliferation, weakens cell attachment to substratum and maintains wound hydration. As collagen deposition proceeds, hyaluronic acid is gradually replaced by proteoglycans (for example chondroitin 4-sulfate and dermatan sulfate) which promote collagen fibril aggregation and polymerization. It is postulated that when a scar is 'rewounded' with abrasion during a time when there is ongoing collagen fibrillogenesis, hyaluronic acid reaccumulates with the re-formation of granulation tissue (Figure 40.1). Proliferating cells produce less proteoglycans as they synthesize more hyaluronic acid. Greater epidermal migration and proliferation may occur with less aggregation of collagen fibrils. Thus cellular output is increased and there is a reduction in collagen maturation.[9] This would result in resurfacing of the wound with a more normal epidermis and less scar tissue. Such a concept is supported by studies of proteoglycan levels and collagen synthesis in hypertrophic scars.[10,11]

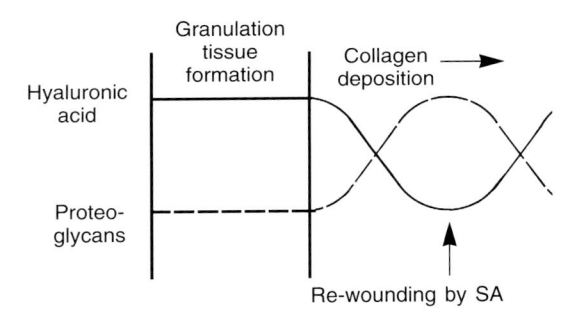

Figure 40.1
Proposed mechanism for the effects of SA on wound healing (from reference 12).

SA OF TRAUMATIC SCARS

The traditional approach to the management of scarring from lacerations or other injuries has been to defer intervention for 6 months to a year after sutures are removed, during which time the scar is allowed to 'mature'. When dermabrasion had been performed at this time, however, there was only marginal improvement.

With the application of SA to traumatic scars at 8 weeks after injury, significant improvement has been achieved in their cosmetic appearance with even complete ablation of the scars[12] (Figure 40.2). A useful modification is to use the small 2.5 × 17 mm or 3 × 13 mm coarse diamond fraises for fine scars. In cases where patients have presented for treatment of mature scars present for several months to years, a different approach is taken. The old scar is excised and then resutured with a double-layer closure. A running subcuticular technique is helpful in avoiding suture 'tracks', and thus allows for abrasion of only a narrow area of scar tissue. Eight weeks later SA is performed on the fresh scar with superior results. Alternatively, if the anatomical location and direction of the scar are appropriate, W-plasty, Z-plasty or geometric broken line closures may be employed and then SA performed 8 weeks later.

PUNCH GRAFTS FOR ICEPICK SCARS

The correction of deep icepick scars is usually not amenable to dermabrasion alone. These fibrotic scars can be removed with a hand-held Stough punch large enough to completely surround the border of the scar. Once the tissue has been excised to subcutaneous fat, and hemostasis has been achieved, grafts measuring 0.25–0.50 mm larger than the defect are harvested from the preauricular or retroauricular skin and kept in place with sterile bandage strips for 1 week. If these grafts are allowed to heal without further intervention, they are often noticeable due to slight elevation and a fine margin of scar tissue between the graft and surrounding skin. It has been found that SA when performed at 8 weeks after placement makes the border of the graft undetectable (Figure 40.3). Care should be taken not to abrade too deeply to avoid dislodging the graft. If a full-face dermabrasion is planned after the repair of icepick scars with punch grafts, the optimal timing for this procedure is also 8

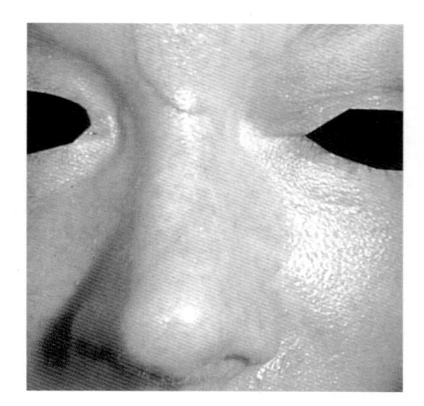

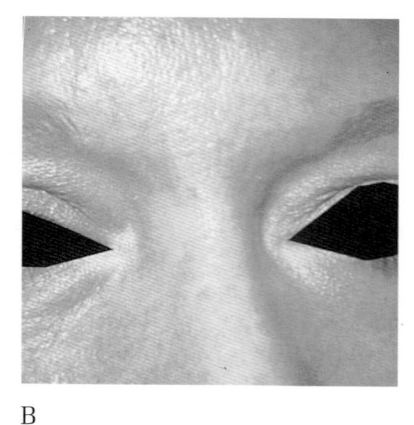

Figure 40.2
(A) Facial scar 8 weeks after trauma and before SA. (B) Four months after SA with complete ablation of scar.

DERMABRASION FOR SCAR REVISION

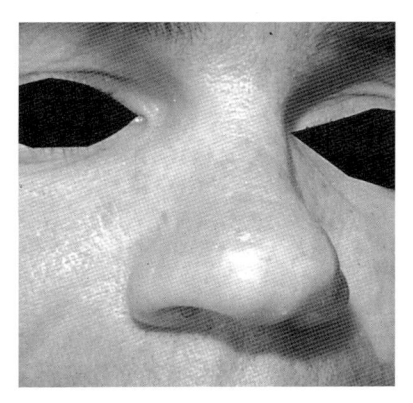

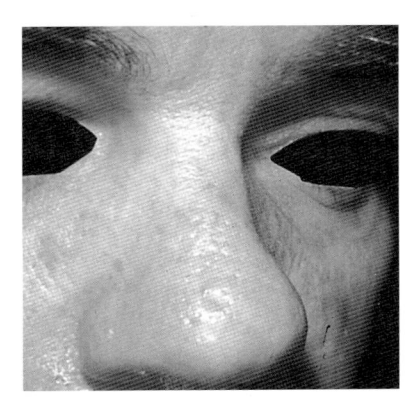

Figure 40.3
(A) Icepick scar of nose before repair with punch graft and SA. (B) Two months after punch graft repair and SA.

weeks after graft placement. Between 20 and 30 icepick scars have been replaced with grafts at one session which was followed by full-face dermabrasion 8 weeks later with excellent results.

VARICELLA SCARS

Facial pox scars resulting from an episode of herpes zoster or chicken pox in aduldhood can be a troubling cosmetic problem for which little has been available therapeutically. A number of patients with both types of scarring have been treated with SA 8 weeks after crusts have fallen off and have achieved excellent cosmetic results. A bullet fraise is the instrument of choice for abrading these small scars. The sharp edges of the pox scar disappear and even the depression appears less evident (Figure 40.4).

For pox scars present for several months or more, one can employ the use of punch grafts in a fashion similar to the repair of icepick scarring. Pox scars have been excised and the defects were filled with retroauricular grafts as large as 5.0 mm in diameter. Scarabrasion is performed

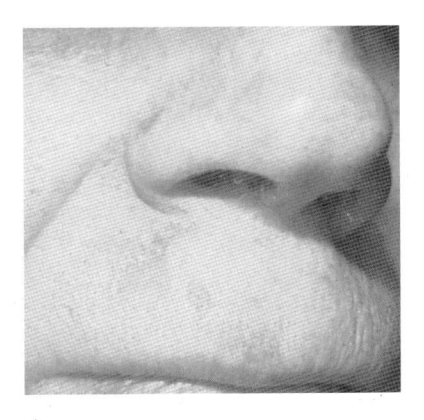

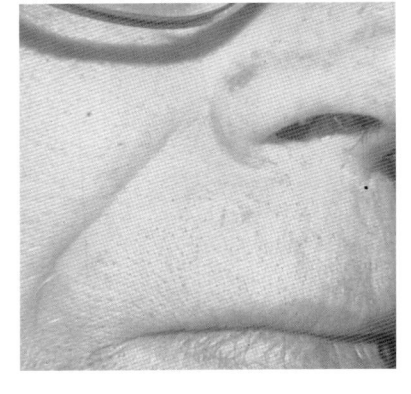

Figure 40.4
(A) Upper lip scar 8 weeks after herpes zoster and before SA. (B) Two months after SA.

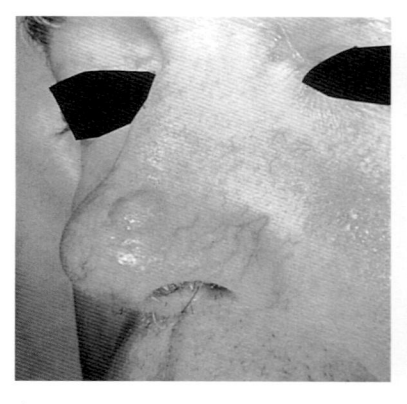

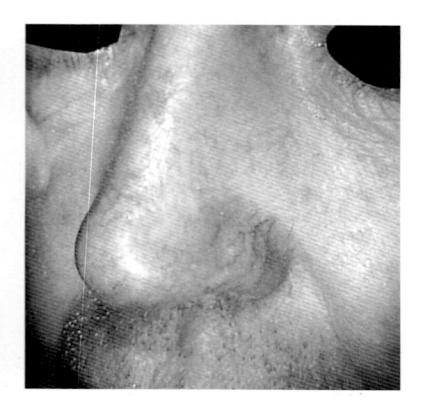

Figure 40.5
(A) Nasal graft 8 weeks after surgery and before SA. (B) Three years after SA of graft.

8 weeks later with impressive results. The appropriate selection criteria for dermabrasion in general should be considered so that abnormalities of pigmentation and keloids are avoided.

FULL-THICKNESS GRAFTS AND FLAPS

The dermatologic surgeon utilizes full-thickness grafts most often to correct defects produced by the excision of basal cell and squamous cell carcinomas from the nose, ear and periorbital areas. Donor sites for grafts include the preauricular, retroauricular, supraclavicular and adjacent tissue areas. Once these defects have healed, the cosmetic appearance of the grafts is often suboptimal. This may be due to differences in skin color and texture between the graft and surrounding skin. In addition, the outline of scar tissue at the margin of the graft or contour deformities allow the graft to be more apparent.

The conventional approach for applying dermabrasion to improve the appearance of full-thickness grafts is to wait at least 6 months from the time of grafting to perform the procedure. When utilized after this interval of time, dermabrasion has been found effective only in adjusting the level of a skin graft when all or part of it is elevated above the surrounding skin.[13]

Since a graft is often conspicuous due to the rim of scar tissue that separates it from the surrounding skin, its appearance was optimized by performing SA 8 weeks after grafting. Abrasion was performed down to the level of the mid-reticular dermis and was extended 2–3 mm onto normal surrounding skin. In addition to there being almost complete blurring of the graft margins, the color and texture match between graft and the surrounding skin improved and any elevation of the graft was also corrected (Figure 40.5). Contour defects due to depression of the graft were not ameliorated.

In certain cases, grafts appeared to heal almost too well when they were abraded at 8 weeks, and thereby remained apparent. On closer inspection, this was found to be due to solar damage of skin in the surrounding cosmetic unit which was characterized by telangiectasias and lentigines. The graft was more noticeable because it contrasted with sun-damaged skin. Careful evaluation of skin contiguous to the graft before abrasion is performed can obviate this problem. If considerable dermatoheliosis is noted, the entire cosmetic unit may be abraded with a better result. This approach works particularly well in the case of nasal grafts.

The outline of surgical flaps may remain visible for reasons similar to those for grafts. If SA is utilized 8 weeks after surgery, an improved cosmetic outcome can be expected.

SILASTIC GEL SHEETING (SGS) AND SCAR REVISION

Conventional treatment of hypertrophic and keloid scars has included steroid injection, surgical revision, radiation, laser, cryotherapy, compression and combination therapy. Many of these techniques have been associated with high rates of recurrence.[14] Scarabrasion had not been applied to this form of scarring due to the possibility of recurrences or worsening of the scars. Preliminary experience with SGS indicates that it may be an effective adjunctive treatment and allow for the use of scarabrasion on hypertrophic and keloid scars.

Silastic gel sheeting (Dow Corning, Valbonne, France), a soft, semi-occlusive scar cover made of crosslinked polydimethylsiloxane polymer, was first reported to be an effective treatment for burn scars and contractures in 1982.[15] Though confirmed in its efficacy for treatment of existing hypertrophic and keloid scars,[16–21] only recently has it been found effective in preventing the development of these scars.[22]

When SGS is applied to longstanding hypertrophic or keloid scars, this author's experience has shown it to be variable in its effect; scars may improve or remain unchanged. However, when it is used on fresh scars, as soon as re-epithelialization occurs, recurrence of hypertrophic scarring has been prevented. Thus, longstanding scars on the chest have been excised and repaired with running W-plasties, and then SGS has been applied for 8 weeks. Scarabrasion was then performed and SGS reapplied again for 8 weeks. After 9 months of follow-up, no recurrences of these hypertrophic scars have been found (Figure 40.6).

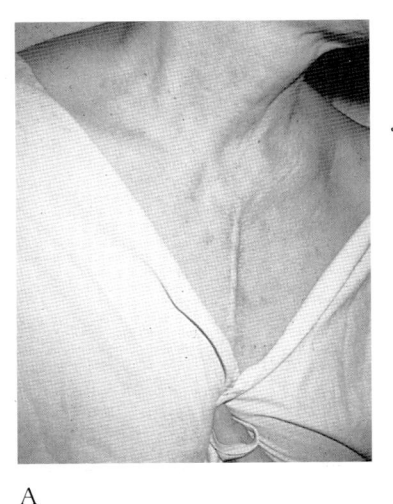

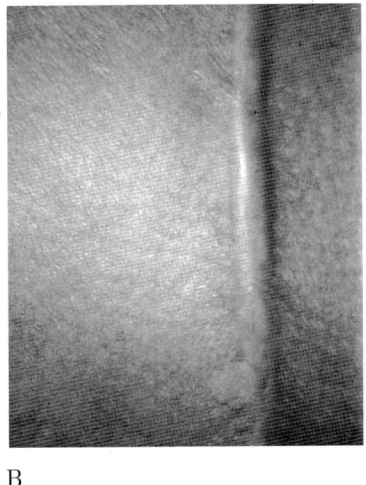

Figure 40.6
(A) Hypertrophic scar of chest before excision, W-plasty repair, SA and application of SGS for 2 months. (B) Close-up of (A). (C) No recurrence of hypertrophic scar 9 months after SGS use was discontinued.

Silastic gel sheeting is packaged in single sterile sheets and is trimmed to fit the specific scar or anatomical site. It may be kept in place with tape, gauze bandage or a compression garment. Avoidance of excessive pressure will prevent maceration of the skin. The sheet should be worn for 12–24 h a day for at least 2 months. Patients are told to wash it once a day with a mild soap and water solution and replace it with a fresh piece every 7–10 days when it begins to crack or crumble.

Various factors have been studied to explain the mechanism of action of SGS.[18] Physical and chemical parameters such as pressure, temperature, oxygen tension, occlusion and particulate release do not appear to be responsible for its therapeutic effect. Since skin water loss by evaporation is reduced by almost half in treated sites, promotion of scar hydration by SGS is thought to be a factor in its mode of action.[19]

SKIN NECROSIS AFTER INJECTION OF ZYPLAST COLLAGEN

Zyplast collagen (Collagen Biomedical, Palo Alto, CA) has been used to correct acne scars, wrinkles and other contour defects. With proper skin testing prior to injection, most allergic reactions can be avoided. Between 1 and 5% of patients have a positive collagen skin test.[23] However, in less than 4% of cases, treatment site reactions may occur even with a negative skin test. These manifest as erythema, induration and occasional pruritus which may persist for 6 months or longer. Such adverse responses resolve without residual scarring.

Skin necrosis after injection of Zyplast collagen has been reported to occur in patients who have previously undergone uneventful injections with this agent[24] and can result in permanent scarring. The incidence of local necrosis was estimated to be 16 cases per 10 000 in 1990.[25] The glabellar area was the site most often affected, with development of depressed crateriform areas of cicatrix.

The strategy used most often when dealing with this form of scarring has been to wait 6 months or more before intervening (Wauk L, personal communication). Surgical revision is then employed to make the scar less apparent.

When a patient seeks treatment to enhance their cosmetic appearance and an untoward side-effect results in a scar, having that individual wait 6 months or more for corrective surgery may lead to a difficult situation. Having had an annoying wrinkle or scar erased, he or she must now

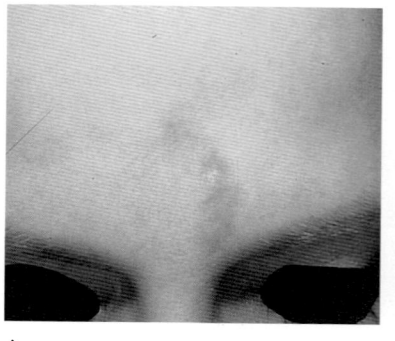

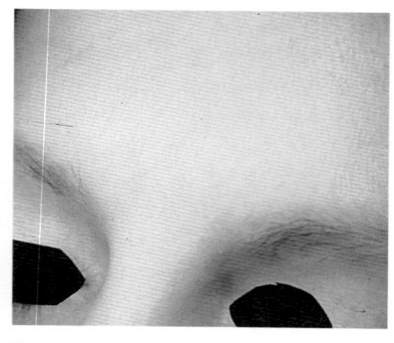

Figure 40.7
(A) Glabellar scar 8 weeks after occurrence of Zyplast skin necrosis and before SA. (B) Four months after SA with no evidence of residual cicatrix.

live for some time with an even more conspicuous cosmetic defect.

This same issue was encountered when a young woman developed Zyplast skin necrosis of the glabellar area. More immediate treatment was considered when the patient insisted that her social commitments would not allow her to wait 6 months for corrective surgery. Since the depressed, sharply demarcated scar that resulted from Zyplast skin necrosis appeared somewhat similar to the scarring from herpes zoster, SA was applied. Eight weeks after the crust cleared, SA was performed on the glabellar scar. Within several months, there was no evidence of any residual cicatrix (Figure 40.7). Scarabrasion may play an important role in the treatment of skin necrosis resulting from Zyplast collagen injection, although more cases need to be studied before conclusions are reached.

SCARABRASION AND ISOTRETINOIN (ACCUTANE)

Atypical scarring may develop in patients undergoing dermabrasion after having recently completed a course of isotretinoin (Accutane, Roche Dermatologics, Nutley, NJ).[26] Recent experience indicates that similar scarring may occur when isotretinoin is taken soon after dermabrasion is performed. Although this has not been a complication in our experience with SA, it seems prudent to elicit any history of isotretinoin use and to weigh carefully its possible impact on the outcome of scar therapy.

REFERENCES

1. Burks J, *Dermabrasion and chemical peeling in the treatment of certain cosmetic defects and diseases of the skin* (Charles C Thomas: Springfield, Ill 1979).

2. Janson P, Eine einfache methode der entfernung, *Dermatol Wochenschr* (1935) **101**:894–5.

3. Iverson PC, Surgical treatment of skin lesions by abrasion, *Plast Reconstr Surg* (1953) **12**:27–31.

4. McEvitt WG, Acne pits, *J Mich Med Soc* (1948) **47**:1234–44.

5. Kurtin A, Corrective surgical planing of the skin, *Arch Dermatol* (1953) **68**(supplement):389–97.

6. Vukas A, Smallpox-induced scars: treatment by dermabrasion. Postsurgical dermabrasion of the nose, *J Dermatol Surg Oncol* (1974) **10**:476–7.

7. Collins PS, Farber GA, Postsurgical dermabrasion of the nose, *J Dermatol Surg Oncol* (1984) **10**:476–7.

8. Yarborough JM, Ablation of facial scars by programmed dermabrasion, *J Dermatol Surg Oncol* (1988) **14**:292–4.

9. Katz BE, Oca AG, A controlled study of the effectiveness of spot dermabrasion ('scarabrasion') on the appearance of surgical scars, *J Am Acad Dermatol* (1991) **24**:462–6.

10. Cohen IK, Keiser HR, Sjoerdsma A, Collagen synthesis in the human keloid and hypertrophic scar, *Surg Forum* (1971) **22**:488–9.

11. Shettar MR, Shettat CL, Chien SF et al, The hypertrophic scar: hexosamine-containing components of burn scars, *Proc Soc Exp Biol Med* (1972) **139**:544–7.

12. Katz BE, Scarabrasion and its application in improving the appearance of scars, *Cosmet Dermatol* (1991) **4**:8–16.

13. Robinson JK, Improvement of the appearance of full-thickness skin grafts with dermabrasion, *Arch Dermatol* (1987) **123**:1340–6.

14. Stucker FJ, Shaw GY, An approach to

management of keloids, *Arch Otolaryngol Head Neck Surg* (1992) **118**:63–6.
15. Perkins K, Davey RB, Wallis KA, Silicone gel: a new treatment for burn scars and contractures, *Burns* (1982) **9**:201.
16. Quinn KJ, Evans JH, Courtney JM et al, Non-pressure treatment of hypertrophic scars, *Burns* (1985) **12**:102.
17. Davey RB, The use of silicone gel and silastic foam in burn scar management—how does it work? Presented at the 7th Congress of the International Society for Burn Injuries, February 1986, Melbourne.
18. Quinn KJ, Silicone gel in scar treatment, *Burns* (1987) **13**:933–40.
19. Ohmori S, Effectiveness of silastic sheet coverage in the treatment of scar keloid (hypertrophic scar), *Aesth Plast Surg* (1988) **12**:95–9.
20. Mercer NSG, Silicone gel in the treatment of keloid scars, *Br J Plast Surg* (1989) **42**:83–7.
21. Ahn ST, Monafo WW, Mustoe TA, Topical silicone gel: a new treatment for hypertrophic scars, *Surgery* (1989) **106**:781–7.
22. Ahn ST, Monafo WW, Mustoe TA, Topical silicone gel for the prevention and treatment of hypertrophic scar, *Arch Surg* (1991) **126**:499–504.
23. Clark DP, Hanke CW, Swanson NA, Dermal implants: safety of products injected for soft tissue augmentation, *J Am Acad Dermatol* (1989) **21**:992–8.
24. Stegman SJ, Chu S, Armstrong RC, Adverse reactions to bovine collagen implant: clinical and histologic features, *J Dermatol Surg Oncol* (1988) **14**(supplement 1):39–48.
25. *Collagen Connection* (1991) **1**:1.
26. Rubenstein R, Roenigk HH, Stegman SJ et al, Atypical keloids after dermabrasion of patients taking isotretinoin, *J Am Acad Dermatol* (1986) **15**:280–5.

Chapter 41

CULTURED EPIDERMAL GRAFTS

Youn H. Kim
David T. Woodley

The optimal replacement of full-thickness surgical wounds has traditionally been full-thickness or split-thickness skin from compatible donor sites of the same patient. However, when the wounds are sufficiently large or multiple, the availability of donor tissue from the same patient can be limited. In such cases, an alternative method for repairing surgical wounds is to replace the defects with grafts derived from in vitro expansion of small skin biopsies. The scope of this chapter will be limited to cultured keratinocyte grafts. The primary focus will be on keratinocyte autografts, although a brief discussion of keratinocyte allografts and composite grafts which combine keratinocyte and dermal components will be included. The technique of keratinocyte graft preparation and transplantation, surgical application of different types of cultured grafts, and the study of structural and functional characteristics of transplanted grafts will be described. Cultured melanocyte grafts will not be discussed in this chapter.

PREPARATION OF EPIDERMAL GRAFTS AND TRANSPLANTATION METHODS

The major technical advances towards the successful culture of keratinocytes from human skin dates back to 1975 when the method of serially expanding keratinocytes from single cell suspensions was established.[1] Currently, there are two major methods of keratinocyte cultivation that are used for the preparation of epidermal grafts. The classical method described by Green involves co-culturing keratinocytes on a mesenchymal (3T3) cell feeder layer with culture medium containing serum and various mitogens.[1,2] The other method involves a two-phase technique where the cells are initially cultivated in serum-free, low-calcium medium without a feeder layer in order to yield large quantities of highly proliferative keratinocytes. The second phase involves the induction of cohesive, stratified sheets of epithelium by changing to high-calcium, serum-containing medium.[3] Raising the calcium concentration of the culture medium causes desmosomes to form between the keratinocytes in culture and allows the cells to stratify into a multilayered epithelium.[4] In either case, the mature epidermal sheets can be released from Petri dishes with dispase, a neutral protease (Figure 41.1).[2] A 1-cm^2 skin biopsy can be expanded to 1 m^2 with serial passaging. Skin from younger patients will expand faster than that from older patients due to the age-related decline of proliferative capacity of keratinocytes in vitro.[5] Cultured

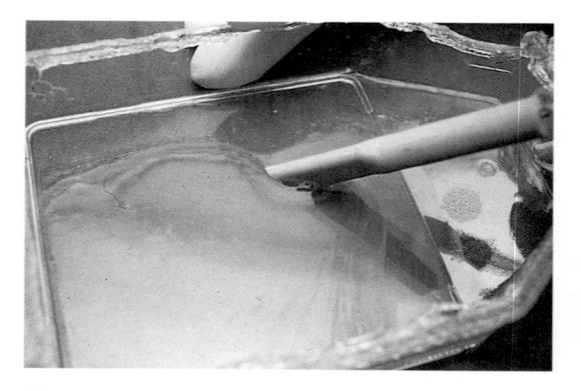

Figure 41.1
The stratified cultured epidermal sheet is released from the Petri dish by treatment with dispase, a neutral protease.

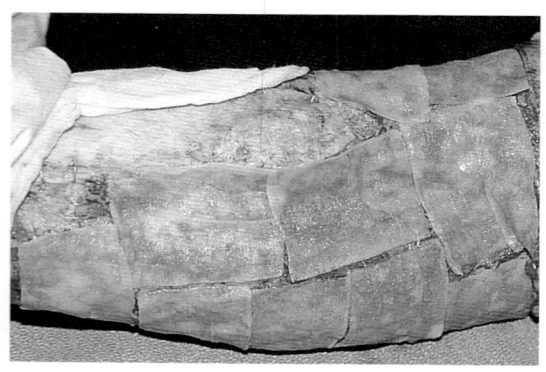

Figure 41.2
The detached keratinocyte sheets are supported with dressing material for ease of handling and placed on the prepared surgical wounds. The basal cell layer of the epidermal grafts faces the wound surface.

epidermal grafts can be available in 2–6 weeks after obtaining the donor tissue.

The detached intact keratinocyte sheets are supported with various dressings for ease of handling and then placed on prepared surgical wounds (Figure 41.2). The epidermal grafts are placed on the wound surfaces with the basal cell layer facing down. The grafts are covered by nonadherent dressings and secured with support or compressible dressings.[6–9]

Proper preparation of the graft bed increases the take rate of cultured grafts. Adequate debridement should be performed prior to grafting, either surgically or using occlusive dressings, to provide healthy granulation tissue. Graft survival is higher with freshly excised wounds than with chronic granulating wounds.[10] Temporary wound coverings may be necessary to maintain healthy graft beds while preparing the cultured grafts. Wounds should be free of clinical infection.[11] Use of common topical antiseptics such as hydrogen peroxide, betadine and chlorhexidine should be avoided since they have been shown to be toxic to keratinocytes in vitro.[12,13]

SURGICAL APPLICATIONS OF CULTURED GRAFTS

Keratinocyte autografts

Epidermal sheets expanded from keratinocyte cultures of autologous donor skin have been used most widely for replacement of extensive burn wounds.[6,10,14–16] The rate of graft take depends on the clinical condition of the graft bed and the method of wound care. In general, treatment with epidermal grafts for these burn patients resulted in decreased morbidity and mortality and enhanced wound healing, although controlled prospective comparisons with conventional treatments have not been performed. One major advantage is that large open wounds can be covered permanently once the cultured sheets are prepared.

Epidermal autografts have been used to treat chronic leg ulcers.[17–19] In the treatment of stasis ulcers, the engraftment rates may be lower due to the chronicity of the wounds, underlying stasis pathology, and the older age of the patients. Other clinical applications have been for the treatment of recalcitrant wounds in epidermolysis bullosa patients[20] and to repair the surgical defects left after excision of giant congenital melanocytic nevi.[21]

Keratinocyte allografts

In the early 1980s, it was thought that keratinocyte grafts prepared with allogeneic donor skin would not be rejected because of the loss of Langerhans cells and HLA-DR expression during in vitro cultivation of keratinocytes.[22,23] The initial trials using cultured epidermal allografts for burn wounds and split-thickness graft donor sites produced good clinical results.[8,24–27] Keratinocyte allografts were also used for the treatment of chronic leg ulcers and allowed wounds to heal that were previously resistant to conventional therapy.[9,27–29] Another clinical use has been to cover chronic wounds of patients with recessive dystrophic epidermolysis bullosa.[30] Hypertrophic scarring was not usually observed. Cryopreserved and fresh keratinocyte allografts have been shown to result in a similar clinical response.[31] Donor tissues and sera are usually screened for HIV, CMV, HSV I and HBs antigens.

In spite of the initial impression that cultured allografts engrafted and were not rejected, it is now well established that the allografts are rapidly rejected or replaced with the host's cells.[15,28,32–34] Use of DNA fingerprinting and sex chromosome probes has firmly demonstrated that there is no persistence of allogeneic keratinocytes. In most cases of keratinocyte allograft treatments, wound healing was observed to initiate from the edges of wounds or from the preserved appendages of the graft beds. The improved clinical healing may be due to induction of inflammatory cytokines, growth factors and matrix proteins involved in stimulating wound healing.

Composite or in vitro reconstituted grafts

A composite or in vitro reconstituted skin can be any combination of keratinocyte sheets, autologous or allogeneic, and a human dermis or dermal equivalent. The human dermis used is usually from an allogeneic source such as cadaver skin. Composite grafts of autologous epidermis from cultured keratinocytes and allogeneic dermis have been used as full-thickness skin replacements for burn wounds.[35–37] In order to create a composite graft, the wounds are initially covered with split- or full-thickness cadaver skin. When the cultured keratinocyte autografts from the patient's skin biopsy are ready, the epidermis of cadaver skin is mechanically removed and the cultured autograft sheets are placed on the exposed cadaver dermis. Thus, the patient's initial wound is now covered with an 'engrafted' cadaver skin dermis covered with a layer of autologous cultured keratinocytes. Implicit in this methodology is that there is engraftment of the cadaver dermis without rejection. An alternative hypothesis is that a low-level, subclinical rejection of the cellular elements in cadaver dermis occurs with subsequent replacement by host cells and connective tissue. Nevertheless, this 'conditions' the wound bed such that it supports the cultured autograft sheets of keratinocytes.

Alternatively, the allogeneic cadaver dermis can be depleted of fibroblasts by repetitive freeze–thaw cycles with or without irradiation. The acellular dermis can be repopulated in vitro with autologous fibroblasts and layered with autologous keratinocytes, creating a full-thickness 'autologous' skin graft.[38] Krejci et al demonstrated good engraftment of these in vitro reconstituted grafts in athymic mice. Future clinical trials on human wounds will determine the effectiveness of such reconstituted skin compared with other wound replacements.

Dermal equivalents composed of collagen lattices embedded with autologous or allogeneic fibroblasts have been combined with autologous or allogeneic keratinocytes. Bell et al and Sher et al reported successful replacement of full-thickness wounds in animals using such skin equivalents. Clinical application of these skin equivalents in burn patients is limited. The clinical results are less impressive than those obtained with composite grafts using human dermis.[39,40]

STRUCTURAL AND FUNCTIONAL CHARACTERIZATION OF GRAFTED WOUNDS

Clinically, the engrafted areas can exhibit spontaneous blistering and/or skin fragility up to 6 months after successful grafting with autologous keratinocyte sheets. Woodley et al used a suction blister device to demonstrate that healed areas that had been engrafted with keratinocyte autografts blistered in 17 min compared with 65 min in an ungrafted area of the same leg.[41] The cleavage plane of the suction blister of grafted skin was below the lamina densa whereas that of the normal skin was above the lamina densa. They further demonstrated that in all four patients studied, the reconstituted basement membrane zone beneath the autografts was incomplete and lacked the collagenase-resistant domain of type IV collagen and had a paucity of anchoring fibrils as late as 5 months after successful engraftment. Thus, the skin fragility with cleavage below the lamina densa zone was thought to be secondary to attenuated anchoring fibrils. Compton et al also observed sparse anchoring fibrils post-transplantation which gradually 'normalized' 1–2 years after engraftment.[42] In both studies, the normal, undulating rete ridge pattern was initially absent and the transplanted autografts had an effaced dermal–epidermal junction. Compton et al found that in children who received cultured autografts, rete ridges developed 5–18 months after grafting.

Peterson et al utilized immunostaining methods to characterize the cellular elements in the healed keratinocyte autografts.[43] Using monoclonal antibodies to cytokeratins, they found that autografted keratinocytes displayed keratin markers similar to hyperproliferative states (for example psoriasis) as late as 5 months after grafting. In contrast, split-thickness grafted skin or re-epithelialized areas using mesh grafts maintained the keratin markers of normal skin. Peterson et al also reported that the transplanted cultured autografts were intially free of Langerhans cells. However, within 3–6 weeks, bone marrow-derived Langerhans cells repopulated the keratinocyte autografts. A neodermis rich in fibronectin formed between the keratinocyte grafts and wound beds within 2 weeks of engraftment. Woodley et al further characterized the neodermis using immunohistochemical methods and ultra-structural analysis.[44] They found that the neodermis contained many of the major connective tissue components such as major collagens, types I, III and VI, and fibronectin early in the post-transplantation period. However, there was a paucity of elastin fibers and poor organization of linkin (microthread-like fibers) in the neodermis as late as 5 months after engraftment. Compton et al reported that in autografted areas of children with burns, considerable 'normalization' of elastic fibers was observed in the neodermis 4–5 years after transplantation.[42]

In the composite grafts consisting of autologous cultured keratinocytes and allogeneic dermis, Langdon et al reported that a normal-appearing basement membrane zone with anchoring fibrils was demonstrated 95 days after completed engraftment using ultrastructural and immunohistochemical analyses.[45] At 47 days, the lamina densa zone was discontinuous and the anchoring fibrils were sparse. The source of the reformed anchoring fibrils is unclear and could be either the autografted keratinocytes or residual anchoring fibrils within the basement membrane zone of the allodermis itself. The pattern of rete ridges 'normalized' 11 months after application of keratinocyte autografts. Normal melanocytes were observed from the outset, indicating persistence from in vitro keratinocyte culture. Suprabasilar epidermal cells staining for S-100 antigen were present within the grafts as early as 7 days after placement of keratinocyte autografts and most likely represent Langerhans cells. The allogeneic dermis was completely revascularized with intact laminin and type IV collagen by 68 days after alloengraftment. Other cellular and connective tissue elements of the cadaveric allodermis were not followed at length. Langdon et al did note that elastic or nerve fibers were not evident at 47 days after application of the keratinocyte autografts.[45] They speculated that most of the cellular elements of the original allodermis are subclinically rejected and gradually replaced by host cells. Subsequently, Young et al demonstrated that the cellular elements of the 'engrafted' allodermis are indeed replaced by host cells using a DNA fingerprinting technique.[46]

Summary

The technical developments enabling clinicians to utilize keratinocyte sheets have provided new alternatives to conventional biological or synthetic wound replacements. Especially in burn patients, cultured grafts have effectively decreased morbidity and mortality. Cultured epidermal grafts have improved healing of certain recalcitrant nonhealing ulcers. Epidermal autografts remain functionally fragile for many months after successful engraftment. Carefully controlled prospective studies have not been performed comparing the effectiveness of different cultured graft techniques, among each other or with other wound treatments, and thus it is difficult to draw conclusions on their comparative efficacy. It is important to emphasize that for routine, relatively small surgical wounds, autologous, full-thickness or split-thickness grafts remain the standard for skin replacement. One must carefully determine the appropriate surgical situations for using cultured grafts and consider the advantages and disadvantages and the risk–benefit ratios. Issues of cost, money and time, and potential transmissible infection from allografts, must be carefully examined.

References

1. Rheinwald J, Green H, Serial cultivation of strains of human epidermal keratinocytes: the formation of keratinizing colonies from single cells, *Cell* (1975) **6**:331–44.

2. Green H, Kehinde O, Thomas J, Growth of cultured human epidermal cells into multiple epithelia suitable for grafting, *Proc Natl Acad Sci USA* (1979) **76**:5665–8.

3. Pittelkow M, Scott R, New techniques for the in vitro culture of human skin keratinocytes and perspectives on their use for grafting of patients with extensive burns, *Mayo Clin Proc* (1986) **61**:771–7.

4. Hennings H, Michael D, Cheng C et al, Calcium regulation of growth and differentiation of mouse epidermal cells in culture, *Cell* (1980) **19**:245–54.

5. Gilchrest B, In vitro assessment of keratinocyte aging, *J Invest Dermatol* (1983) **81**:184S–9S.

6. Gallico G, O'Connor N, Compton C et al, Permanent coverage of large burn

wounds with autologous cultured human epithelium, *N Engl J Med* (1984) **331**:448–51.

7. Eisinger M, Monden M, Raaf J et al, Wound coverage by a sheet of epidermal cells grown in vitro from dispersed single cell preparations, *Surgery* (1980) **88**:287–93.

8. Hefton J, Madden M, Finkelstein J et al, Grafting of burn patients with allografts of cultured epidermal cells, *Lancet* (1983) **2**:428–30.

9. Phillips T, Kehinde O, Green H et al, Treatment of skin ulcers with cultured epidermal allografts, *J Am Acad Dermatol* (1989) **21**:191–9.

10. O'Connor N, Mulliken J, Banks-Schlegel S et al, Grafting of burns with cultured epithelium prepared from autologous epidermal cells, *Lancet* (1981) **1**:75–8.

11. Eldad A, Burt A, Clark J et al, Cultured epithelium as a skin substitute, *Burns* (1987) **13**:173–80.

12. Tatnall F, Leigh I, Gibson J, Comparative toxicity of antimicrobial agents on transformed human keratinocytes, *J Invest Dermatol* (1987) **89**:316A.

13. Tatnall F, Leigh I, Gibson J, Comparative study of antiseptic toxicity on basal keratinocytes, transformed human keratinocytes and fibroblasts, *Skin Pharm* (1990) **3**:157–63.

14. Teepe R, Ponec M, Kreis R, Improved grafting method for the treatment of burns with autologous cultured human epithelium, *Lancet* (1986) **1**:385.

15. De Luca M, Albanese E, Bondanza S et al, Multicentre experience in the treatment of burns with autologous and allogeneic cultured epithelium, fresh or preserved in a frozen state, *Burns* (1989) **15**:303–9.

16. Bettex-Galland M, Slongo T, Hunziker T et al, Use of cultured keratinocytes in severe burns, *Z Kinderchir* (1988) **43**:224–8.

17. Hefton J, Caldwell D, Biozes D et al, Grafting of skin ulcers with cultured autologous epidermal cells, *J Am Acad Dermatol* (1986) **14**:399–405.

18. Leigh I, Purkis P, Culture grafted leg ulcers, *Clin Exp Dermatol* (1986) **11**:650–2.

19. Hunyadi J, Farkas B, Bertenyi C et al, Keratinocyte grafting: a new means of transplantation for full thickness wounds, *J Dermatol Surg Oncol* (1988) **14**:75–8.

20. Carter D, Lin A, Varghese M et al, Treatment of junctional epidermolysis bullosa with epidermal autografts, *J Am Acad Dermatol* (1987) **172**:246–50.

21. Gallico G, O'Connor N, Compton C, Cultured epithelial autografts for giant congenital naevi, *Plast Reconstr Surg* (1989) **84**:1–9.

22. Morhenn V, Benike C, Cox A et al, Cultured human epidermal cells do not synthesize HLA-DR, *J Invest Dermatol* (1982) **78**:32–7.

23. Hefton J, Amberson J, Biozes D et al, Loss of HLA-DR expression by human epidermal cells after growth in culture, *J Invest Dermatol* (1984) **83**:48–50.

24. Thivolet J, Faure M, Demidem A et al, Long term survival and immunological tolerance of human epidermal allografts produced in culture, *Transplantation* (1986) **42**:274–80.

25. Thivolet J, Faure M, Demidem A, Cultured human epidermal allografts are not rejected for a long period, *Arch Dermatol Res* (1986) **287**:252–4.

26. Madden M, Finkelstein J, Staiano-Coico L et al, Grafting of cultured allogeneic epidermis on second and

third degree burn wounds on 26 patients, *J Trauma* (1986) **26**:955–60.

27. Phillips T, Gilchrest B, Cultured allogeneic keratinocyte grafts in the management of wound healing, *J Dermatol Surg Oncol* (1989) **15**:1169–76.

28. Leigh I, Purkis P, Navsaria H, Treatment of chronic venous ulcers with sheets of cultured allogeneic keratinocytes, *Br J Dermatol* (1987) **117**:591–7.

29. Shehade S, Clancy J, Blight A et al, Cultured epithelial allografting of leg ulcers, *J Dermatol Treat* (1989) **548**:262–70.

30. McGuire J, Birchall N, Cuono C et al, Successful engraftment of allegeneic keratinocytes in recessive dystrophic epidermolysis bullosa, *Clin Res* (1987) **35**:702A.

31. Teepe R, Koebrugge E, Ponec M et al, Fresh versus cryopreserved cultured allografts for the treatment of chronic skin ulcers, *Br J Dermatol* (1990) **122**:81–9.

32. Brain A, Purkis P, Coates P et al, Survival of cultured allogeneic keratinocytes transplanted to deep dermal bed assessed with probe specific for Y chromosome, *Br Med J* (1989) **298**:917–19.

33. Burt A, Pallet C, Sloane J et al, Survival of cultured allografts in patients with burns assessed with probe specific for Y-chromosome, *Br Med J* (1989) **298**:915–17.

34. Phillips T, Bhawan J, Leigh I et al, Cultured epidermal autografts and allografts: a study of differentiation and allograft survival, *J Am Acad Dermatol* (1990) **23**:189–98.

35. Heck E, Bergstresser P, Baxter C et al, Composite skin graft: frozen dermal allografts support the engraftment and expansion of autologous epidermis, *J Trauma* (1985) **25**:106–12.

36. Cuono C, Langdon R, McGuire J, Use of cultured epidermal autografts and dermal allografts as skin replacement after burn injury, *Lancet* (1986) **1**:1123–4.

37. Cuono C, Langhdon R, Birchall N et al, Composite autologous-allogeneic skin replacement: development and clinical application, *Plast Reconstr Surg* (1987) **980**:626–35.

38. Krejci N, Cuono C, Langdon R et al, In vitro reconstitution of skin: fibroblasts facilitate keratinocyte growth and differentiation on acellular dead reticular dermis, *J Invest Dermatol* (1991) **97**:843–8.

39. Wassermann D, Schlotterer M, Toulon A et al, Preliminary clinical studies of a biological cultured skin equivalent in burned patients, *Burns* (1988) **14**:326–30.

40. Hull B, Finley R, Miller S, Coverage of full thickness burns with bilayered equivalents: preliminary clinical trial, *Surgery* (1990) **107**:496–502.

41. Woodley D, Peterson H, Herzog S et al, Burn wounds resurfaced by cultured epidermal autografts show abnormal reconstitution of anchoring fibrils, *JAMA* (1988) **259**:2566–71.

42. Compton C, Gil J, Bradford D et al, Skin regenerated from cultured epithelial autografts on full thickness burn wounds from 6 days to 5 years after grafting, *Lab Invest* (1989) **60**:600–12.

43. Peterson M, Lessane B, Woodley D, Characterization of cellular elements in healed cultured keratinocyte autografts used to cover burn wounds, *Arch Dermatol* (1990) **126**:175–80.

44. Woodley D, Briggaman R, Herzog S et al, Characterization of 'neo-dermis'

formation beneath cultured human epidermal autografts transplanted on muscle fascia, *J Invest Dermatol* (1990) **95**:20–6.

45. Langdon R, Cuono C, Birchall N et al, Reconstitution of structure and cell function in human skin grafts derived from cryopreserved allogeneic dermis and autologous cultured keratinocytes, *J Invest Dermatol* (1988) **91**:478–85.

46. Young D, Langdon R, Kahn R et al, Analysis of the fate of allografted dermis using a DNA fingerprinting technique, *Proc Am Burn Assoc* (1989) **21**:71A.

Chapter 42

ADVANCES IN FLAPS AND GRAFTS IN DERMATOLOGIC SURGERY

Eckart Haneke

The treatment of skin tumors has become more surgical and dermatologists have refined their skills accordingly. A great number of dermatologic surgery textbooks and atlases has appeared during recent years, evidence of dermatologists' mastery of all surgical techniques needed to treat tumors, skin disease and aesthetically embarrassing conditions. Flaps and grafts are a major means to reconstruct defects after tumor surgery when primary wound closure is not possible. The principles of virtually all flaps and grafts have been well known for about a century and a half, but some refinements and new combinations have been described during the last few decades. Apart from microsurgical techniques, progress in dermatologic plastic surgery is mainly due to increased expertise, new drugs and materials. Nevertheless, even with the best drugs, the surgeon has to adhere to common surgical rules and must not be careless.[1-15]

Although illustrations often demonstrate marvellous results, the live situation is frequently different. The dermatologic surgeon must be able to react adequately to altered conditions.

Flaps are classified according to:

A. Donor region
   1. local
   2. regional
   3. distant flaps
B. Movement
   1. advancement
   2. rotation
   3. transposition
   4. island flaps
C. Tissue layers
   1. skin only
   2. composite flaps
D. Blood supply
   1. random pattern
   2. axial flaps

Dermatologic surgeons commonly use local flaps obtained from adjacent skin especially on the face, where the aesthetic and functional result has serious physical and psychological implications for the patient. Flaps offer optimal color and skin texture match. The use of flaps is essential for full-thickness defects of the nose, eyelids, lips and ears.[5,10,16] They require experience and planning, and it is not always possible to adhere to the preoperative flap design when the defect turns out to be different from what had been anticipated.

Local flaps are easier to perform in older people and difficult in children because of skin laxity or elasticity. Functional problems to consider preoperatively include ectropion, nasal obstruction and dislocation of the lips. The flap may be too thick and bulky, be hairbearing, or have the wrong color and texture. Anatomical landmarks have to be preserved to avoid obvious asymmetry. Flap failure is a serious sequela and ultimately leads to more scarring and poor functional and cosmetic results.

Complications may result from errors in judgment, planning and performance. The most serious complication is tumor persistence inevitably leading to recurrence. Although textbooks prefer to show neoplasms and the corresponding defects as geometric figures such as circles, ovals, rectangles or lozenges, no tumor will respect any of these fine figures and therefore the real flap design has to be different from the ideal one. Noticeable scarring, bulkiness and tissue distortion are usually due to design faults, whereas hematoma, damaged blood supply, and sutures under tension are mainly technical errors.[5] However, a design fault frequently leads to technical errors and often no clear-cut distinction is possible.

IMPROVEMENT OF FLAP SURVIVAL

Flaps are limited by the amount of movable skin available to cover the primary and donor defects. Technical errors such as a large flap extending beyond its blood supply may result from an initially good flap design. Imminent tip necrosis of the flap may be reversed by calcium channel blockers, drugs improving blood fluidity, hemodilution, progesterone, scavengers of free radicals plus allopurinol, repeated high doses of corticosteroids, and prostaglandin E_1 and prostacyclin.[16–19] Iloprost, a new stable carbaprostacycline derivative, has proved, in my experience, to improve blood supply, reduce cyanosis, and accelerate the disappearance of edema.[16]

Smoking has been shown not only to cause poor scars but also to significantly increase the risk of flap and full-thickness skin graft failure.[20] Smoking must be prohibited from the day before until at least 5 days postoperatively. However, even former smokers have an increased risk of developing flap necrosis.[20]

Hematoma is another risk factor for flap survival. Apart from meticulous hemostasis, a hemovac suction drainage may be necessary; its advantage is coaptation of tissues without exerting external pressure or obscuring the flap. Concentrated human fibrinogen may also be used, particularly for large defects. It seals minute vessels, thus reducing wound secretion, and 'glues' the flap to its new bed, thereby relieving tension from the sutures.[16] Fibrin glue even allows us to perform flaps in patients under anticoagulation.[21]

FACILITATION OF FLAP MOVEMENT

Even when classical areas of skin availability[5,10] are used, the flap skin may be relatively stiff and rigid. Both the flap and the skin of the donor area can be made more movable by blunt cannula dissection. Since suction has been shown to damage blood vessels of the subcutaneous septa, the strokes with the cannula should initially be performed without aspiration,[22] but may be repeated with light syringe suction.

The donor defect in areas with abundant subcutaneous fat tissue can usually be closed much more easily when the subcutaneous fat has been worked loose by gently inserting scissors and cautiously opening the blades vertically and by subsequent massage of the wound margins. The same is true for subcutaneous pedicle flaps; loosening of the stiff pedicle by making small channels through it, and a gentle massage, not only makes flap movement easier, but also greatly diminishes postoperative bulking. Another way to facilitate closure of large skin defects is presuturing. Preoperative stretching for 12–14 h increases the amount of skin available by stretch tension.[23,24] Intraoperative skin expansion is similarly effective.[25,26]

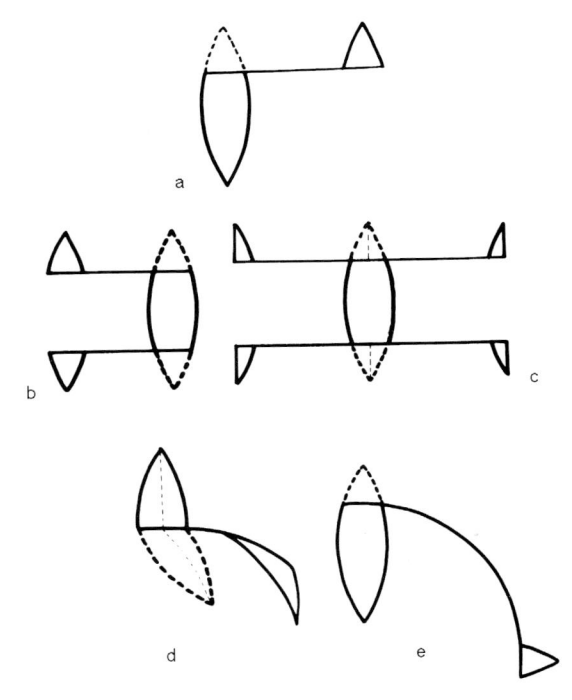

Figure 42.1
Idealized schematic illustration of advancement flaps. (a) Burow's advancement flap. (b) Rectangular advancement flap. (c) Double rectangular advancement flap. (d) Crescentic advancement flap. (e) Rotation flap.

Flaps frequently result in wounds of unequal lengths. In rotation flaps, this may be overcome by using the rule of halves or a running (locked) suture evenly distributing the excess tissue over the entire length of the wound. Burow's triangles are the most frequently used way of solving this problem. A triangle is excised from the longer side, enabling equal wound suture. One may also use a back cut, a V-Y advancement or a Z-plasty.

How can flaps be moved?

There are only three basic principles of flap design. The most frequently used flap is basically a fusiform excision divided into portions perpendicular to its long axis. The excision segments may be shifted linearly to yield simple advancement flaps or around a circular line to form a rotation flap (Figure 42.1). The crescentic flaps, although usually presented with sophisticated schematic drawings, are simply modifications of advancement flaps in which the long axis of the shifted portion has been curved.

The second basic movement is to take skin from an area of adjacent laxity and to transpose it into the defect. The various transposition flaps—bilobed, rhombic, Z-plasty etc.—are examples of this technique.

The third type of movement is sliding of tissue into a defect without Burow's triangles. The most simple technique is the V-Y advancement, which employs the principle of 90° shift of skin tension (Figure 42.2). If one cuts the skin between the defect and the V, the skin is converted into a subcutaneous pedicle island flap.

Although some flaps may include more than one principle of flap movement, and there is still some debate (for example on how to classify a bilobed flap) it is important to know the major types of flap movement and how to use each flap for a given defect and region.[16,27]

Forehead and Temple

Due to the underlying bone, only small and medium-sized defects can usually be closed primarily.[2,3] The median forehead, suprabrow and temple have skin available for direct closure or flap elevation.[5,10] Undermining should be done in the subcutis below the subdermal vascular plexus, since this yields more skin than the easier subfascial dissection.[28,29] However, the central forehead portion is nourished by vertically ascending arteries which have to be preserved to avoid flap necrosis. Large defects of the forehead should therefore, if possible, be closed by flaps not cutting the afferent vessels. Many

SURGICAL DERMATOLOGY

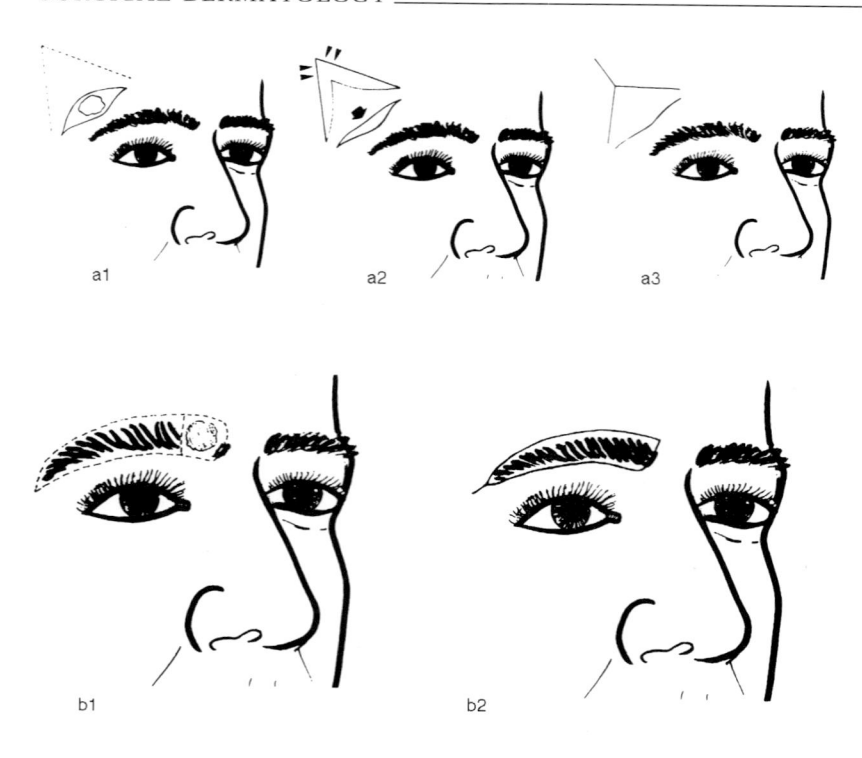

Figure 42.2
V-Y advancement and subcutaneous pedicle flap. (a) V-Y advancement of a skin bridge allows us to virtually avoid distortion of the contralateral wound margin: a1, design; a2, skin undermined and mobilized; a3, suture lines. (b) Subcutaneous pedicle (island) flap: b1, flap includes entire eyebrow; the design allows meticulous preparation of flap pedicle, leaving the arteries which cross it intact; b2, suture lines indicating good cosmetic result.

defects can be transformed into roughly triangular shape, allowing rotation flaps or two Burow advancement flaps to form an A-T-plasty (Figure 42.3).

Many textbooks recommend the bilateral H-plasty advancement flap.[2,3] This cuts horizontally through the forehead, leaving large flaps at risk for necrosis, and the scar is usually quite obvious, even when there are deep frown lines. The double rotation flap has one incision at the frontal hairline and one in suprabrow skin which risks cutting the arterial blood supply. Furthermore, the incision when performed as a circle line will be visible and should therefore be modified according to Figure 42.3. This will hide the scar much better. A major concern is to avoid eyebrow asymmetry which may occur after removal of tumors above the eyebrow. Defects includ-

ing the median eyebrow portion may be closed using a subcutaneous pedicle flap. This incorporates the eyebrow and replaces its paramedian origin, which is cosmetically more important than its lateral end (Figure 42.2B).[30] Rhomboid flaps and different modifications such as the LLL flap[31] or the Webster 30° flap[32] are quite useful for reconstruction since incisions can be placed into frown lines. More detailed approaches are described by Jackson,[5] Dzubow[13,28] and many other authors.

EYELIDS

The periocular region includes the eyelids and lateral and medial canthi. The eyelid skin is very thin and usually pale. The subcutaneous tissue is thin and loose, usually does not contain much fat and has

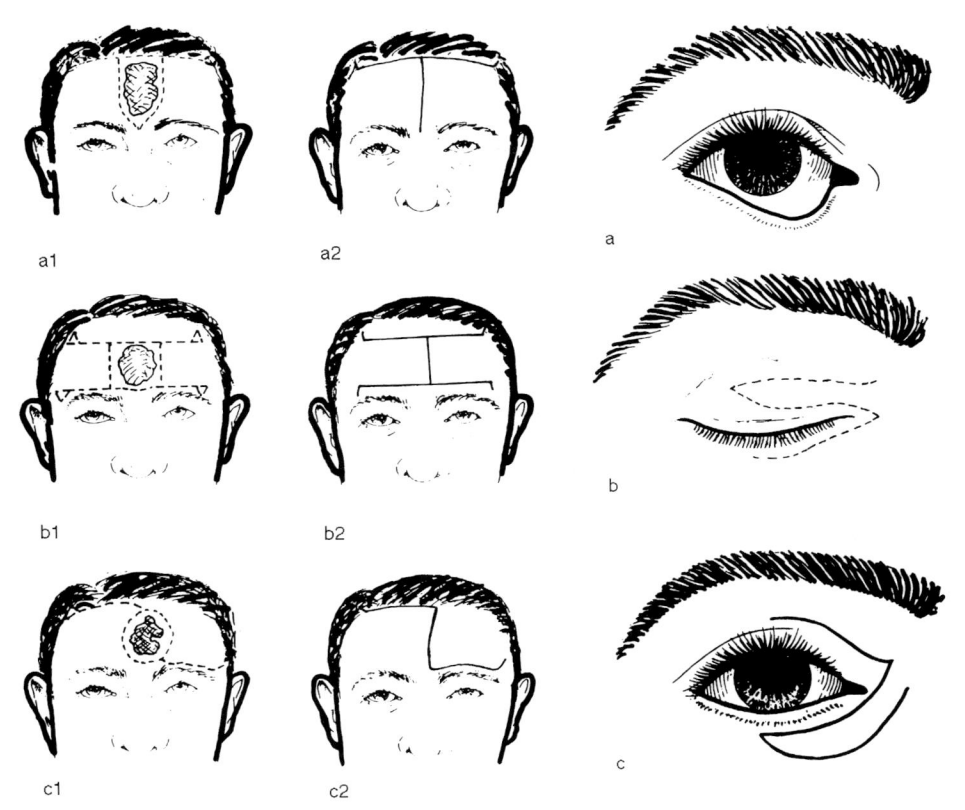

Figure 42.3
Advancement flaps for mid-forehead repair. (a) A-T closure (double Burow's advancement): a1, incision lines; a2, suture lines. (b) Double rectangular advancement flaps (H-plasty): b1, incision lines; b2, suture lines. (c) Double rotation flaps: c1, incision lines slightly modified to avoid grossly visible areas; c2, suture lines.

Figure 42.4
Ectropion repair with medial Tripier flap. (a) Ectropion. (b) Incision lines. (c) Suture lines.

a tendency to swell and become lax. A vertical excess of skin develops with age that may be used for defect closure. Symmetry of the palpebral openings is of utmost aesthetic importance and both ectropion and entropion must be avoided.

Whenever possible eyelid defects which cannot be closed primarily should be repaired using skin from the opposing lid. This is known as the Tripier flap[33] and is essentially a bridge flap from the upper lid to restore the entire surface of the lower lid. It may also be used as a single pedicle transposition flap to cover up to two-thirds of the eyelid. The medially based Tripier flap is an excellent technique to avoid an ectropion after tumor resection of the medial aspect of the lower lid as well as to repair a postoperative ectropion (Figure 42.4).

Large defects of the lower lid may be closed with a cheek rotation flap. Almost all schematic illustrations[5] show flap designs which do not demonstrate the

SURGICAL DERMATOLOGY

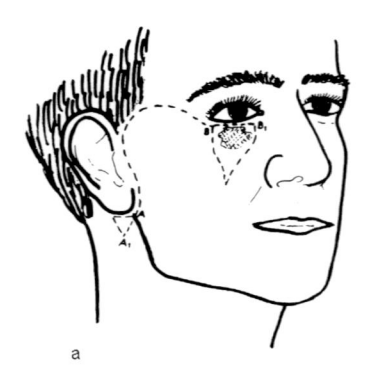

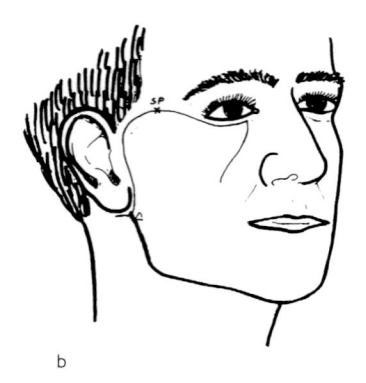

Figure 42.5
Cheek rotation flap for defect of lower eyelid. (a) Flap design with incision line going up over the zygomatic arch; the flap is sutured here to the temporal fascia which acts as a suspension point (SP). (b) Suture lines showing that suspension of cheek flap to temporal fascia and lateral wall of nasal bridge avoids ectropion.

relatively heavy cheek skin which is pulled up, thus risking lower lid ectropion. The incision line for the cheek rotation flap should go up over the palpebral line on the temple. When the flap is rotated, preauricular skin will be suspended to the superficial temporal fascia, avoiding tension to the lower lid. The innermost tip of the flap is sutured to the periosteum of the lateral aspect of the root of the nose. The cheek flap has a large wound surface which should be sealed with human fibrinogen glue to avoid seroma formation[21] otherwise a suction drain is mandatory (Figure 42.5).

NASAL ROOT AND GLABELLA

The side of the nasal root and the medial canthus are frequently the site of skin tumors. Depending on the size of the defect primary closure, grafts or flaps may be used; however, this area gives surprisingly good cosmetic results after second intention healing. The flaps most commonly used are the glabella rotation flap, the glabella median forehead transposition flap, or the subcutaneous pedicle flap from the paranasal area.

The glabella rotation flap is the time-honored approach but care must be taken not to include eyebrows. This can usually be prevented by changing the direction of rotation. By staying away from the eyebrow, one avoids bringing the thick glabella skin directly adjacent to the fine eyelid skin. However, the glabella rotation flap has fixed dimensions and does not allow closure of large defects.

Large defects can be closed using a median glabella transposition flap. The design is easy and avoids the transfer of eyebrows if the glabella is not hirsute. The secondary defect can usually easily be closed by direct suture. The older the patient, the easier this flap is to carry out, since the glabella skin becomes softer and more movable with age.

Defects at the inner aspect of the lower lid and medial eye corner can also be closed with subcutaneous pedicle flaps. This flap has to be adapted to the thinner skin by gently loosening its pedicle through multiple tunnels achieved by a round-tipped cannula. Suction should not be instituted to avoid damage to its vessels. The advantage of this flap is the ease with which it is raised and moved into the defect. When properly sutured and suspended it will gently tighten the medial aspect of the cheek and prevent ectropion formation. This is possible since the vertical tension from the flap movement can be transformed into horizontal tension in the

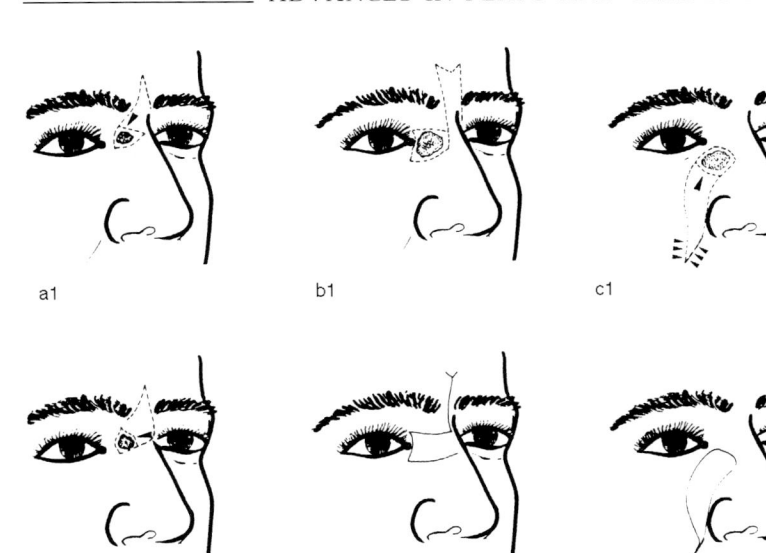

Figure 42.6
Closure of defects in inner eye corner. (a) Glabella rotation flap: a1, with contralateral base; a2, with ipsilateral base. (b) Median forehead transposition flap with M-plasty at donor site: b1, flap design; b2, suture lines. (c) Subcutaneous pedicle flap: c1, incision lines; c2, flap sutured in place.

cheek and since the flap can be suspended to the periosteum of the side of the nasal bridge (Figure 42.6).

NOSE

The nose is one of the most complicated aesthetic structures of the face. More than 40% of all nonmelanoma skin cancers are located on the nose and a plethora of different flaps has been described to repair nasal defects. However, sometimes a combination of two or more flaps or grafts may be necessary to cover large defects or those going beyond the limits of an aesthetic unit.[34,35] Skin color, texture and appearance vary in the different subunits of the nose. Thus moving skin from 'far away' may not be cosmetically better than using a full-thickness skin graft. The method ultimately used should provide the best form, contour, color and skin texture and not cause deformity in the donor area.

Defects on the nose are usually round. U-shaped or rhombic flaps may be raised from nasal areas with lax skin or from the cheek nearby. For the nasal tip and ala, adjacent skin should be used to avoid differences in color and texture. If this is not possible a bilobed flap may be used[36,37] to gradually adapt the flap skin to its new surroundings. If the pivot point of the bilobed flap is near the tip of the nose, the skin is rather stiff and rotation may be difficult. To compensate for an apparent loss of flap length with rotation the second portion of the bilobed flap has to be longer than the first one.[34,37] The second flap may be taken from an area which is less conspicuous so that the excess of scar lines will not be cosmetically embarrassing.

The heminose flap is an extended glabella flap and may be used to close defects on the tip of the nose. This flap can be designed as a random pattern[38] or an axial pattern flap.[39] The latter has recently been described in detail.[40]

The cascade flap separates the heminose flap into a Marchac rotation flap and a glabella flap. This allows the lower nasal flap to be transposed down more readily. The secondary defect is closed with the glabella flap using a V-Y slide or a transposition to the upper portion of the

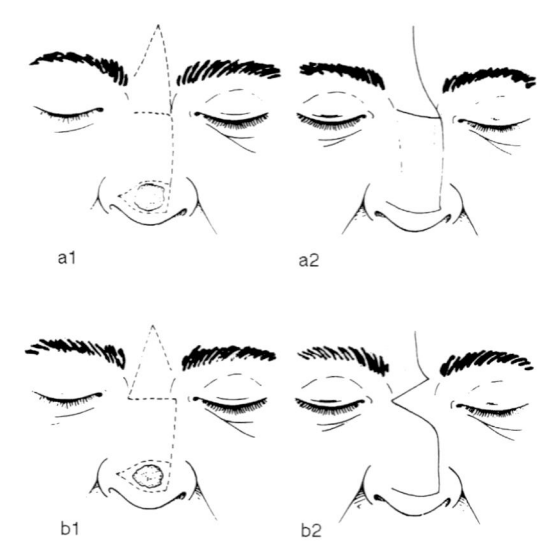

Figure 42.7
Emmett's cascade flap for defects of the nasal tip and dorsum: a1, a2, flaps with ipsilateral bases; b1, b2, contralaterally based flaps.

nasal bridge. The glabella flap is based on the supratrochlear artery and the nasal flap is supplied by the vascular pedicle to the dorsum of the nose originating from the angular artery. Both arteries are connected by the dorsal nasal artery, which is fed by the ophthalmic and angular arteries (Figure 42.7).[41]

Alternatives for nasal tip repair are the nasolabial transposition flap, the Rintala flap, the pinch modification of the linear advancement flap, and a bilateral rotation flap with its pivot point being placed into the columella. The nasolabial flap is not difficult and allows coverage of relatively large defects. Pincushioning almost never occurs and, in males, hair-bearing skin must not be transposed to the tip of the nose. This flap allows one to reshape pronounced convexities and concavities of nasal ala and tip and is suitable for full-thickness alar defects since its distal tip can be turned in to repair the mucosal defect.

The Rintala advancement flap is a long narrow random pattern advancement flap.[42] It provides matching skin for the nasal tip, but it is often difficult to achieve sufficient advancement. The nose may be shortened, the frontonasal angle may be flattened and, above all, the distal end is at risk of ischemia. Scarring may also be relatively conspicuous.

A bilateral rotation flap technique[43] was proposed to repair the nasal tip. Its major advantages are the use of immediate adjacent skin with an optimal match, short incision lines, and confinement to only two cosmetic units. This flap is easy to execute but it is not suitable for medium-sized and large defects. A round to oval defect is transformed into a triangular one with its tip pointing to the columella. A small rotation flap is designed on each side and the defect closed by moving the flaps towards each other.

The pinch modification of the linear advancement flap[44] is a technique for defect closure where insufficient skin is available right next to the wound. It combines the features of an advancement flap with those of a bilateral rotation flap. The wound margins are pinched together to allow final suture of the defect.

Defects of the paramedian aspect of the nasal tip may be repaired using the perialar crescentic rotation flap,[37,45] the nasalis myocutaneous sliding flap[46,47] and again the various modifications of the extended glabella flap. The perialar rotation flap is a versatile technique for the repair of small defects near the ala nasi. The incision line is placed into the natural alar groove and a crescentic portion of skin is removed laterally. The major part of the incision is hidden in the alar groove (Figure 42.8). The horizontal J rotation flap is essentially a variation of the perialar crescentic rotation flap with a classical Burow's triangle

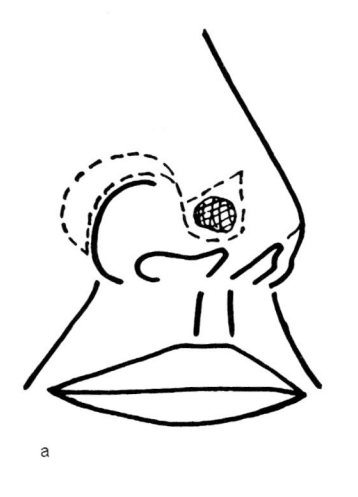

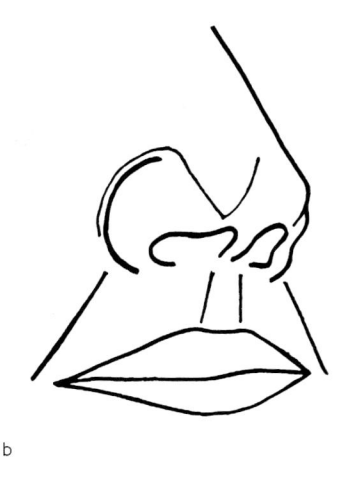

Figure 42.8
Perialar crescentic rotation flap. (a) Design. (b) Suture lines.

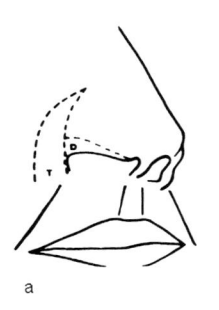

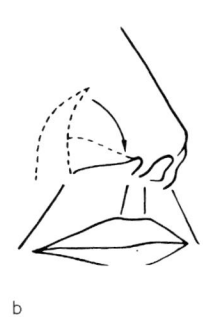

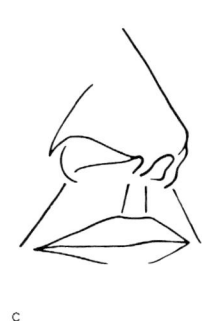

Figure 42.9
Reconstruction of alar rim defect with the hinged turn-down flap (Field).[49] (a) Defect and flap design. Width of transposition flap T is double that of defect width D. (b) Hinged turn-down flap raised. (c) Perinasal transposition sutured on turn-down flap of alar rim.

instead of a crescent.[48] The nasalis myocutaneous sliding flap is an axial subcutaneous pedicle flap based on the lateral nasal artery, which is a branch of the angular artery supplying the nasal muscle.

Nasal rim deformities are not uncommon, especially after tumor excision and trauma. An interesting approach to repair the alar rim was proposed utilizing a perinasal transposition flap overlying a hinged 'turn-down' flap. A supradefect incision is made, measuring as much as the entire defect makes up. The skin is carefully dissected to half the alar thickness and opened. This provides a base for a thin transposition flap from the perinasal cheek skin. The flap is trimmed to match the thickness of the ala, the donor defect is closed after undermining its lateral side and the flap is sutured on to the hinged alar turn-down flap. The flap base (T) is double the width of the alar defect (D) (Figure 42.9). This allows reconstruction of a normal alar rim.[49]

The columella is difficult to reconstruct because there is no excess skin immediately adjacent to it. Lesions up to 10 mm wide may be closed by simple or double advancement with a V-Y closure (Figure 42.10).

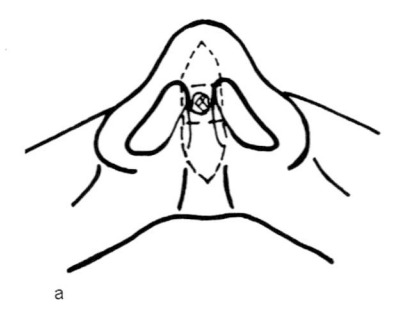

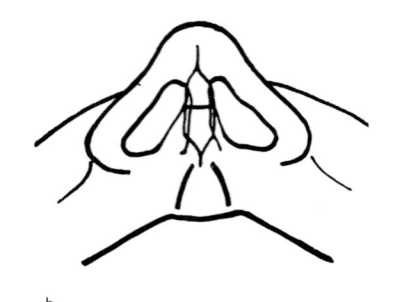

Figure 42.10
Double subcutaneous pedicle flap technique for defect of the columella. (a) Flap design. (b) Suture lines.

CHEEK

The cheeks are made up of skin exhibiting different color, texture, thickness and hair growth. These differences have to be kept in mind when one plans a flap. Under the skin, there is a superficial musculo-aponeurotic system (SMAS) which is continuous with the platysma of the neck. The facial nerve has to be respected when incisions are performed in the lateral cheek–preauricular area.

Depending on the size and site of the defect, as well as skin laxity and movability, cheek rotation, advancement, transposition, bilobed or rhombic flaps may be used. The perialar crescentic advancement flap is a particularly useful technique for cheek defects adjacent to the ala nasi. Although it produces long scars, these are placed in natural folds and soon become virtually invisible. When the defect is created, two gently curved fusiform pieces of skin are excised along the alar groove and in the nasolabial fold. Starting from the superior incision point the flap is advanced with the suture through an approximation of the longer lateral wound edge to the shorter medial one (Figure 42.11).

UPPER LIP

The upper lip is a very delicate structure without bony support. The philtrum and cupid's bow are extremely difficult structures to reconstruct. There are a great number of flaps available dating back to the mid-1800s. Only the crescentic perialar advancement flap will be mentioned here since it is a very elegant and time-honored method. It may be performed as a unilateral or bilateral flap for defects of labial skin or full-thickness lip defects. This technique can be combined with a typical

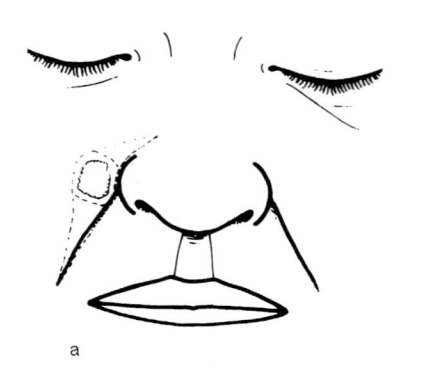

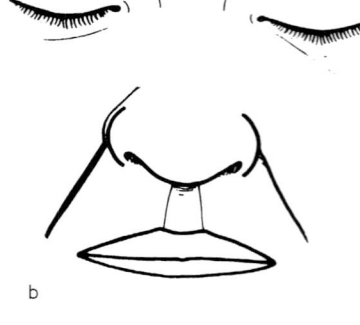

Figure 42.11
Perinasal cheek advancement flap. (a) Incision lines. (b) Suture lines.

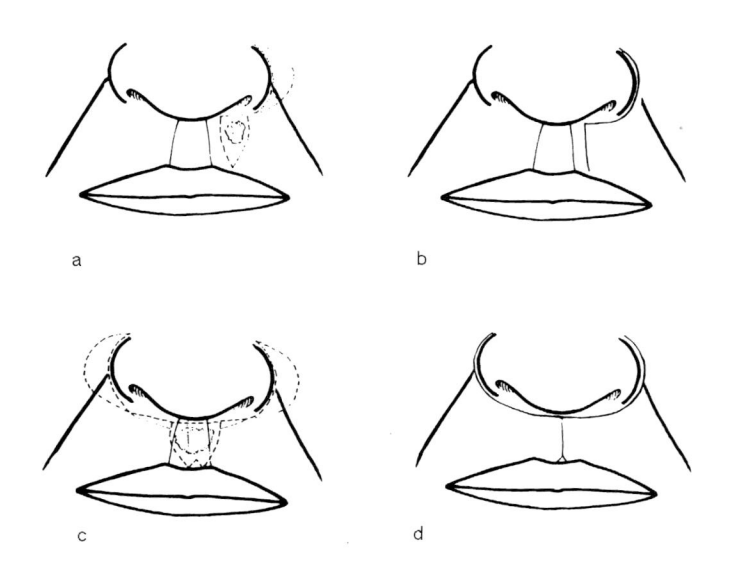

Figure 42.12
Perinasal crescentic advancement flap for small to medium-sized defect of upper lip. (a) Incision and suture lines of simple advancement flap. (b) Incision and suture lines of double advancement flap. A broad base will result in vertical wound margins which are considerably longer than the height of the upper lip; to avoid distortion of the vermilion border; narrow horizontal skin wedges have to be removed.

wedge excision. Problems may arise when skin wedges are sutured and the new suture line is longer than the initial height of the lip. This will result in a protuberance at the vermilion border which usually remains visible. It should be corrected while bearing in mind the natural scar shrinkage. Suturing has to begin at the superior tips of the perialar crescents, which automatically advances the flaps; it is then continued at the tip of the wedge. This shows the excess in scar length which can be trimmed to avoid a lip protuberance (Figure 42.12). It sometimes helps give the impression of a philtrum when situated favorably. Sketches in textbooks show a preserved philtrum and cupid's bow. In reality, this is not possible in most cases. Extensive loss of lip and reconstruction with any advancement flap will also flatten the nasolabial fold, sometimes necessitating a second operation on the other side of the mouth. In the case of a centrally located defect, a bilateral advancement flap may be used.

Relatively large defects can be closed in elderly people using a subcutaneous pedicle flap. While the size of the defect determines the width of the flap base, its length can be selected to reach the area of skin availability without risk of distortion of the labial commissure (Figure 42.13).

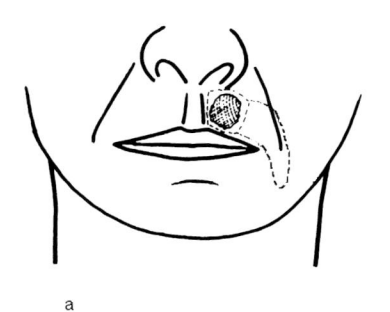

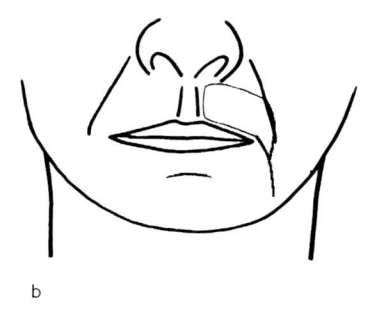

Figure 42.13
Subcutaneous pedicle island flap for large defect of lateral aspect of upper lip. (a) Flap design. (b) Flap sutured in place.

SURGICAL DERMATOLOGY

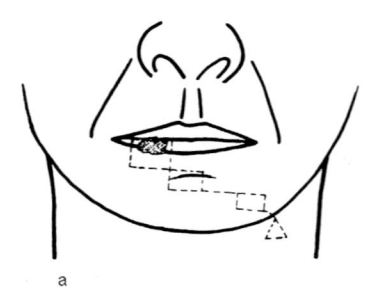

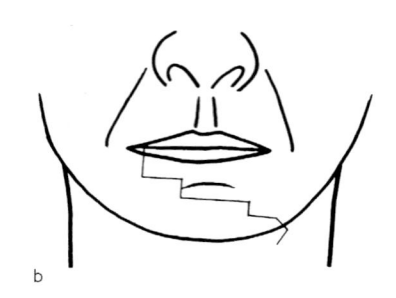

Figure 42.14
Step technique for closure of lower lip defect. (a) Incision lines. (b) Suture lines.

LOWER LIP

Squamous cell carcinomas are frequently found on the lower lip and sometimes require large excisions. Reconstructive techniques are described in many textbooks.[2,5] Wedge excisions are commonly performed and are often found to be entirely satisfactory for lesions measuring up to a quarter of the lip. Usually, a W-plasty instead of a simple V is advantageous since the closure better matches the natural contour lines of the labiomental fold. For defects measuring up to a third of the lip, a step advancement flap has been found to be very useful. It divides long incision lines and allows an excellent approximation of the wound edges. A transverse 1–2-cm incision is made from the base of the postexcisional defect on one side, then a vertical incision of about 1 cm and again a transverse incision of 1–2 cm. A rectangular tissue block of about three-quarters of the width of the original defect is excised at the end of the first transverse excision, and then three-quarters of the second defect at the end of the second transverse excision, etc. The last tissue block to be excised is a triangle to allow easy wound closure.[50] This procedure may also be performed as a bilateral step flap or be combined with Gillie's fan flap or other techniques[51] (Figure 42.14).

LIP COMMISSURE

Repair of commissure defects is delicate since the normal contralateral commissure remains for comparisons. Most textbook

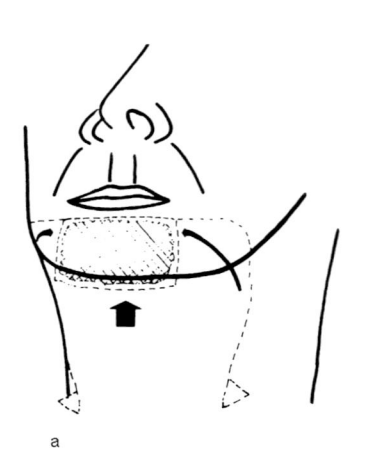

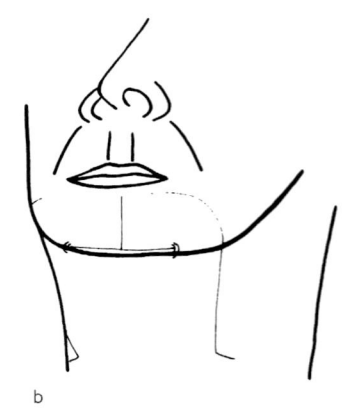

Figure 42.15
Advancement flap with double rotation flaps to reconstruct chin.[53] (a) Flap design. (b) Flap sutured in place.

sketches of major upper and lower lip reconstruction show symmetrical commissures. In most cases, this is impossible to obtain. The A-T approach may be a valuable technique for the reconstruction of medium-sized defects from skin tumors of the commissure. A triangular defect is created with its tip pointing to the commissure and its base parallel to the nasomental fold. An incision is performed along or parallel to this fold and the defect is sutured from its tip to its base. The secondary crescentic defect is easily closed by the rule of halves or by a crescentic advancement procedure. The final result is a scar which is hardly visible.[52]

CHIN

Most textbooks do not specifically describe reconstructive techniques for the chin. This probably reflects the relative rarity of tumors in this area. Large skin tumors may occur on the chin and pose reconstructive problems. Any inferiorly based flap on the chin may pull the lower lip down. We have designed a technique combining an advancement flap carrying bilateral rotation flaps at its tip.[53]

For the replacement of virtually the entire chin, incisions are made transversely from the top of the defect on both sides. They extend semicircularly around the mandibular arch to the submental area. Two Burow's triangles are cut at the level above the larynx and the entire flap is moved up. The two rotation flaps are sutured end to end. Since their upper part is tighter than the lower one, the flap rests on the chin and does not pull down the lower lip (Figure 42.15).

GLANS PENIS

Erythroplasia of Queyrat and superficial squamous cell carcinoma of the glans do not need amputation of the glans or distal third of the penis as is usually done by urologists. Defects extending right into the corpus cavernosum glandis and of virtually the entire glans surface can adequately be covered using the external sheet of the foreskin.[54,55] If the lesion to be excised is large, this operation should be done under general anesthesia since a penis block does not normally last long enough. It is wise to infiltrate the sublesional area with a mixture of bupivacaine, a very long-acting local anesthetic, and ornipressin (POR 8), a vasoconstrictor without the epinephrine-typical postvasoconstriction hyperemia. Once the lesion is completely removed, a modified circumcision is performed, leaving a part of the external preputial lamina corresponding to the size of the glans defect. This preputial flap is fixed to the base of the defect with human fibrinogen glue to avoid postoperative bleeding and hematoma, and sutured using 5-0 chromic or 6-0 monofilament sutures. This technique allows coverage of the entire glans, providing optimal cosmetic and functional results.[54–57] Although penile lesions are exceptional in circumcised men they may occur and can be treated with a modified transposition flap using penile shaft skin.[55]

DIGITS

Defects of the fingers and toes that cannot be primarily closed may be left for second intention healing, grafting or flaps. Small flaps such as those needed for repair after excision of myxoid pseudocysts may be designed as a transposition, rotation or advancement flap with V-Y closure. Large defects of nearly an entire phalanx may need a regional or distant flap; for example, the defect resulting from extirpation of the entire nail organ can be reconstructed by a muff plasty with temporary implantation of the finger under abdominal skin[58] or by a cross-digit flap which is applicable both for fingers and the lesser toes. The latter technique is less uncomfortable since the hand does not need to be fixed to the abdomen for 3 weeks and it is much easier to splint the two digits together as needed. A template is made of the future defect and transferred to the other digit, keeping in mind the distance from the donor digit to the defect. The flap is incised all around but not fully raised. This delay enhances its survival, which otherwise would not be optimal.[16] About a week later the flap is raised and sutured in place, and the donor defect is closed with a full-thickness skin graft. Utmost care has to be taken to splint the digits together without tension to the flap and without impairing the blood circulation of the digits and the flap pedicle. This can be cut after 18–21 days and the digits remodeled. This flap is particularly useful for defects of the terminal phalanx.

Z-PLASTIES AND V-Y ADVANCEMENT

The Z-plasty is an exchange of triangular flaps resulting in an increase in length in the central limb axis of the Z. Multiple Z-plasties may be used to release a long scar contracture. These are usually done with the Zs in the same direction. A combination of two Zs in opposite direction and a central V-Y advancement, also called the five-flap technique, has been shown to be useful for the release of scars in finger webs and of epicanthal folds.[59] It gives maximal vertical elongation and avoids fluctuation of perpendicular advancement needed for the exchange of triangular flaps. The V-Y advancement between two alternating Z-plasties reduced this fluctuation and gives further elongation. A series of alternating five-flap designs has been proposed instead of a multiple Z-plasty.[60] This technique avoids the long limbs created by the latter technique which itself may give rise to scar contracture.

NEW FLAPS

A meshed advancement flap was described by Motley and Holt[61] for defects of the lower leg that cannot be closed primarily. The skin adjacent to the defect was undermined circumferentially for about 3 cm in the superficial fat. The most favorable axis of closure was chosen by gently pulling the wound edges with skin hooks. Tension-relieving incisions were made, each about 1 cm in length, 1 cm from the margin and 1 cm apart, in the axis of the wound closure. The wound margins were then approximated and sutured without tension, leaving a grossly diminished primary and several small secondary defects. Second intention healing is favored using dressings with antimicrobial ointments. Healing time depends on the size of the defects, but is considerably shorter. In our experience this technique is also useful for defects of the forearm.

Round and oval defects usually yield dog-ears when sutured primarily. An O-to-Z closure can be performed or the dog-ears may be used to create kite flaps, subcutaneous pedicle flaps, or transposition flaps.[62] The latter is executed after undermining and intentionally producing dog-ears with a central holding pully suture. The dog-ears are picked up with fine hooks and pulled laterally to opposite sides. Transposition flaps are marked and cut. The descending limbs of the transposition flaps are extended to the origin of the descending ones. The flaps are undermined, raised, and transposed 90° into the defect. If necessary the descending limb is lengthened obliquely to increase flap mobility and widen its pedicle. The holding suture is released and the donor defects are closed primarily. The two transposition flaps are sutured to each other and to the surrounding tissue. Since the lengths of the wound margins are not equal the sutures should evenly distribute excess lengths. The final scar will have an S shape with two verticle lines.

MODIFICATION OF THE ROTATION FLAP TO AVOID TIP AND MARGIN NECROSIS[63]

Tips and margins of rotation flaps are at risk of necrosis when they are sutured into the defect under tension. This risk is particularly high when the tip has an angle below 90°. Rotation flaps should therefore be designed with rounded tips to shorten the distance of blood circulation from the base to the tip. A V-shaped skin point is thus created (Figure 42.16a). The flap is then rotated into the defect and a short incision is made into the flap opposite the point (Figure 42.16b). Expanding the flap creates a V-shaped defect fitting into the point. This also prolongs the rotation flap along its transverse axis thereby reducing the tension by decreasing the rotation angle (Figure 42.16c). Furthermore, the wedge-shaped fixation adds to the support of the flap (Figure 42.16d).

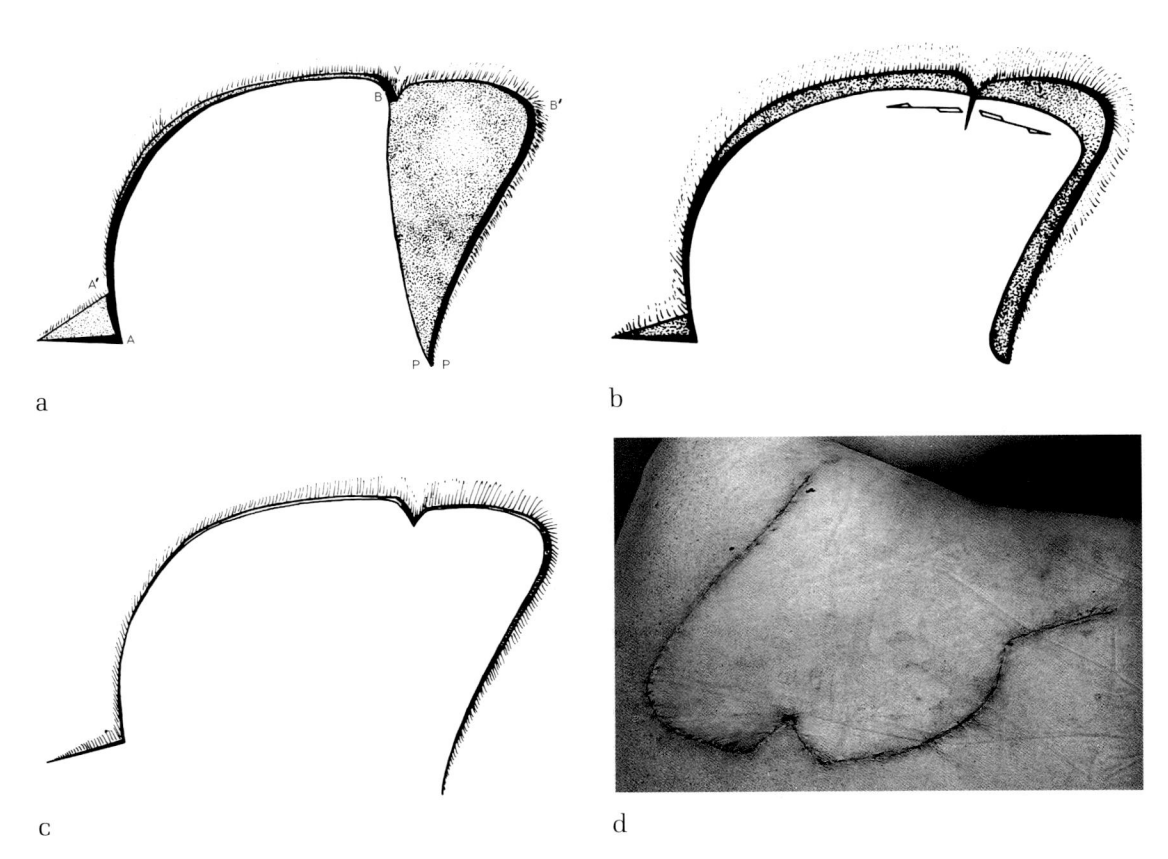

Figure 42.16
Modification of the rotation flap to avoid tip and margin necrosis. (a) Rounding the excision defect and the tip of the rotation flap creates a V-shaped point (V) on the rotation circumference. (b) An incision in the flap opposite the V-shaped point allows us to expand the rotation flap; this makes AB almost as long as A'B'. (c) Flap sutured in place. (d) Flap repair of a defect on scapular region. AB is considerably shorter than A'B' which will become the line of maximal tension. V, V-shaped point. pp, pivot point. (From ref. 63, by permission of the author.)

Grafts

Skin grafts are standard procedures in dermatologic surgery and there are only a few new facts. Graft survival is enhanced when alcoholic beverages are prohibited for 1 week, starting 2 days prior to the operation. Alcohol was found to interfere with neutrophil functions.[64] Smoking also impairs circulation of the recipient wound and decreases the survival changes of free grafts.[20]

Delayed grafting is more frequently used. Large deep defects left from melanoma surgery are first allowed to granulate. When the granulation tissue has reached the surface level it is grafted with split- or full-thickness skin. This technique avoids deep holes which inevitably remain when there is considerable adipose tissue and the defect extends down to the fascia.

A major disadvantage of grafts is a permanent patch appearance which is often due to the distant donor area having a different skin color and texture. This can be partly overcome by using facial skin for facial defects: preauricular[65] or subauricular skin[66] is sun-exposed, readily available and easy to prepare, and the defect can be closed with a running intracutaneous suture or a V-Y advancement technique.

Round defect margins may interfere with cosmetic subunits of the donor area and make the graft appear more conspicuous. The addition of W-plasties on the lateral margins of nasal defects may suffice to obscure the scar line between the graft and the donor area.[67]

There are several clever proposals to use skin immediately adjacent to the defect. Dog-ears have often been used, but Burow's triangles may also be suitable for covering residual defects.[68] They fulfill the criteria of color and texture match although even this type of graft may retain a patch appearance. Salasche et al[69] proposed using residual flap tissue as a delayed graft when detaching a median forehead flap from its recipient site.

Improvement of Flap Appearance

Some authors routinely use dermabrasion to enhance the appearance of skin grafts. This greatly obscures the sharp border between the graft and the surrounding skin and can also smooth a step formation.[70] (See Chapter 40.)

Reversed Dermal Graft

Dermal grafts have not frequently been used in dermatologic surgery although they can be a powerful tool in certain difficult areas.[71,72] Dermal grafts are now often used in orthopedic surgery as a substitute for facia lata and dura mata because of the mechanical resistance of dermis. The connective tissue is cell-poor, best quality, virtually nonshrinking and may even be grafted on bone without periosteum. First, a thin split-thickness graft is taken, leaving its pedicle intact. It is reflected back, exposing the superficial dermis with its abundant fine vessels. A portion of the dermis is incised according to the size of the defect to be covered and the graft is harvested in the same manner as a full-thickness skin graft. The fat is stripped from the base and the graft is laid on the defect upside down. It contains viable connective tissue with natural orientation of its collagen and elastic fibers, but relatively few cells, and therefore it is not demanding. It is sewn into the defect with slight tension and a cotton or rubber-foam stent is fixed over it; care has to be taken to avoid drying of its surface. The graft usually takes after about 7–10 days, depending on the quality of the recipient site. Hair follicles degenerate within a few weeks. Remnants of sweat glands and all pilo-arrector muscles remain. Surprisingly, cyst formation has not been observed. The graft gradually develops granulation tissue on its surface and may epithelialize from the cut follicles; however, at that stage, it can be overgrafted with split- or full-thickness skin grafts. Especially on the soles, the reversed dermal graft provides an excellent base for a skin graft, enhancing its mechanical properties. If considered useful, it may be overgrafted with a second dermal graft before it is covered with a skin graft. Dermal grafts in the oral cavity may take on the appearance of oral mucosa.

The reversed dermal graft can also be used as a mesh graft,[73] reducing the size of the donor area. Recently a composite reversed dermal and split-thickness skin graft has been described[74] which combines the excellent take and the advantages of a full-thickness skin graft.

PREPARATION OF MESH GRAFTS

Mesh grafts are indicated for covering large wound areas and leg ulcers. There are several costly instruments available for different mesh sizes. However, in many cases no sophisticated machine is necessary. Bertényi[75] takes a strip of firm paper about 1.5–2 cm wide, rolls the split-thickness skin graft over it and cuts it alternately on each side at regular intervals. A similar method was described by Yanai and Hiraga[76] but they fold the skin in a zig-zag manner.

REFERENCES

1. Epstein E, Epstein E Jr, *Skin surgery*, 7th edn (Saunders: Philadelphia 1987).
2. Petres J, Hundeiker M, *Korrektive Dermatologie. Operationen an der Haut* (Springer: Berlin–Heidelberg–New York 1975).
3. Petres J, Hundeiker M, *Dermatosurgery* (Springer: Berlin–Heidelberg–New York 1978).
4. Harahap M, *Skin surgery* (WH Green: St Louis 1984).
5. Jackson IT, *Local flaps in head and neck reconstruction* (CV Mosby: St Louis 1985).
6. Kaufmann R, Landes E, *Dermatologische Operationen* (Thieme: Stuttgart–New York 1987).
7. Schulz H, *Operative Dermatologie im Gesicht* (Diesbach: Berlin 1988).
8. Harahap M, *Principles of dermatologic plastic surgery* (PMA Publishing Corp: New York 1988).
9. Bennett RG, *Fundamentals of cutaneous surgery* (CV Mosby: St Louis 1988).
10. Salasche SJ, Bernstein G, Senkarik M, *Surgical anatomy of the skin* (Appleton & Lange: Norwalk CN 1988).
11. Tromovitch TA, Stegman SJ, Glogau RG, *Flaps and grafts in dermatologic surgery* (Year Book: Chicago 1989).
12. Roenigk RK, Roenigk HH Jr, *Dermatologic surgery. Principles and practice* (Marcel Dekker: New York–Basel 1989).
13. Dzubow LM, *Facial flaps: biomechanics and regional application* (Appleton & Lange: Norwalk, CN 1990).
14. Moy RL, *Atlas of cutaneous facial flaps and grafts: a differential diagnosis of wound closures* (Lea & Febiger: Philadelphia 1990).
15. Fewkes JL, Cheney ML, Pollack SV, *Illustrated atlas of cutaneous surgery* (Gower: New York–London 1991).
16. Haneke E, Indications for skin flaps and mechanism of flap survival. In: Harahap M, ed., *Principles of dermatologic plastic surgery* (PMA Publishing Corp: New York 1988).
17. Yessenow RS, Garner SL, Bauer CA et al, The effects of calcium channel blockers on random skin flap survival in the pig model, *Eur J Plast Surg* (1991) **14**:3–6.
18. Ata Uysal O, The effect of progesterone hormone on the viability of flaps, *Eur J Plast Surg* (1991) **14**:192–6.

19. Salemark L, Wieslander JB, Dougan P et al, Infusion of prostacyclin reduces in vivo thrombus formation following arteriotomy/intimectomy in small arteries. An experimental study in the rabbit, *Eur J Plast Surg* (1991) **14**:89–93.

20. Goldminz D, Bennett RG, Cigarette smoking and flap and full-thickness graft necrosis, *Arch Dermatol* (1991) **127**:1012–15.

21. Staindl O, Indikationen der Fibrinklebung zur lokalen Blutstillung und Gewebssynthese in der Dermatochirurgie, In: Petres J, ed., *Aktuelle Behandlungsverfahren*, Fortschritte der Operativen Dermatologie 3 (Springer: Berlin–Heidelberg–New York 1987) 36–47.

22. Ozcan G, Shenag S, Baldwin B et al, The trauma of suction-assisted lipectomy cannula on flap circulation in rats, *Plast Reconstr Surg* (1991) **88**:250–8.

23. Liang MD, Briggs P, Heckler FR et al, Presuturing—a new technique for closing large skin defects: clinical and experimental studies, *Plast Reconstr Surg* (1988) **81**:694–702.

24. Hedén P, Presuturing in rhytidectomy: a case report, *Aesthet Plast Surg* (1991) **15**:161–5.

25. Sasaki GH, Intraoperative sustained limited expansion (ISLE) as an immediate reconstructive technique, *Clin Plast Surg* (1987) **14**:563–73.

26. Greenbaum SS, Greenbaum CH, Intraoperative tissue expansion using a Foley catheter following excision of a basal cell carcinoma, *J Dermatol Surg Oncol* (1990) **16**:45–8.

27. Haneke E, Criteria and techniques of flaps. In: Panconesi E, ed., *Dermatology in Europe* (Blackwell: Oxford 1991) 22–4.

28. Dzubow LM, Flap dynamics, *J Dermatol Surg Oncol* (1991) **17**:116–30.

29. Siegle RJ, Forehead reconstruction, *J Dermatol Surg Oncol* (1991) **17**:200–4.

30. Hartschuh W, Kohl PH, Kisiel U et al, Das mikrozystische desmoplastische Adnex-Karzinom. In: Meigel W, Lengen W, Schwenzer G, eds, *Diagnostik und Therapie maligner Melanome*, Fortschritte der Operativen Dermatologie 6 (Diesbach, Berlin 1991) 95–7.

31. Dufourmentel C, La fermeture des pertes de substance cutanées limitées. Le lambeau de rotation en L pour losange, dit 'LLL', *Ann Chir Plast* (1962) **7**:61.

32. Webster RC, Davidson TM, Smirk RC, The thirty degree transposition flap, *Laryngoscope* (1978) **88**:85.

33. Tripier L, Du lambeau musculocutané en forme de pont appliqué à la restauration des paupières, *Rev Chir* (1890) **4**.

34. Dzubow LM, Zack L, The principle of cosmetic junctions as applied to reconstruction of defects following Mohs surgery, *J Dermatol Surg Oncol* (1990) **16**:353–5.

35. Dzubow LM, Defect subdivision as a technique to repair defects following Mohs surgery, *J Dermatol Surg Oncol* (1990) **16**:526–30.

36. Esser JFS, Gestielte lokale Nasenplastik mit zweizipfligem Lappen, Deckung des Sekundärdefektes vom ersten Zipfel durch den zweiten, *Dtsch Z Chir* (1918) **143**:385–90.

37. Fratila A, Bertlich R, Kreysel HW, Aesthetic repair of soft triangle defects, *Skin Cancer* (1991) **6**:205–10.

38. Rieger RA, A local flap for repair of the nasal tip, *Plast Reconstr Surg* (1967) **40**:147–9.

39. Marchac D, Toth B, The axial frontonasal flap revisited, *Plast Reconstr Surg* (1985) **76**:686–94.

40. Fratila A, Bertlich R, The 'heminose flap': the classical and modified variant, *J Dermatol Surg Oncol* (1992) in press.

41. Emmett AJJ, The cascade flap for nasal tip repair, *Eur J Plast Surg* (1991) **14**:69–72.

42. Rintala AE, Asko-Seljavaara S, Reconstruction of midline skin defects of the nose, *Scand J Plast Reconstr Surg* (1969) **3**:105, 147–9.

43. Greenbaum SS, Greenbaum SH, An alternative for nasal tip reconstruction: the bilateral rotation flap, *J Dermatol Surg Oncol* (1991) **17**:455–9.

44. Peng VT, Sturm RL, Marsch TW, 'Pinch modification' of the linear advancement flap, *J Dermatol Surg Oncol* (1987) **13**:251–3.

45. Hill TG, The perialar arc rotation skin flap, *J Dermatol Surg Oncol* (1989) **15**:78–83.

46. Rybka FJ, Reconstruction of the nasal tip using nasalis myocutaneous sliding flaps, *Plast Reconstr Surg* (1983) **71**:40–4.

47. Constantine VS, Nasalis myocutaneous sliding flap: repair of nasal supratip defects, *J Dermatol Surg Oncol* (1991) **17**:439–44.

48. Snow SN, Mohs FE, Olansky DC, Nasal tip reconstruction: the horizontal 'J' rotation flap using skin from the lower lateral bridge and cheek, *J Dermatol Surg Oncol* (1990) **16**:727–32.

49. Field LM, Alar rim reconstruction utilizing a perinasal transposition flap overlying a hinged 'turn-down' flap, *J Dermatol Surg Oncol* (1991) **17**:281–4.

50. Johanson B, Aspelund E, Breine U et al, Surgical treatment of non-traumatic lower lip lesions with special reference to the step technique, *Scand J Plast Reconstr Surg* (1974) **8**:232–40.

51. Sebastian G, Funktionelle und ästhetische Spätergebnisse nach operativer Behandlung von Unterlippentumoren. In: Haneke E, ed., *Gegenwärtiger Stand der operativen Dermatologie*, Fortschritte der Operativen Dermatologie 4 (Springer: Berlin–Heidelberg–New York 1988) 108–21.

52. Haneke E, Klinik und Therapie benigner und semimaligner Tumoren im Lippenbereich. In: Müller RPA, Friederich HC, Petres J, eds, *Operative Dermatologie im Kopf-Hals-Bereich*, Fortschritte der Operativen Dermatologie 1 (Springer: Berlin–Heidelberg–New York–Tokyo 1984) 143–9.

53. Haneke E, Ulzeriertes Radioderm—eine einfache Methode zum Ersatz der Kinnhaut. In: Petres J, Müller R, eds, *Präkanzerosen und Papillomatosen der Haut* (Springer: Berlin–Heidelberg–New York 1981) 223–6.

54. Happle R, Zur operativen Behandlung des Morbus Bowen an der Glans penis, *Hautarzt* (1972) **23**:125–8.

55. Haneke E, Preputial flaps for defects of the glans penis. First Int. Cong. Dermatol. Surg., Lisbon 1979.

56. Mato J, Vilalta A, Mascaró JM, Decorticación de glande. First Int Cong. Dermatol. Surg., Lisbon 1979.

57. Haneke E, Operative Therapie im männlichen Genitalbereich, *Z Hautkr* (1989) **64**:1089–92.

58. Haneke E, Binder D, Subunguales Melanom mit streifenförmiger Nagelpigmentierung, *Hautarzt* (1978) **29**:389–91.

59. Hirshowitz B, Karev A, Rousso M, Combined double Z-plasty and V-Y

advancement for thumb web contracture, *Hand* (1975) **7**:291.

60. Kasai K, Ogawa Y, Alternating-pattern Z-plasties in association with multiple V-Y advancements: a new idea of multiple Z-plasties, *Plast Reconstr Surg* (1991) **88**:353–6.

61. Motley RJ, Holt PJA, Meshed advancement flap for lower leg lesions, *J Dermatol Surg Oncol* (1990) **16**:346–8.

62. Arnold AJ, Bennett RG, The bilateral dog-ear transposition flap, *J Dermatol Surg Oncol* (1990) **16**:667–72.

63. Groth WE, Modifikation am Rotationslappen zur Vermeidung von Lappenspitzen-/Lappenrandnekrosen: abgerundete Ecken, VY-Plastik, *Zbl Haut Geschlkr* (1992) **160**:255–6.

64. Hill TG, Enhancing the survival of full-thickness grafts, *J Dermatol Surg Oncol* (1984) **10**:639–42.

65. Welke S, Das präaurikuläre Vollhaut-transplantat zur Defektdeckung im Nasenbereich—eine Methode für die Praxis, *Akt Dermatol* (1977) **3**:105–13.

66. Field LM, The infra-auricular full-thickness donor site with V-Y closure, *J Dermatol Surg Oncol* (1984) **10**:345–6.

67. Field LM, Skin grafts to the distal parts of noses using dual vertical W-plasties, *J Dermatol Surg Oncol* (1982) **8**:735.

68. Chow W, Adjacent tissue full-thickness skin grafts, *Zbl Haut-Geschlkr* (1991) **159**:331.

69. Salasche SJ, Grabski WJ, Mulvaney MJ, Delayed grafting of midline forehead flap donor defect: utilization of residual flap tissue, *J Dermatol Surg Oncol* (1990) **16**:633–5.

70. Robinson JK, Improvement of the appearance of full-thickness skin grafts with dermabrasion, *Arch Dermatol* (1987) **123**:1340–5.

71. Haneke E, Versatility of dermal grafts, *J Méd Esthét* (1981) **88**:122–3.

72. Haneke E, Das umgekehrte Koriumtransplantat zur Defektdeckung im Schädelbereich, *Z Hautkr* (1981) **56**:84–7.

73. Pleier R, Schwantes H, Balda B-R, Das 'gemeshte' umgedrehte Koriumtransplantat. In: Haneke E, ed., *Gegenwärtiger Stand der operativen Dermatologie,* Fortschritte der Operativen Dermatologie 4 (Springer: Berlin–Heidelberg–New York 1988) 126–9.

74. Fratila A, Bertlich R, Kreysel HW, Das umgekehrte Koriumtransplantat—die Originaltechnik und unsere Modifikation. Vth Cong Int Ass Maxillo-Facial Surg, Kassel 1991. *Zbl Haut-Geschlkr* (1991) **158**:951(abstr.).

75. Bertényi C, Zur Technik der lokalen Exzision. In: Weidner F, Tonak J, eds, *Das maligne Melanom der Haut* (Perimed: Erlangen 1981) 115–18.

76. Yanai A, Hiraga Y, Method for preparing meshed skin grafts without using skin-graft meshers, *Plast Reconstr Surg* (1991) **88**:524–6.

Section V

COSMETIC SURGERY

43. SCLEROTHERAPY: ADVANCES IN TREATMENT
    Mitchel P. Goldman

44. SOFT TISSUE AUGMENTATION: NEW TECHNIQUES AND RECENT CONTROVERSIES
    Jeffrey L. Melton, C. William Hanke

45. MICROLIPOINJECTION
    Kevin S. Pinski, Henry H. Roenigk Jr

46. NEW TRENDS IN LIPOSUCTION
    William P. Coleman III

47. FACIAL CHEMICAL PEEL WITH TRICHLOROACETIC ACID
    Randall K. Roenigk, David G. Brodland

48. CHEMICAL PEEL WITH PHENOL
    Thomas H. Alt

49. DERMABRASION: REJUVENATION AND SCAR REVISION
    Henry H. Roenigk Jr

50. MINIGRAFTS IN HAIR REPLACEMENT
    Jean Arouete

51. NEWER TECHNIQUES IN HAIR REPLACEMENT
    Pierre Bouhanna

Chapter 43

SCLEROTHERAPY: ADVANCES IN TREATMENT

Mitchel P. Goldman

INTRODUCTION

Sclerotherapy as a treatment for varicose and telangiectatic leg veins is becoming increasingly popular in the USA. This treatment originates from the mid-1800s when various solutions were injected into varicose veins.[1] Unfortunately, because of aseptic techniques and solutions, these early treatments often resulted in major complications and the procedure was abandoned. At the turn of the century, intravenous treatment for syphilis was noted to produce sclerosis in injected veins and physicians once again thought of injecting varicose veins.[2]

Early reports on this treatment were enthusiastic and the basic principles of treatment were established. Linser in 1916 first recommended postsclerotherapy compression to limit thrombosis and excessive phlebitic reactions.[3] McAusland in 1939 promoted injection into 'empty veins'.[4] He described the necessity for beginning treatment by closing the saphenofemoral junction before treating distal varicosities. He also developed the concept of 'minimal sclerosing concentration', using sodium morrhuate froth to treat venulectases and telangiectasia and more concentrated sodium morrhuate to treat larger veins.

However, general surgeons who had previously been practicing sclerotherapy became disenchanted with this technique because of allergic reactions to sclerosing solutions, difficulty in accurately diagnosing reflux points, and difficulty in applying compression dressings for long periods. In addition, with the onset of World War II the surgeon's expertise was directed towards more serious problems and less to cosmetic concerns. Arterial surgery was rapidly evolving and sclerotherapy of varicose veins, indeed the treatment of venous disease in general, became less glamorous and, perhaps more importantly, less financially rewarding.

However, primarily in Europe and to some extent in the USA, both surgeons and medical physicians, including dermatologists, continued refining sclerotherapy techniques. Less toxic synthetic sclerosing solutions (sodium tetradecyl sulfate, described by Reiner in the USA[5]) were being used with greater efficacy and less morbidity. The concept of prolonged compression was advanced by Sigg,[6] Orbach[7] and Fegan.[8] Also, more accurate methods for diagnosing points of high-pressure reflux (Doppler ultrasound) were developed. The foundation for proper technique was established.

Why then is sclerotherapy treatment becoming popular now? Present-day interest has arisen through the publication of many articles in the dermatologic literature and, more importantly, from publication in the lay press. Only within the past few years have patients begun to take an active role in their medical care. Patients are unwilling to submit to the morbidity and scarring process of ligation and stripping operations of the past. They are demanding cosmetic treatment. They are also unwilling to accept a physician's advice that they should not worry about 'minor' leg pains. Sclerotherapy offers the vast majority of those who suffer from both the symptoms and cosmetic embarrassment of varicose veins an affordable and practical treatment. This chapter will describe three 'advances' in sclerotherapy treatment. These are advances not because they are new, but because they are newly popular—proper diagnosis prior to treatment, optimal choice of sclerosing solutions and concentrations, and ideal compression techniques to limit sclerophlebitis, recanalization and complications.

PRESCLEROTHERAPY EVALUATION

To appreciate the fundamentals of noninvasive diagnostic techniques, an understanding of the anatomy and pathophysiology of varicose and telangiectatic veins is required. Since this is beyond the scope of this chapter the reader is referred to a recent textbook.[9] In short, the venous system is just that—a 'system' of veins. Flow through the venous system is directed towards the heart by one-way valves which are present in all veins below the dermal–epidermal junction.[10] Under external compression through various muscle pumps, especially the calf and foot pumps, blood is propelled through the veins. Respiratory actions which decrease intra-abdominal pressure suck blood into the abdominal veins. Vis-a-tergo and osmotic gradients propel blood through venulectases. This orchestrated flow can only occur if the valvular system is competent. With valvular destruction or venous dilatation, one-way flow is replaced by retrograde flow, resulting in venous hypertension. Because veins are intricately connected, venous hypertension is distributed throughout the venous system, resulting in a cascading breakdown of one-way flow.

Dermal and superficial venulectases have anastomotic connections with larger subcutaneous veins (Figure 43.1). An elegant radiographic study of cadaver veins illustrates the intricate connections between superficial and deep veins

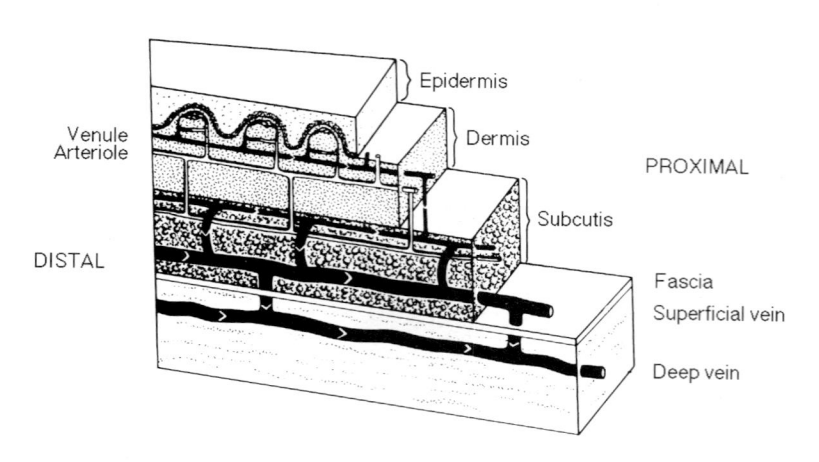

Figure 43.1
Schematic diagram of the cutaneous and subcutaneous vascular plexus. (Reproduced with permission from Goldman MP, Sclerotherapy treatment of varicose and telangiectatic leg veins, Mosby-Yearbook Inc., St Louis, 1991.)

SCLEROTHERAPY: ADVANCES IN TREATMENT

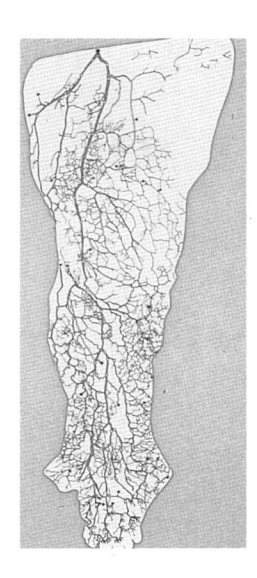

Figure 43.2
Radiographic demonstration of the superficial venous system. (Reproduced with permission from Taylor et al.[11])

through multiple perforator veins[11] (Figure 43.2): 'perforator' because connections between the superficial and deep system occur through veins which perforate the fascial covering of the deep venous system. Therefore, to alleviate venous hypertension, one must first cut off the most proximal point of abnormal reflux. Various physical and noninvasive diagnostic techniques have been developed to find this point. It is here that treatment should begin.

Physical examination

Visual observation and palpation are the obvious first steps in presclerotherapy evaluation. Patients' legs should be exposed in their entirety. At times, a bulging dilatation of an incompetent junction between the deep and superficial system can be missed (Figure 43.3). A diagram of the visual varicosities and telangiectasias is made on a standard form with notation of bulges and fascial defects (Figure 43.4).

Although fascial defects usually overlie incompetent perforator veins,[12] these defects may only be associated with perforator veins 50–70% of the time.[13–15] To detect fascial defects it is best to have the patient lie on their back and elevate the leg. After a few minutes the medial leg is massaged distal to proximal. With practice the examiner's finger will fall into depressions within the subcutaneous tissue.

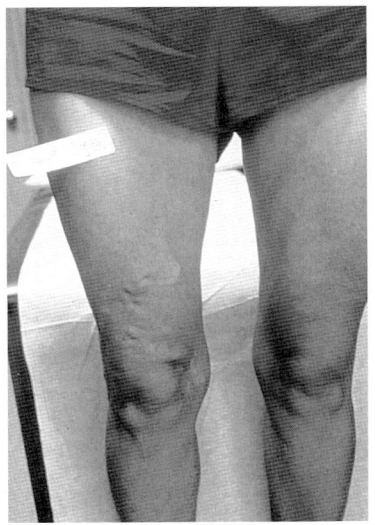

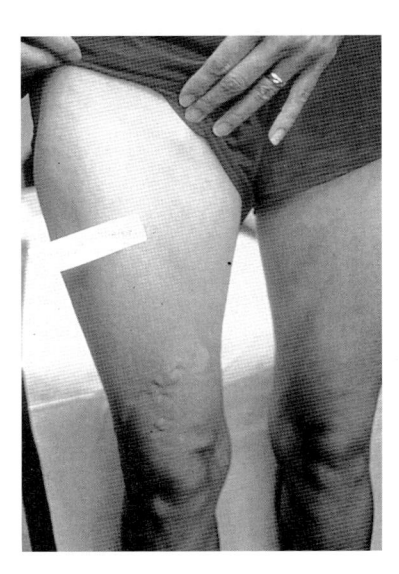

A   B

Figure 43.3
(A) This patient sought treatment because of an obviously enlarged varicose vein in her thigh. (B) Further inspection revealed a varix at the saphenofemoral junction (arrow) indicative of insufficiency. (Courtesy Anton Butie.) (Reproduced with permission from Goldman MP, Sclerotherapy treatment of varicose and telangiectatic leg veins, *Mosby-Yearbook Inc., St Louis, 1991.*)

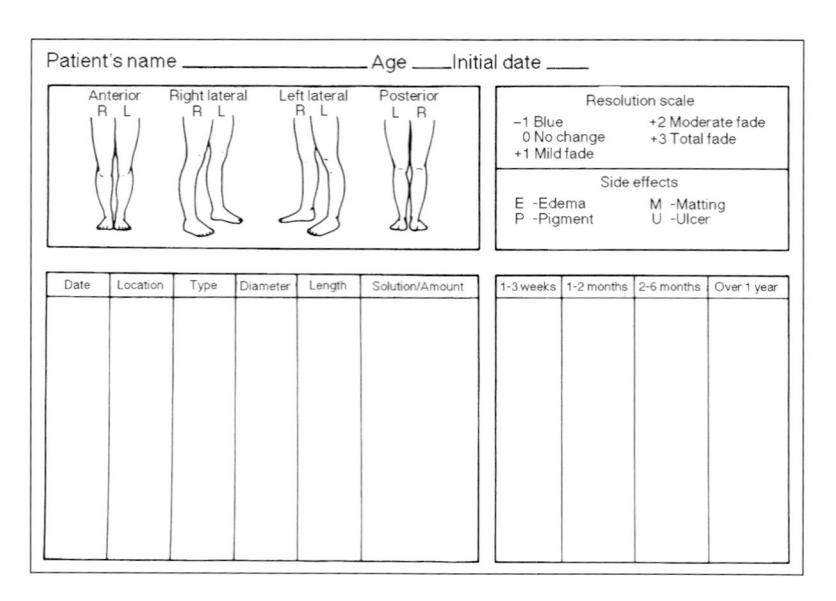

Figure 43.4
Diagrammatic chart notes and follow-up notes. (Reproduced with permission from Goldman MP, Sclerotherapy treatment of varicose and telangiectatic leg veins, Mosby-Yearbook Inc., St Louis, 1991.)

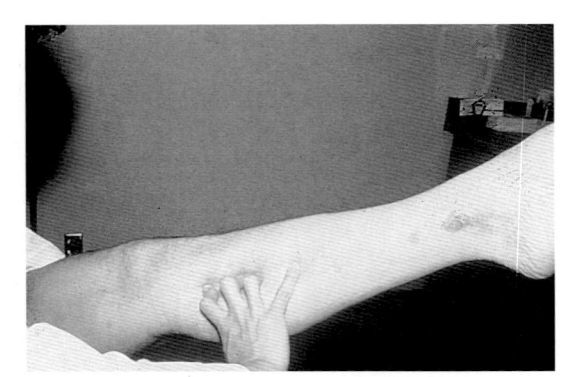

Figure 43.5
(A) Compression of fascial defects indicating 'points of control' of incompetent perforating veins with the leg elevated. (B) When the patient stands, the varicose vein remains collapsed while pressure is maintained over control points and distends when the control points are released. (Courtesy Helane Fronek.) (Reproduced with permission from Goldman MP, Sclerotherapy treatment of varicose and telangiectatic leg veins, Mosby-Yearbook Inc., St Louis, 1991.)

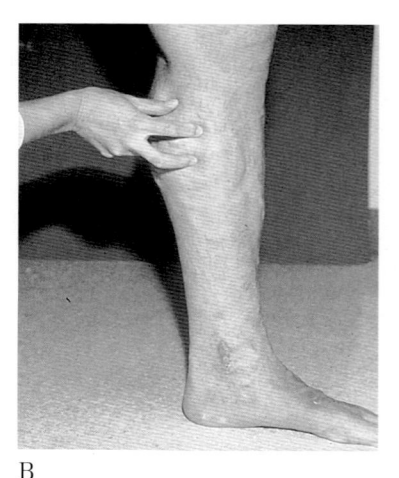

These defects are marked. If only a few depressions are felt one then allows the patient to stand while holding pressure on these points. If the varicose vein fails to reappear the examiner then releases each finger one at a time, distal to proximal, and notes the point at which the vein recurs. This point represents the site of the most distal incompetent perforating vein (Figure 43.5). In the patient with an incompetent saphenofemoral junction, the test is just as simple.

Trendelenburg first described a physical examination technique for diagnosing incompetence at the saphenofemoral

Figure 43.6
Interpreting the Brodie–Trendelenburg test. (A) Nil—no distension of the veins for 30 s both while the tourniquet remains on and also after it is removed implies a lack of reflux. (B) Positive—distension of the veins only after the tourniquet is released implies reflux only through the saphenofemoral junction (SFJ). (C) Double positive—distension of the veins while the tourniquet remains on and further distension when it is removed implies reflux through perforating veins as well as the SFJ. (D) Negative—distension of the veins while the tourniquet remains on and no additional distension once it is removed implies reflux only through perforating veins. (Courtesy Helane Fronek.) (Reproduced with permission from Goldman MP, Sclerotherapy treatment of varicose and telangiectatic leg veins, Mosby-Yearbook, Inc, St Louis, 1991.)

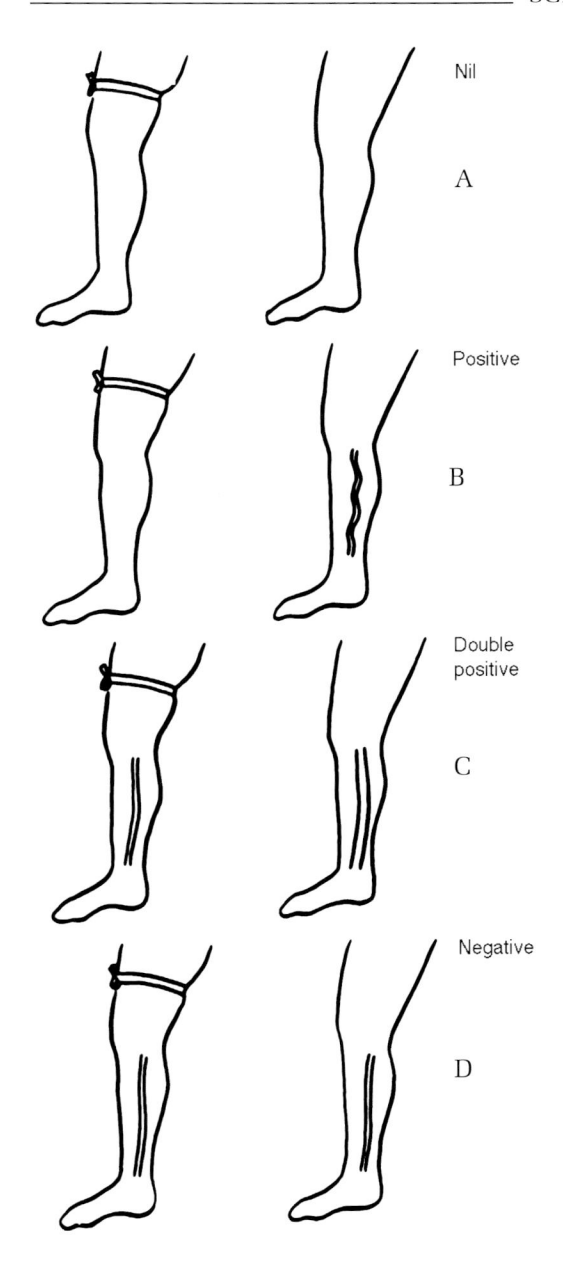

junction (SFJ).[16] In short, the superficial veins of the leg are emptied by raising the leg 60° above the horizontal. A tourniquet is placed at the proximal thigh to occlude superficial veins and the patient stands. If the superficial varicosity fails to refill within 20 s the test is positive and the etiology of venous reflux is at the SFJ. If the vein refills within 20 s one should look for incompetent perforating veins in the distal calf, knee and thigh (Figure 43.6).

Another physical examination technique is a modified Perthe's test.[17] To determine if superficial varicosities are necessary for venous return, the patient is fitted with a 30–40-mmHg graduated compression stocking and/or a tourniquet is applied at the proximal thigh. This degree of compression will occlude the superficial veins. If the leg feels better or does not become painful after walking for 15–30 min, adequate flow is present in the deep venous system.

Noninvasive diagnostic techniques

The venous Doppler is as indispensable for the phlebologist as the stethoscope is for the cardiologist. The Doppler ultrasound transmits sound waves to a recorder or audio system which are reflected off blood cells traveling through a specific vein. This provides information on both the direction of blood flow and its velocity. By performing various physical maneuvers one can then determine the presence of deep venous thrombosis, deep venous valvular insufficiency, and superficial venous valvular insufficiency. A complete description of this examination technique is found elsewhere.[18,19]

Patients who should be evaluated with Doppler ultrasound are those with varicose veins large enough to be hemodynamically significant. Since spider telangiectasia commonly occurs over an incompetent perforating vein, a radiating flare of telangiectasia from a central point may also indicate an incompetent perforator vein. Although there is no substitute for sound clinical judgment, recommendations for performing a venous Doppler examination include:

1. Patients with varicosities greater than 4 mm in diameter.
2. Any varicosity over 2 mm in diameter extending throughout the calf or thigh.
3. Any varicosity extending into the groin or popliteal fossae.
4. When a 'star-burst' cluster of telangiectasia is present, especially if it is over the usual points of perforating veins (mid-posterior calf, medial knee, medial mid-thigh, medial distal calf).
5. Patients with a history of deep vein thrombosis and/or thrombophlebitis.
6. Patients who have undergone previous venous surgery or sclerotherapy with poor results or recurrence of varicosities.

The deep venous system is evaluated at three sites for the presence of acute or chronic damage to the valvular system by thrombosis or phlebitis. One listens for normal one-way flow at the junction of the femoral and iliac veins in the groin, in the popliteal vein in its fossae, and in the posterior tibial vein in the medial malleolar region. Patients are best examined in a warm room lying down. A spontaneous continuous venous signal near the arterial signal should be heard over all of the above-mentioned veins unless venoconstriction is present from low temperature or emotional excitation. Augmentation of the venous signal is performed by applying pressure distal to the Doppler probe. Lack of augmentation should be heard if pressure is applied proximal to the probe.

The first point in examining the superficial system is the saphenofemoral junction (SFJ). The Doppler probe is placed on the anterior medial thigh a few centimeters below the groin crease. The long saphenous vein (LSV) is located by moving the probe along the thigh while performing a short series of compressions on the medial distal thigh to augment flow. When it is located, competence of the LSV is established by eliciting one-way flow through augmentations. The patient then performs a valsalva maneuver. If significant flow occurs down the LSV lasting longer than a few seconds the SFJ is incompetent. This can be confirmed through duplex examination (described below). A wide range of accuracy for venous Doppler examination of SFJ incompetence has been reported, which probably reflects the experience of the examiner. At times, competent iliac vein valves or occlusion with valsalva from the inguinal ligament may give a false-negative examination. Overall, the accuracy ranges between 80 and 100%.[19,20]

A similar sequence of augmentation and release is then performed over any other visible varicose veins to determine if they are competent and if the incompetence arises from the SFJ. In addition, Doppler examination permits a fairly accurate tracing of the varicose vein origin which aids in determining if reflux comes from the LSV or short saphenous vein. Atypical reflux may also occur through incompetent pelvic varicosities or anatomical anomalies described elsewhere.[21] Finally, fascial defects are examined for evidence of perforator vein incompetence. Augmentation maneuvers will produce the loudest amplitude changes over the pathological perforator veins. These points should be treated first with sclerotherapy.

Light reflection rheography ((LRR), photoplethysmography) offers a simple technique for 'physiologically' evaluating the efficiency of the calf muscle pump. With this instrument, a light source illuminates a small area of skin, which by convention is located 8–10 mm above the medial malleolus. An adjacent photoelectric sensor measures light reflectance, which correlates with cutaneous blood volume. The patient sits with the knee bent at a 80–70° angle and raises the toe 10 times in synchrony with the machine to empty the superficial venous plexus through the calf pump. The photoelectric cell measures the time until cutaneous blood volume returns to baseline (refilling time (RF)). By convention, a RF <25 s indicates venous valvular insufficiency. If a shortened RF occurs, the test is repeated after applying a tourniquet above or below the knee at 40–60 mmHg. This effectively prevents reflux from the superficial venous system. If the RF normalizes, a presumptive diagnosis of hemodynamically significant incompetent superficial veins can be made. If the RF remains abnormal, the deep venous system may be damaged and sclerotherapy should not be performed without further evaluation.

The LRR can also be used to assess the efficacy of sclerotherapy treatment. Successful treatment will normalize the LRR RF. An abnormal RF after sclerotherapy treatment should alert the physician to more closely evaluate the superficial venous system for additional incompetent perforator veins, or recanalized sclerosed veins. Figure 43.7[22] is a useful guide to LRR evaluation and treatment.

Duplex sonography is the most advanced (and expensive) modality for evaluating the patient prior to sclerotherapy. This modality combines the utility of venous Doppler with pictorial information from sonography. As a screening tool, duplex sonography evaluates the deep venous system for evidence of thrombosis. Most perforating veins can be accurately localized, and the degree of junctional reflux can be quantified. During treatment, duplex sonography can aid the physician in placing the sclerosing solution accurately within the desired vein. In addition, augmentation maneuvers can be used to determine if effective sclerosis occurs with injection. Posttreatment, duplex sonography can be used to evaluate the degree of endofibrosis and recanalizations in sclerosed veins. Although duplex sonography is not indicated for the majority of varicose vein patients, its availability enhances the quality of a sclerotherapy practice.

Sclerosing solutions

The goal of sclerotherapy treatment is to destroy the endothelium producing endosclerosis with resorption of the resulting fibrotic process. The key event is endothelial destruction. Too little destruction leads to thrombosis without fibrosis and early recanalization. Too much destruction leads to vascular dehiscence with resulting extravasation of red blood cells and sclerosing solution into perivascular tissues. This produces hyperpigmentation through hemosiderin-laden macrophages and may also produce cutaneous necrosis through direct toxic effects on dermal tissue. In addition, excessive inflammation may stimulate angiogenic and vasodilatory effects which may lead to telangiectatic matting. Therefore, one must choose the appropriate sclerosing solution and, most importantly, the appropriate concentration of solution. Sadick has coined the term minimal sclerosant concentration (MSC) through an evaluation of the effectiveness of different concentrations of hypertonic

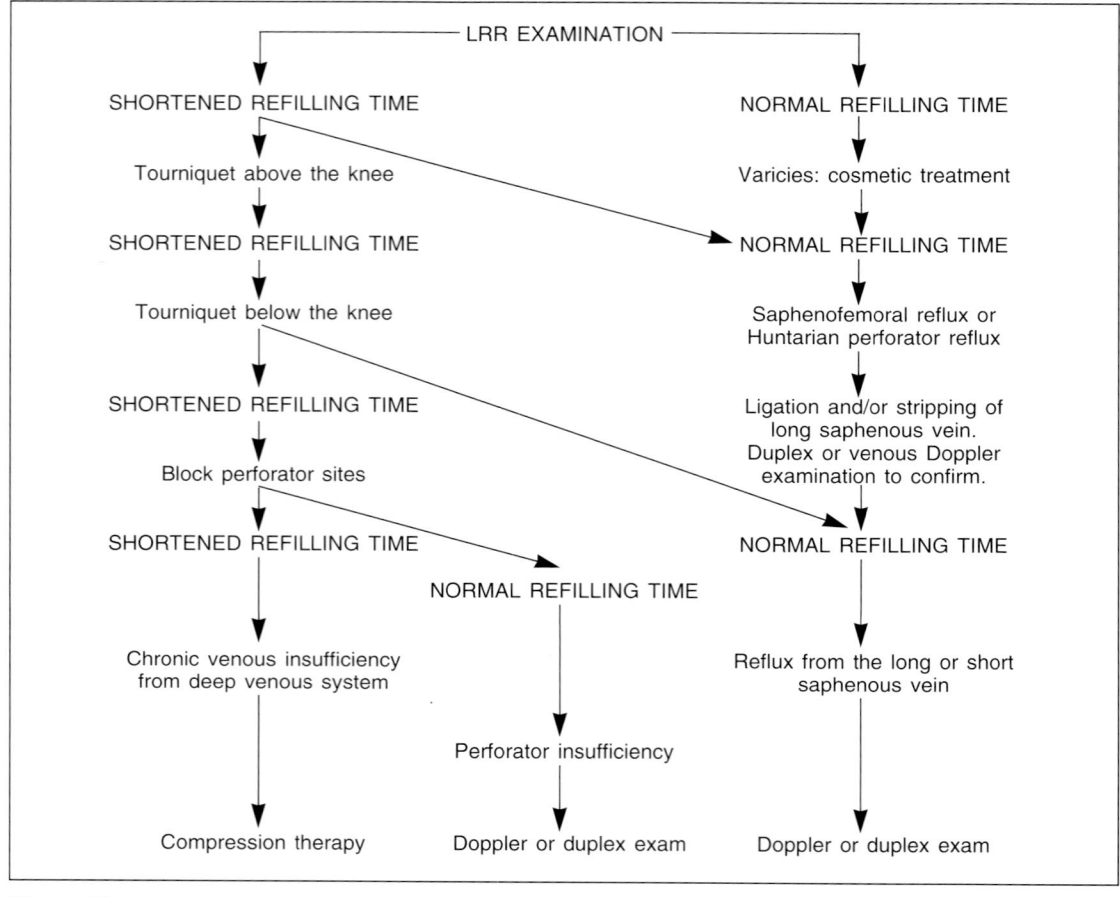

Figure 43.7
Flow diagram for light reflection rheography as an aid to planning treatment. (Modified from Neumann HAM, Boersma I, Light reflection rheography: a non-invasive diagnostic tool for screening venous disease, J Dermatol Surg Oncol *(1992)* **18**:425–30.)

saline (HS).[23] Studies utilizing the rabbit ear vein have also determined MSCs for a variety of sclerosing solutions.[24–26] Table 43.1 summarizes recommended MSCs for various vessel diameters.

Every sclerosing solution has its own inherent advantages and disadvantages (Table 43.2). Although the author personally utilizes four different sclerosing solutions at various concentrations in his practice to tailor treatment to the particular patient, excellent results can be achieved with any sclerosing solution. Space does not permit a complete discussion of each type of sclerosing solution; this appears elsewhere.[1] It is also inappropriate to discuss the rationale for using FDA-approved versus non-FDA-approved solutions. This section will present a summary of the three types of sclerosing solutions—detergent solutions, osmotic agents and chemical irritants.

Table 43.1
Relative potency of sclerosing solutions (minimal sclerosant concentrations)

Vein diameter (mm)	Sclerosing solution
<0.4 mm	Scleremo 1:1 Polidocanol 0.25% Sodium tetradecyl sulfate 0.1% Scleremo 100% Polidocanol 0.5% Variglobin 0.1% Hypertonic saline 11.7% Sclerodex Ethanolamine oleate 2% Sodium morrhuate 1%
0.6–2 mm	Sodium tetradecyl sulfate 0.25% Polidocanol 0.75% Variglobin 1.0% Hypertonic saline 23.4% Ethanolamine oleate 5% Sodium morrhuate 2.5%
3–5 mm	Polidocanol 1–2% Sodium tetradecyl sulfate 0.5–1.0% Variglobin 2% Sodium morrhuate 5%
>5 mm	Polidocanol 3–5%
Perforating vessels Saphenopopleteal and saphenofemoral junction	Sodium tetradecyl sulfate 2–3% Variglobin 3–12%

Reproduced from Goldman.[9] By permission of Mosby-Yearbook, Inc.

Table 43.2
Sclerosing agents

	Active ingredient	Allergic reaction	Necrosis	Pain
Osmotic agents				
Hypertonic saline	18–30% saline	None	Occasional[b]	Moderate
Sclerodex[a]	10% saline + 5% dextrose	None	Occasional	Mild
Chemical irritants				
Scleremo	Chromated glycerin	Rare	Very rare	Moderate
Variglobin	Polyiodinated iodine	Rare	Frequent	Moderate
Detergents				
Sodium morrhuate[a]	Fatty acids in cod liver oil	Occasional	Frequent[b]	Moderate
Sotradecol[a]	Sodium tetradecyl sulfate	Occasional	Occasional[b]	Mild
Aethoxysklerol[c]	Polidocanol	Very rare	Very rare[b]	None
Etholamin	Ethanolamine oleate	Occasional	Occasional	Mild

[a]Approved for use by the Food and Drug Administration.
[b]Concentration dependent.
[c]Not approved for use in the USA.
Reproduced from Goldman.[9] By permission of Mosby-Yearbook, Inc.

Detergent solutions

Sodium morrhuate (SM) (Scleromate, Palisades Pharmaceuticals Inc., Tenafly, NJ) is a mixture of sodium salts of the saturated and unsaturated fatty acids present in cod liver oil. As with all detergent solutions, SM acts to damage endothelial membranes through alterations of cell surface lipids. The disadvantages of SM consist primarily of extensive cutaneous necrosis when it is inadvertently injected perivascularly and allergic reactions. Anaphylactic reactions have occurred within a few minutes of injection or more commonly when injections are repeated after a few weeks. Anaphylactic reactions have rarely been fatal.[27,28] Of note is that there have been no reports of allergic reactions involving SM in the recent medical literature. Gallagher describes treating 20 000 patients over 25 years with one anaphylactic reaction 15 years ago and 20 anaphylactoid reactions, all with favorable outcomes.[29] Sodium morrhuate is approved by the FDA for sclerosis of varicose veins. However, because of its extremely caustic nature, it is not recommended for treating telangiectasias.

Ethanolamine oleate (EO) (Etholamin, Block Drug Company, Piscatawy, NJ) is a synthetic mixture of ethanolamine and oleic acid with an empirical formula of $C_{20}H_{41}NO_3$. The oleic acid component is responsible for the inflammatory action. Oleic acid may also activate coagulation in vitro by release of tissue factors and Hageman factor XII. Although EO is mainly used in the USA for sclerosis of esophageal varices, it is commonly used in Australia for sclerotherapy of varicose veins.

Ethanolamine oleate is thought to have a decreased risk of allergic reactions compared to SM or sodium tetradecyl sulfate.[30] Anaphylactic shock has been reported following injection in a number of patients.[31–33] Generalized urticaria occurred in about 1 out of 400 patients, clearing with antihistamines.[34]

Some degree of nonspecific red blood cell hemolysis may also occur with its use. A hemolytic reaction occurred in 5 out of 900 patients with injection of over 12 ml 0.5% EO per patient per treatment session.[34] Acute renal failure with spontaneous recovery followed injection of 15–20 ml EO in two women.[35]

Sodium tetradecyl sulfate (STS) (Sotradecol, Elkins Sinn, Cherry Hill NJ, sodium 1-isobutyl-4-ethyloctyl sulfate plus benzoyl alcohol 2% (as an anesthetic agent)) is a synthetic long-chain fatty acid salt of an alkali metal with detergent properties. It is commonly used worldwide as a sclerosant for varicose and telangiectatic veins. Sodium tetradecyl sulfate, presently approved for use by the FDA for vein sclerosis, has a number of disadvantages. Epidermal necrosis frequently occurs if concentrations over 0.5% are even slightly extravasated. Occasional anaphylactic shock and, more commonly, generalized urticaria and edema or diffuse maculopapular eruptions have been noted.[36–41]

Polidocanol (POL) (hydroxypolyethoxydodecane, Aethoxysklerol, Chemische Fabrik Kreussler & Co GmbH, Wiesbaden-Biebrich, Germany) is a urethane anesthetic (compounds with an $-NHCO_2-$ linkage). Unlike the two main groups of local anesthetics, the esters (procaine, benzocaine and tetracaine) and the amides (lidocaine, prilocaine, mepivacaine, procainamide and dibucaine), POL lacks an aromatic ring. The actual active substance is an aliphatic molecule composed of a hydrophilic chain of polyethylene glycolic ether and a liposoluble radical of dodecylic alcohol. Polidocanol is a weaker detergent type of sclerosant than STS. Experimental studies indicate that its sclerosant power is about 50% that of STS.[25,26] Polidocanol is unique among sclerosing agents in that it is painless to inject (when the solution, which contains 5% alcohol, is diluted) and will not produce cutaneous ulcerations even with intradermal injection of a 1% solution.[42] Allergic reactions have only been reported in four patients with an estimated incidence of 0.01%.[36] In addition, patients who are allergic to STS do not develop an allergic reaction with POL.[43]

Osmotic solutions

Hypertonic saline (HS) (sodium chloride 23.4%, Lymphomed Inc., Rosemont, IL), unlike detergent sclerosing solutions, acts nonspecifically to destroy all cells (intra- and extravascular) within its osmotic gradient. Therefore, osmotic agents are very damaging to all cellular tissues, readily producing ulceration if injected (or with seepage) extravascularly. In addition, osmotic agents are rapidly diluted in a blood-filled vein, losing potency within a short distance of injection. Thus, these agents are not recommended for treating veins larger than 1–2 mm in diameter. Unadulterated HS is not an allergen. An annoying adverse effect with its use is unpleasant stinging on injection and 5 min or so of muscle cramping immediately following injection. Pain and cramping can be minimized by using MSC.[23]

Heparsol (20% hypertonic saline, 100 units/ml heparin, and 1% procaine) was patented by Foley in 1975 for microinjection of 'venous blemishes'.[44] He believed that adding heparin helped prevent thrombi in larger vessels, with procaine decreasing the immediate pain and cramping from injection. Recently, Sadick,[45] in a randomized, blinded, 800-patient study, found no benefit for adding heparin to HS.

Sclerodex (SX) (Dextroject, Ondee Laboratory Ltd, Montreal, Quebec, Canada) is a mixture of dextrose 250 mg/ml, sodium chloride 100 mg/ml, and phenethyl alcohol 8 mg/ml (as a local anesthetic/preservative) and is mainly used in Canada for sclerosis of telangiectasias. It is essentially a mid-potency hypertonic solution with a mechanism of action similar to that of HS. It is best reserved for vessels less than 1 mm in diameter. Mantse[46] notes one allergic reaction in 500 patients treated with SX, an incidence of 0.2%. Like HS, it is slightly painful on injection and occasionally produces superficial necrosis.

Chemical irritants

Polyiodide iodide (PII) (Varigloban, Chemische Fabrik Kreussler & Co., Wiesbaden-Biebrich, Germany; Variglobin, Globopharm, Switzerland; Sclerodine, Omega, Montreal, Canada) is a stabilized water solution of iodide ions, sodium iodine and benzyl alcohol. The active sclerosing ingredient is iodine, with sodium and potassium increasing its water solubility. Benzyl alcohol is added as a preservative/stabilizer. The sclerosing effect is from direct destruction of endothelium. The entire vessel wall is destroyed through defusion at the point of injection. It is neutralized within a few seconds by binding to different blood components, especially proteins, and thus its sclerosing effect is lost within a centimeter or two.[47] Polyiodide iodide is primarily used for large varicosities including the saphenofemoral junction. Paravenous injections produce extensive tissue necrosis. Fortunately, PII is painful when injected outside a vein so that improper injection technique is immediately apparent. To prevent nonspecific damage, the concentration, not the volume, of solution is increased to enhance sclerosing power.

Chromated glycerin, 72% (SCL) (Scleremo, Laboratories E Bouteille, Limoges, France) is a polyalcohol with a mechanism of action similar to that of PII. It provokes endothelial lesions without desquamation of endothelial cells in plaques.[48] Its clinical efficacy has been shown to be dose dependent with a very low incidence of adverse sequelae.[49,50] In the dorsal rabbit ear vein,[26] undiluted SCL appears to be equivalent in potency to 0.25% polidocanol. The relatively weak sclerosing power of SCL corresponds to its promotion as a mild sclerosant. Pigmentation and cutaneous necrosis are exceedingly rare.[51,52] The disadvantages of SCL include its high viscosity and local pain with injection. These drawbacks can be partially overcome by dilution with 1% lidocaine without epinephrine. Hypersensitivity is very rare.[53,54] Hematuria accompanied by ureteral colic can occur transiently following injection of over 10 ml undiluted SCL. Ocular complications, including blurred vision and partial visual field loss, have been reported by a single author with resolution in less than 2 h.[55]

POSTSCLEROSIS COMPRESSION

Postsclerosis compression is perhaps the most important advance in sclerotherapy treatment of varicose veins since the introduction of relatively safe synthetic sclerosing agents in the 1940s. Primarily, compression eliminates a thrombophlebitic reaction and substitutes a 'sclerophlebitis' with the production of a firm fibrous cord.[56] For compression to be effective it must be given in a graduated manner to prevent a tourniquet effect. Higher proximal external pressures will cause retrograde blood flow with further dilatation of distal superficial veins. However, localized increase in pressure can be given with foam pads or cotton balls which will increase pressure under the pad by 15–50%[57,58] (Figure 43.8). A complete discussion of graduated compression appears elsewhere.[59]

Compression serves at least five purposes. First, compression, if adequate, may result in direct apposition of the treated vein walls to produce more effective fibrosis.[36] Therefore, sclerosing solutions of lesser strength may be successfully utilized. Second, compressing the treated vessel will decrease the extent of thrombus formation which inevitably occurs with the use of all sclerosing agents,[25,60,61] thereby decreasing the risk for recanalization of the treated vessel.[54,62,63] Third, a decrease in the extent of thrombus formation may also decrease the incidence of postsclerosis pigmentation.[36,64,65] Fourth, the limitation of thrombosis and phlebitic reactions may prevent the appearance of telangiectatic matting.[54] Finally, the function of the calf muscle pump is improved by the physiological effect of a graduated compression stocking.[66] This

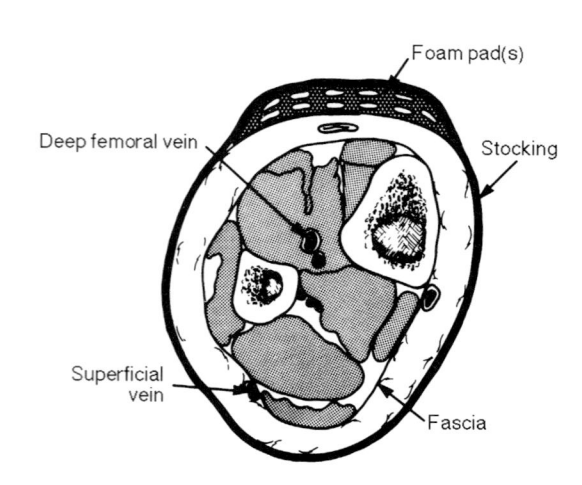

Figure 43.8
Schematic cross-section of a superficial varicose vein compressed with a foam rubber pad under a compression stocking. Note that superficial varicosities lateral to the foam rubber pad are only slightly compressed, and veins deep to the fascia are not compressed. (Reproduced with permission from Goldman MP, Sclerotherapy treatment of varicose and telangiectatic leg veins, Mosby-Yearbook Inc., St Louis, 1991.)

improved efficiency promotes emptying of the superficial veins into the deep system, thereby decreasing their diameter. In addition, by externally supporting untreated large veins, compression stockings will narrow vein diameters, restoring valve function and decreasing retrograde blood flow.[67] External pressure will also retard the reflux of blood from incompetent perforating veins into the superficial veins. In short, compression sclerotherapy is now the standard practice for the treatment of varicose veins.

Compression is also advocated for treating leg telangiectasia. Although one study has found that superficial telangiectasias require up to 80 mmHg for complete closure,[68] graduated compression has a number of potential benefits. First, since telangiectasias are fed by veins of larger diameter, compression (via Laplace's law)

Table 43.3
Sclerotherapy of varicose veins—sequence of events

1. Physical examination
2. Venous Doppler/light reflection rheography
3. If abnormal, consider duplex scanning or varicography
4. Eliminate high-pressure inflow points
   (a) Saphenofemoral–popleteal junction
   (b) Incompetent perforators
5. Sclerotherapy of large-diameter varicose veins
6. Sclerotherapy of communicating or reticular veins which feed 'spider' telangiectasias
7. Sclerotherapy of 'spider' telangiectasias
8. Yellow light laser treatment of remaining fine telangiectasias and arteriolar telangiectasias

Modified from Goldman.[9] By permission of Mosby-Yearbook, Inc.

will produce a greater decrease in luminal diameter of larger feeding veins, decreasing inflow into distal telangiectasias. In addition, if a direct connection exists between telangiectasias and the deep venous system, which has been demonstrated in 13% of patients radiographically,[69] compression will ensure rapid dilution of sclerosant from deep veins, thereby preventing endothelial or valvular damage with subsequent thromboembolic complications. Finally, graduated compression, while not totally closing telangiectasia luminal diameter, will decrease the lumen.[68] A decreased luminal diameter will limit thrombus formation and its resulting complications as demonstrated in a multicenter study.[70]

Summary

The treatment of varicose and telangiectatic leg veins can be approached in a logical, systematic fashion (Table 43.3). Instead of merely the injection of as many veins as possible in a given period of time, 'venous regions' or entire abnormal superficial venous networks on the leg can and should be injected in a single session. Although patients will require differing amounts of time with this systematic approach, with experience, accurate estimations can be made ensuring optimal productivity. It is illogical for physicians to only treat large veins or small veins. A phlebologist (sclerotherapist) should strive to appreciate the venous system as a complete 'system'. With this understanding, we will be best able to render optimal care. Hopefully, this will prevent present-day enthusiasm for sclerotherapy to disappear as it did in the 1940s so that the wheel will not have to be 'reinvented' in the future.

References

1. Pravas C-G, *CR Acad Sci* (1853) **236**:88.
2. Stemmer R, *Sclerotherapy of varicose veins* (Anzoni & Cie AG: St Gallen, Switzerland 1990) 6–8.
3. Linser P, Ueber die konservative behandlung der varicen, *Med Klin* (1916) **12**:897.
4. McAusland S, The modern treatment of varicose veins, *Med Press* (1939) **201**:404–10.
5. Reiner L, The activity of anionic surface active compounds in producing vascular obliteration, *Proc Soc Exp Biol Med* (1946) **62**:49.
6. Sigg K, The treatment of varicosities and accompanying complications, *Angiology* (1952) **3**:355.
7. Orbach EJ, A new approach to the sclerotherapy of varicose veins, *Angiology* (1950) **1**:302.
8. Fegan WG, Continuous compression technique of injecting varicose veins, *Lancet* (1963) **2**:109.
9. Goldman MP, *Sclerotherapy treatment of varicose and telangiectatic leg veins* (Mosby-Yearbook: St Louis 1991).
10. Braverman IM, Ultrastructure and organization of cutaneous

10. microvasculature in normal and pathologic states, *J Invest Dermatol* (1989) **93**:28.
11. Taylor GI, Caddy CM, Watterson PA et al, The venous territories (venosomes) of the human body: experimental study and clinical implications, *J Plast Reconstr Surg* (1990) **86**:185–213.
12. Fegan WG, Compression sclerotherapy, *Ann R Coll Surg Engl* (1967) **41**:364.
13. Beesley WH, Fegan WG, An investigation into the localization of incompetent perforating veins, *Br J Surg* (1970) **57**:30.
14. O'Donnell TF Jr, Burhand KG, Clemenson G et al, Doppler examination vs clinical and phlebologic detection of the location of incompetent perforating veins, *Arch Surg* (1977) **112**:31.
15. Townsend J, Jones H, Williams JE, Detection of incompetent perforating veins by venography at operation, *Br Med J* (1967) **3**:583.
16. Trendelenburg F, Uber die unterdindung der vena saphena magna bei unterschendelvaricen, *Beitr Z Klin Chir* (1891) **7**:195.
17. Perthes G, Uber die operation der unterschelkenvaricen nach trendelenburg, *Dtsh Med Wehrschr* (1895) **21**:253.
18. Fronek H, Noninvasive examination of the patient before sclerotherapy. In: Goldman MP, ed., *Sclerotherapy treatment of varicose and telangiectatic leg veins* (Mosby-Yearbook Publishers: St Louis 1991) 108–57.
19. Hoare MC, Royle JP, Doppler ultrasound detection of saphenofemoral and saphenopopleteal incompetence and operative venography to ensure precise saphenopopleteal ligation, *Aust NZ J Surg* (1984) **54**:49–52.
20. Schultz-Ehrenburg U, Hubner H-J, *Reflux diagnosis with Doppler ultrasound.* (FK Schattauer Verlag: New York 1989).
21. McIrvine AJ, Corbett CRR, Aston NO et al, The demonstration of saphenofemoral incompetence; Doppler ultrasound compared with standard clinical tests, *J Surg* (1984) **71**:509–10.
22. Neumann HAM, Boersma I, Light reflection rheography: a non-invasive diagnostic tool for screening venous disease, *J Dermatol Surg Oncol* (1992) **18**:425–30.
23. Sadick NS, Sclerotherapy of varicose and telangiectatic leg veins: minimal sclerosant concentration of hypertonic saline and its relationship to vessel diameter, *J Dermatol Surg Oncol* (1991) **17**:65–70.
24. Goldman MP, A comparison of sclerosing agents: clinical and histologic effects of intravascular sodium morrhuate, ethanolamine oleate, hypertonic saline (11.7 percent), and sclerodex in the dorsal rabbit ear vein, *J Dermatol Surg Oncol* (1991) **17**:354–62.
25. Goldman MP, Kaplan RP, Oki LN et al, Sclerosing agents in the treatment of telangiectasia: comparison of the clinical and histologic effects of intravascular polidocanol, sodium tetradecyl sulfate, and hypertonic saline in the dorsal rabbit ear vein model, *Arch Dermatol* (1987) **123**:1196–201.
26. Martin DE, Goldman MP, A comparison of sclerosing agents: clinical and histologic effects of intravascular sodium tetradecyl sulfate and chromated glycerin in the dorsal rabbit ear vein, *J Dermatol Surg Oncol* (1990) **16**:18–22.
27. Dick ET, The treatment of varicose veins, *NZ Med J* (1966) **65**:310–13.

28. Lewis KM, Anaphylaxis due to sodium morrhuate, *JAMA* (1936) **107**:1298.

29. Gallagher PG, Varicose veins—primary treatment with sclerotherapy: a personal appraisal, *J Dermatol Surg Oncol* (1992) **18**:39–42.

30. Miyake H, Kauffman P, de Arruda Behmer O et al, Mechanisms of cutaneous necrosis provoked by sclerosing injections in the treatment of microvarices and telangiectasias: experimental study, *Rev Ass Brasil* (1976) **22**:115–20.

31. Glaxo Pharmaceuticals, Product insert, Research Triangle Park, NC, 1989.

32. Foote RR, Severe reaction to monoethanolamine oleate, *Lancet* (1944) **2**:390–1.

33. Hughes RW Jr, Larson DE, Viggiane TR et al, Endoscopic variceal sclerosis: a one-year experience, *Gastrointest Endosc* (1982) **28**:62.

34. Reid RG, Rothine NG, treatment of varicose veins by compression sclerotherapy, *Br J Surg* (1968) **55**:889–95.

35. Ethanolamin Injection 5%, Product Information, Glaxo Inc., December, 1988.

36. Goldman MP, Bennett RG, Treatment of telangiectasia: a review, *J Am Acad Dermatol* (1987) **17**:167–82.

37. Fegan WG, The complications of compression sclerotherapy. *The Practitioner* (1971) **207**:797–9.

38. Stother IG, Bryson A, Alexander S, The treatment of varicose veins by compression sclerotherapy, *Br J Surg* (1974) **61**:387–90.

39. Passas H, One case of tetradecyl-sodium sulfate allergy with general symptoms, *Soc Franc Phlebol* (1972) **25**:19–26.

40. Clinical Drug Safety Surveillance Group, Correspondence from Minicozzi P, Wyeth-Ayerst Laboratories, 1991.

41. Fronek H, Fronek A, Saltzbarg G, Allergic reactions to sotradecol, *J Dermatol Surg Oncol* (1989) **15**:684.

42. Jaquier JJ, Loretan RM, Clinical trials of a new sclerosing agent, aethoxysklerol, *Soc Fran Phlebol* (1969) **22**:383–5.

43. Heberova V, Treatment of telangiectasias of the lower extremities by sclerotization. Results and evaluation, *Cs Dermatol* (1976) **51**:232–5.

44. Foley WT, The eradication of venous blemishes, *Cutis* (1975) **15**:665–8.

45. Sadick N, The treatment of varicose and telangiectatic leg veins with hypertonic saline: a comparative study of heparin and saline, *J Dermatol Surg Oncol* (1990) **16**:24–8.

46. Mantse L, A mild sclerosing agent for telangiectasias, *J Dermatol Surg Oncol* (1985) **11**:9.

47. Wenner L, Anwendung einer mit athylalkohol modifizerten polijodidjonenlosung bei skleroseresistenten varizen, *VASA* (1983) **12**:190–2.

48. Imhoff E, Stemmer R, Classification and mechanism of action of sclerosing agents, *Soc Franc Phlebol* (1969) **22**:143–8.

49. Ouvry PA, Telangiectasia and sclerotherapy, *J Dermatol Surg Oncol* (1989) **15**:177–81.

50. Scleremo Product Information, Laboratoires E. Bouteille, 7, rue des Belges, 8100 Limoges, France, 1987.

51. Hutinel B, Esthetique dans les scleroses de varices et traitement des varicosites, *La Vie Medicale* (1978) **20**:1739–43.

52. Nebot F, Quelques points tecniques sur le traitement des varicosites et des telangiectasies, *Phlebologie* (1968) **21**:133–5.

53. Ouvry P, Arlaud R, Le traitement sclerosant des telangiectasies des membres inferieurs, *Phlebologie* (1979) **32**:365–70.

54. Ouvry P, Davy A, Le traitement sclerosant des telangiectasies des membres inferieurs, *Phlebologie* (1982) **35**:349–59.

55. Wallois P, Incidents et accidents de la sclerose. In: Tournay R, ed., *La sclerose des varices*, 4th edn (Expansion Scientifique Francaise: Paris 1985) 297–319.

56. Reid RG, Rothnie NG, Treatment of varicose veins by compression sclerotherapy, *Br J Surg* (1968) **55**:889–95.

57. Fentem PH, Goddard M, Godden BA et al, Control of distension of varicose veins achieved by leg bandages as used after injection sclerotherapy, *Br Med J* (1976) **2**:725.

58. Raj TB, Goddard M, Makin GS, How long do compression bandages maintain their pressure during ambulatory treatment of varicose veins? *Br J Surg* (1980) **67**:122.

59. Goldman MP, Compression hosiery and elastic bandages. In: Goldman MP, ed., *Sclerotherapy treatment of varicose and telangiectatic leg veins* (Mosby-Yearbook: St Louis 1991) 158–82.

60. Lufkin H, McPheeters HQ, Pathological studies on injected varicose veins, *Surg Gynecol Obstet* (1932) **54**:511–17.

61. Harridge H, The treatment of primary varicose veins, *Surg Clin North Am* (1960) **40**:191–202.

62. Fegan WG, Continuous compression technique of injecting varicose veins, *Lancet* (1963) **2**:109–12.

63. Fegan WG, Continuing uninterrupted compression technique of injecting varicose veins, *Proc R Soc Med* (1960) **53**:837–40.

64. Wenner L, Sind endovarikose hamatische ansammlungen eine normalerscheinung bei sklerotherapie? *VASA* (1981) **10**:174–6.

65. Goldman MP, Kaplan RP, Duffy DM, Postsclerotherapy hyperpigmentation: a histologic evaluation, *J Dermatol Surg Oncol* (1987) **13**:547–50.

66. Struckmann J, Christensen SJ, Lendorf A et al, Venous muscle pump improvement by low compression elastic stockings, *Phlebology* (1986) **1**:97–103.

67. Somerville JJ, Brown GO, Byrne PJ et al, The effect of elastic stockings on superficial venous pressures in patients with venous insufficiency, *Br J Surg* (1974) **61**:979–81.

68. Allan JC, The micro-circulation of the skin of the normal leg, in varicose veins and in the post-thrombotic syndrome, *S African J Surg* (1972) **10**:29.

69. Bohler-Sommeregger K, Karnel F, Schuller-Petrovic S et al, Do telangiectases communicate with the deep venous system? *J Dermatol Surg Oncol* (1992) **18**:403–6.

70. Goldman MP, Beaudoing D, Marley W et al, Compression in the treatment of leg telangiectasia, *J Dermatol Surg Oncol* (1990) **16**:322–5.

Chapter 44

SOFT TISSUE AUGMENTATION: NEW TECHNIQUES AND RECENT CONTROVERSIES

Jeffrey L. Melton
C. William Hanke

INTRODUCTION

Augmentation of soft tissues by injection has long been an attractive notion for both physicians and patients. Surgically placed implants have long been used for tissue augmentation, but the simplicity and elegance of an injectable material has an even broader appeal. This is reflected in the illustrious history of tissue augmentation by injection. Silicone was one of the first substances used. From early on, its use has attracted controversy. Such controversy recently intensified, with increased regulatory activity by the United States Food and Drug Administration (FDA) in this area. Fortunately other injectable substances have been developed for soft tissue augmentation. These include the injectable collagens, which are the only injectable materials presently approved by the FDA for soft tissue augmentation. Other newer techniques and materials, such as microlipoinjection and autologous collagen, are increasingly used options open to the practitioner and patient. Microlipoinjection is discussed in Chapter 45.

ZYDERM/ZYPLAST

History and development

Zyderm I was the first injectable filler substance to be approved by the Food and Drug Administration (FDA), in 1981. Zyderm (Collagen Corporation, Palo Alto, CA) is pepsin-digested purified bovine dermal collagen. Thus, it is a xenograft. Pepsin digestion removes the telopeptide regions of the collagen molecule; this renders the molecule less antigenic. Three forms of bovine collagen are available: Zyderm I, Zyderm II, and Zyplast. The concentration of collagen in Zyderm I is 35 mg/ml. Zyderm I is 95% type I collagen and 1–5% type III collagen. The product is suspended in a phosphate-buffered saline solution, and also contains 0.3% lidocaine to minimize the discomfort of injection. Zyderm II is a similar product, but with a higher concentration of collagen, 65 mg/ml. Zyderm II was approved by the FDA in 1983. Zyplast, FDA approved in 1985, is crosslinked with glutaraldehyde during processing. The concentration of collagen in Zyplast is the same as for

Zyderm I, 35 mg/ml. However, the crosslinking renders Zyplast a more stable product, with less short-term shrinkage from syneresis than Zyderm I or Zyderm II.

Indications, contraindications and skin testing

Zyderm and Zyplast are indicated for the correction of contour deficiencies of the dermis. The particular material chosen and duration of correction are in part site dependent (Table 44.1).

A past history of autoimmune disease, such as systemic lupus erythematosus, dermatomyositis or rheumatoid arthritis, is a contraindication to treatment, as is a positive skin test to Zyderm. Allergy to other bovine products or to lidocaine also contraindicates treatment with Zyderm or Zyplast. Patients with an atopic background or multiple allergies should be treated with caution. Patients allergic to or undergoing desensitization to meat products should not be treated with Zyderm or Zyplast.

Recommendations regarding skin testing prior to bovine collagen treatment are changing. When they are used for the general population, a single skin test is recommended on the current Zyderm and Zyplast package inserts, except in patients with a history of beef allergy. In those patients, a second skin test is recommended. A second skin test identifies a small group of patients who react only to the second test. This process of double skin testing is now recommended by Elson,[1] Klein,[2] Hanke[3] and others for all new patients receiving Zyderm or Zyplast. Approximately 2% of patients who are initially skin test negative will be positive on the second skin test. It is felt that these patients are at increased risk for treatment site reactions. However, patients who test positive on only the second or subsequent tests may have a tendency for milder treatment site reactions than those who are positive on the first test.[2] Double skin testing decreases but does not eliminate treatment site reactions, since reactions to later injections may occur even after two negative tests. Nevertheless, we feel that the consensus among practitioners currently favors double skin testing. In our practice, double skin testing is performed as follows: 0.1 ml Zyderm is placed intradermally on the volar forearm. The patient is evaluated at 48–72 h, and at 4 weeks. If no reaction occurs, a second test is placed on the opposite arm at 4 weeks. The patient is again evaluated at 48–72 h, and at 4 weeks. If no reaction has occurred on either arm, treatment is initiated. If a patient has had multiple treatments

Table 44.1
Indications and duration of correction for Zyderm/Zyplast

Indication	Recommended product	Duration of correction (months)
Crow's feet	Zd I	6–12
Glabellar frown lines	Zd I or II	6–12
Transverse forehead lines	Zd I or II	6–12
Secondary cheek wrinkles	Zd I or II	12–18
Marionette lines	Zd I or II, Zp	4–6
Perioral lines	Zd I or II, Zp	4–6
Nasolabial furrows	Zd I or II, Zp	4–6
Undulating scars	Zd I or II, Zp	6–18

Zd, Zyderm; Zp, Zyplast.

without difficulty from another physician, we may treat without additional testing. However, if 2 years have elapsed since any testing or treatment, we perform a single skin test. A positive skin test manifests as local induration and/or erythema at the treatment site which persists more than 6 h (Figure 44.1).

Injection technique and results

Before treatment, the skin should be washed with soap and water and wiped with an alcohol pad. Patients should be treated in the sitting position to allow for gravitational effects on facial contours. A mirror should be given to the patient to facilitate the discussion of areas of interest. Patients should avoid taking aspirin or other nonsteroidal anti-inflammatory agents for 10 days prior to treatment. Tangential lighting is optimal for accentuating depressed areas to be treated.

Zyplast is best suited for deeper placement in the reticular dermis (Figure 44.2). Thus it is appropriate for deeper wrinkles and furrows such as the nasolabial groove. Zyderm is preferred for superficial defects and is placed in the papillary dermis (Figures 44.3 and 44.4). If Zyderm is placed too deeply (that is, in the deep reticular dermis) the correction will be minimal; if Zyplast is placed too superficially, an unattractive, slowly resolving 'beading' will occur. Beading can also occur with Zyderm if it is placed superficially in thin skin, such as the lateral canthus. For defects

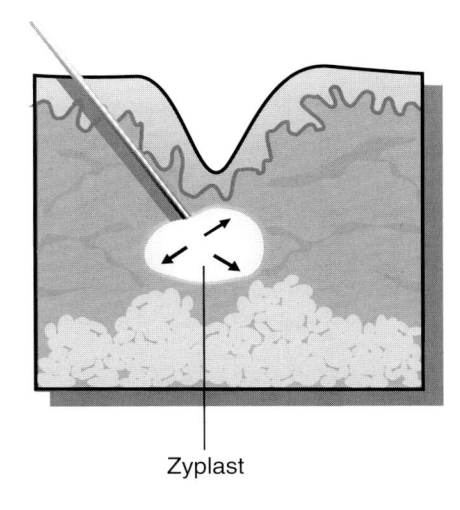

Figure 44.2
Zyplast is placed in the mid-to-lower reticular dermis.

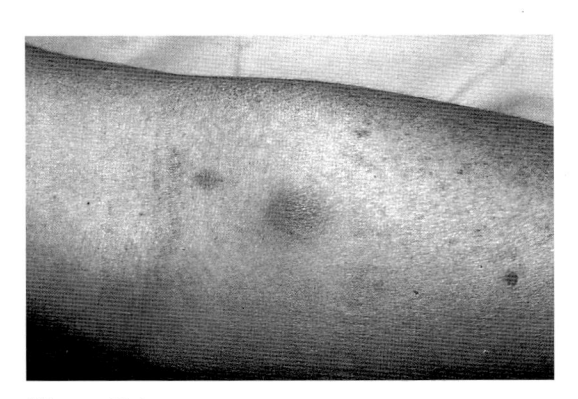

Figure 44.1
A positive Zyderm skin test is characterized by swelling and erythema.

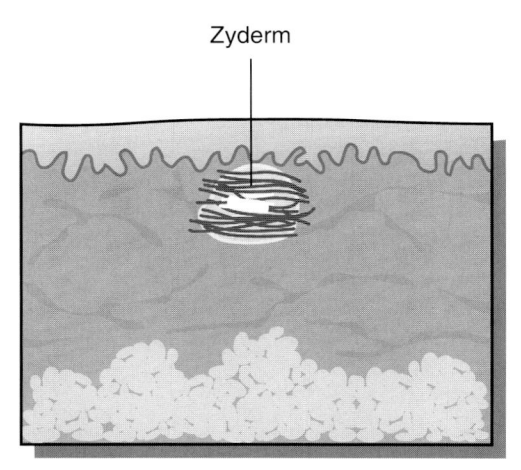

Figure 44.3
Zyderm is placed in the papillary or superficial reticular dermis.

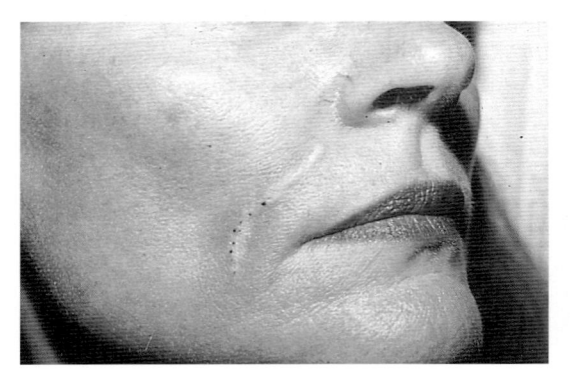

SURGICAL DERMATOLOGY

Figure 44.4
A white blanch is observed immediately following papillary dermal placement of Zyderm I.

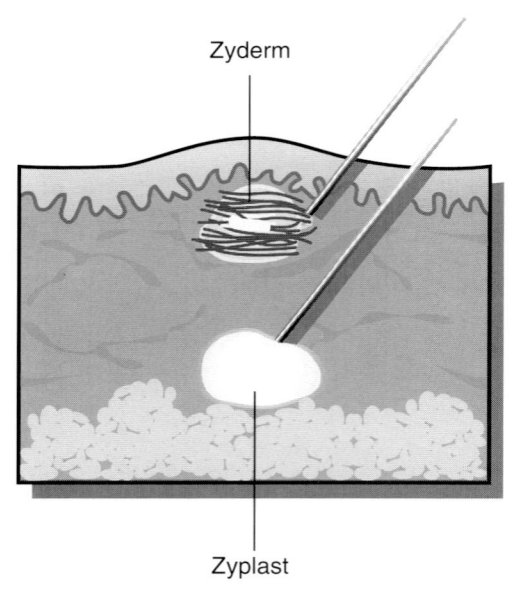

Figure 44.5
The 'layering technique' is used for defects involving both papillary and reticular dermis. Zyplast is placed in the deeper reticular dermis, followed by placement of Zyderm in the superficial dermis.

Figure 44.6
(A) A 50-year-old woman with superficial creases and deep furrows in the nasolabial fold areas. (B) Correction with 'layering technique' with Zyplast placed deeply and Zyderm I superficially.

involving the superficial and deeper dermis, the 'layering technique', using both Zyderm and Zyplast, can be helpful (Figures 44.5 and 44.6). Superficial wrinkle lines are treated by the serial puncture technique using Zyderm I (Figure 44.7).

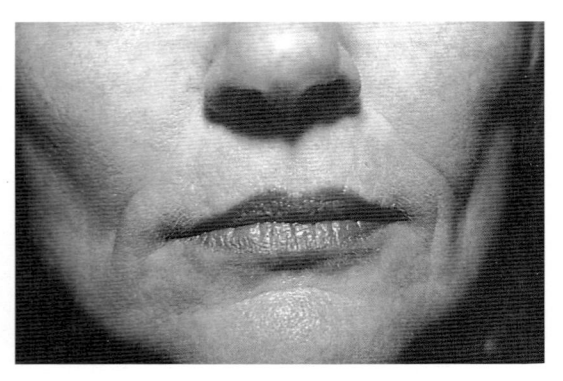

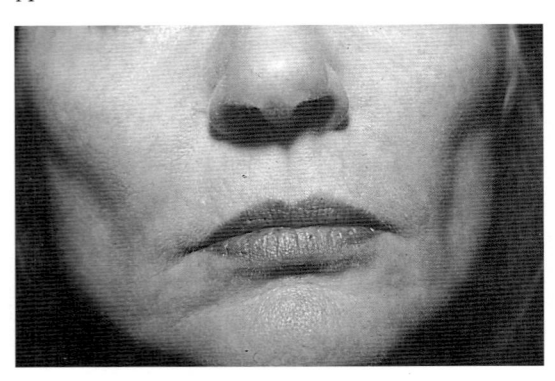

The duration of the implant depends upon the material used and the patient's movement at the site of the implant (Table 44.1). Zyderm and Zyplast correction is lost as implants gradually migrate from the dermis into the subcutaneous tissue.[4,5] Dynamic wrinkles and folds lose correction relatively quickly; nasolabial folds may require retreatment every 6 months. Scars subject to little motion can maintain correction up to 18–24 months.

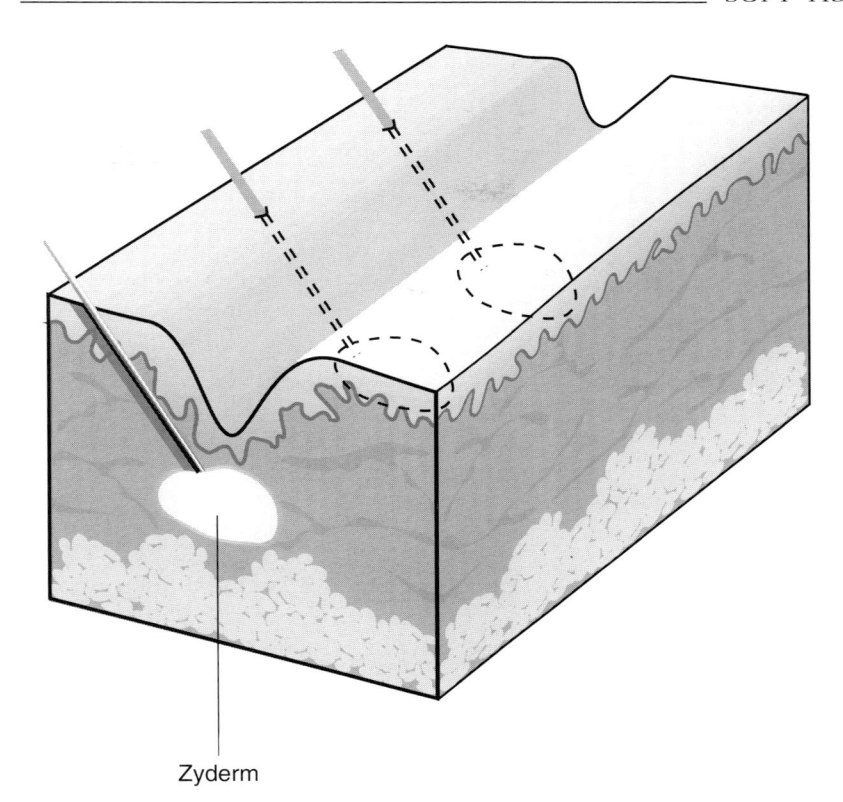

Figure 44.7
The serial puncture technique for superficial wrinkle lines involves the superficial placement of small amounts of Zyderm via multiple punctures.

Zyderm

Adverse reactions

Adverse reactions to Zyderm and Zyplast injections can be divided into allergic and nonallergic types. Nonallergic reactions include bruising, surface irregularity, necrosis, infection, and intermittent swelling. Bruising occurs easily in some patients. Aspirin, other nonsteroidal anti-inflammatory agents or anticoagulants predispose to bruising. In patients not taking these medications, bruising is usually minimal and resolves quickly.

Surface irregularities, such as beading, usually occur with placement that is too superficial for the product or site. Thus, it is more common with Zyplast but can occur with Zyderm in the lateral canthal area or very thin skin. This beading resolves very slowly.

Local necrosis most commonly occurs with Zyplast, and the glabella is a particularly susceptible site. Necrosis may result from intravascular or juxtavascular placement. Infection is quite rare following collagen injection. Allergic reactions to Zyderm and Zyplast can be minimized by double skin testing. Allergic reactions most commonly occur after the first or second treatment, and are uncommon after several successful treatments. Allergic reactions usually manifest as erythematous papules or linear streaks localized to the site of placement (Figure 44.8). The reaction usually resolves spontaneously over a 6-month period. Rarely, this reaction may last up to 2 years. Topical, intralesional or systemic corticosteroids are not usually helpful. Excision of the allergic reaction site is best avoided, since spontaneous resolution

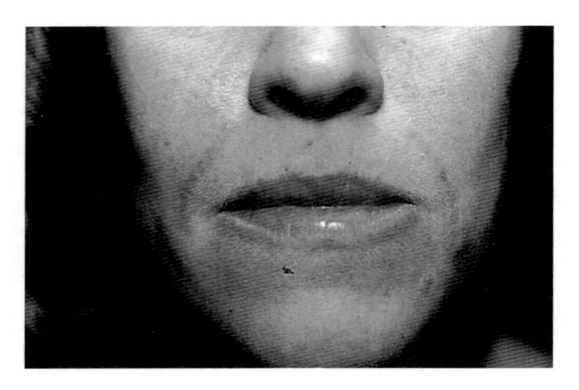

Figure 44.8
This 30-year-old woman has an allergic treatment site reaction to Zyderm I in the nasolabial fold area. The reaction resolved over 6 months.

without scarring is the rule. Rarely, a painful abscess-like reaction may occur.[6] This reaction is similar to the standard allergic reaction, except that nodules and draining abscesses occur. Incision and drainage is the treatment of choice.

A small subgroup of patients treated with Zyderm or Zyplast have been reported to develop connective tissue diseases, including polymyositis/dermatomyositis, rheumatoid arthritis, or systemic lupus erythematosus. Although patients with no such previous history have manifested these disorders subsequent to collagen injection, no causal relationship has been established. An 'FDA Collagen Public Meeting' was held at Rockville, Maryland on 25 October 1991. A panel of seven experts concluded that there was not significant statistical or biological evidence for increased risk of connective tissue disease in patients receiving bovine collagen implants.

Fibrel

History and development

Fibrel (Serono Laboratories, Randolf, MA) was the second collagen-based injectable material to be approved by the FDA for the correction of soft tissue defects. Fibrel was approved by the FDA for scars in 1988, and for age-related lines in 1990. Fibrel developed from the work of Spangler,[7] who in 1957 published his first results with a mixture of fibrin foam (Gelfoam), human plasma and thrombin. This technique was later refined by Gottlieb, who dubbed the technique the GAP (gelatin foam, epsilon-aminocaproic acid, plasma) technique. The Fibrel kit is sterile and contains all components necessary for treatment except the patient's plasma. One hundred and twenty-five milligrams of epsilon-aminocaproic acid are mixed with 100 mg gelatin powder, 0.5 ml normal saline, and 0.5 ml serum. Thus, a centrifuge is required to spin blood drawn from the patient. Preparing the material takes approximately 15 min. The gelatin powder is composed of porcine collagen (types II and III) that has been denatured.

Indications, contraindications and skin testing

Fibrel is indicated for the treatment of depressed cutaneous scars and for age-related lines. Scars ideal for treatment are distensible and improve with manual stretching or pinching.

Age and sun-related lines and wrinkles such as nasolabial grooves and glabellar frown lines can be improved by Fibrel. However, very superficial lines and wrinkles are difficult to treat as it is difficult to place the product superficially with a 27-gauge needle. The viscosity of Fibrel usually precludes using a smaller-gauge needle. Scars, particularly undulating acne scars, are also treated with Fibrel. The ideal acne scar for treatment is a dish-shaped scar which becomes less obvious when tension is applied across it. Deeper 'ice-pick' scars are difficult to improve with injectable augmentations. Depressed skin grafts can also be elevated with Fibrel injections (Figure 44.9).

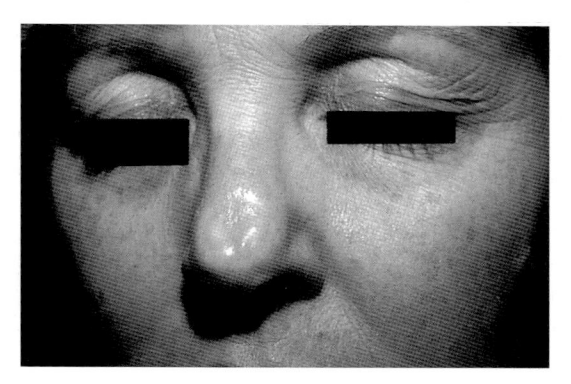

SOFT TISSUE AUGMENTATION

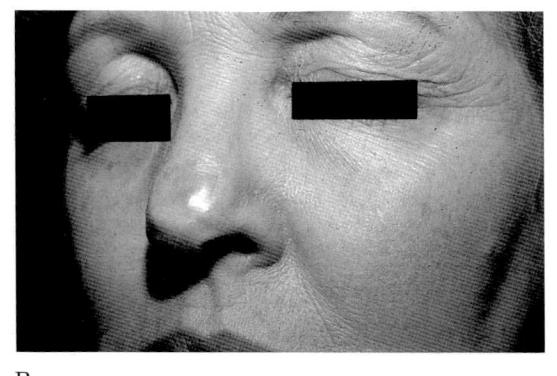

A

B

Figure 44.9
(A) A 36-year-old woman with a depressed full-thickness skin graft on the nose following excision of a basal cell carcinoma. (B) The contour of the graft is much improved following Fibrel injections.

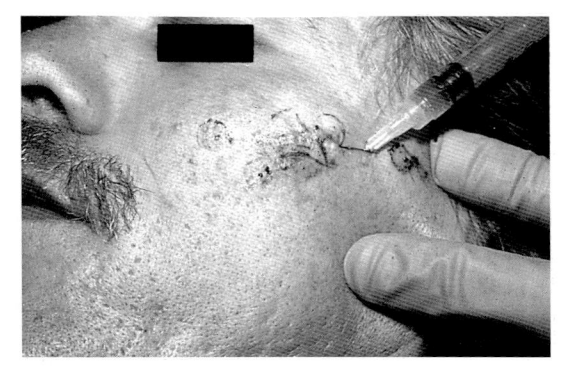

Figure 44.10
A 30-year-old man with acne scars on the cheeks. The areas to be treated with Fibrel are outlined before local anesthetic is injected. A white blanche is evidence that the implant is in the upper dermis.

Fibrel is contraindicated in patients who have a history of keloids, anaphylactoid reactions, previous hypersensitivity to Fibrel, or a history of autoimmune disease. Patients who are allergic to epsilon-aminocaproic acid, gelatin foam or benzyl alcohol should likewise not be treated with Fibrel. A Fibrel skin test is done before treatment. An intradermal injection of 0.05 ml Fibrel is administered on the volar forearm. For the skin test, the gelatin powder is mixed with normal saline only (the patient's plasma is not used). A positive skin test is characterized by erythema, induration or inflammation lasting more than 5 h. The patient should return for evaluation of the skin test 4 weeks later, but no evaluation at 24–72 h is required. Of patients undergoing skin tests with Fibrel, 1.9% have a positive response. Patients who are allergic to Zyderm or Zyplast may be skin tested to and treated with Fibrel.

Injection technique

In our experience, patients cannot tolerate Fibrel injection without prior local anesthesia. This is due to both the burning upon injection and the need to use a 27-gauge needle, which is painful. Prior to treatment, the face is washed with soap and water and then an alcohol wipe. The scars to be treated are outlined (Figure 44.10). After marking, each scar is anesthetized with 1% lidocaine with 1:200 000 epinephrine, using a 30-gauge needle. The scars are injected with Fibrel 15 min later, using the 27-gauge needle. An overcorrection of 100–200% is desired. Fibrotic scars can sometimes be released with the custom undermining needle in the Fibrel kit. This creates a pocket for the Fibrel implant.

Placement of Fibrel too superficially can result in prolonged surface irregularities. Therefore, Fibrel should be placed in the mid-to-deep reticular dermis. It is also important to minimize the number of needle punctures through the skin during treatment so that the material does not leak back onto the skin surface through excessive puncture wounds. Therefore, a linear threading technique is preferred for treating wrinkles.

In animal studies, Fibrel is completely replaced by collagen 90 days after implantation in the dermis. The original Fibrel multicenter trial included 288 patients with 840 scars treated. At 1 year follow-up the percentage of scars showing correction was 65% by patient evaluation, 63% by physician evaluation, and 86% by photogrammetric measurements.[8] In a subsequent study,[9] 111 patients with 302 scars were treated and followed for 2 years. At 2 years 65% improvement was still present. In another series,[10] 78 patients were followed for 5 years. More than 50% of the scars maintained significant correction, with an average loss of only 35% of their original correction.

Adverse reactions

Mild swelling of the treated area is common and occurs immediately following injection. Swelling usually lasts for 1–3 days, but may take as long as 1–2 weeks before resolving spontaneously. Swelling may occur to a greater degree if placement of the implant is too superficial or if correction is too aggressive. Local necrosis has also occurred after Fibrel injection, as with Zyplast, and the glabella is the most likely site. Allergic treatment site reactions are rare with Fibrel. Spangler has observed no allergic treatment site reactions in over 17 years of experience with fibrin foam.[7]

AUTOLOGOUS COLLAGEN

Liposuction and lipoinjection, discussed elsewhere in this book (Chapter 45), have brought to the forefront yet another source of collagen for soft tissue augmentation. This was originally described by Fournier,[11] who used fibrous septae, discarded from liposuction, for injection into soft tissue defects. At present, the viscosity of autologous collagen necessitates a fairly large needle for injection. A 15–18-gauge needle is usually needed with prior local anesthetic. Unfortunately, the larger needle results in significant bruising and also makes superficial placement difficult.

LIQUID SILICONE

Although solid silicone implants have been extensively used as medial prostheses for a long time, use of liquid silicone for soft tissue augmentation has always been controversial. Opponents of liquid silicone assert that the material is inherently unsafe. Proponents maintain that when pure silicone is used with proper technique, the side-effects are minimal. There is support for the safety of liquid silicone in the literature.[12,13] However, the FDA has recently increased its regulatory interest with respect to liquid silicone. On 13 February 1992, FDA commissioner David Kessler, speaking before the Utah International Medical Device Congress, stated that liquid silicone injections 'cannot legally be used in this country. We are investigating certain clinicians who practice this procedure, and will investigate others as violations are detected'.[14] Since the FDA's interpretation is that the use or promotion of liquid silicone is illegal, most if not all clinical use of liquid silicone has stopped.

Editors' note: Patient safety comes first. 'Physician do no harm.' This philosophy sufficiently justifies the FDA's position on silicone. However, it does not justify the fear of recrimination that the FDA has instilled in American physicians who wish to discuss new or unapproved therapies in an academic forum. Injectable silicone is discussed in great detail elsewhere,[15] but is not discussed further in this book.

REFERENCES

1. Elson ML, The role of skin testing in the use of collagen injectable materials, *J Dermatol Surg Oncol* (1989) **15**:301–3.

2. Klein AW, In favor of double skin testing, *J Dermatol Surg Oncol* (1989) **15**:263.

3. Hanke CW, Coleman WP, Collagen filler substances. In: Coleman WP, Hanke CW, Alt TH et al, eds, *Cosmetic surgery of the skin* (BC Decker: Philadelphia 1991) 89–103.

4. Grosh SK, Hanke CW, DeVore DP et al, Variables affecting the results of xenogenic collagen implantation in an animal model, *J Am Acad Dermatol* (1985) **13**:792–8.

5. Robinson JK, Hanke CW, Injectable collagen implant: histopathologic identification and longevity of correction, *J Dermatol Surg Oncol* (1985) **11**:124–30.

6. Hanke CW, Higley HR, Jolivette DM et al, Abscess formation and local necrosis after treatment with Zyderm or Zyplast collagen implant, *J Am Acad Dermatol* (1991) **25**:319–26.

7. Spangler AS, Treatment of depressed scars with fibrin foam—seventeen years of experience, *J Dermatol Surg Oncol* (1975) **1**:65.

8. Millikan LE, Rosen T, Monheit G et al, Treatment of depressed cutaneous scars with gelatin matrix implant: a multicenter study, *J Am Acad Dermatol* (1987) **16**:1155–62.

9. Millikan L, Alexander AM, Chungi VS et al, Long-term safety and efficacy with Fibrel in the treatment of cutaneous scars—results of a multi-center study, *J Dermatol Surg Oncol* (1989) **15**:837–42.

10. Millikan LE, Banks K, Parkail B et al, A 5-year safety and efficacy evaluation with Fibrel in the correction of cutaneous scars following one or two treatments, *J Dermatol Surg Oncol* (1991) **17**:223–9.

11. Fournier P, Facial recontouring with fat grafting, *Dermatol Clin* (1990) **8**:523–37.

12. Clark DP, Hanke CW, Swanson NA, Dermal implants, safety of products injected for soft-tissue augmentation, *J Am Acad Dermatol* (1989) **21**:992–8.

13. Webster RC, Fuleihon MP, Gaunt JM, Injectable silicone for small augmentations: twenty year experience in humans, *Am J Cosmet Surg* (1984) **1**:1–10.

14. Schwartz RM, Action on silicone injection marks busy regulatory period for the FDA. *Cosmet Dermatol* (1992) **5**:48–51.

15. Orentreich DS, Orentreich N, Injectable fluid silicone. In: Roenigk RK, Roenigk HH Jr, eds, *Dermatologic surgery—principles and practice* (Marcel Dekker: New York 1989) 1349–95.

Chapter 45

MICROLIPOINJECTION

Kevin S. Pinski
Henry H. Roenigk Jr

INTRODUCTION

Fat transplantation surgery began almost one century ago when, in 1893, Neuber[1] reported on his technique of free fat transplantation. He utilized 1-cm pieces of free fat from the upper arm to reconstruct depressed facial defects. In 1911, Bruning[2] was the earliest to report the technique of fat injection. He placed small pieces of fat into a syringe and by injecting this adipose tissue corrected post-rhinoplasty deformities. Free fat transplants were then neglected because most surgeons preferred to use pedicle flaps which preserved the blood supply to the fat, thus making the outcome more predictable. In addition, artificial substances such as paraffin and silicone became available and were used to fill defects in the skin at that time.

Peer[3] reported a series of experiments in 1950 with autologous human fat transplants in which over 50% of the fat remained as a viable transplant 1 year following grafting. The current phase of fat transplantation began in 1976 when Fischer and Fischer[4] performed fat extraction with the cellusuctiotome. Two years later, Illouz[5,6] introduced the simplified and safer method known today as liposuction. This has provided the cosmetic surgeon with an abundant supply of viable adipose tissue which can be used to augment soft tissue deformities.

TECHNIQUE

Microlipoinjection involves extracting and reimplanting adipose tissue by a closed technique. The instrument used can be a needle, cannula or trocar, all of variable caliber and mounted on a syringe. This allows the extraction, preparation and reinjection of adipose tissue in a closed space while respecting the integrity and sterility of the extracted tissue.

Initially the donor and recipient sites should be marked, and then under sterile conditions the fat is removed. The surgeon must respect the extracted tissue and minimize the hydraulic and chemical trauma. Anesthesia of the donor area should be performed first. Several possibilities exist: a nerve block, local anesthesia, external cryoanesthesia, or general anesthesia. The authors prefer local anesthesia with the tumescent technique[7] (Table 45.1).

Anesthesia of the recipient area is then performed. The skin should be anesthetized as a priority as the subcutaneous fat is less sensitive. If local anesthe-

Table 45.1
Tumescent formula

Lidocaine	500 mg (50 ml 1% lidocaine solution)
Epinephrine	1 mg (1 ml 1:1000 solution of epinephrine)
Sodium bicarbonate	12.5 mmol (12.5 ml 8.4% NaH$_2$CO$_3$ solution)
Normal saline	1000 ml 0.9% NaCl solution

sia is used, care should be taken not to distort the recipient sites. This is successfully accomplished by placing only a small bleb of 1% lidocaine at the proposed entry points of the needle.

After waiting 10–15 min for the maximum hemostatic effect of epinephrine, extract the fat with a 5–60-ml syringe, using either a 1½-inch 14-gauge needle or a 6- or 9-cm microlipoextractor. There are other microcannulas with different diameters and tips that are equally effective.

It is important to fill the dead space in the syringe tip and cannula lumen in order to create the hydraulic action of the syringe vacuum. Fill the syringe with normal saline and then expel all but enough to fill the dead space in the cannula.

Next, a 2-mm incision is made in the skin with a No. 11 blade. Incision sites should be kept to a minimum as multiple incisions create an open atmosphere and diminish the benefits of a closed system. After the needle or the microcannula attached to the syringe is inserted in the fat, the plunger of the syringe is pulled to create a negative pressure within it. This relative vacuum will be sufficient to aspirate the fat as the needle is maneuvered back and forth within the fat. During the entire procedure, the skin is constantly palpated by the surgeon's free hand. The hand is held flat over the treated area and the skin is pinched to feel the thickness of the fat.

The needle/cannula is moved back and forth five or six times in the same area, after which the maneuver is repeated in a radial fashion until the entire donor area is used or sufficient fat has been aspirated. During the whole extraction the plunger will be kept in the same position. When the extraction is complete the extracting needle or microcannula is removed and the syringe capped.

The syringe is placed vertically in a test tube holder, plunger up. This will cause separation and the excess fluid (local anesthetic and blood) to accumulate in its dependent part, near its tip. This fluid should be expelled by gently pushing the plunger after it stands for approximately 10 min. The syringe will also contain a turbid, pale yellow supernatant fluid from the broken adipocytes. This should be drained by removing the plunger and pouring it out.

An 18- or 16-gauge needle is attached to the filled syringe. This is inserted at the anesthetized recipient sites, into the subcutaneous layer, until it reaches its most distal point. As the plunger is gently pushed in, the needle is slowly withdrawn in a retrograde fashion until it almost reaches its point of insertion. It is then introduced in different areas until the defect is completely corrected. The injected material should be gently molded with thumb and index finger.

LONG-TERM FOLLOW-UP

Recently, the technique of fat transfer by injection, after syringe or cannula suction, has found many clinical applications. Despite this, many questions remain to be answered. The most basic of these include: which factors influence the survival of fat grafts? What is the morbidity of this procedure? What is the best donor site? Do the grafts survive and for how long? In an attempt to answer these questions, the authors were prompted to review their long-term experience with autologous fat transplantation.[8]

There really is no scientific way to objectively quantify the amount of fat remaining in long-term follow-up studies of fat transplantation. All attempts to mark the injected fat with dyes and radioactive elements have failed because this kills the adipose cells.[9] Optical profilometry to quantitatively analyze augmentation therapy has also been tried.[10] This is an excellent technique for assessing the volume of superficially injected materials like collagen, but it is limited in measuring subcutaneously placed filler substances such as fat. Therefore, in this study we have chosen to determine long-term results by using a clinical evaluation scale together with patient assessments, despite the inherent subjectivity of this method. We are currently undertaking a second project utilizing magnetic resonance imaging to evaluate fat injections.[11]

Our study[8] involved 43 patients (24 women and 19 men), mean age 34.5 years (range 22–69 years). These patients had previously undergone autologous fat transplantations for the correction of cosmetic defects (Table 45.2). The recipient sites of the fat transplant (or the sites of the cosmetic defects) were the cheeks, forehead, nasolabial folds, and earlobe (Table 45.3). The donor sites of the adipose tissue were the abdomen, thigh, and buttocks (Table 45.4). Our duration of follow-up ranged from 3 to 48 months, with a mean of 26 months. These 43 patients were evaluated clinically and with serial photographs and patient questionnaires.

Graft longevity was examined in relation to the cosmetic defect treated (Figure 45.1). Four specific time intervals were studied: 3, 6, 9 and 12 months postoperatively. Because we corrected only one case of trauma-induced scarring, this datum is omitted. Lesions of linear morphea tended to have the least amount of fat resorption (55% of fat graft remaining at 12 months). There was greater fat resorption for expression lines/wrinkles, which initially had slightly better results than acne scars. However, both had only 30% fat remaining at 12 months. The treatment of discoid lupus erythematosus scars was suboptimal, with 50% fat resorption at 3 months and only 10% of the transplanted material remaining at 12 months.

Table 45.2
Cosmetic problems treated with autologous fat transplantation

Cosmetic problem	No. of cases
Acne scars	23
Linear morphea	9
Expression lines	8
Discoid lupus erythematosus scars	2
Post-traumatic scarring	1
Total	43

Table 45.3
Recipient sites of autologous fat transplants

Recipient site	No. of cases
Cheeks	26
Forehead	10
Nasolabial folds	6
Earlobe	1
Total	43

Table 45.4
Donor sites for autologous fat transplantation

Donor site	No. of cases
Abdomen	24
Thigh	10
Buttock	9
Total	43

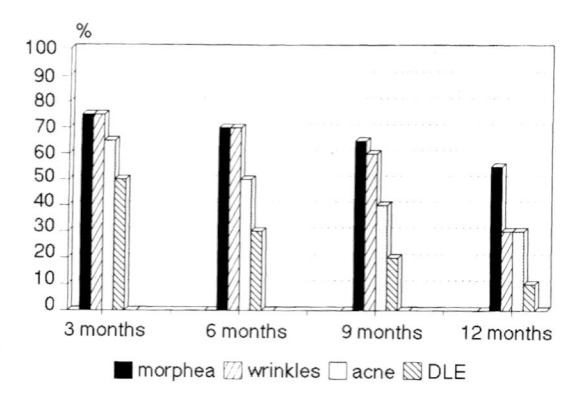

Figure 45.1
Northwestern University—fat transplant study. Graft longevity in relation to cosmetic defect.

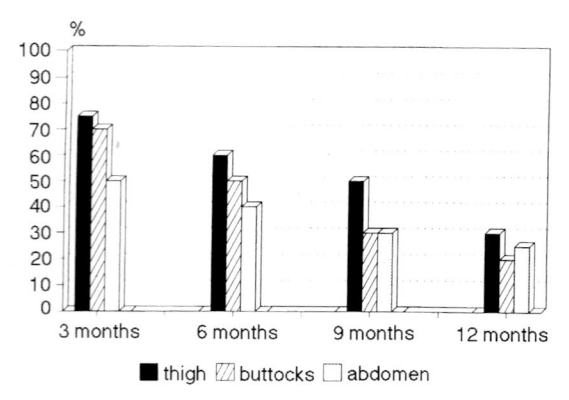

Figure 45.2
Northwestern University—fat transplant study. Graft longevity in relation to donor site.

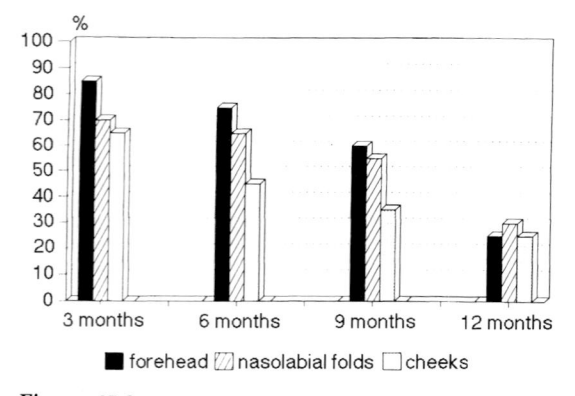

Figure 45.3
Northwestern University—fat transplant study. Graft longevity in relation to recipient site.

Fat graft longevity was assessed in relation to the donor site. Obtaining adipose tissue from the thigh resulted in less fat resorption throughout all four time intervals (Figure 45.2). In comparing the buttocks and abdomen as donor sites, the difference in fat resorption was not as distinct. Both resulted in only 30% of the fat graft remaining at 9 months after fat transplantation.

Graft longevity in relation to the recipient site revealed that the forehead allowed less fat resorption during the first 9 months postoperatively (Figure 45.3). Similarly, the nasolabial folds were a better recipient site than the cheeks. However, at the 12-month interval all three recipient sites had only 25–30% of the original fat transplant remaining (Figure 45.3).

Our postoperative complications included minor bruising, pain, edema and erythema, which persisted from 12 to 24 h, and rarely up to 72 h. None of our 43 cases experienced any long-term complications. Representative cases from the study group are shown (Figures 45.4–45.18).

Surgeons have used fat grafting to cover bone defects, nerve tissue exposure, ocular enucleation, mastoid defects, ears, etc. Dermatologists are now using fat grafts to fill in depressed scars and modify the contours of the face and body, some of which are the results of photoaging.[1,12–19]

The clinical use of autologous fat obtained by liposuction for transplantation has progressed at a much faster pace than basic research. Survival rates for transplanted fat have been reported from 30%[20] to as much as 80%.[21] Methods of assessing adipose tissue viability are usually performed on either a volumetric basis or from histological study.[3,20,22,23]

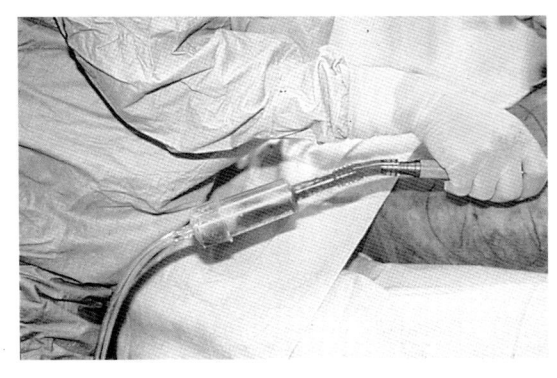

Figure 45.4
Filter trap for fat connected to standard liposuction machine and cannula.

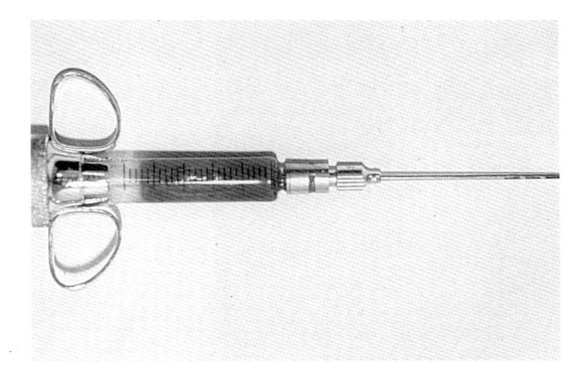

Figure 45.5
Syringe and small cannula for direct removal of fat into syringe.

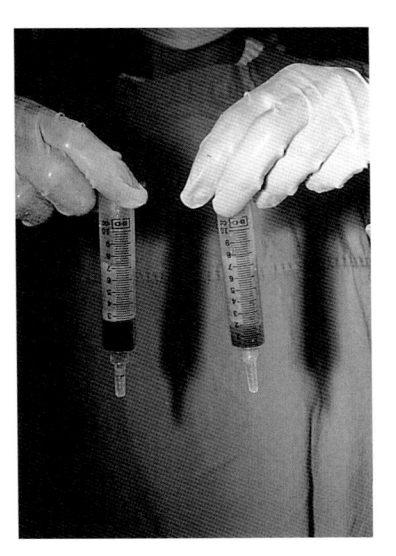

Figure 45.6
Syringes with fluid separated and then drained off, leaving pure fat in syringe.

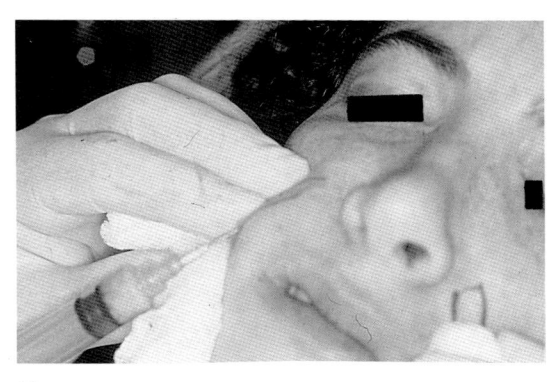

Figure 45.7
Injection of fat into face using other hand to direct the fat placement.

After reviewing our compiled data we conclude that the nature of the cosmetic defect being treated is most important in determining graft longevity. For example, fat transplantations to lesions of linear morphea resulted in the least amount of fat resorption. This has held true not only for the initial 1-year period, but also in long-term assessment over the past 68 months. The greatest amount of fat resorption was encountered in treating fibrotic acne scars and atrophic discoid lupus erythematosus scars. Perhaps the impaired vascularity of these fibrotic and scarred lesions contributed to the decreased viability of the fat grafts. The importance of adequate vascularization of the recipient site has been previously reported.[9,14,24-26] However, since the blood vessels may also be affected in lesions of morphea, this reasoning is purely conjecture. One may also

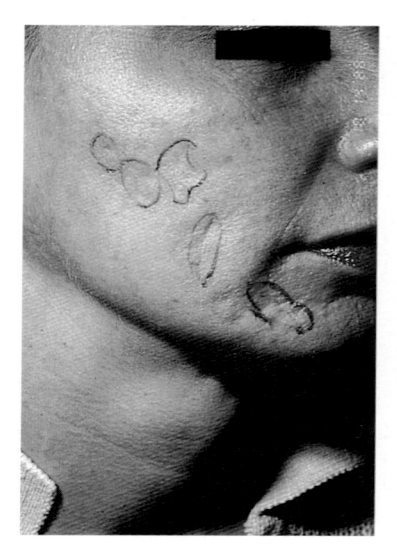

Figure 45.8
Deep acne scars before fat transplant.

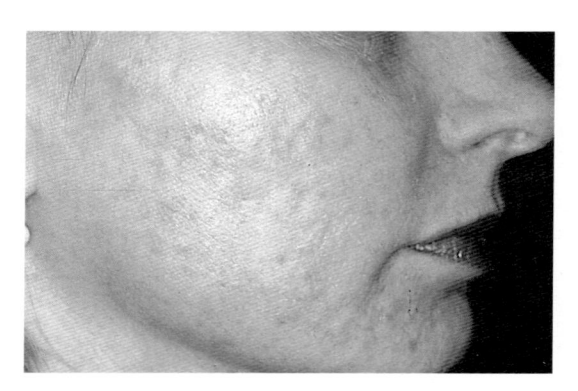

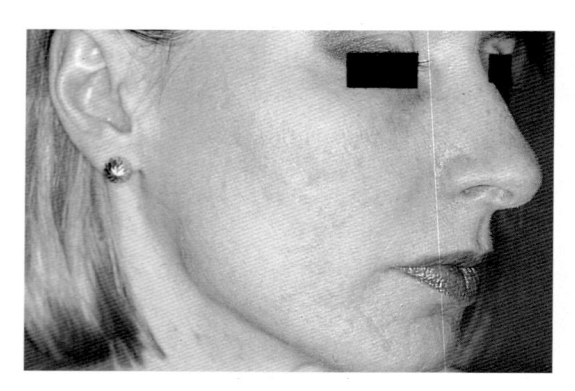

Figure 45.10
Six months after fat transplant into acne scars. Still has good retention.

Figure 45.9
One month after fat transplant into acne scars.

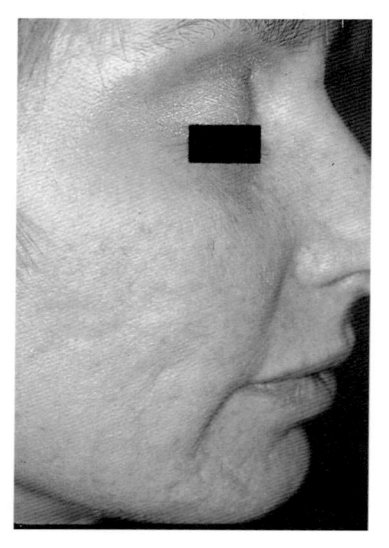

Figure 45.11
Two years after fat transplant.

hypothesize that since we were injecting clinically inactive sclerotic patches of linear morphea, the cellular degradation may have been altered in some way so as to slow down the resorption of transplanted adipocytes.

We feel that the forehead provided better results initially due to its decreased mobility. Fat transplantation may be likened to collagen injections in this regard. For example, collagen augmentation of highly mobile areas, such as the lips, requires more frequent maintenance injections than do less mobile zones (for example nasolabial or glabellar folds). As the majority of linear morphea lesions were located in areas of

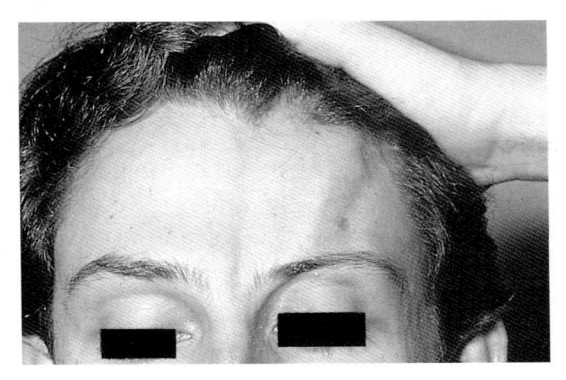

Figure 45.12
Linear scleroderma of forehead with two different areas of atrophy.

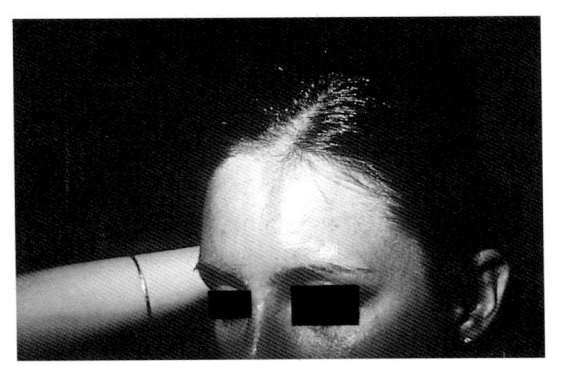

Figure 45.14
Facial hemiatrophy with involvement of scalp.

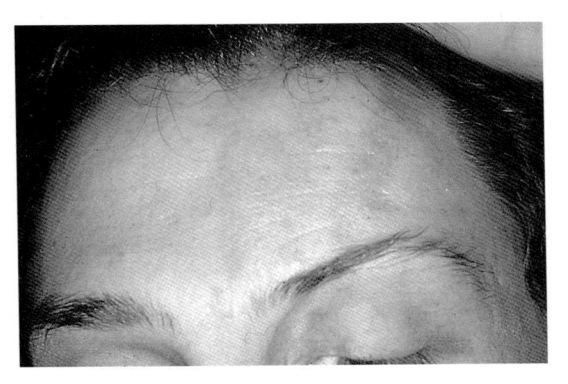

Figure 45.13
Two years after fat transplant with long-term retention of transplanted fat.

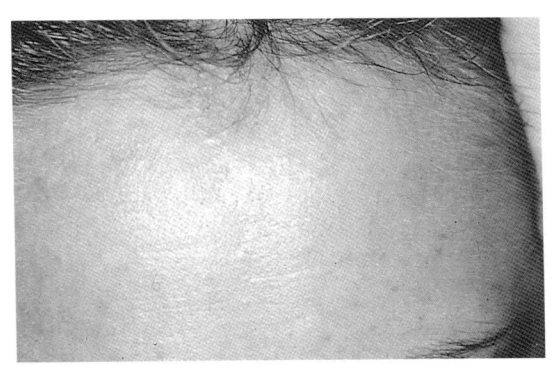

Figure 45.15
Four-year follow-up after scalp reduction and two fat transplants.

low mobility, this may have contributed to the durability of their fat transplants.

Lipoextraction from the thigh was also less discomforting and more longlasting than removing adipose tissue from the buttocks or abdomen. These findings support previous claims that the thigh is the ideal donor site.[27–29] Asken reported that the thigh has less fibrous tissue than the flanks or abdomen, and less postoperative tenderness than the abdomen, and that its fat has the highest antilipolytic activity.[27] Hudson et al[28] measured adipocytes from various regions of the body and also measured their lipogenic activity. They found that cells from the gluteal–femoral areas are the largest and have the greatest lipogenic activity, thus making these adipocytes the site of choice for donor fat. In addition, by using the thigh as the donor site one avoids the risk of abdominal herniation (ventral, incisional or umbilical) and more discomfort postoperatively.

Our study,[8] as well as others,[29,30] has shown few complications from the proce-

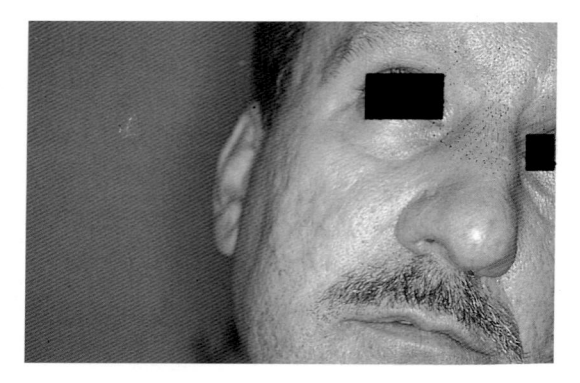

Figure 45.16
Deep acne scars of right cheek.

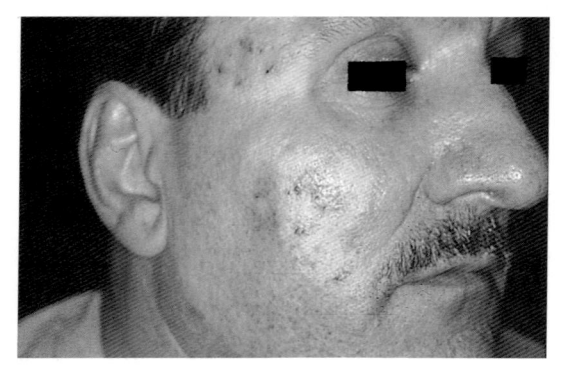

Figure 45.17
Immediately after the fat transplants.

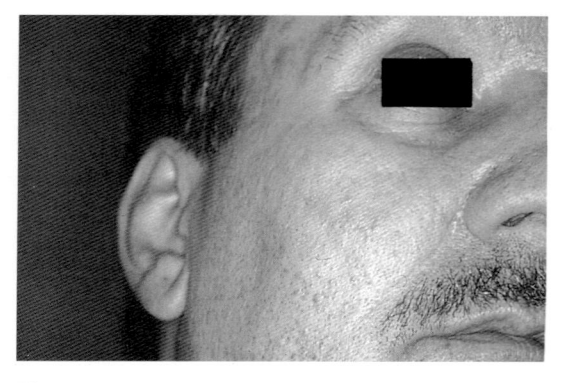

Figure 45.18
One week after fat transplant to right cheek.

dure of fat transplantation. Temporary swelling and very minor bruising at the recipient site and mild tenderness at the donor site have occurred. There has also been a report of unilateral blindness following transplantation of autologous fat to the glabella.[31] However, due to the large size of these particles, intravascular penetration of fat is a rare occurrence.

CONCLUSIONS

Autologous fat transplantation is a safe and effective procedure. Long-term results are still variable but are becoming more predictable as further follow-up studies are presented. One difficulty in evaluating results, as has been pointed out by Glogau,[30] is the limitation of two-dimensional photography. The correction of subcutaneous defects is three-dimensional and often subtle. It is difficult to translate results onto the printed page or photograph even though the surgeon and patient may be able to appreciate the improvement.

The current hypothesis regarding fat graft transfer supports the cell survival theory.[32-34] The volume of fat, when surgically removed from the donor site, becomes ischemic. After transfer into the recipient site, some cells may die, some survive as adipocytes and others dedifferentiate into preadipocyte cells.[35,36] The preadipocyte cell, after recovery from the transfer process, can accumulate fat and mature into an adipocyte. Ultimately, the fat graft regains its blood supply from the periphery and those cells which have survived will remain and function. Those which die will be cleared and replaced by the normal process of fibrosis.[12,34]

Due to the resurgence of autologous fat transplantation and limited documentation of long-term results, many pertinent questions regarding fat graft survival need to be addressed. Is it possible that the fibrosis process and not true fat cell survival is responsible for the contour improvement seen after fat transplantation? If this is true, then perhaps transplanting living fat cells is less important than having an autologous substance or procedure that will cause volume-producing fibrosis.[34,35]

REFERENCES

1. Neuber F, Fat grafting, *Cuir Kongr Verh Otsum Ges Chir* (1893) **20**:66.
2. Bruning P, Cited by Broeckaert TJ, Contribution a l'etude des greffes adipeueses, *Bull Acad R Med Belg* (1919) **28**:440.
3. Peer LA, Loss of weight and volume in human fat grafts, *Plast Reconstr Surg* (1950) **5**:217.
4. Fischer A, Fischer GM, Revised technique for cellulitis fat. Reduction in riding breeches deformity, *Bull Int Acad Cosm Surg* 1977) **2**:40.
5. Illouz Y-G, Communications at the Societe Francaise de Chirurgie Esthetique, June 1978 and 1979.
6. Illouz Y-G, L'Avnir de la reutilisation de la graisse apres liposuction, *Rev Chir Esthet Lang Franc* (1985) **10**.
7. Klein JA, The tumescent technique for liposuction surgery, *Am J Cosmet Surg* (1987) **4**:263–7.
8. Pinski K, Roenigk HH Jr, Autologous fat transplantation—long term follow up, *J Dermatol Surg Oncol* (1992) **18**:179–84.
9. Illouz YG, Present results of fat injection, *Aesth Plast Surg* (1988) **12**:175.
10. Gormley DE, Eremia S, Quantitative assessment of augmentation therapy, *J Dermatol Surg Oncol* (1990) **16**:1147.
11. Horl HW, Feller AM, Biemer E, Technique for liposuction fat reimplantation and long-term volume evaluation by magnetic resonance imaging, *Ann Plast Surg* (1991) **26**:248.
12. Billings E Jr, May JW Jr, Historical review and present status of free graft autotransplantation in plastic and reconstructive surgery, *Plast Reconstr Surg* (1989) **83**:368.
13. Shore JW, Burks R, Leone CR Jr et al, Dermis-fat graft for orbital reconstruction after subtotal exenteration, *Am J Ophthalmol* (1986) **102**:228.
14. Guberina C, Hornblass A, Meltzer MA et al, Autogenous dermis-fat orbital implantation, *Arch Ophthalmol* (1983) **101**:1586.
15. Smith B, Bosma KS, Nesi F et al, Dermis-fat orbital implantation: one hundred eighteen cases, *Ophthalmic Surg* (1983) **14**:941.
16. Weisz GM, Gal A, Long-term survival of a free fat graft in the spinal canal: a 40-month postlaminectomy case report, *Clin Orthop* (1986) **205**:204.
17. Bryant MS, Bremer AM, Nguyen TQ, Autogenic fat transplants in the epidural space in routine lumbar spine surgery, *Neurosurgery* (1983) **13**:367.
18. Chajchir A, Benzaquen I, Liposuction fat grafts in face wrinkles and hemifacial atrophy, *Aesth Plast Surg* (1986) **10**:115.
19. Roenigk HH, Rubenstein R, Combined scalp reduction and autologous fat implant treatment of localized soft tissue defects, *J Dermatol Surg Oncol* (1988) **14**:67.
20. Gurney CE, Experimental study of the behavior of free fat transplants, *Surgery* (1938) **3**:680.
21. Fischer G, Autologous fat implantation for breast augmentation. Workshop on liposuction and autologous fat reimplant. Isola d'Elba, September 1986.
22. Dolsky RL, Adipocyte survival. Presented at the Third Annual Scientific Meeting of the American Academy of Cosmetic Surgery and the

American Society of Lipo-suction Surgery, Los Angeles, California, February 1987.

23. Johnson G, Body contouring by macroinjection of autogenous fat, *Am J Cosmet Surg* (1987) **4**:103.

24. Agris J, Autologous fat transplantation: a 3-year study, *Am J Cosmet Surg* (1987) **4**:95.

25. Illouz Y-G, Aspiration: resultats a long terme et commentaries, *Rev Chir Esthet Lang Franc* (1985) **10**.

26. Saunders MC, Keller JT, Dunsker SB et al, Survival of autologous fat grafts in humans and in mice, *Con Tis Res* (1981) **8**:81.

27. Asken S, Autologous fat transplantation: micro and macro techniques, *Am J Cosmet Surg* (1987) **4**:111.

28. Hudson DA, Lambert EV, Bloch CE, Site selection for autotransplantation: some observations, *Aesth Plast Surg* (1990) **14**:195.

29. Matsudo PKR, Toledo LS, Experience of injected fat grafting, *Aesth Plast Surg* (1988) **12**:35.

30. Glogau RG, Microlipoinjection, *Arch Dermatol* (1988) **124**:1340.

31. Temourian B, Blindness following fat injections. Correspondence and brief communications, *Plast Reconstr Surg* (1988) **80**:361.

32. Gurney CE, Studies on the fate of free transplants of fat, *Proc Staff Meet Mayo Clin* (1937) **12**:317.

33. Clark ER, Clark EL, Microscopic studies of the new formation of fat in living adult rabbits, *Am J Anat* (1940) **67**:255.

34. Nguyen A, Pasyk KA, Bouvier TN et al, Comparative study of survival of autologous adipose tissue taken and transplanted by different techniques. Discussion by May JW Jr, *Plast Reconstr Surg* (1990) **85**:387.

35. Van RL, Bayliss CE, Roncari DA, Cytological and enzymological characterization of adult human adipocyte precursors in culture, *J Clin Invest* (1976) **58**:699.

36. Van RLR, Roncari DAK, Isolation of fat cell precursors from adult rat adipose tissue, *Cell Tissue Res* (1977) **181**:197.

Chapter 46

NEW TRENDS IN LIPOSUCTION

William P. Coleman III

Liposuction has evolved as a multispeciality procedure performed chiefly by cosmetic dermatologic surgeons, plastic surgeons, and otolaryngologists. Input from all three of these medical specialties has given liposuction a special flavor, but with the bad aftertaste of controversy.[1] Obviously the unique training of each of these medical specialties increases the opportunity to develop innovative approaches to each procedure that overlaps their practice spectrums.

LOCAL ANESTHESIA

The development of practical approaches to performing liposuction under local anesthesia has been the biggest breakthrough in this procedure since its introduction in the 1970s.[2] Obviously simplification of anesthetic technique provides a greater degree of safety for any surgical procedure. Local anesthesia is safer than general anesthesia and is therefore more desirable whenever possible.[3] However, early attempts at employing local anesthesia for liposuction proved frustrating since limitations on the volume of lidocaine that could be safely employed prevented the use of this agent for medium to large cases.[4] Although various innovations were developed to get the most out of commercial preparations of lidocaine, they all proved unsatisfactory. In 1987, Klein's development of the tumescent technique changed forever the way dermatologists would look at local anesthesia.[5] Klein's breakthrough was based on the instillation of large volumes of very dilute lidocaine and epinephrine. He was able to demonstrate that this approach resulted in improved lidocaine absorption kinetics.[6] Because lidocaine was absorbed less readily using the tumescent technique, increased amounts could be safely employed, enabling the surgeon to perform larger liposuction surgeries than were formerly possible using commercial preparations.[7]

In a series of studies, Klein demonstrated that 35 mg/kg lidocaine could be safely instilled into the fat using the tumescent anesthetic approach without exceeding safe plasma levels.[8] Older studies of lidocaine in human tissue had recommended a maximum dose of 7 mg/kg.[9] Consequently surgeons are now able to perform liposuction safely using five times the quantity of lidocaine than was formally thought prudent.

In addition to more efficient use of lidocaine, the tumescent technique achieves better vasoconstriction than with any other approach developed before.[10] Consequently blood loss during liposuction is dramatically reduced. Using the older approach of general anesthesia with little attention to thorough instillation of epinephrine, the typical liposuction aspirate contained 25% or more of blood.[11] This severely restricted the surgeon's ability to perform larger surgery without blood transfusion. In fact autologous blood transfusion became quite popular in the mid-1980s.[12] Using the tumescent technique, the dilute epinephrine solution is delivered thoroughly throughout the operative site, resulting in a yellow aspirate nearly devoid of blood. The typical liposuction aspirate using this technique contains less than 5% whole blood. This, of course, allows the liposuction surgeon to approach larger cases without the added risk of blood transfusion. Postoperative bruising, bleeding and hemotomas are rarely seen using the tumescent technique.

After the instillation of large volumes of anesthetic fluid, a firm operative site is achieved. The surgeon can then more easily pass cannulas through the subcutaneous tissue. Forceful grasping of the skin is not required and the cannula is more easily controlled than when the operative site is flaccid. However, tactile feedback is not compromised as one might expect. As the liposuction proceeds it is quite easy to assess the amount of remaining fat as the tissue becomes softer.

Interestingly, the most superficial fat and the dermis are not well anesthetized using the tumescent technique. Consequently, pain may result if the surgeon inadvertently tunnels too superficially. This provides an excellent safety benefit, since superficial tunneling may result in skin waviness postoperatively. Furthermore, muscular tissue below is also not well anesthetized, providing instant feedback to the surgeon from the patient if he inadvertently tunnels too deeply.

The tumescent technique works well in concentrations of 0.05 or 0.1%. Generally, those who use the dilute formula supplement the anesthetic with intramuscular and/or sublingual sedation. Sensitive areas such as the central infraumbilical region require the higher concentration for adequate anesthesia. The use of fresh epinephrine at a 1:1 000 000 concentration has become standard and no untoward side-effects have been reported even though several milliliters in total of 1:1000 epinephrine are routinely used for larger cases.

Some controversy, however, has developed over the appropriate concentration of sodium bicarbonate. Although Klein recommended 12.5 mEq/l, tumescent solutions containing 5 mEq/l of bicarbonate result in a more physiological pH of 7.4.[13] However, the physiological concentration of bicarbonate is 25 mEq/l. It is conceivable that using several liters of tumescent fluid containing 12.5 mEq/l or lower of bicarbonate could lead to metabolic acidosis. However, in spite of these theoretical concerns, the author has seen no difference clinically using tumescent solutions varying from 5 mEq/l up to 25 mEq/l. There also appears to be no difference in burning on injection or the degree of anesthesia or vasoconstriction between these various concentrations.

Delivery of the local anesthetic solution in such high volumes is time-consuming. Although the original Klein needle and Klein apparatus were popular, this involved the surgeon constantly emptying and refilling a syringe, which can be quite tiresome if several liters of fluid are required. Furthermore, the Klein needle is painful to advance through tissue. Small-diameter injection needles in the 12–14-gauge range with multiple injection ports are more efficient and less painful to pass through the adipose layer. These can be attached directly via intravenous tubing to the sterile bag containing the tumescent

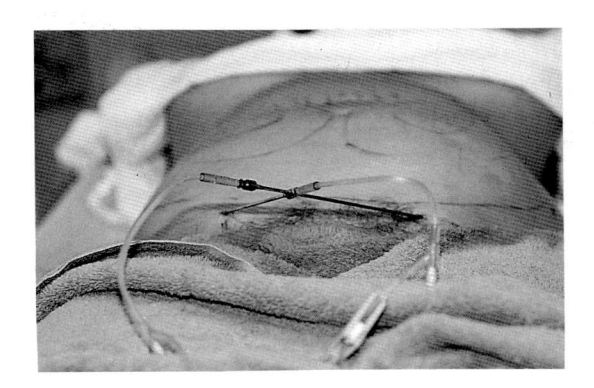

Figure 46.1
A closed tumescent anesthetic delivery system with the intravenous bag connected directly to the injection needle.

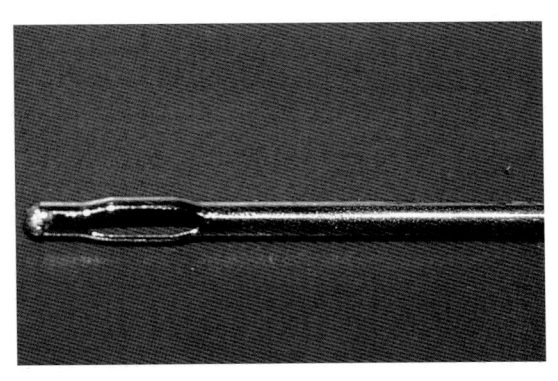

Figure 46.2
A basket-style cannula.

mixture. This creates a sterile closed system (Figure 46.1). By the use of a blood pump or blood pressure cuff around the intravenous bag the fluid can be pumped directly into the operative site.[14] It is most efficient to use several injection needles so that multiple areas can be anesthetized simultaneously. A peristaltic pump is also available for this purpose. However, if multiple infusions are performed simultaneously then multiple pumps need to be purchased, which can be quite expensive.

CANNULA DESIGN

The original liposuction cannulas used were large (8–10 mm in diameter) and contained one to three apertures located on the deep-facing facade of the instrument. There has been a gradual trend over the last decade to use smaller and smaller instruments for liposuction. Six-millimeter cannulas are now used for bulk fat removal and 3–4-mm and smaller instruments are used for sculpting.

Although cannulas have always been available in varying lengths and either straight or curved, there are now hundreds of options in aperture design. Most aperture variations make very little difference clinically, but a few designs are worth mentioning.

Both Klein and Becker have developed basket-style cannulas with apertures located near the tip of the instrument (Figure 46.2). With the tip of the instrument larger than its shaft, tunneling is more efficient. This design, however, proves to be quite aggressive at cutting as well as aspirating fat. It is most useful as a 3- or 4-mm instrument, where its aggressiveness is tempered by the small size of the tunnel. Larger instruments of this sort may produce dimpling or skin waviness if not used extremely carefully.

Cannulas with an 'open' aperture design perform more like a curette and are the most aggressive cannulas. These variations of the 'cobra' design are excellent for tunneling through fibrotic areas such as the male flanks or breasts (Figure 46.3). However, such instruments cause increased bleeding and therefore are less suitable for the usual liposuction areas (thighs, abdomen and neck). As with the open basket designs, some of the negative features of these cannulas can be tempered by using them only in smaller diameters (4 mm or less).

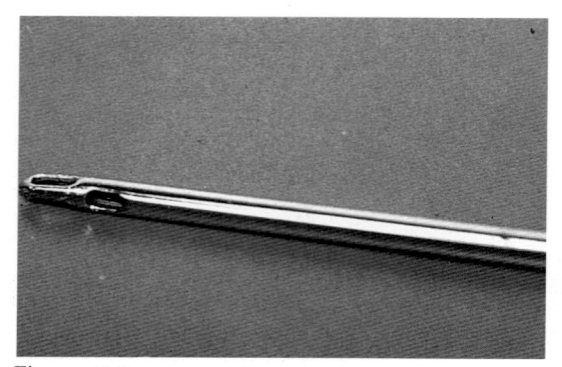

Figure 46.3
A cobra-style cannula.

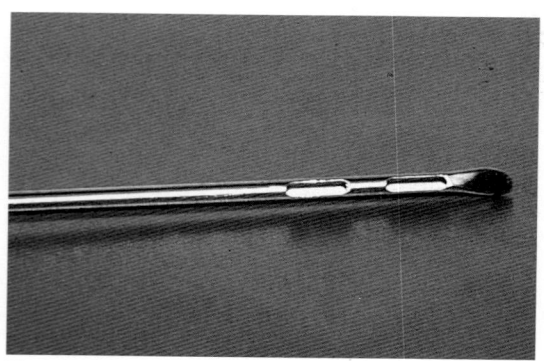

Figure 46.4
Klein minicannula.

Minicannulas are available in an increasing array of designs. One minicannula is available with a wider closed tip and the apertures located behind on a narrower shaft (Figure 46.4). This instrument is very useful for lipoaspiration for fat transfer. It is also quite delicate and works nicely on the inner thighs where aggressive liposuction can result in skin waviness.

Cannulas of all sorts are now available with luerlock attachments for fitting on a separate handle. This enables the surgeon to clean the instruments very efficiently. Also their shorter length allows them to fit into an autoclave more readily. Some manufacturers also design an attachable handle with a variation on the luerlock design. Unfortunately true luerlock cannulas from other manufacturers do not fit on their handle. This makes them less flexible.

A separate handle which contains a thumb control for suction is quite handy (Figure 46.5). The surgeon can simply occlude a small hole in the handle with his thumb to re-establish pressure in the system. This allows the surgeon to clear the tubing of fat without turning the machine on or off or removing the cannula from the tunnel. Cannulas of various sizes and shapes can be attached to the handle via a luerlock arrangement. A variety of dispos-

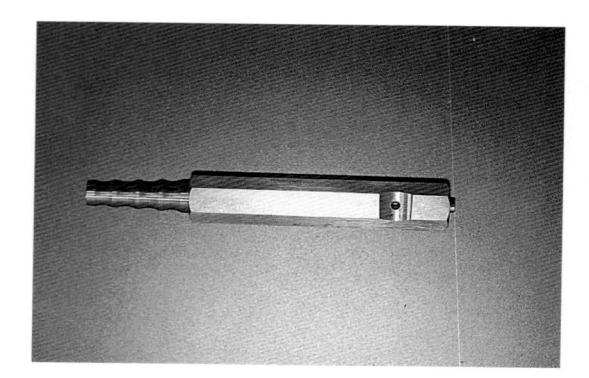

Figure 46.5
The Klein cannula handle.

able liposuction cannulas are now available from several manufacturers. The advantages of assured sterilization is obvious.

LIPOSCULPTURE

In many patients seeking liposuction each adiposity contains a central area where the fat is the thickest with decreasing amounts of subcutaneous tissue radiating out from this (Figure 46.6). This can be demonstrated with a series of circles similar to a topographic map. Consequently most liposuction involves two phases: a debulk-

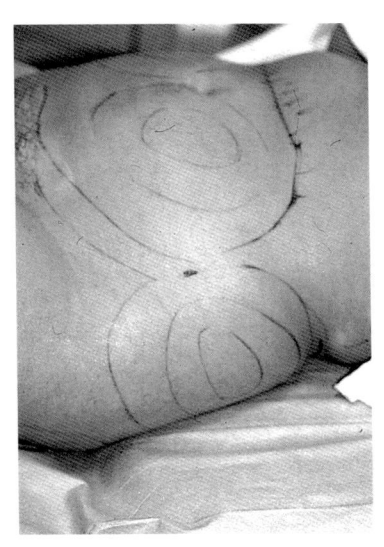

Figure 46.6
Smaller circles indicate areas of thicker fat.

ing phase and a sculpting phase. Debulking is used to remove the thickest parts of the adiposity, whereas sculpting is used to thin out the less fatty areas and to blend the area of liposuction into the surrounding areas to avoid an obvious transition zone.

Debulking usually involves the use of larger cannulas and more aggressive technique. The purpose of this step is to remove the fat in the centralmost part of the adiposity where it is the thickest. Larger adiposities may require several layers of tunnels. It is often less painful and more efficient to perform this step after the sculpting phases of the liposuction because pretunneling with smaller cannulas enables the surgeon to insert larger cannulas more easily.

The sculpting phase of liposuction involves developing one or two layers of small tunnels throughout the adiposity. Less aggressive cannulas and a gentle technique are mandatory. Using very small cannulas (3 mm in diameter or smaller) the surgeon can tunnel more superficially without fear of skin waviness. Smaller cannulas should also be used on the periphery of the adiposity to 'feather' the liposuction and decrease the difference between the treated and untreated areas. Fournier has advocated a peripheral mesh dissection which involves tunneling with the suction power turned off at the end of the procedure.[15] This is usually unnecessary if the surgeon feathers the periphery of the adiposity using smaller instruments with fewer passes through the tunnels. There is no benefit to reinserting cannulas through all of the suction tunnels at the end of the procedure with the power turned off as some advocate.

CONTROVERSY IN POSTOPERATIVE CARE

Originally the French inventors of liposuction recommended the use of special adhesive tape as a postoperative splint.[16] Later, various surgical girdles and other compression garments were added over the tape. Many liposuction surgeons have gradually evolved their postoperative regimen to include using only the garment without tape. All forms of tape are skin irritants and they impede the patient's ability to bathe normally.

However, the use of adhesive compression tape allows the surgeon to directly mold the postoperative area and splint the wounded tissue. Furthermore, the surgeon is certain that the compression is constant with the use of tape. Some patients are not reliable about postoperative care and tend to remove their girdles for long periods of time, compromising the desired compression. Furthermore, postoperative bruising appears to be decreased by careful taping. Quite often there is no bruising in the areas that are taped and only an occasional bruise where the tape may have slipped or curled.

It should be noted that some liposuction surgeons do not feel that postoperative compression is important. Most, however, advocate compression garments for 1–2 weeks postoperatively. I find that many patients appreciate the support of the compression garment and usually continue using it at least part time for up to a month postoperatively. Any elastic garment can be used as an alternative to surgical compression dressings. Recently, stretch shorts have become quite popular and provide excellent compression as well as being more stylish than a surgical girdle. Tight garments can be taken on and off more easily if they are used in double layers with a looser garment applied first. Then it is very easy to slide the second tighter one on top.

HYPERHIDROSIS AND HIDRADENITIS

Liposuction has been performed for hyperhidrosis of the axillae in the last several years.[17] This approach is far superior to surgical axillectomy because it avoids the large unsightly scar and hair loss associated with the more radical technique. Furthermore, liposuction in a patient with hyperhidrosis tends to provide a normalization of sweating rather than a cessation of sweating.

The tumescent technique has simplified liposuction of the axilla for hyperhidrosis. The ballooning of the tissue afforded by this technique allows easy penetration by the cannula and provides a buffer of swollen fat, allowing the surgeon to maintain the cannula at a safe distance from the underlying axillary structures (Figure 46.7). Using the tumescent technique it is easy to find the proper subdermal plane. Because of the superficial lipodissection required to remove the sweat glands (Figure 46.8) there is increased bruising compared to liposuction performed strictly for removal of fat. However, most patients recover quite well within 1 week and the contralateral axilla can usually be treated safely within 2 weeks after the first.

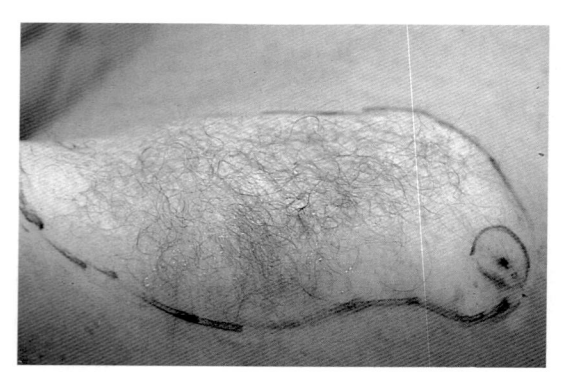

Figure 46.7
Tumescent anesthesia provides a buffer of swollen fat to protect the underlying axillary structures.

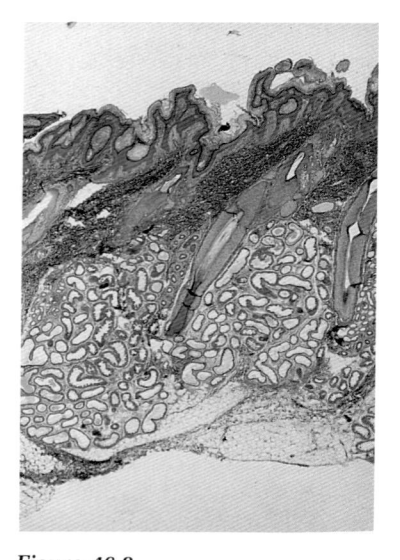

Figure 46.8
Histology of axillary hyperhidrosis with hyperplasia of apocrine glands between the hair follicles in the deep dermis with hypoplastic collagen and interfacing with subcutaneous fat. (Courtesy of RK Roenigk, MD)

Recently the author has begun to perform liposuction on young patients with early signs of apocrine hidradenitis. Hopefully, removal of some of the offending apocrine glands will minimize the severity of their disease in later years.

Results

Liposuction patients definitely obtain better results than 10 years ago when the procedure was rarely performed. Dermatologic surgeons now understand the parameters for performing safe, effective liposuction. It is also quite common to suggest 'touch-up' liposuction 1 year after the initial surgery. This, of course, must be discussed prior to the original surgery so that the patient understands that it is being performed to 'fine tune' the liposuction. In general, patients who have had touch-up liposuction get better results.

Liposuction in the early 1990s has become a predictable, safe procedure. Dermatologic surgeons who perform liposuction uniformly find it extremely gratifying. The patients are among the happiest of all cosmetic surgery patients. Liposuction has expanded the horizons of dermatologic cosmetic surgery.

References

1. Newman J, Liposuction surgery: past, present, future, *Am J Cosmet Surg* (1984) **1**:1.
2. Coleman WP III, The history of dermatologic liposuction, *Dermatol Clin* (1990) **8**:381.
3. Coleman WP III, Liposuction and anesthesia, *J Dermatol Surg Oncol* (1987) **13**:1295.
4. Klein J, Anesthesia for liposuction in dermatologic surgery, *J Dermatol Surg Oncol* (1988) **14**:1124.
5. Klein JA, The tumescent technique for liposuction surgery, *Am J Cosmet Surg* (1987) **4**:263.
6. Klein J, The tumescent technique. Anesthesia and modified liposuction technique, *Dermatol Clin* (1990) **8**:425.
7. Lillis PJ, Liposuction surgery under local anesthesia: limited blood loss and minimal lidocaine absorption, *J Dermatol Surg Oncol* (1988) **14**:1145.
8. Klein JA, Tumescent technique for regional anesthesia permits lidocaine doses of 35 mg/kg for liposuction: peak plasma lidocaine levels are diminished and delayed 12 hours, *J Dermatol Surg Oncol* (1990) **16**:248.
9. Malamed S, *Handbook of local anesthesia*, 2nd edn (Mosby: St Louis 1986) 44.
10. Lillis PJ, The tumescent technique for liposuction surgery, *Dermatol Clin* (1990) **8**:439.
11. Chrisman B, Coleman WP III, Determining safe limits for untransfused outpatient liposuction: personal experience and review of the literature, *J Dermatol Surg Oncol* (1988) **14**:1095.
12. Gargon T, Courtiss E, The risks of suction lipectomy: their prevention and treatment, *Plast Reconstr Surg* (1984) **11**:457.
13. Smith S, Hodge J, Lawrence N et al, Lidocaine/bicarbonate ratios: revisiting the tumescent anesthesia formula, *J Derm Surg Oncol* (1992) **18**:973–5.
14. Coleman WP III, Badame A, Phillips H, A new technique for injection of tumescent anesthetic mixtures, *J Dermatol Surg Oncol* (1991) **17**:535.
15. Fournier P, *Liposculpture: Ma technique* (Arnette: Paris 1989).
16. Ottani F, Fournier P, A history and comparison of suction techniques until their debut in North America. In: Hetter G, ed., *Lipoplasty: the theory and practice of blunt suction lipectomy* (Little, Brown: Boston 1984) 19–23.
17. Lillis P, Coleman WP III, Liposuction for treatment of axillary hyperhidrosis, *Dermatol Clin* (1990) **8**:479.

Chapter 47

FACIAL CHEMICAL PEEL WITH TRICHLOROACETIC ACID

Randall K. Roenigk
David G. Brodland

Trichloroacetic acid has been used for the treatment of extensive actinic keratoses and other dermatoses for many years.[1,2] Ayres[3] delineated the use of TCA as therapy for aging skin. There are many cosmetic and therapeutic indications for TCA chemexfoliation, and various application techniques and combinations with other methods have been used (Table 47.1).

TCA chemically destroys the epidermis and upper dermis, causing a sluff of dead skin within 5–7 days.[4,5] New epidermis migrates from the cutaneous adnexa within 7 days. Dermal regeneration is evident in 2–3 weeks, but remodeling of the collagen normally continues for 6 months. The resultant histologic changes in skin are homogenization of the superficial dermal collagen and increased elastic staining in the dermis—changes that are essentially permanent. In addition, cytologically atypical keratinocytes are replaced by normal cells derived from the adnexae (Figure 47.1).

Treatment of premalignant lesions and actinic damage has been recognized as a principal indication for chemical peeling.[6–8] Treatment of actinic keratoses may decrease the incidence of basal and squamous cell carcinoma. Although other common methods such as cryotherapy are effective, in some cases the number of actinic keratoses is such that more aggressive treatment may be warranted. Trichloroacetic acid chemical peel also compares favorably with 5-fluorouracil cream for extensive actinic damage because of the severe reaction to 5-fluorouracil cream, which may last 4–7 weeks and is often repeated. The secondary benefit of decreasing mild to moderate wrinkling of facial skin through

Table 47.1
Some variations of the trichloroacetic acid (TCA) facial chemical peel

---

Superficial peel with 20% TCA

Intermediate peel with 35% TCA

Deep peel with 50% or 60% TCA

Tape occlusion

TCA plus tretinoin cream preoperatively and postoperatively

TCA plus 5-fluorouracil

TCA plus dermabrasion or chemabrasion

TCA plus phenol

TCA plus solid CO_2

Focal treatment with 50–100% TCA

Other agents sometimes added: lactic acid, glycolic acid, resorcinol, salicylic acid.

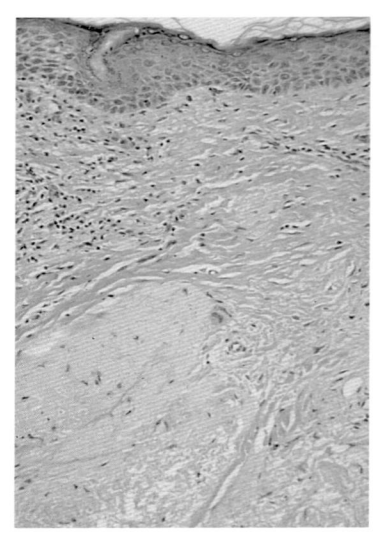

Figure 47.1
Histology 6 months after 50% TCA chemical peel for extensive actinic keratoses on male facial skin. Note bands of new hypercellular basophilic collagen that overlie a nodule of solar elastosis.

Table 47.2
Formulation of TCA

Concentration (%)	Formulation
60	TCA USP (crystals) 60 g per 100 ml distilled H_2O
50	TCA USP (crystals) 50 g per 100 ml distilled H_2O
35	TCA USP (crystals) 35 g per 100 ml distilled H_2O
20	TCA USP (crystals) 20 g per 100 ml distilled H_2O

USP, United States Pharmacopeia.

replacement and rejuvenation of actinically damaged, elastotic dermis is pleasing (Figures 47.2 and 47.3).

Trichloroacetic acid is also used for the treatment of fine crosshatched facial wrinkles. Moderately deep wrinkles and perioral wrinkles may also respond well to this procedure. The deepest creases of facial expression will not respond to chemical peeling with TCA.

Indications for TCA chemical peel also include sun pigmentary disorders, especially lentigo simplex. Other pigmentary problems such as postinflammatory hyperpigmentation or melasma may respond, but the results are highly variable and the condition may be worsened. Test patch is suggested in these cases, and patients should be cautioned about the variable results.

Chemical peeling with TCA is a versatile and elegant procedure because the concentration of TCA is easily adjusted by the operator and the depth of dermal damage is regularly reproducible. The authors prefer standard concentrations of 20, 35 and 50% TCA, occasionally using concentrations up to 60% (Table 47.2). Clearly, 80% TCA causes unacceptable scarring in facial skin and animal models. Gynecologists routinely use 70% TCA to treat vaginal and cervical condyloma. However, this moist mucosal surface probably reduces the effect at a given concentration of TCA so scar does not result. Scarring might occur if 70% TCA were applied to the face.

Two techniques are generally used for the treatment of severely sun-damaged skin.[6,8–10] The first is intermediate or deep chemical peeling in a single session with 35–60% TCA. The choice of concentration depends on the amount of solar damage and the thickness of the skin (usually higher concentrations are used on the cheek, nose and forehead; lower concentrations are used on the lips and eyelids). The second method is to repeat a superficial chemical peel using 20% TCA 1–2 weeks apart for three to four treatments. In both approaches, the skin may be pretreated with topical tretinoin, and some clinicians use 5–fluorouracil cream.

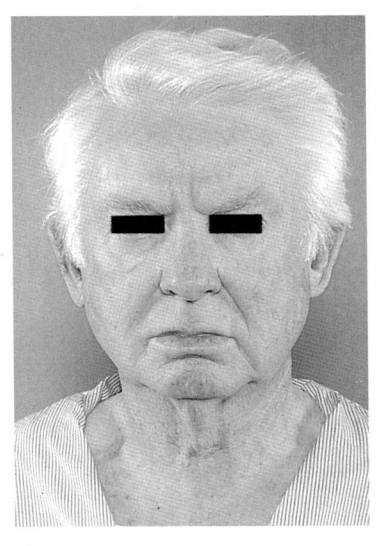

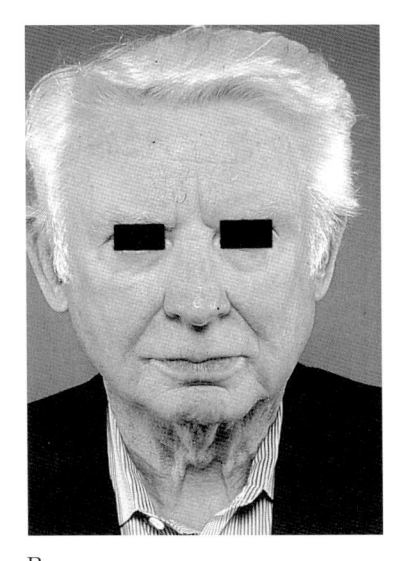

Figure 47.2
(A) Patient with photoaging preoperatively, front view. (B) Six months postoperatively (20, 35 and 50% TCA acid), front view. (C) Side view preoperatively. (D) Side view 6 months preoperatively.

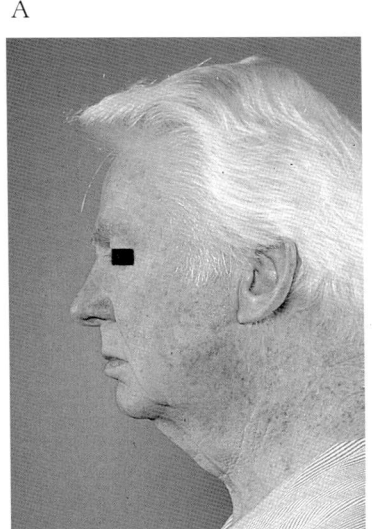

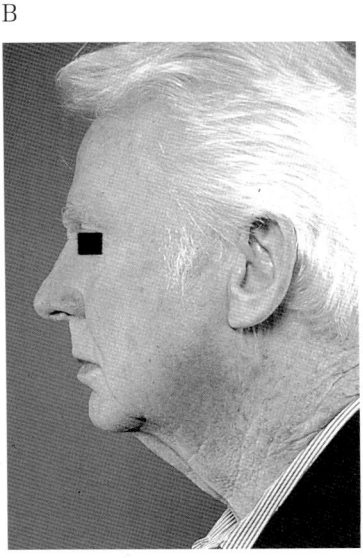

HISTOLOGICAL EFFECTS OF TRICHLOROACETIC ACID ON THE SKIN

The depths of wounds created by various concentrations and application techniques of TCA were evaluated by Stegman[4,5] and Brodland et al[10] in human and animal models (Tables 47.3 and 47.4). The therapeutic effects of TCA are destruction of the epidermis and dermis with subsequent re-epithelialization from epidermal appendages and stimulation of new collegen formation. The depths of the wounds caused by various dilutions of TCA are of paramount importance in its therapeutic efficacy.

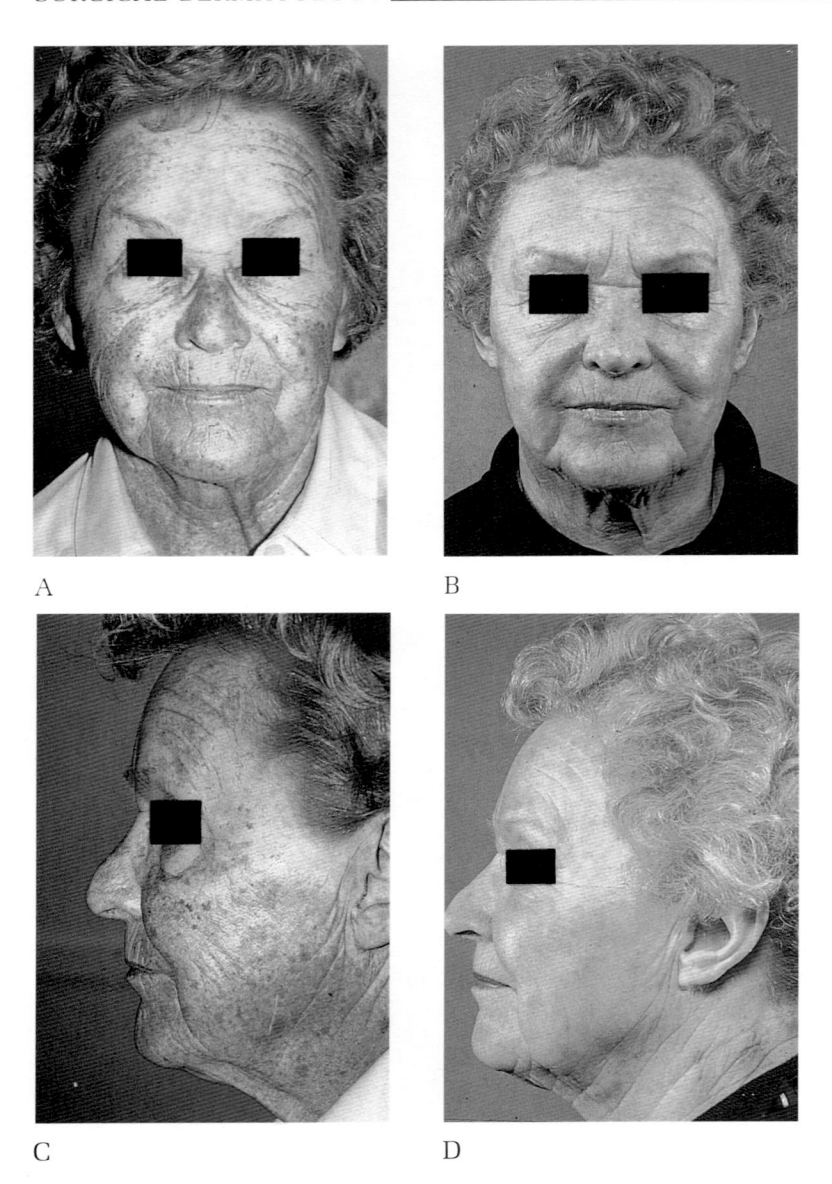

Figure 47.3
(A) Patient with photoaging and lentigo simplex, front view. (B) Three months postoperatively (20, 35 and 50% TCA). (C) Side view preoperatively. (D) Side view 3 months postoperatively.

Immediate histological effects of trichloroacetic acid

In studies undertaken by the authors, as expected, the depth of tissue necrosis increased with the concentration of TCA (Table 47.4).[10] The concentration of TCA used for actinic keratoses should be at least 35–50% because this is what is required for complete removal of the epidermis and superficial dermis to allow re-epithelialization by normal appendageal keratinocytes. Concentrations of TCA used for facial rejuvenation depend on the desired effect. A concentration of 20% TCA results in epidermal exfoliation; this is well toler-

Table 47.3
Depth of dermal necrosis produced by treatment with 60% TCA, 100% phenol, or Baker's formula with and without tape occlusion

	Wound thickness (mm)		Depth of scar at 60 days (mm)	
	Not occluded	Occluded	Not occluded	Occluded
Non-sun damaged skin				
60% TCA	0.27	0.36	0.35	0.25
100% phenol	0.41	0.41	0.38	0.41
Baker's mix	0.6	0.65	0.41	0.40
Sun-damaged skin				
60% TCA	0.5	0.4	0.5	0.45
100% phenol	0.55	0.4	0.5	0.53
Baker's mix	0.63	0.85	0.57	0.9

Modified from Stegman.[5]

Table 47.4
Depth of necrosis (mm) porcine model

TCA concentration (%)	Depth of necrosis (mm)[a] Unoccluded technique	Occluded technique	Difference
20	0.044	0[b]	—
35	0.255	0.075	0.180
50	0.500	0.178	0.322
80	0.983	0.633	0.350

[a]Mean ± SD.
[b]No measurable necrosis.
From Brodland et al.[9] By permission of Elsevier Science Publishing Company, Inc.

ated, but the degree of rejuvenation is less and relatively short term and superficial. Serial applications, weekly or biweekly, of 20% TCA may directly or indirectly induce remodeling of the papillary dermis because of the repeated caustic damage to a temporarily thinned epidermis.

Concentrations of 35 and 50% TCA cause not only replacement of the epidermis but also longer-lasting dermal changes histologically (0.3–0.5 dermal necrosis), in association with the reduction of fine and medium wrinkles. There are no reports of the clinical use of 80% TCA for facial rejuvenation procedures; however, because dermal necrosis (0.8–0.9 mm) is deeper, scarring would result and be cosmetically unacceptable.

Tape occlusion for chemical peeling has been thought to increase the depth of penetration of TCA. Increased penetration and a deeper peel after skin occlusion with tape may occur with phenol. However, in the authors' studies with TCA, it was found that tape occlusion reliably decreases the depth of dermal necrosis. In a porcine model, at all TCA concentrations tested, the occluded technique produced significantly less necrosis than the unoccluded technique (Figures 47.4 and 47.5). Hypothetically, less dermal necrosis in the occluded specimen could be the result of interstitial humidification (Figure 47.6). Occlusion accomplishes this by the prevention of transepidermal water loss, which leads to increased interstitial water content in the epidermis and dermis. Therefore, the effective concentration of TCA is decreased or more rapidly 'neutralized'.

In addition, the authors showed why there is benefit to pretreating the skin with tretinoin cream for 2 weeks and acetone preoperatively. Although both drugs degrease the skin, they also affect the thickness of the epidermis, making it flatter, especially by thinning the stratum corneum.[11] The depth of damage in the skin is most dependent on the concentration of TCA and is constant. Thinning the epider-

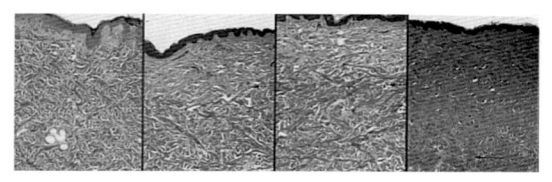

Figure 47.4
In the hairless minipig, 20, 35, 50 and 80% TCA (left to right) was applied by the open (no tape) technique. At 24 h, necrosis is delineated by arrows. As expected, higher concentrations resulted in deeper dermal necrosis.

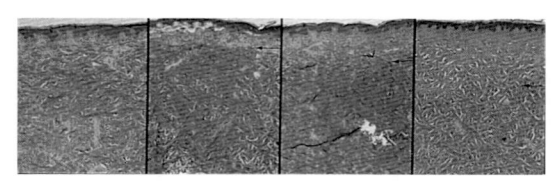

Figure 47.5
In these specimens of the hairless minipig, 20, 35, 50 and 80% TCA (left to right) were applied with tape occlusion. Histology at 24 h consistently demonstrated less depth of dermal necrosis at a given concentration (arrows). Occlusion may cause interstitial humidification that decreases ('neutralizes') the effective concentration.

mis causes relatively deeper dermal necrosis at a given concentration. The effect on the epidermis is relatively short-lived, although a longer-lasting dermal effect is usually preferable. Higher concentrations of TCA might be used in place of preparing the skin with tretinoin and acetone. Tretinoin thins the epidermis and acetone debrides the stratum corneum, which may contain hypertrophic actinic keratoses preoperatively. Pretreatment with tretinoin results in a more effective, longer-lasting chemexfoliation with use of 35–50% TCA for photoaged skin (Figure 47.7).

Long-term histological effects

The authors also studied the long-term histological effects of TCA in a porcine model. Test sites were treated with 20, 35, 50 and 80% TCA and either tape-occluded or unoccluded techniques. In addition, two sites were treated serially with 20% TCA on six occasions over 9 weeks. Biopsy specimens were obtained over a 28-week period from all sites. Each specimen was stained with

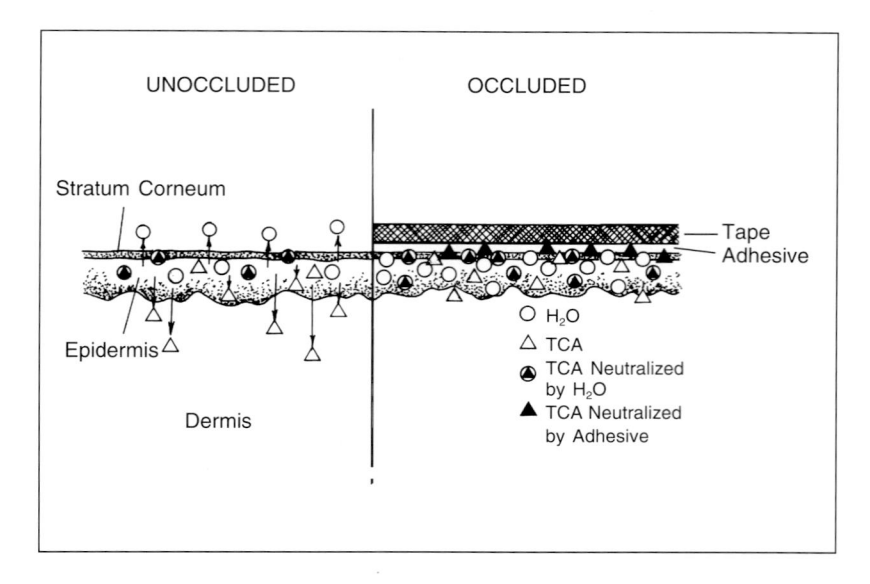

Figure 47.6
Occlusion on skin with silk tape after application of TCA may cause decreased water loss, and therefore increased interstitial humidification and relative decrease in the effective concentration of TCA.

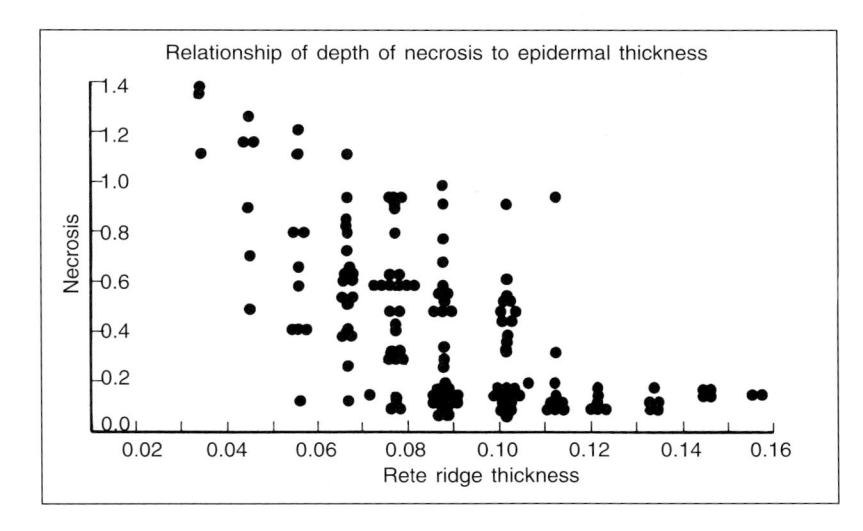

Figure 47.7
The thicker the epidermis, the less dermal damage for a given concentration of TCA. Therefore, pretreating to decrease the thickness of the stratum corneum (i.e. tretinoin cream and acetone) is more likely to result in a more even chemexfoliation.

hematoxylin and eosin and sel Giemsa and was microscopically evaluated. For each specimen, the epidermal thickness and the depth of dermal necrosis were measured with a micrometer. Qualitative and semiquantitative determinations were made of several histological factors, including changes in collagen, fibroblast and elastic tissue.

The epidermal changes included thinning and orthokeratosis of the stratum corneum at 4 weeks after treatment with TCA. This change was transient, and at 8 and 28 weeks the stratum corneum was similar to its baseline status. The change in the epidermal thickness was variable, depending on the concentration of TCA, the time of the biopsy, and the application technique (Figure 47.8).

At 24 and 4 weeks, collagen was distinctly basophilic, which represented the zone of necrosis. The collagen was altered at 8 and 28 weeks. The staining of the collagen tended to be much more pale in the superficial dermis, and the level of dermal necrosis was much less distinct. The bundles were noted to be haphazardly organized, smaller, and fragmented with less well-defined borders.

The number of fibroblasts was increased in the superficial dermis at 4, 8 and 28 weeks in the specimens treated with 35% TCA or higher concentrations. These fibroblasts appeared histologically to be metabolically active and were characterized by abundant basophilic cytoplasm. High concentrations of TCA induced a greater number of fibroblasts than low concentrations. At 28 weeks, the number of fibroblasts remained greater than that at baseline.

The elastic fibers were histologically unchanged in the specimens treated with 20% TCA and the serial application technique. However, the specimens treated with higher concentrations consistently had a decrease in the quantity of elastin (stained with sel Giemsa) at 4 and 8 weeks. At 28 weeks, the amount of elastin was actually increased, compared with the amount at baseline. The depth of these alterations in elastin corresponded roughly to the depth of basophilic necrosis. The morphology of new elastic fibers at 28 weeks showed no characteristic pattern and ranged from short, thin fragments to long, branching, thick fibers.

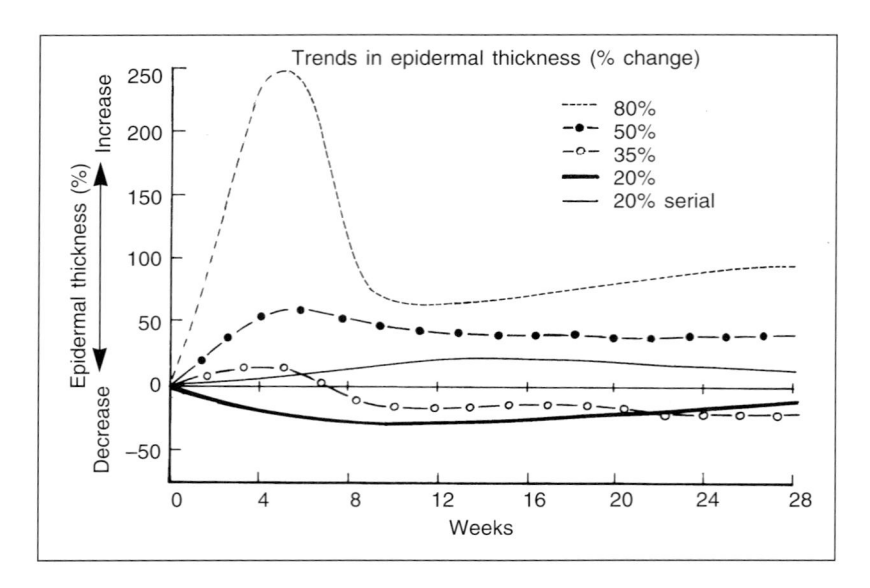

Figure 47.8
Damage to the dermis with edema followed by new collagen formation provide much of the long-term clinical benefits of chemexfoliation with TCA. The highest concentrations have the greatest long-term effects. Serial 20% peels are also effective, however.

In summary, the long-term (28 weeks) histological effects vary depending on the concentration used and the application technique. Serial applications of 20% TCA have very little long-term effect. However, further clinical investigation of the serial application of 20% TCA is warranted because there were some short-term histological changes.

Specimens treated with 35, 50 and 80% TCA had definite alterations, which persisted for at least 7 months (the end of the study). Generally, the degree of histological alteration increased in proportion with the increase in TCA concentration. The histological effects were most intense with 80% TCA. Scar and pigmentary alteration were clinically evident in some of the sites treated with 80% TCA but not in those treated with 35% and 50% TCA.

Perhaps the most surprising finding in this study involves the assumption that tape occlusions of TCA enhances its penetration and results in enhanced histological and clinical effects. When the long-term histological effects of tape-occluded and unoccluded techniques were compared, the tape-occluded specimens had significantly less long-term histological alteration than the unoccluded specimens. This finding is consistent with what is seen at 24 h after treatment.

SUMMARY

Variations of facial chemical peel are employed as each clinician tries to achieve better results. If possible, variations from standard techniques should be studied scientifically to establish their safety and efficacy. The goal of chemical face peeling, however, is not just to get a deeper peel. Higher concentrations of TCA and phenol may cause full-thickness chemical burns, leaving long-lasting scars.

Table 47.5
Advantages of TCA peels

Few medical contraindications
Elegant (adjust depth of necrosis by concentration of TCA)
No allergic reactions
No systemic toxicity
Scarring rare (perioral, eyelids, jawline)
Wound healing time shorter than with 5-fluorouracil cream (better compliance)
More practical than repeated cryotherapy for patients with extensive actinic keratoses

Facial chemical peel encompasses a plethora of procedures and techniques. Although sometimes confusing, this should not blunt one's enthusiasm for what chemexfoliation can achieve. With the use of TCA, facial chemical peel is a safe, effective and elegant method for treating common problems associated with photoaged fair skin (Table 47.5). When standardized techniques are used, it is also possible to quantify the therapeutic effects and reliably predict the outcome.

REFERENCES

1. Monash S, The uses of diluted trichloroacetic acid in dermatology, *Urol Cutan Rev* (1945) **49**:119.
2. Resnik SS, Chemical peel with trichloroacetic. In: Roenigk HH, Roenigk RK, eds, *Dermatologic surgery: principles and practice* (Marcel Dekker: New York 1989) 979–95.
3. Ayres S III, Superficial chemosurgery in treating aging skin, *Arch Dermatol* (1962) **85**:385–93.
4. Stegman SJ, A study of dermabrasion and chemical peels in an animal model, *J Dermal. Surg Oncol* (1980) **6**:490–7.
5. Stegman SJ, A comparative histologic study of the effects of three peeling agents and dermabrasion on normal and sun damaged skin, *Aesth Plast Surg* (1982) **6**:123–35.
6. Brodland DG, Roenigk RK, Trichloroacetic acid chemexfoliation (chemical peel) for extensive premalignant actinic damage of the face and scalp, *Mayo Clin Proc* (1988) **63**:887–96.
7. Lober CW, Chemexfoliation—indications and cautions, *J Am Acad Dermatol* (1987) **17**:109–12.
8. Matarasso SL, Salman SM, Glougau RC et al, *J Dermatol Surg Oncol* (1990) **16**:945–54.
9. Brody HJ, Hailey CW, Medium-depth chemical peeling of the skin: a variation of superficial chemosurgery, *J Dermatol Surg Oncol* (1986) **12**:1268–75.
10. Brodland DG, Cullimore KC, Roenigk RK et al, Depths of chemexfoliation induced by various concentrations and application techniques of trichloroacetic acid in a porcine model, *J Dermatol Surg Oncol* (1989) **15**:967–71.
11. Zelickson AS, Mottaz JH, Weiss JS et al, Topical tretinoin in photoaging: an ultra structural study, *J Cutan Aging Cosmet Dermatol* (1988) **1**:41–7.

Chapter 48

CHEMICAL PEEL WITH PHENOL

Thomas H. Alt

Chemical peeling is an effective method to regenerate the epidermis and upper layers of the dermis for the purpose of improving changes due to aging, pigmentary disorders, keratoses of actinic and seborrheic origin and conditions of abnormal epidermal turnover. In particular, the phenol peel in its various formulas is the most effective preparation and provides the longest-lasting results of all peels commonly performed by physicians.

HISTORY

Baker and Gordon are credited with the introduction of a modified chemical peel which has become the most popular deep peeling agent.[1] They have written numerous articles since that time.[2-6] Baker and Gordon credit Mackee, an American dermatologist, with the introduction of phenol as an agent in chemical peeling.[7] Mackee, in 1952, reported on his 50 years of experience with the use of phenol to correct a variety of facial defects.[8] It is interesting to note that Baker and Gordon, in their most recent textbook, list only three major references, all of which were by dermatologists, demonstrating that dermatologists played a major role in developing and understanding this treatment for aging skin.[9-11] In addition to those listed by Baker and Gordon, the phenol preparation developed by Litton has also been used since its first publication in 1962.[12]

Table 48.1
Indications

1. Aging skin, fine to medium wrinkling
2. Actinically damaged skin (Chataigne skin)
   (a) Actinic keratoses
   (b) Superficial basal cell epithelioma
3. Pigmentary changes
   (a) Melasma
   (b) Ephelis
   (c) Lentigines, lentigo maligna
   (d) Postinflammatory hyperpigmentation
       (i) Dermatitis
       (ii) Compulsive excoriation
       (iii) Acne vulgaris
   (e) Periorbital hyperpigmentation
   (f) Nevoid conditions

INDICATIONS (TABLE 48.1)

The effects of aging are the primary reason to perform phenol chemical peel (Figures 48.1 and 48.2). These changes occur in light-complexioned individuals who have little or no actinic damage. Baker and Gordon describe the ideal patient as a fair-skinned, English woman who spends most of her time indoors in a London

SURGICAL DERMATOLOGY

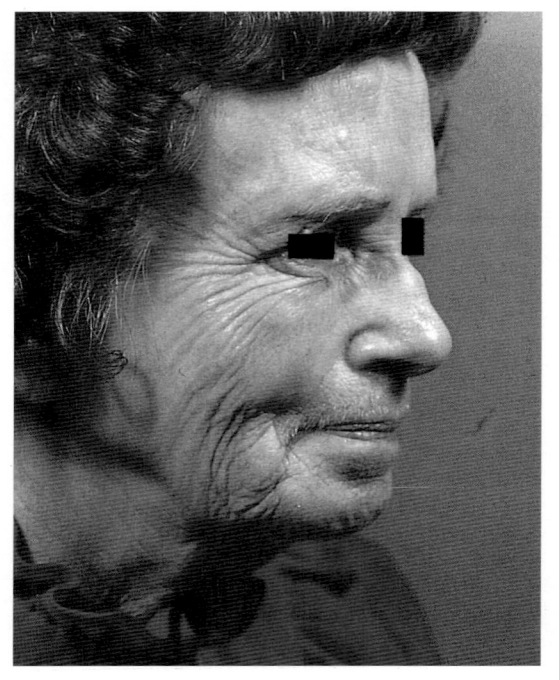

Figure 48.1
A red-headed, fair-skinned woman of 72 years of age with many fine and medium wrinkles but very little actinic damage. She represents an ideal patients for this procedure.

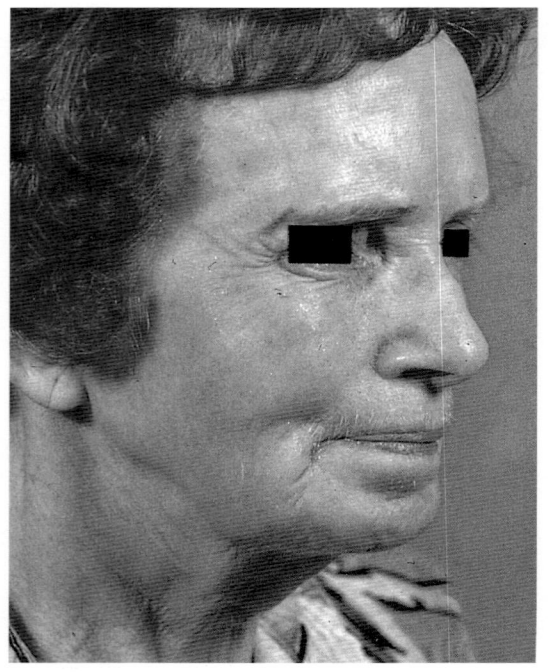

Figure 48.2
Same patient as in Figure 48.1 6 months following a taped Baker–Gordon phenol peel. Virtually all of the medium and fine wrinkles have been removed with the exception of her periorbital area. Note that the neck is unchanged since this area was untreated.

climate with very little exposure to the sun.[13] Most practitioners, particularly dermatologic surgeons, would consider the changes seen in actinically damaged skin, particularly in light-complexioned individuals, as a more common indication since both aging and actinic damage will accelerate wrinkling. The phenol peel works best in individuals with fine to medium wrinkles and is less effective on skin severely damaged as a result of long-term, unprotected sun exposure. In addition to fair complexion, many authors consider blue eyes and light hair to be additional characteristics of the ideal patient. This author feels that these criteria are invalid since it is the skin and its response to the chemical peel which is the critical factor. Patients with medium to dark complexions and even blacks may be treated. Extensive experience using this technique on 'olive' complexion or Mediterranean-type skin without any unacceptable results is referred to by Baker and Gordon.[7] Although Baker and Gordon caution against the use of phenol in black patients,[13] Pierce has experience with patients who have successfully undergone the Baker–Gordon peel with good results.[14] McCullough and Langsdon caution that dark-skinned individuals

480

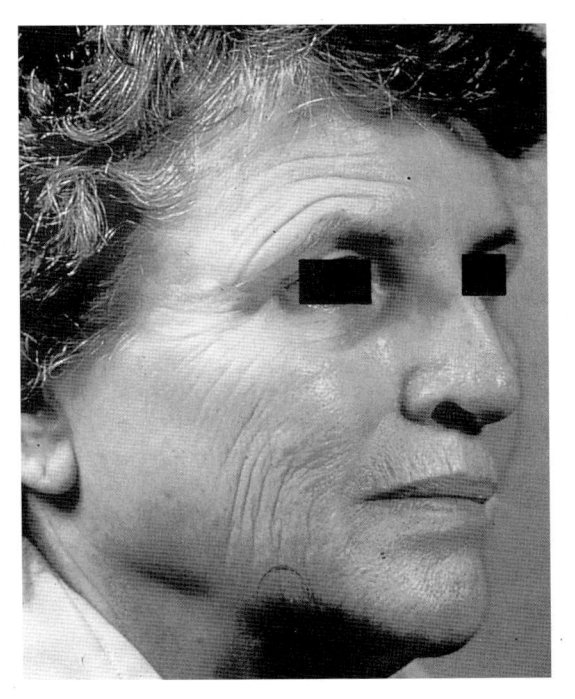

Figure 48.3
A fair-complexioned female of 62 years of age with dark brown and gray hair and many medium-sized wrinkles. There is very little actinic damage evident.

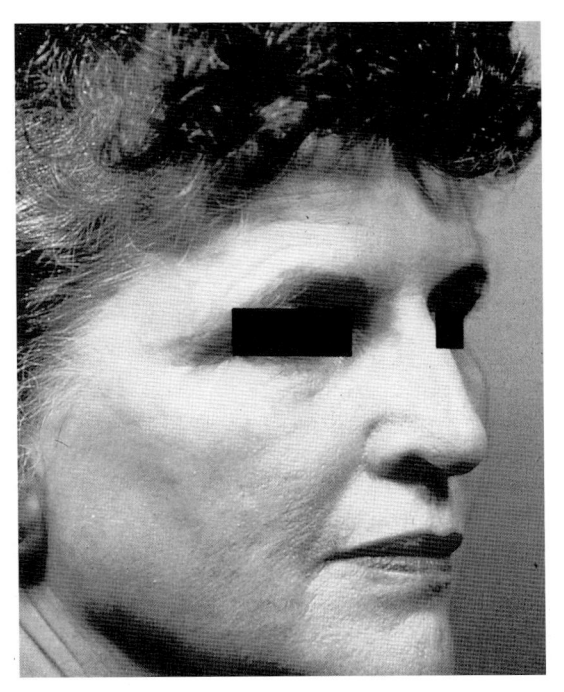

Figure 48.4
Same patient as in Figure 48.3 shown 10 years following a taped Baker–Gordon peel. Note that despite this time span virtually all of her rhytides continue to be eliminated. There is excellent blending of skin color.

are more likely to have pigmentary problems since phenol produces some degree of hypopigmentation in almost all cases.[15] The author's personal experience is that patients rarely notice any color change when a full facial peel is performed.

The most severely affected areas and, therefore, the most difficult regions to treat, are the rhagades radiating from the perioral area, the crow's feet of the periorbital region, the glabellar folds and the horizontal rhytides of forehead. Although all of these wrinkles will not be completely eliminated, there is significant and long-lasting improvement when these areas are treated using the deep phenol peel (Figures 48.3 to 48.6).

Elastotic skin resulting from long-term actinic exposure, known as Chataigne skin, occurs in farmers, and is an excellent indication for this procedure.[7,15–17] Sunbathers may comprise our largest number of candidates: sunscreens and an awareness of the accumulated damage created by sun exposure have only become apparent in the past two decades. Patients with coarse-textured, thick seborrheic skin in addition to those with severe actinic damage will not obtain the results which can be expected in fair-complexioned thin-

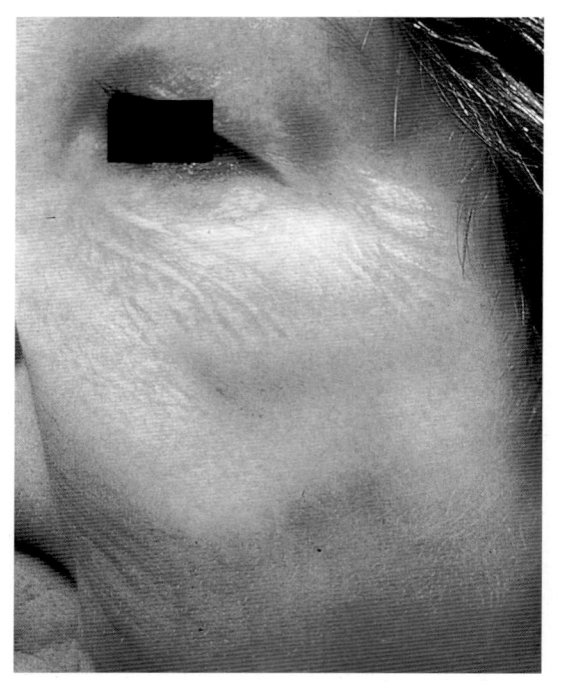

Figure 48.5
A medium-complexioned woman of 57 years of age with many fine wrinkles and excess skin of her eyelids and face. This patient is an excellent candidate for a blepharoplasty and rhytidectomy to be followed 3–6 months later with a Baker's phenol chemical peel.

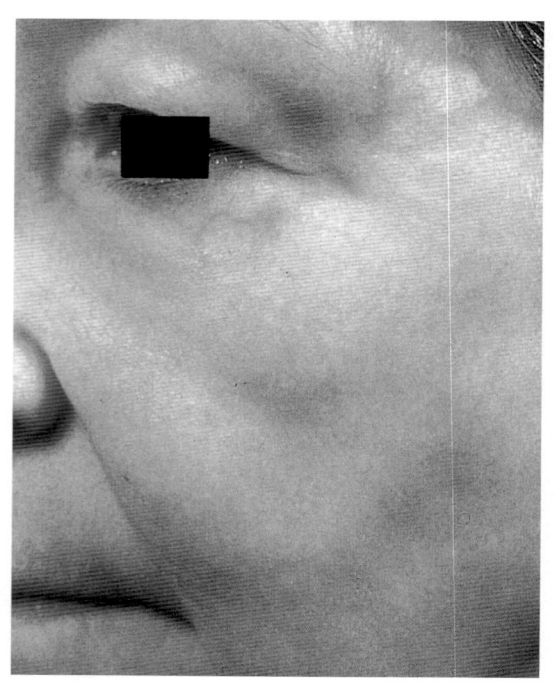

Figure 48.6
The same patient as in Figure 48.5 1 year following a taped Baker's phenol peel. This patient opted for a chemical peel only despite the fact that blepharoplasty and rhytidectomy would have been appropriate procedures to perform. Note that the excess skin of the lids and face persists.

skinned individuals who have mild to moderate sun damage.

Actinic keratoses are also a major indication for the use of phenol chemical peeling.[7,13,14,18,19] Thick and hyperkeratotic actinic keratoses do not respond as adequately unless the thickened keratin layer is removed mechanically by curettage or some other method prior to the application of the phenol peel. Basal cell epitheliomas of the superficial variety which do not invade deeply into the dermis do respond well to phenol peel.[19] Basal cell epitheliomas of the nodular or sclerosing type are not appropriate indications for phenol chemical peeling. However, the presence of multiple superficial basal cell epitheliomas is an indication. Skin damage secondary to radiation therapy is an indication mentioned by Baker and Gordon.[13] The author presumes that this is ionizing radiation for benign and malignant disease. Most dermatologists would question this indication if there is significant atrophy of the adnexal structures, particularly when malignant disease has been treated. Because of this epidermal defect, adequate healing following an injury by phenol may not be possible.

Pigmentary changes are also an indication for the use of deep phenol peeling (Figures 48.7 and 48.8). Estrogen therapy

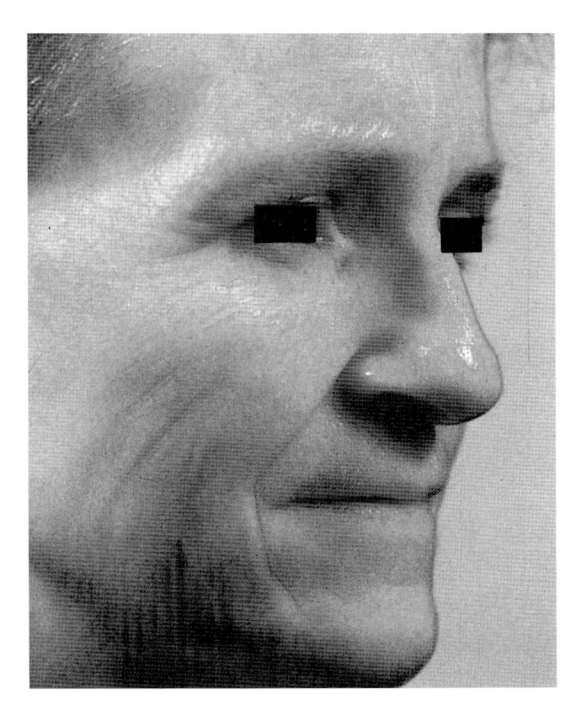

Figure 48.7
A 46-year-old woman with medium to dark complexion and many medium to deep rhytides resulting from premature aging.

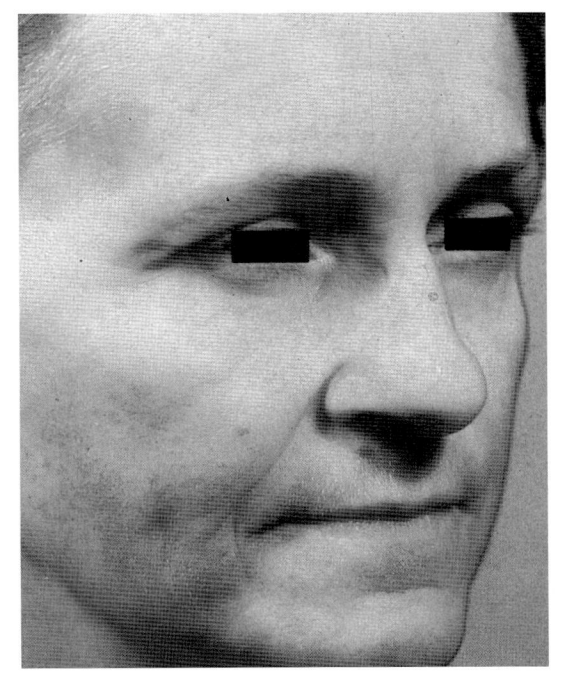

Figure 48.8
Same patient as in Figure 48.7 4 months after a taped Baker–Gordon phenol peel. Some mild postinflammatory hyperpigmentation persists but no mottled hyperpigmentation is present despite the fact that the patient spent 2 weeks in Hawaii during her third postoperative month.

and pregnancy resulting in melasma are accepted indications. Baker and Gordon[7] consider this as a major indication for the procedure and Wood-Smith and Rees[16] consider the procedure as a prologue to a permanent cure. Stegman and Tromovitch,[18] recognizing that the depth of the pigmentary changes in melasma may vary, report the response as variable. Ephelis or freckling is usually eliminated by this peel. This is advantageous in the patient who demonstrates only facial freckling but may be disadvantageous for the patient who undergoes a regional peel of the perioral or periorbital areas if the remaining freckles are still apparent on the unpeeled regions of the face. Many patients with facial freckling have little or no changes on their neck and, therefore, the elimination of freckles on the face is not disadvantageous when a full facial peel is performed. Although Baker and Gordon[7] and the author have observed that the elimination of ephelis is permanent, McCullough and Langsdon[15] state that they reappear only a few months later. This may be the result of a more superficial peel since the latter authors do not occlude the peel with tape.

Chronically sun-damaged epidermal melanocytes produce benign lentigines such as lentigo simplex, lentigo senilis and lentigo maligna. All of these conditions respond well to deep phenol peeling. An increase of epidermal melanin occurs in chronic inflammatory states such as dermatitis, compulsive excoriation and superficial acne. This type of hyperpigmentation also responds well to chemical peeling. However, these forms differ from that seen in chronic postinflammatory hyperpigmentation in which the melanin is frequently found in the subepidermal melanophage such as that in lichen planus, lupus erythematosus and fixed drug eruptions. Chemical peeling is less effective when pigmentation is found subepidermally. In periorbital hyperpigmentation in which the melanin is commonly increased in the epidermal layer, the effect of deep chemical peeling is excellent.[13] Although the author is not aware of any reported cases, nevoid conditions such as nevus spilus, nevus of Ota and Becker's nevus all produce hyperpigmentation in the epidermal layer and, therefore, one would expect these conditions to improve with deep phenol peel.

Although superficial acne scarring (Table 48.2) is listed by a number of authors as an appropriate indication,[7,12,15,16,19] Mackee[8] stated that in his 50 years' experience phenol had very little effect on acne scarring and dermabrasion was a much better procedure to remove scars (Figures 48.9 and 48.10). Baker and Gordon now agree with this assessment, stating that phenol peeling is of little value in acne scarring.[13] The author concurs with this evaluation.

Litton[20] and Wood-Smith and Rees[16] have stated that telangiectasias are improved with chemical peeling. The author's own experience is that there is very little change following a phenol peel. Baker and Gordon agree with the author's conclusion.[7] Telangiectasia is a dermal defect and, therefore, would respond less than defects which are found in the epidermal layers. Baker and Gordon[7,13] state that

Table 48.2
Conditions with Variable Response

1. Radiation dermatitis
2. Superficial acne scarring
3. Telangiectasia
4. Enlarged adnexal pores
5. Postsurgical scarring

large adnexal pores frequently become larger after phenol peeling. The author disagrees with this observation: close-up photographs of patients who have undergone deep phenol peeling using the occluded method in the author's hands show that adnexal pores are usually decreased in size when long-term results are evaluated.[21]

Histological Changes

Baker et al[22] have outlined the microscopic changes seen in long-term evaluation of treated and untreated skin. Specimens were obtained from the neck in an area that included a section of tissue containing both treated and untreated skin obtained at the time of rhytidectomy. Specimens ranged from 3 months to 13 years postpeel. Three significant changes were noted.

1. A broad band of well-orientated dermal fibers measuring 2–3 mm was present in the upper layers of the dermis. By contrast, the orientation of the deeper collagen layers was irregular. This new dermal band contained normal vessels without any perivascular lymphocytic inflammatory response. Telangiectatic vessels were only seen in the deeper portions of the dermis which were unaffected by the phenol.
2. There was a significantly increased amount of elastic fibers present in the altered skin as shown by special staining techniques.

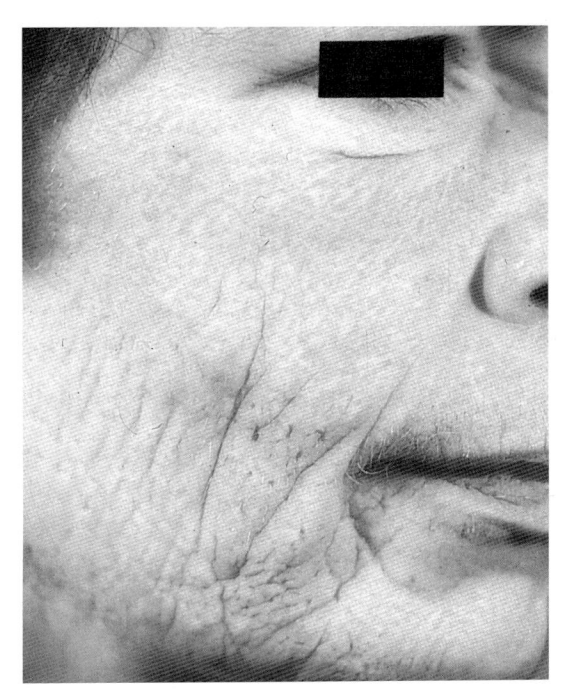

Figure 48.9
This patient has marked wrinkling, excess skin and severe scarring of chronic cystic acne. She subsequently underwent a facelift and blepharoplasty prior to a taped Baker–Gordon phenol peel.

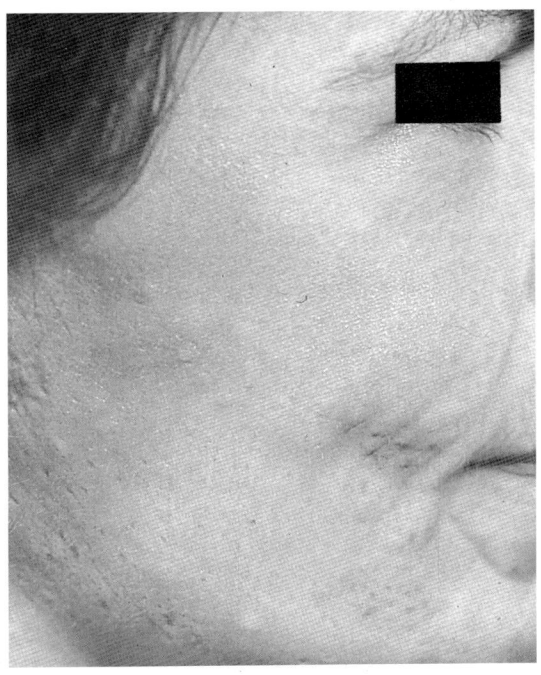

Figure 48.10
Same patient as in Figure 48.9 following a taped Baker–Gordon phenol peel. Although the contour and excess skin have improved, there is virtually no improvement in the scar formation, particularly on the chin, which resulted from earlier acne.

3. In the epidermis keratinocytes stained evenly, were of uniform size and shape, and had returned to their normal polarity. Microscopic actinic keratoses and lentiginous downgrowths were either not seen or rarely seen. Melanocytes were present in normal amounts but the melanin granules appeared to be decreased.

Stegman[23] evaluated the effects of numerous chemical peeling agents on the neck of a severely actinic-damaged adult male. Multiple biopsies performed during the early and late postpeeling period showed that the Baker–Gordon formula wounded deeper than full-strength (88%) phenol which, in turn, wounded deeper than 60% trichloroacetic acid. The study showed that occlusion using tape increased the depth of the wound with the phenol peels. The depth of penetration was greater in sun-damaged skin than in non-sun-damaged skin and the healing period was directly proportional to the depth of the wound. When re-epithelialization was completed, the thickness of the regenerated papillary dermis was directly related to the strength of the agent applied.

Technical Factors

The formula for the Baker–Gordon peel is:

3 ml USP liquid phenol, 88%
2 ml tap water
8 drops liquid soap (Septisol)
3 drops croton oil

Phenol (C_6H_5OH) is suspended in water by the use of a saponifying agent such as Septisol or any liquid soap. The phenol attacks the sulfide bonds in the epidermis, causing keratocoagulation and keratolysis. There is also denaturization because of its acidic properties. Phenol in a 45–55% concentration is the most effective agent in chemical peeling. As this concentration is increased, the absorption of phenol will decrease; therefore, the use of a diluted phenol will have a greater effect upon the skin. Croton oil is a vesicant and increases absorption by acting as a keratolytic agent. The author mixes this formula by drawing the ingredients into individual identical 3-ml plastic syringes onto which an 18-gauge needle has been attached. The formula is posted on a placard during mixing, which is carefully monitored by at least two reliable office personnel. It is better to substitute sterile water for tap water to decrease the possible contamination of adulterants, which will vary from community to community. Croton oil, which is difficult to obtain from local suppliers,[1] is added last so that any mistake which occurs during the mixing of the formula will not cause loss of this ingredient. (Croton oil may be obtained from Polysciences Inc., Warrington, PA 18976.)

The ingredients are placed in a clear glass medicine cup which allows the surgeon to see if the mixture has remained in suspension or has separated (Figure 48.11). Since the formula is a suspension, frequent stirring is necessary (Figure 48.12). McCullough and Langsdon[15] have recommended that an amber glass bottle be used, but the author disagrees with this since the layering of the suspension cannot be readily observed and the rolling of a soaked cotton-tipped applicator in the neck of the bottle is more difficult than it is on the side of a medicine cup. The author agrees with the recommendation of Baker and Gordon[7] that the preparation should be freshly mixed before each case. However, many surgeons state that they use their mixture on multiple occasions. The author discards the preparation immediately at the conclusion of each procedure by diluting it with water while wearing a protective rubber glove.

Preoperative Preparation

Since phenol can have toxic effects, all patients undergo a careful preoperative history, physical examination and extensive laboratory examination (Table 48.3).

Particular attention is directed toward the cardiac, renal and hepatic systems. All patients over the age of 40 years undergo EKG and chest radiographic examinations. Special care should be taken by the patient to avoid facial or eye makeup at least 1 day prior to the chemical peel since it is very difficult to remove waterproof eyeliner from the edge of the upper and lower eyelids. The face is washed with ordinary soap and water the night before and on the morning of the procedure to begin the degreasing process.

Some authors[15] avoid pHisoHex and pHisoderm (Winthrop-Breon Laboratories, New York, NY) as a surgical scrub since it deposits an oil residue on the skin which they feel will retard the absorption of the phenol mixture. The author uses Technicare (Care-Tech Laboratories, St Louis, MO) since its producer states that 99.9% of the bacteria are destroyed within a 30-s exposure and the product is not an oil-based suspension. Most surgeons use ether, acetone or a combination of acetone and

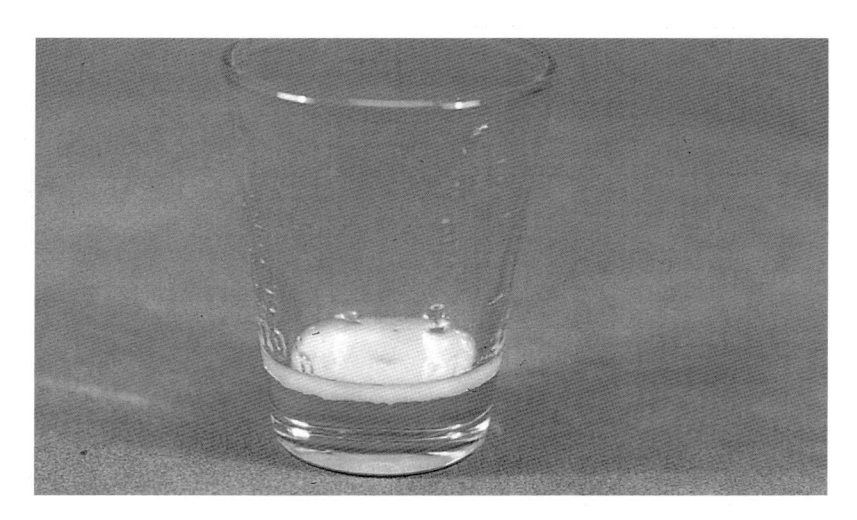

Figure 48.11
The Baker–Gordon formula produces an emulsion which if not stirred regularly will separate into layers.

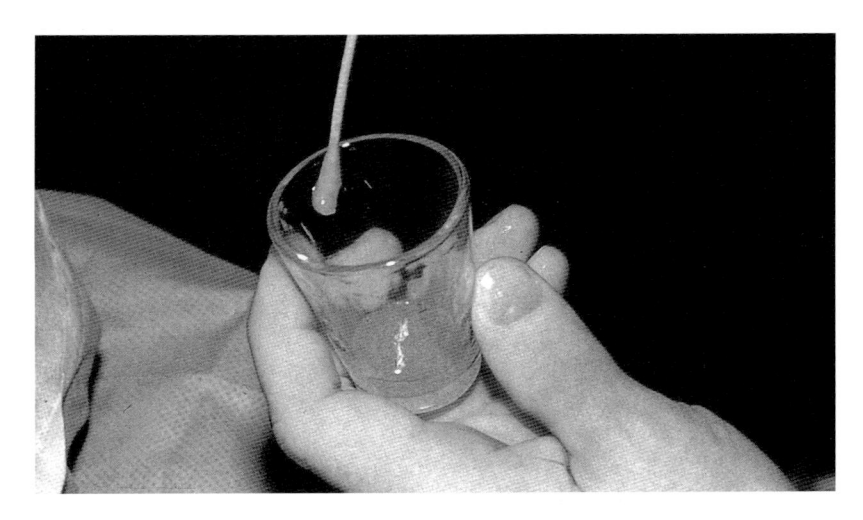

Figure 48.12
The emulsion must be stirred thoroughly and regularly to suspend the phenol in the water.

alcohol to degrease the skin immediately prior to the peeling. Stegman and Tromovitch[18] feel that this is unnecessary and state that there is no proof that facial oils retard the penetration of the phenol solution. The author feels that it is very important to degrease the face and does so immediately before the peeling agent is applied to each segment of the skin. The author further believes that no pressure or excessive scrubbing should be applied to the skin during the degreasing. McCullough and Langsdon[15] recommend that the skin should be thoroughly cleansed using a folded 2 × 2 inch gauze sponge grasped in a hemostat. They state that the acetone is applied repeatedly until a sandpaper-like sound is heard as the sponge is rubbed across the skin. The author believes that this is unnecessarily aggressive and will

Table 48.3
Preoperative Laboratory Evaluation

1. Complete blood count
2. Differential
3. Prothrombin time
4. Partial thromboplastin time
5. SMA 12 including, glucose, creatinine, uric acid, cholesterol, triglycerides, sodium, potassium, chlorides, carbon dioxide, calcium, SGOT and alkaline phosphatase
6. Urinalysis
7. Platelet count
8. HIV
9. Hepatitis B surface antigen
10. Pregnancy test, urine or serum

cause an abrasive stripping of the keratin layer in an irregular fashion. Tissue overlying bony structures will offer a greater amount of resistance and, therefore, the abrasion would be deeper than that which would occur in areas of skin that do not overlay areas of bony structures such as the central cheeks. The author further believes that this aggressive scrubbing can lead to a significant difference in the absorption of the peeling substance. At least one physician who has used this technique consulted the author, requesting assistance for a patient who developed scars over the bossing of the forehead and malar prominences.

The patient is placed in a sitting position prior to the administration of any preanesthetic sedatives or analgesics. A line of small dots of aqueous gentian violet is placed approximately 1 cm below the mandibular ramus. The chemical peel is extended to this area so that permanent color changes will fall into the shadow cast by the mandible. The Baker–Gordon formula is not recommended for use on the neck but trichloroacetic acid of 25–35% can be safely used in patients in whom a blending chemical peel would be helpful on the neck.

Every surgeon has their own preference for preoperative sedation and analgesia. The author's preference is the use of monitored anesthesia care (MAC) employing the assistance of an anesthesiologist or a nurse–anesthetist using an analgesic, i.e. meperidine (Demerol, Winthrop-Breon Laboratories, New York, NY) or fentanyl citrate (Elkins-Sinn, Cherry Hill, NJ) in combination with the sedative midazolam (Versed, Roche Laboratories, Nutley, NJ). Although in the past many surgeons personally administered these intravenous preparations, most guidelines now recommend that no intravenous medications be administered without the assistance of an anesthetist or anesthesiologist. Regional block anesthesia using long-acting local anesthetics such as bupivacaine (Marcain, Winthrop-Breon Laboratories) or etidocaine (Duranest, Astra Pharmaceutical Products, Westboro, MA) can also be employed.[18] The author removes all fine facial hair using an electric or safety razor to avoid the discomfort which occurs when these hairs are traumatically removed during the tape removal following surgery.

CHEMICAL AGENT APPLICATION

Small segments are treated immediately following degreasing with acetone. No fixed pattern is necessary; however, the surgeon should develop a routine which will assure that all areas are adequately treated (Figures 48.13 to 48.16). Most surgeons begin by painting one-half or all of the forehead. The preparation is stirred thoroughly to allow for an even suspension of the ingredients. The author's technique is to use one cotton-tipped applicator to apply the mixture in a sweeping or brushing motion. Variations from other authors include the use of three applicator sticks[18] or one large proctology swab.[19] The author strongly urges that the latter method not be used since a proctology swab can deliver a very large bolus of the chemical, which can

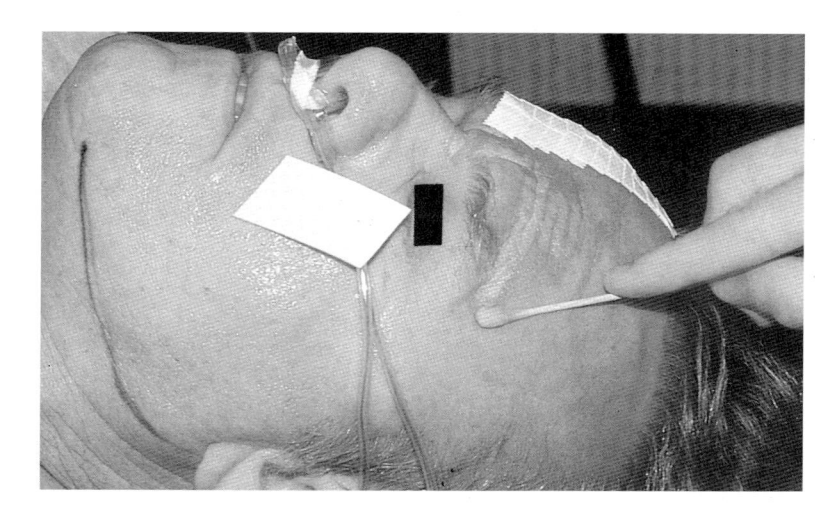

CHEMICAL PEEL WITH PHENOL

Figure 48.13
Small segments of the face, such as half the forehead, are treated individually. The area is gently cleansed with a degreasing agent such as acetone, following which the wrinkles are spread with the thumb and forefinger and the Baker–Gordon preparation applied to the depth of the deep wrinkles. The solution is then applied over the entire area, with a second layer over the deeper wrinkles. One or two cotton-tipped applicators are used to limit the amount of preparation applied.

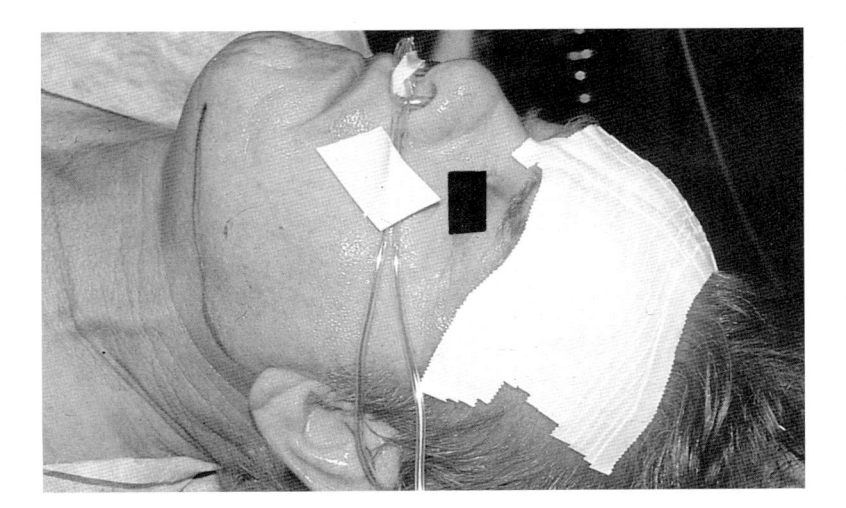

Figure 48.14
Small pieces of Curity Brand waterproof adhesive tape are placed in two layers over the treated skin after several minutes of drying. This delay allows the phenol and water to evaporate, providing an adequate base to which the tape may adhere. Small narrow tapes work better than long wide tapes since they allow for a hinge effect with movement of the underlying skin.

precipitate arrhythmia; the author has personally witnessed this. The preparation is first applied to the deepest wrinkles, which are separated using digital pressure by the nondominant hand. A distinct white frosting appears. The segment may then be treated in toto during which the original deep wrinkles are retreated. If the patient remains awake without the use of MAC they will experience an almost immediate burning sensation which may be moderate to severe, depending upon the patient's tolerance. The author's use of MAC is based primarily on the advantage of having an attending anesthetist or anesthesiologist to monitor the cardiopulmonary response rather than the need to relieve this discomfort. Usually after 15–30 s this discomfort begins to subside. The chemical must evaporate completely from the segment

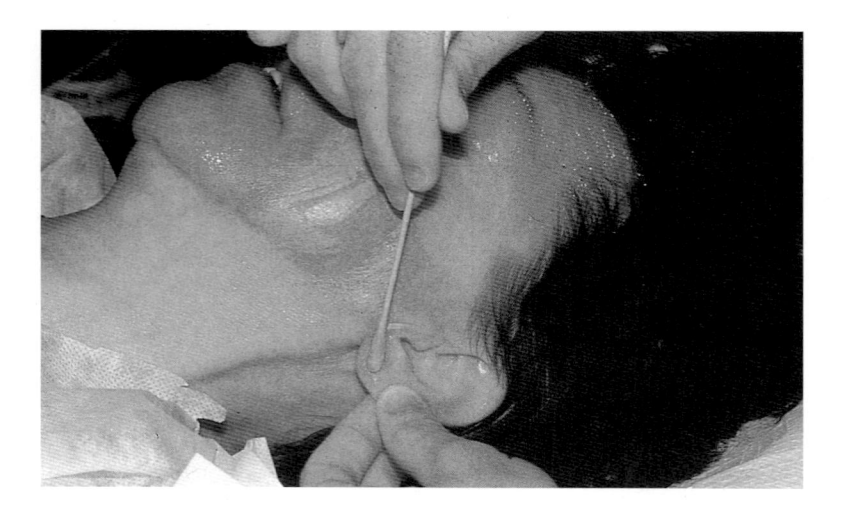

Figure 48.15
The cheek is degreased using acetone and the deep wrinkles are treated. Note that this patient is undergoing an untaped Baker phenol peel since the amount of skin damage is only moderate.

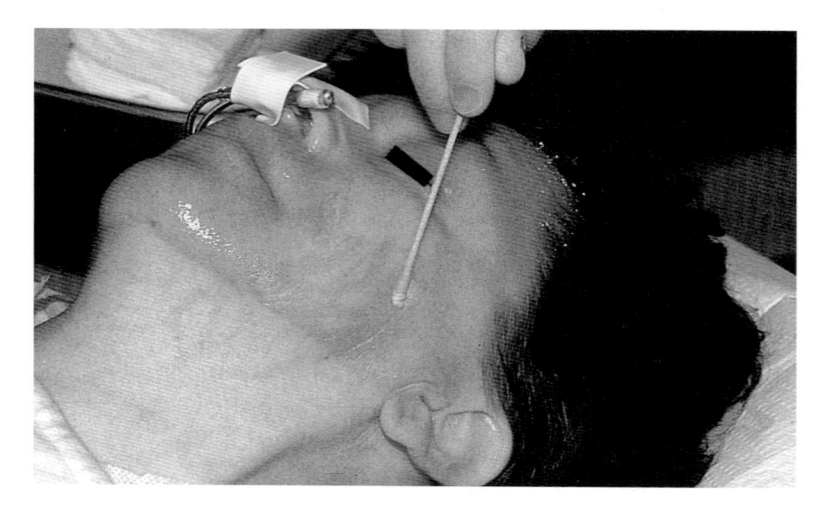

Figure 48.16
The earlobe is also treated since color changes and wrinkles are frequently apparent. Although the cheek is routinely taped, the earlobe is usually left untaped.

prior to the application of the tape or the tape will not adhere satisfactorily. The skin will usually retain a mild frosted color until the tape is applied.

APPLICATION OF TAPE

The tape is applied to each segment as the application of the peeling agent progresses. It is known that occlusion using a waterproof substance increases the absorption of materials placed on the human skin. Waterproof zinc oxide tape is applied as an occlusive agent. The author prefers 1/2-inch Curity brand tape (Colgate-Palmolive Co., New York, NY) because it is more adhesive and pliable than the Johnson & Johnson brand. Strips are cut in varying lengths of 1.5–4 cm and are lined on the edge of a Mayo stand so that the surgeon may select the appropriate length. As the pieces are removed, the assistant immediately cuts and replaces the size that has been used so that a ready supply is always available. Tapes of shorter length have an advantage over longer pieces since overlapping of the ends will act as a hinge, allowing for a slight amount of motion which will favor the tape remaining adherent to the treated skin. At least two layers of tape cover each treated area of skin (Figure 48.17). Stegman and Tromovitch[18] feel that two or even three layers as recommended by Pierce[14] are unnecessary and they recommend only one layer of occlusive tape. They also differ from most other surgeons in that they apply the active chemical to the entire face prior to initiating the taping process. The author has found that this is not the optimum method of application since a greater amount of the chemical will evaporate in the areas which are last taped and, therefore, a peel of lesser depth will occur.

When the tape does not remain adherent to the skin the occlusion will be incomplete and a skip area will appear in which the peeling is less effective. Most of these skip areas will blend after several months. If, after 6 months, blending has not been satisfactory, then repeeling of the skip area is advisable.

The peeling agent is extended into the hairline, sideburns and eyebrows, although these areas are not taped. Taping is carried to the area immediately adjacent to the hair-bearing skin to avoid traction alopecia at the time of the tape removal. If areas such as the eyebrow or scalp skin are not peeled, an obvious line of demarcation may appear where the treated skin meets the aged, sun-damaged, untreated skin.

Following completion of the forehead, the temple region, preauricular area and half of the cheek are degreased with acetone and treated. The tragus and earlobe are also treated. It is not necessary to tape the earlobe. Longer strips of tape may be used in areas where there is less curvature such as the central cheek.

On the lips the chemical should be applied to at least 2 or 3 mm of the vermilion to treat the perioral rhagades which extend from the glabrous skin onto the vermilion. If this is not done these furrows remain on the lip and allow lipstick to bleed onto the adjacent skin. The use of waterproof zinc oxide tape is often inadequate in the perioral area because motion of the mouth will prevent adhesion of the tape. The author now uses Microfoam tape (3M, St Paul, MN) to occlude this area. This tape is elastic and will stretch and contract during motion of the lips. Since this area is commonly the most severely damaged area, with excessive wrinkling, the author recommends that patients do no talking during the 48-h period of taping. They are given a writing pad and pencil for communication and a squeeze bottle used by cyclists for the administration of a liquid diet.

The author prefers to treat and tape a segment of skin measuring 1–2 cm inferior to the border of the mandible. This line corresponds to the line most women produce when applying facial cosmetics. In contrast, Stegman and Tromovitch[18] recommend the use of a sawtooth taping method along the mandibular region because they feel an irregular line is less easily noticed than a straight line.

Baker's solution is applied to the eyelid usually at the conclusion of the procedure since considerable edema and discomfort are produced (Figures 48.18 and 48.19). The chemical is applied to the superior border of the tarsal plate on the upper lid to minimize this edema. Application of the chemical on the lower lid is carried to within 1 mm of the lid margin using a relatively dry applicator stick (Figure 48.20). After rolling the cotton applicator stick on the side of the glass medicine cup the author then additionally blots the cotton applicator with a gauze pad, thus

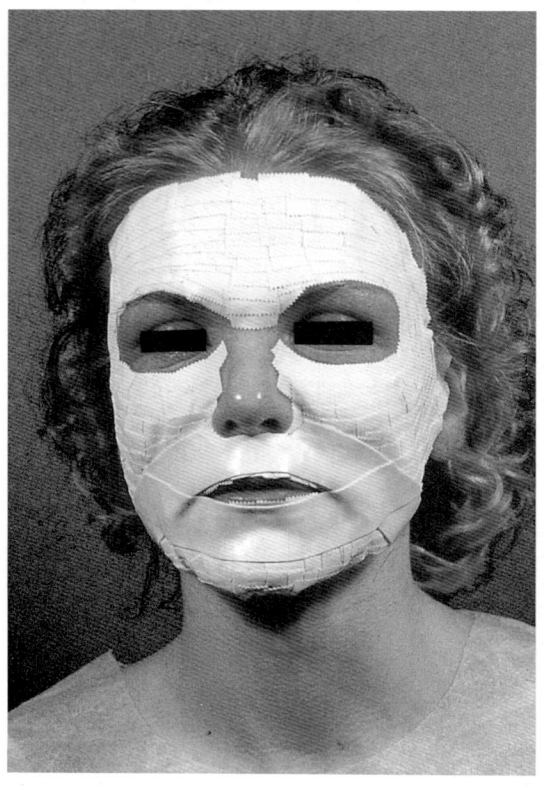

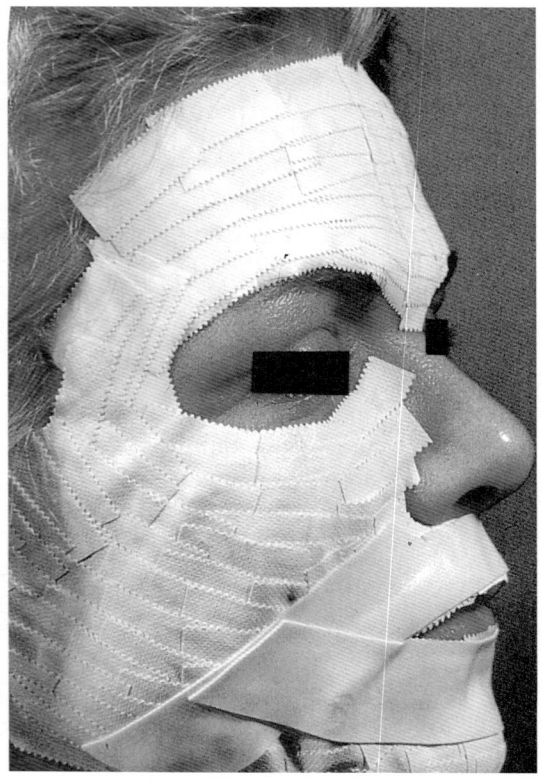

Figure 48.17
A double layer of short-tapes is used over areas of increased contour and high motion. Longer tapes can be used in areas of decreased motion and flat surfaces. The use of 3M Microfoam tape in the perioral area will allow some motion to occur without the tape lifting since it has some elasticity. Note that it is not necessary to tape the nose in most patients since there are no wrinkles in this area. In patients with severe actinic damage of the nose it would be beneficial to tape this structure.

assuring that there is only a minimal amount of Baker–Gordon solution on the cotton applicator. The applicator is then carefully rolled in the direction of the globe until the lower lid margin becomes frosted. The motion is then reversed so that the rolling action is away from the globe: this allows the surgeon to apply the agent to within 1 mm of the lid margin. When applying the chemical to the eyelid, a squeeze bottle containing mineral oil should be held by an assistant so that lavage of the globe and conjunctival sac can occur immediately if any of the chemical is inadvertently placed on the ocular apparatus (Figure 48.21). If the patient is awake and responsive some surgeons place them in a sitting position or elevate the head to decrease the likelihood of chemical entering the conjunctival sac. If a wide band (3 mm) of untreated skin is left on the lower lid, this will usually leave a line of

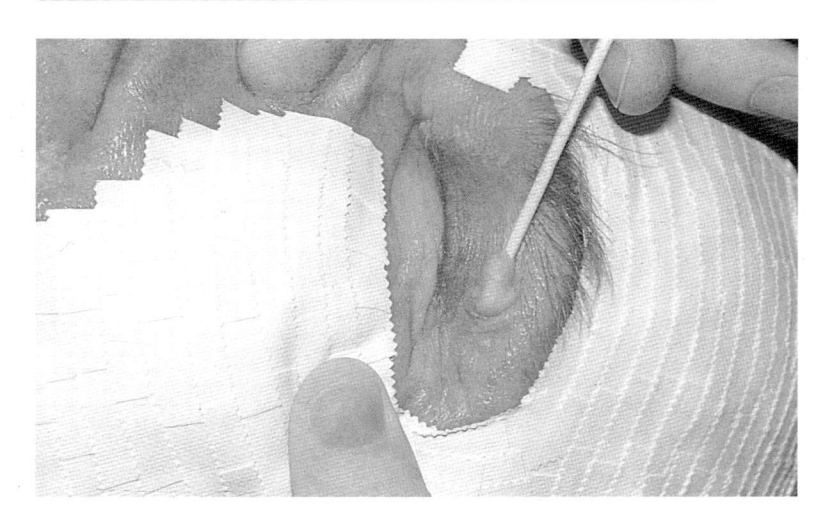

Figure 48.18
The eyelids are treated last since this areas creates the most discomfort. With the use of monitored anesthesia care (MAC) the patient is lightly sedated and will generally tolerate this quite well. The application is made to the superior border of the tarsal plate to avoid excessive edema of the upper lids.

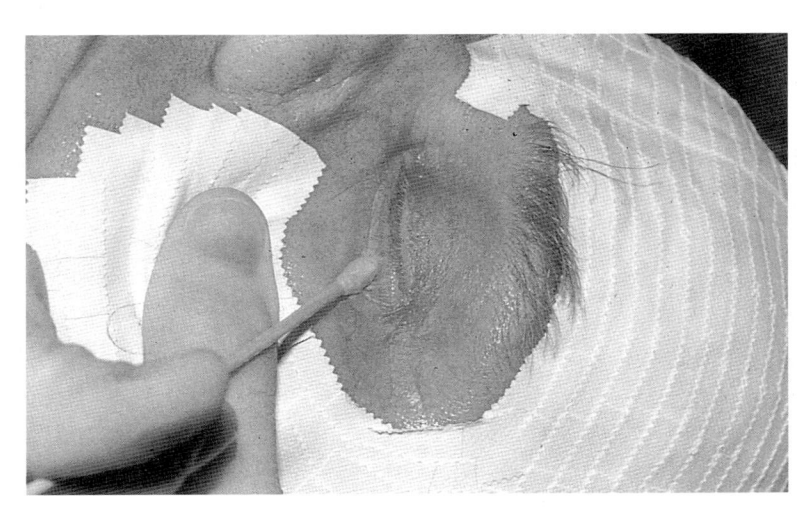

Figure 48.19
The solution on a relatively dry applicator stick is applied to within 1 mm of the lid margin on the lower lid. The applicator stick is rotated away from the lid margin with the lid closed. The motion is then reversed with the direction toward the lid margin with the eye open.

demarcation which is perceptible and permanent. The eyelids are not taped and no occlusive agent such as petrolatum is applied to them for at least the first 24 h. The tape is applied to an area several millimeters below the infraorbital rim. Extending the tape closer to the eyelid will usually restrict movement and is unnecessary. Most surgeons do not apply the Baker–Gordon formula to the anterior neck for fear that this area has a greater tendency to scar. The author now routinely uses 25% trichloroacetic acid for a blending peel in this area (Figure 48.22). Other surgeons have applied concentrations of up to 35% TCA without scar formation.

There is general agreement among authors concerning the time during which the agent should be applied. Baker and Gordon,[7] Litton,[12] Pierce,[14] Stegman and Tromovitch[18] and the author[21] all agree that 1½ –2 h is an acceptable amount of time. The author prefers

SURGICAL DERMATOLOGY

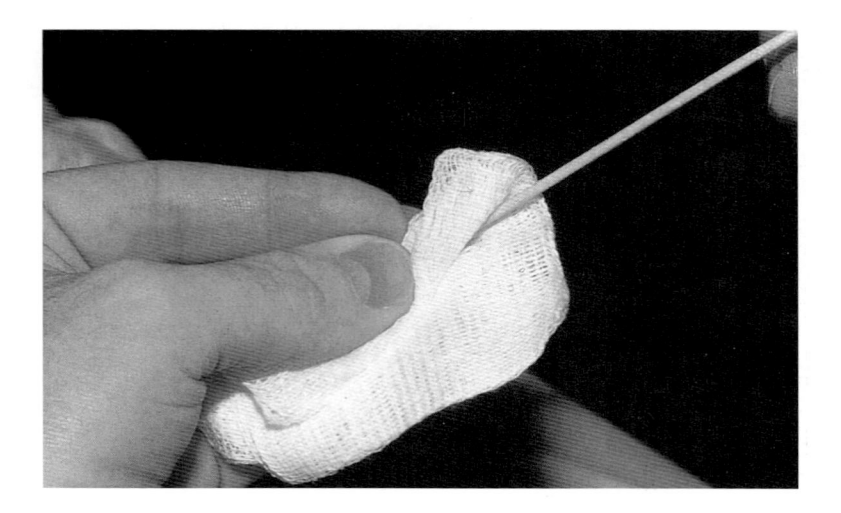

Figure 48.20
When applying the solution to the eyelids, particularly the lower lid, the solution should be applied in scant amounts to avoid contaminating the conjunctival sac with this caustic agent. This can be done by gently drying the soaked cotton applicator tip in a 3 × 3 gauze. Note that gloves are not worn during this procedure since the adhesive tape will adhere to the gloves during application.

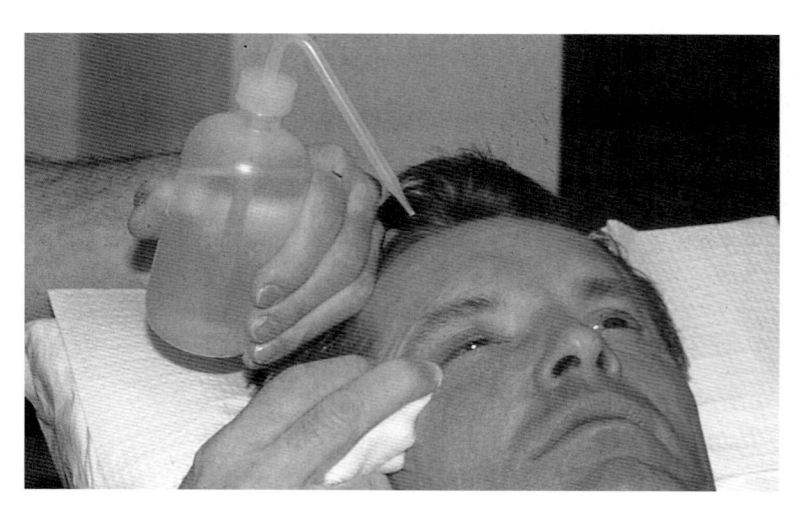

Figure 48.21
In all patients who undergo chemical peeling in the periorbital area an appropriate preparation should be immediately available for lavage of the conjunctival sac and globe if any of the caustic agent comes in contact with these structures. Because water dilutes phenol and makes it become more active, it should not be used when this substance is used. Mineral oil is the appropriate flushing agent for phenol.

the use of short tapes since this is an inducement to slow the procedure. Careful monitoring of the time is the responsibility of the surgeon, the surgical assistant and the attending anesthetist or anesthesiologist.

Mask Removal

Patients return at 24 h for an examination and evaluation. This is an important visit because it provides the psychological support necessary to assure the patient that the progress is within normal limits. At 48 h the patient returns for the removal of the tape (Figure 48.23). These visits must be accompanied by a responsible adult who can drive a vehicle since the mask and edema will cause obstruction of vision. Meperidine (Demerol) is given 30 min prior to mask removal. The mask is readily separated from the treated skin, leaving the exudate on both the face and the tape.

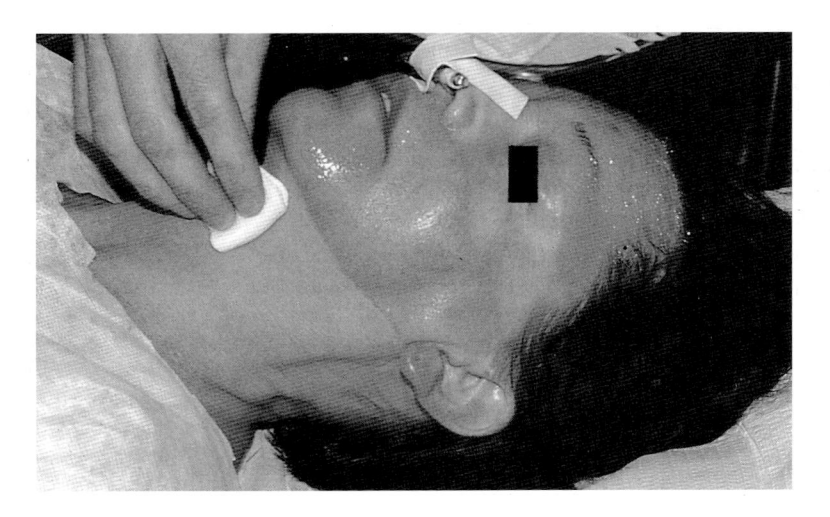

CHEMICAL PEEL WITH PHENOL

Figure 48.22
The neck is cleansed with acetone, following which a solution of 25–35% trichloroacetic acid is applied using a cotton ball. Phenol is not applied to the neck since some feel it will result in scarring. Note that this patient is undergoing an untaped Baker phenol peel since only moderate skin damage is present.

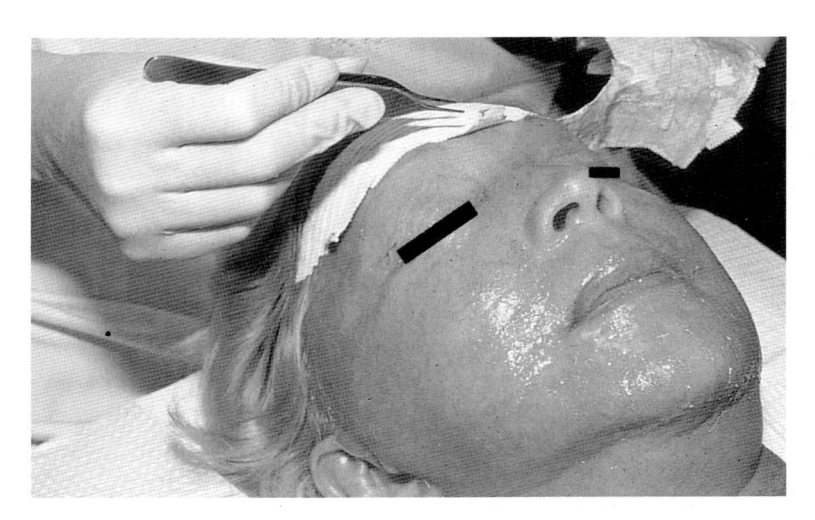

Figure 48.23
The tape is removed at 48 h. The exudate which has accumulated under the tape makes the removal considerably easier than that at 24 h. The patient is sedated with meperidine to decrease discomfort although this is not always necessary. It is helpful to remove all of the vellus hairs prior to the chemical peel so that the tape may be removed without discomfort.

Mask removal is considerably more difficult if the fine vellus hairs of the face have not been removed prior to the peel. These hairs act as hundreds of small anchors which are attached to the tape and cause discomfort upon removal. The treated skin is denuded, edematous and erythematous (Figures 48.24 to 48.28). Surgical sites are cleansed with sterile saline and petrolatum (Vaseline, Cheseborough-Ponds, Greenwich, CT) is applied to all surgical sites. Half-strength boric acid solution is used for wetpacking which is applied continuously during the daytime until the crust is removed. The duration of wetpacking is then decreased from 8 h to 6 h, progressing to 1 h three times a day until complete re-epithelialization occurs. When wetpacking is not performed, the treated areas are covered with petrolatum over which Saran Wrap (The Dow Chemical Company, Indianapolis, IN) is placed. Numerous

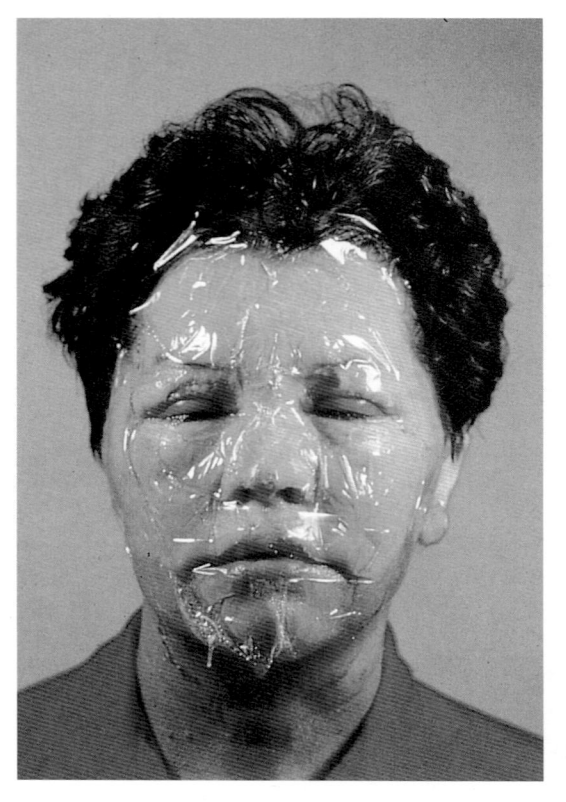

Figure 48.24
When the patient is not wetpacking with half-strength boric acid solution, petrolatum is applied to the skin over which Saran Wrap is placed to decrease desiccation. This patient shows the usual edema and is 24 h postpeel using an untaped Baker–Gordon technique.

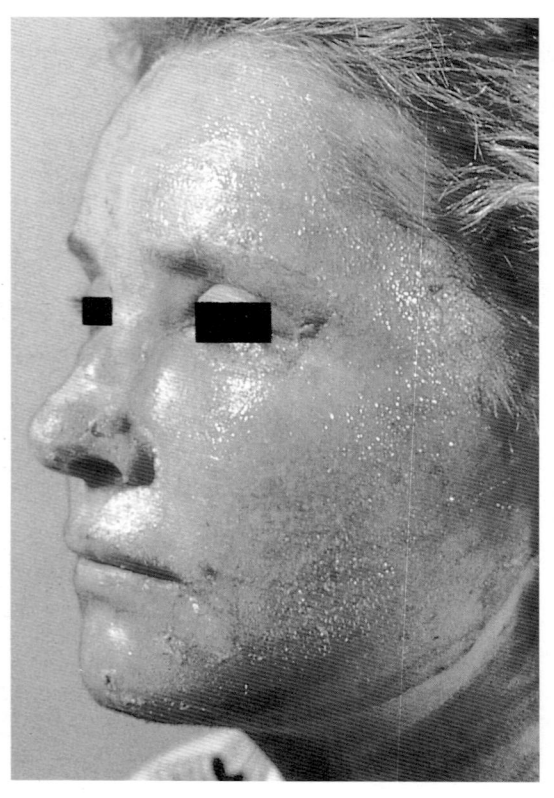

Figure 48.25
The patient is 48 h postpeel using a taped Baker–Gordon technique. The tape has been removed and the skin may be cleaned with hydrogen peroxide and water or saline. Note the moderate amount of crust which remains adherent to the face.

showers, beginning with four per day, will soften the crust and allow it to be removed more readily with gauze and unscented shaving cream such as Edge (S.C. Johnson & Son, Inc) or Gillette (The Gillette Company, Boston, MA).

Drying techniques for wound care such as the use of thymol iodide powder, initially recommended by Baker and Gordon,[1-6] are no longer recommended. Hinman et al[24] showed that wound healing is retarded when dry techniques are employed and is improved when occlusion or wet techniques are used. Dermatologists routinely employ wet techniques or occlusion which not only decreases the healing time but will also diminish the postoperative bacterial growth and decrease the expected inflammatory response. Occlusive dressings also greatly reduce postoperative pain. Showers are helpful to hydrate the crust and facilitate its removal. The use of

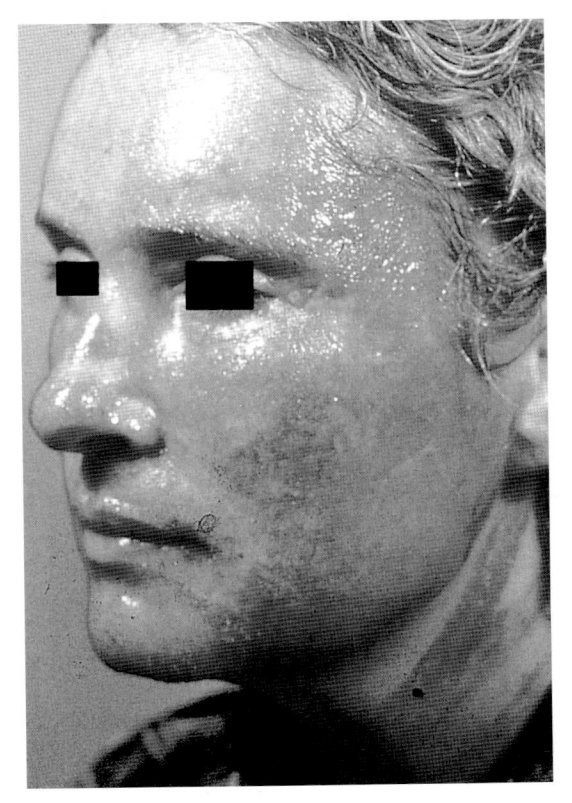

Figure 48.26
Three days postpeel, same patient as in Figure 48.25. The use of half-strength boric acid wetpacks and vaseline covered with Saran Wrap has decreased the crusting. Note that the patient has undergone a 25% trichloroacetic acid peel on the neck.

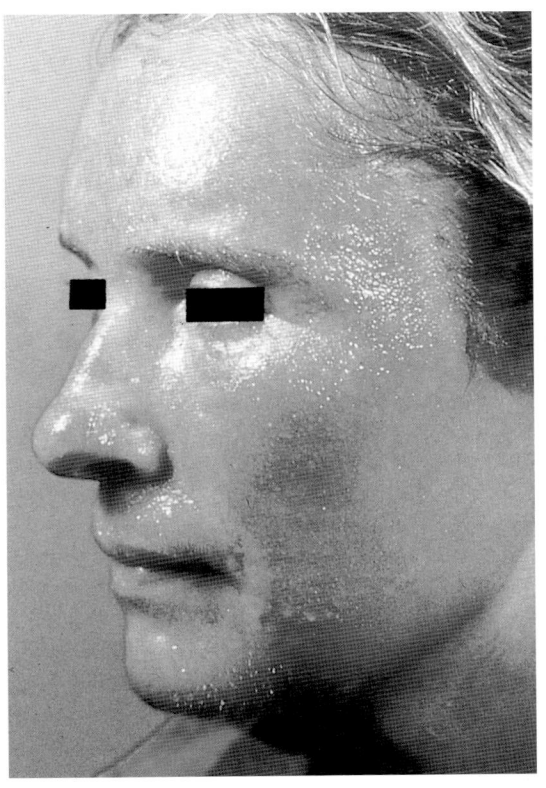

Figure 48.27
The same patient as in Figure 48.25, now 4 days postpeel. Vaseline and Saran Wrap have softened the facial crusting and allowed the showers and half-strength boric acid wetpacks to remove all the detritus. Very little edema persists at this stage.

thymol iodide powder by Baker and Gordon may be the reason why surgeons employing this technique comment on the considerable hypopigmentation which occurs after the procedure. The author presumes that because of this drying technique the depth of injury is greater, resulting in more damage to the melanocyte and subsequent melanin production.

Moisturizing creams which are non-comedogenic and hydrocortisone cream (2.5%) are used to rehydrate the skin and decrease pruritus. Systemic steroids are not used since the author believes that the inflammatory response which stimulates the regeneration of collagen and elastic fibers should not be diminished through their use. As soon as re-epithelialization is complete, cosmetics may be applied. A list of acceptable cosmetics which are noncomedogenic and hypoallergenic should be provided to the patient. Custom compounded cosmetics

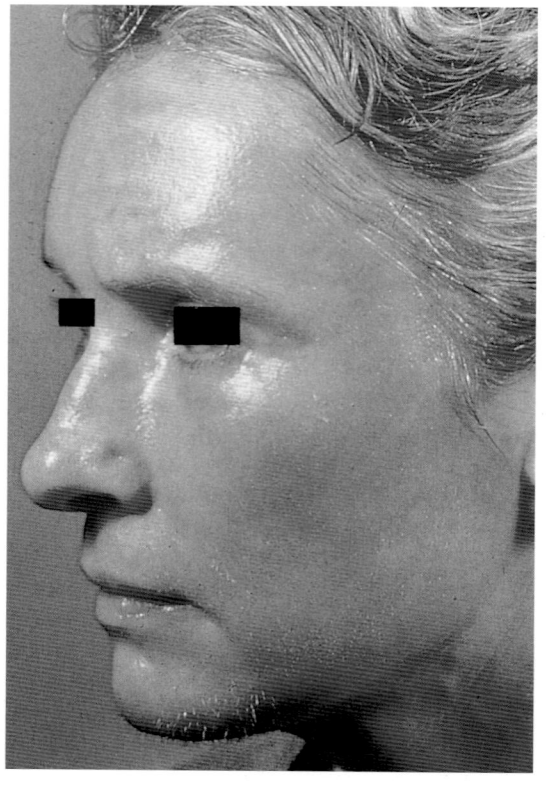

Figure 48.28
Same patient as in Figure 48.25, now 7 days after chemical peel, with no crusting and almost complete re-epithelialization. Very little edema persists although erythema is quite apparent. Re-epithelialization is normally complete by the ninth to eleventh day, at which time noncomedogenic moisturizers and cosmetics may be used.

containing a green base may be necessary to mask the intense erythema that patients may experience. Sun exposure is avoided until the postinflammatory erythema is completely resolved, usually within a 3-month period.

The author recommends that sunscreens of SPF factor 25 and above be used on a regular basis to avoid actinic hyperpigmentation. Since the skin has recently re-epithelialized and its normal epidermal barrier is not yet present, sunscreens are tested in small areas of the preauricular region at the beginning of the fourth week. If no irritant or allergic response occurs, the sunscreen is then applied at least twice daily to the surgical sites during seasons when sunlight is prevalent. For patients who have indoor occupations, sunscreens are not used on a routine basis or during the winter in cold cloudy regions.

Activities which produce a Valsalva maneuver such as lifting, straining and strenuous physical exercise should be avoided since small-vessel damage will occur, leading to multiple petechiae. Contact sports and facial trauma from whisker burn will cause similar result. The torsional effect on the upper layer of epidermis, which has not yet formed an adequate depth of rete ridges, causes the epidermis to slide on the dermis, causing microscopic bleeding at the interface.

VARIATIONS

McCullough has popularized the untaped technique with the Baker–Gordon formula.[15] The advantages are that an anesthetic is not necessary for the removal of the tape mask, there is a reduced risk of postoperative scarring and the patient enjoys the increased convenience and comfort of the open technique. Certainly the first and last advantages exist, but have very little long-term impact on the chemical peel technique. The author has been unable to find any statistical evidence showing that untaped peels have less complications than taped peels. However, this may be correct since untaped peels do not achieve the depth of penetration that is possible with the taped variety. As a result, the therapeutic and cosmetic effects are diminished when compared with the taped method.

Stough has popularized a second version, which is the staged taped peel.[25,26]

Areas of the face, including the forehead and temple regions along with the perioral area, are treated and taped for 48 h. The mask is then removed and the patient is allowed a 24-h rest period. The remainder of the face is then treated and taped for an additional 48 h. The stated advantages of this technique are that less discomfort occurs during the application of the chemical and a significantly lower level of systemic phenol is reached, which provides a greater margin of safety against phenol toxicity. The author has employed this method and has found that it provides excellent results despite the temporary color changes which may occur at the junction of the areas which were treated at different settings.

Repeat Peeling

In Litton's first article,[12] he recommended that peeling could be employed in 6–8 weeks. Most authors would disagree with this recommendation, with Wood-Smith and Rees recommending a waiting period of 12–18 months.[16] The author recommends waiting a minimum of 6 months between applications.[21]

Postoperative Events

Most patients, if treated awake, will experience discomfort prior to the completion of the chemical peel. Edema occurring underneath the taped areas will create a burning sensation which usually lasts between 4 and 6 h. The use of analgesics such as meperidine and the use of crushed ice in a plastic bag applied directly over the tape will usually decrease this discomfort, allowing the patient to have a restful night of sleep on the evening of treatment. Hypnotics are also helpful during the first to third nights, during which the patient is advised to sleep in a sitting or semireclining position to decrease the edema. The exudate which is yellow–green in color, is evident after the first 24 h and will begin to exude from the edges of the taped area. Patients undergoing the untaped technique will have edema erythema and microvesiculation with exudation occurring usually on the second postoperative day. After the removal of the tape the exudate will form crusts, particularly if wetpacking is inadequate. An emollient such as petrolatum, wetpacking and frequent showering will soften and remove the exudate and crusts. Minimal bleeding at pinpoint sites will frequently occur and is expected when wetpacking is adequate since a mild abrasive action must be used with the moistened gauze pads to manually remove the crust and exudate. The treated areas are deeply erythematous, much more so than following a facial dermabrasion. This erythema, along with the edema, begins to subside during the second week. Edema can be marked in many patients and will migrate to the neck area during the first week.

The intermediate effects of the postoperative period occur between 10 days and 6 months. Most patients are completely re-epithelialized by the tenth to eleventh postoperative day. Some healing may not be complete in the area of thin skin which surrounds the periorbital region. The author has seen one patient in whom this area was not completely healed until 4 weeks but no scar was evident upon the completion of healing. It is important to keep these areas moist with petrolatum to prevent the formation of a scar. Stegman and Tromovitch[18] comment on a similar delay in healing, also leading to no apparent scarring. If erythema is intense during this intermediate phase, custom cosmetics can be compounded which include a green- or blue-colored base, which will assist in neutralizing the red color. Pruritus is a common symptom early in this phase and may be improved by the application of mild steroid creams such as hydrocortisone cream 2.5%. McCullough and Langsdon[15] recommend aspirin as a mild analgesic and for this pruritus. Occasionally the author recommends the use of ice packs during periods of more severe pruritus. Dryness of the skin is also a frequent complaint in this early phase. Moisturizing creams and lotions that are noncomedogenic should be provided in addition to the hydrocortisone cream to diminish any pruritus and subsequent excoriation. If the pruritus is persistent and severe, the use of petrolatum or Eucerin (Beiersdorf, Norwalk, CT) at bedtime may be helpful. Milia are a less common event in chemical peeling than in dermabrasion and either will resolve spontaneously or can be extracted by excision and drainage.

COMPLICATIONS (TABLE 48.4)

Complications of chemical peels have been thoroughly reviewed by Brody.[27] Patients with lighter complexions (Fitzpatrick skin types I–III[28]) are less likely to show contrast between the treated and untreated areas. Type IV skin may produce color changes which are perceptible. Therefore, the use of 25% trichloroacetic acid to blend can be beneficial in masking this color change. Most authors feel that type V skin, such as that of Orientals, southern Europeans, American Indians and Latins, has a high likelihood of pigmentary changes. Often, however, these are patients who have very little sun damage because of their natural pigmentary protective system and therefore do not need chemical peeling.

Spira et al[29] cautioned that pigmented nevi may increase in color following phenol chemical peeling. The author has seen these changes occur and does advise patients prior to phenol chemical peeling. However, this is not a universal response and occurs in a small number of cases.

Hyperpigmentation can also be a postoperative complication and is most commonly the result of sun exposure. Oral contraceptives, estrogen therapy, photosensitizing drugs and pregnancy are much less common causes. Hyperpigmentation is treated using a compounded cream of equal parts of retinoic acid cream 0.1% (Retin-A Cream, Ortho Pharmaceutical Corporation, Raritan, NJ) and hydroquinone cream 4% (Eldoquin Forte, ICN Pharmaceuticals Inc., Costa Mesa, CA) applied to the affected areas of hyperpigmentation. If the patient routinely uses a sunscreen of SPF 25 or above, the likelihood of hyperpigmentation is decreased significantly. When this bleaching cream is used within 1 week after the onset of hyperpigmentation pigmentary changes are usually controlled within 2–4 weeks. It is important to recognize that 30 min of exposure to sunlight can produce perceptible hyperpigmentation.

Patients do not become depigmented but rather show hypopigmentation as proven by Kligman et al.[30] These studies confirm Baker and Gordon's earlier reports that melanocytes were not decreased in number. The cells do produce melanin, with melanin granules found evenly distributed in the epidermal cells. The author has found that these patients do tan following surgery, although to a lesser degree than

Table 48.4
Complications and Side-effects of Chemical Peeling

1. Pigmentary changes
2. Scarring
3. Infection
4. Persistent erythema
5. Cutaneous atrophy
6. Textural changes
7. Cardiac arrhythmias
8. Laryngeal edema
9. Toxic shock syndrome
10. Transient erythema
11. Pruritus
12. Milia
13. Acne vulgaris

preoperatively. Aging skin usually increases in color with increased actinic damage. The author feels that criticisms of the phenol peel based upon postoperative hypopigmentation have been unwarranted since younger skin is naturally lighter in color. Therefore, when actinically damaged skin is resurfaced it becomes lighter, which is a normal response. Since the neck is generally untreated, that skin retains its darker color and therefore contrasts with the face. Surgeons who use the dry treatment employing thymol iodide powder will increase the depth of the damage and will presumably destroy more melanocytes because of the deeper wound. A mottled result, which is a combination of hyperpigmentation and hypopigmentation, can be attributed to various causes, including inadequate skin preparation, uneven application of the chemical peeling agent and inadequate mask application or skip areas resulting from the tape becoming detached before the end of the first 24-h period.

The author agrees with Brody's statement that test spot peels do not guarantee that the skin of the remainder of the face will respond in a similar manner to the test area. As a result, this author does not perform a spot test either for dermabrasion or chemical peeling unless the patient has a past history of keloid formation or isotretinoin therapy (Accutane, Roche Laboratories, Nutley, NJ). The author has commented on the use of dermabrasion and chemical peeling in individuals who have undergone Accutane therapy.[31] Current recommendations by the author caution against using a deep phenol peel for a minimum of 24 months after cessation of Accutane therapy.

Scarring

Scarring is the second most feared complication following that of cardiac toxicity. In the author's experience of 15 years of performing taped Baker–Gordon phenol peels, no patients have experienced scar formation. However, Litton and Trinidad, in a questionnaire returned by 588 plastic surgeons, showed that 21% reported scarring when using phenol as the active ingredient in facial chemical peeling.[32] The most common sites were found around the oral cavity, specifically the lips, chin and perioral region. It was proposed that constrictive taping, previous rhytidectomy, excessive mastication or talking might be factors which predisposed patients to this complication. No scientific evidence was given by the authors to support these suppositions. Spira et al[29] have reported that most scars appear within the first 3 months of the postoperative period. The peel should not be performed over an area of recent undermining or flap surgery either for correction of neoplasia or a rhytidectomy. Spira et al recommend that secondary healing is the best approach if this complication occurs. However, Lober[33] recommends excision of the area with the use of a flap or graft to correct the defect. Litton has noted that deep phenol peeling done at the time of rhytidectomy increases the risk of skin slough.[34] Most surgeons wait at least 3 months to perform the deep phenol peel in areas of recent rhytidectomy flap creation. Litton has also reported that phenol peeling can be performed 2–3 months prior to rhytidectomy without untoward results.[35] Ectropion of the lower lid may also occur if the peel is performed in conjunction with a blepharoplasty. Litton and Trinidad have recommended that a period of at least 6 months elapse between the treatment of lower lids using a phenol chemical peel and blepharoplasty.[36] Some cases of cicatricial ectropion have been noted in individuals who have undergone phenol peeling without previous blepharoplasty.[37] Careful examination of the eyelids should be performed to evaluate the muscular and tarsal suspension of the lower lid by performing a snap test, retraction test and pinch test. These tests will show the presence of laxity in the inferior sling which can predispose to ectropion.

Treatment of postpeel scarring should include early and aggressive application of mild topical steroid creams. Caution should be used to avoid telangectasia and excessive atrophy. It is recommended that the patients be seen on a semi-monthly basis to establish the effectiveness of the topical therapy. Fluocinonide-impregnated tape (Cordran, Dista Products, Indianapolis, IN) is also effective in these scars. The tape is cut to the shape of the scar and applied at bedtime, and removed the following morning. This is used 3–5 days per week until significant changes have been noted. Dilute amounts of intralesional triamcinolone diacetate (Aristicort Forte, Lederle, Carolina, Puerto Rico) in doses of 2.5–5.0 mm/ml can be injected every 4–6 weeks if the above measures are not satisfactory.

Postoperative Infection

The most common postoperative infection is that of pre-existing herpes simplex reactivated by the act of peeling the skin[38] (Figure 48.29). Almost every surgeon who performs chemical peel or dermabrasion has experienced this complication. A thorough past history should be performed prior to the surgery and patients who have a history of facial herpes should be treated prophylactically with 200 mg acyclovir (Zovirax, Boroughs-Wellcome, Research Triangle Park, NC) three to five times per day, beginning 24–48 h prior to surgery and continuing until the re-epithelialization process is completed. Collins uses a less aggressive approach, with therapy twice per day and the completion of treatment 4–5 days after the chemical peel.[39] The author also feels that it is important to treat any individual in the family who has a past history of herpes simplex to prevent an exacerbation during the time of re-epithelialization by the patient. If pre-existing herpes simplex is reactivated it is rare that scarring occurs. However, if the infection is primary in nature, usually being contracted from a family member who develops an exacerbation during the postoperative phase, the patient may experience considerable scarring because of no pre-existing personal immunity. If this condition appears to exist, it is wise for the surgeon to seriously consider hospitalization with intravenous acyclovir therapy, topical wetpacks and the topical application of acyclovir.

Persistent Erythema

Erythema is expected to persist for an average of 60–90 days. Very few patients have a cessation of erythema in a shorter period of time, with the exception of those who have undergone peeling without occlusion. The author has seen patients who continue to have erythema for over 6 months. This persistent inflammatory response usually results in an excellent therapeutic and cosmetic result because the stimulation of collagen and elastic fiber regeneration occurs over a longer period of time and is therefore greater in extent. Brody reports that, in his experience, some patients have persisted in having erythema for up to 2 years following a deep phenol peel.[27]

The author cautions that persistent erythema associated with induration, even when subtle, is the precursor of an impending cicatrix. It is at this time that the surgeon should treat with mild topical steroids which, when introduced early, will often resolve the induration within several weeks.

Cutaneous Atrophy

Brody states that atrophy or loss of normal skin markings in the absence of scarring may occur after multiple deep

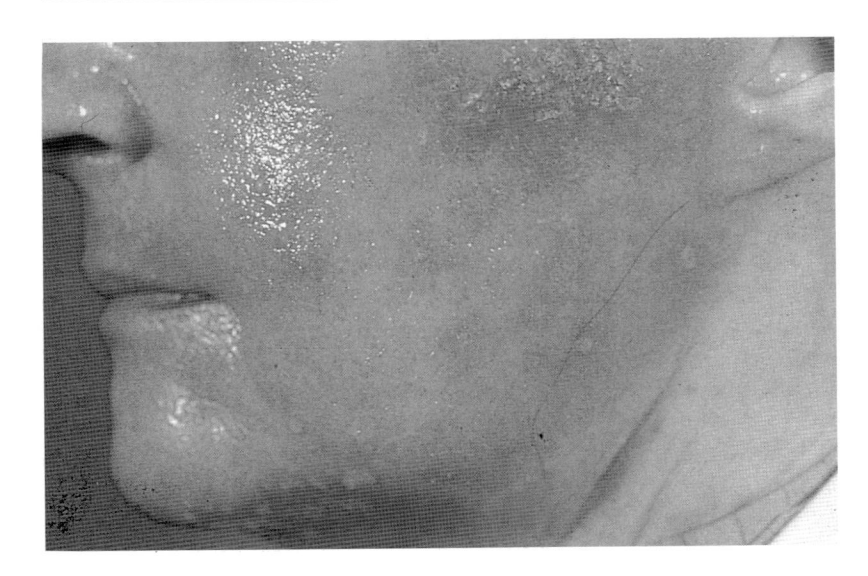

Figure 48.29
This patient who is 5 days post-chemical peel shows reactivation of pre-existing herpes simplex. In secondary cases, adequate wetpacking and occlusive therapy will usually prevent any scar formation. It is wise to prophylactically treat patients with known herpes simplex using Zovirax.

peels with phenol but is usually not seen after superficial or medium-depth peels even after multiple applications of agents such as trichloroacetic acid.[27] This, however, can occur with a single application of phenol in individuals with very thin skin.

Although shortly after chemical peeling the skin appears atrophic, Kligman et al have shown that, histologically, the skin ultimately attains its normal thickness.[30] Kligman also notes that there is a phase of hypertrophy which occurs and can persist for as long as 6 months in the postoperative period.

Changes in Texture

Stegman and Tromovitch state that pores may enlarge during the postpeel period secondary to removal of the stratum corneum but that this change is temporary.[18] The author has not found this to be true and in fact most patients with enlarged pores will experience a diminution in pore size which is a most pleasing secondary effect of deep chemical peeling.[21]

Cardiac Arrhythmia

The most serious complication of phenol peeling is cardiac arrhythmia. Although hepatotoxic and nephrotoxic complications have been proposed, neither of these has ever been reported. Wixler has reported that 70% of the phenol applied to the skin will be absorbed within 30 min.[40] Truppman and Ellenby[41] report that 23% of their patients developed cardiac arrhythmias when more than 50% of the face was treated with phenol in less than 30 min. No arrhythmias occurred when 50% or more of the face was peeled in 60 min or greater. The questionnaire of Litton and Trinidad[32] showed that only 13% of 588 plastic surgeons had encountered cardiac complications. In individuals who were deliberately peeled in less than 30 min the first symptom was usually tachycardia, followed by premature ventricular contractions, bigeminy, paroxysmal atrial tachycardia and ventricular tachycardia.[40] Gross[42] also reported atrial fibrillation.

There is no reliable past history which can assist the surgeon in predicting which patient might develop these complications. Techniques which reduce the likelihood of arrhythmias include preloading with 500 ml lactated Ringer's solution, with the administration of 1000 ml during surgery and an additional 500–1000 ml during the immediate postoperative phase. This will induce a brisk diuresis which decreases the systemic level of phenol. The face should also be peeled in small segments, preferably using one or two cotton stick applicators to avoid overdosage such as that seen with the use of proctology swabs or cotton balls. The author now allows 2 h for the completion of this procedure to avoid the likelihood of phenol toxicity. Cardiac monitoring and regular monitoring of blood pressure and pulse are imperative. The surgeon or accompanying staff should be trained in advanced cardiac support and emergency equipment capable of cardiopulmonary resuscitation should be on hand. McCullough and Langsdon[43] recommend that if arrhythmias occur, the application of phenol should cease until a normal sinus rhythm returns for a minimum of 15 min. Upon resuming the peel, intervals should be extended by an additional 15 min per segment. Stagnone et al have shown that phenol is toxic to the cardiac muscle, producing slow electrical activity and absence of contraction as demonstrated in laboratory rats.[44] They did point out that there was a wide variety of phenol levels when these cardiac effects occurred.

Laryngeal Edema

Klein and Little[45] have reported an interesting and uncommon complication which they attributed to phenol. Stridor, hoarseness and tachypnea resulting from laryngeal edema developed in three patients within 24 h of phenol peeling. These patients were described as heavy smokers. Resolution occurred within 48 h with warm mist therapy. The author has proposed that an antihistamine prior to peeling may be of value.

Toxic Shock Syndrome

Toxic shock syndrome, also a rare condition, has also been reported in three cases.[46,47] This condition has occurred with both occluded and unoccluded techniques, and begins with fever, syncope, hypotension, vomiting or diarrhea occurring 2–3 days after the surgical procedures. A scarlatiniform rash also occurs 2–6 days following the peel. *Staphylococcus aureus* was cultured from the exudate. Other symptoms found with this condition may include myalgia, mucosal hyperemia, and hematologic, hepatorenal or central nervous system symptoms. The treatment consists of beta-lactamase-resistant antibiotics in high levels in combination with large volumes of parenteral fluid to maintain adequate blood pressure.

SIDE-EFFECTS OF PHENOL PEELS

1. Erythema
2. Pruritus
3. Milia
4. Acne vulgaris

All patients should expect erythema, which is a normal part of the postoperative phase. This will persist for an average of 2–3 months but, as mentioned earlier, may remain for 12–24 months in unusual patients. Therapy consists of mild topical steroids such as hydrocortisone cream 2.5%. Pruritus is also a common symptom which can lead to excoriation if measures are not taken. McCullough and Langston[43] recommend the use of aspirin to decrease this mild pain sensation. Hydrocortisone cream is also of value, as are moisturizing creams which are noncomedogenic. Occasionally it is necessary to use short-acting systemic steroids either in oral or injectable form. Milia is very common but occurs less often than following a facial dermabrasion. A mild abrasive substance such as a Buf-Puf can be used at 4–6 weeks to gently open and drain these milia. If this is not effective, Retin-A Cream may be used or incision may be necessary. Mild acne is also a common occurrence, particularly in those individuals with pre-existing acne. This is considerably less common than following dermabrasion, presumably because most patients are older and have outgrown their tendency towards acne. Systemic therapy with antibiotics is usually ineffective with patience being the most common mode of therapy.

Relative Contraindications

Brody has recently compiled a list of relative contraindications with which the author agrees.[27] If the surgeon keeps these conditions in mind during the preoperative evaluations, complications can often be avoided. Most of these conditions have been referred to earlier in this chapter. Patients who are HIV-positive are at a greater risk of secondary infection which would cause delayed healing and chronic inflammatory impairment. Also, the virus will be present in the exudate which occurs during the postoperative recuperative phase. Special care must be taken to avoid contamination of non-infective individuals.

References

1. Baker TJ, Gordon HL, The ablation of rhytides by chemical means: a preliminary report, *J Fla Med Assoc* (1961) **49**:451.

2. Baker TJ, Chemical face peeling and rhytidectomy, *Plast Reconstr Surg* (1962) **29**:199.

3. Baker TJ, Gordon HL, Chemosurgery of the face: some warnings and misconceptions, *J Fla Med Assoc* (1962) **48**:218.

4. Baker TJ, Gordon HL, Chemical face peeling: an adjunct to surgical face lifting, *South Med J* (1963) **56**:412.

5. Baker TJ, Gordon HL, Seckinger DL, A second look at chemical face peeling, *Plast Reconstr Surg* (1966) **37**:487.

6. Baker TJ, Gordon HL, Chemical face peeling and dermabrasion, *Surg Clin North Am* (1971) **51**:387.

7. Baker TJ, Gordon HL, *Surgical rejuvenation of the face* (CV Mosby: St Louis 1986) 38–100.

8. Mackee GM, Karp FL, The treatment of post-acne scars with phenol, *Br J Dermatol* (1952) **64**:456.

9. Burks JW, Marascalo J, Clark HW, Half-face planing of precancerous skin after five years, *Arch Dermatol* (1963) **88**:140.

10. Kligman AM, Early destructive effects of sunlight in human skin, *JAMA* **210**:2377.

11. Ayres S III, Dermal changes following application of chemical cauterants to aging skin, *Arch Dermatol* (1960) **82**:578.

12. Litton C, Chemical face lifting, *Plast Reconstr Surg* (1962) **29**:371.

13. Baker TJ, Gordon HL, Chemical peel with phenol. In: Epstein E, Epstein E Jr, eds, *Skin surgery*, 2nd edn (WB Saunders: Philadelphia 1987) 423–38.

14. Pierce HE, Chemexfoliation. In: Harahap M, ed., *Skin surgery* (Warren H. Green: St Louis 1985) 881–9.

15. McCullough EG, Langsdon PR, *Dermabrasion and chemical peel, a*

guide for facial plastic surgeons (Thieme Medical Publishers: New York 1988) 53–112.
16. Wood-Smith D, Rees TD, Chemabrasion and dermabrasion. In: Rees TD, Wood-Smith D, eds, *Cosmetic facial surgery* (WB Saunders: Philadelphia 1973) 213–31.
17. Brown AM, Kaplan LM, Brown ME, Phenol-induced histological skin changes: hazards, technique and uses, *Br J Plast Surg* (1960) **13**:158.
18. Stegman SJ, Tromovitch TA, *Cosmetic dermatologic surgery* (Year Book Medical Publishers: Chicago 1984) 27–46.
19. Farber GA, Chemical peeling. In: Burks JW, ed., *Dermabrasion and chemical peeling* (Charles C Thomas: Springfield, IL 1979) 209–26.
20. Litton C, Followup study of chemosurgery, *South Med J* (1966) **50**:1007.
21. Alt TH, Occluded Baker–Gordon peel, *J Dermatol Surg Oncol* (1989) **15**:980–93.
22. Baker TJ, Gordon H, Mosienko P et al, Long term histological study of skin after chemical face peeling, *Plast Reconstr Surg* (1974) **53**:522.
23. Stegman SJ, Histologic changes on normal sun-damaged skin produced by various chemical peeling agents, *Aesthetic Plast Surg* (1982) **6**:123.
24. Hinman CC, Maibach H, Winter GD, Effect of air exposure and occlusion on experimental skin wounds, *Nature* (1963) **200**:377.
25. Stough DB, The chemical face peel, *Cutis* (1976) **18**:239.
26. Stough DB, Irwin B, Chemical peel for facial wrinkles, *J Am Fam Prac* (1974) **10**:106.
27. Brody HJ, Complications of chemical peeling, *J Dermatol Surg Oncol* (1989) **15**:1010–19.
28. Fitzpatrick TB, The validity and practicality of sun-reactive skin types I through VI, *Arch Dermatol* (1988) **124**:869–71.
29. Spira M, Gerow FJ, Hardy SB, Complications of chemical face peeling, *Plast Reconstr Surg* (1974) **54**:397–403.
30. Kligman AM, Baker TJ, Gordon HL, Long-term histologic followup of phenol face peels, *Plast Reconstr Surg* (1985) **75**:652–9.
31. Alt TH, Dermabrasion. In: Krause CJ, Mangat DS and Pastauk N, eds, *Aesthetic facial surgery* (J.B. Lippincott Company 1991) 623–40.
32. Litton C, Trinidad G, Complications of chemical face peeling as evaluated by a questionnaire, *Plast Reconstr Surg* (1981) **67**:738–44.
33. Lober CW, Chemexfoliation—indications and cautions, *J Am Acad Dermatol* (1987) **17**:109–12.
34. Litton C et al, A survey of chemical peeling of the face, *Plast Reconstr Surg* (1973) **51**:645–9.
35. Litton C, Observations after chemosurgery of the face, *Plast Reconstr Surg* (1963) **32**:554–6.
36. Litton C, Trinidad G, Chemosurgery of the eyelids. In: Aston SJ, Hornblass A, Meltzer MA et al, eds, *Third International Symposium of Plastic and Reconstructive Surgery* (Williams & Wilkins: Baltimore 1982) 341–5.
37. Wojno T, Tenzel R, Lower eyelid ectropion following chemical face peeling, *Ophthalmic Surg* (1984) **15**:596–7.
38. Rapaport MJ, Kamer F, Exacerbation of facial herpes simplex after phenolic face peels, *J Dermatol Surg Oncol* (1984) **10**:57–8.
39. Collins PS, The chemical peel, *Clin Dermatol* (1987) **5**:57–74.

40. Wixler MR et al, The prevention of cardiac arrhythmias produced in an animal model by the topical application of a phenol preparation in common use for face peeling, *Plast Reconstr Surg* (1984) **73**:595–8.

41. Truppman F, Ellenby J, The major electrocardiographic changes during chemical face peeling, *Plast Reconstr Surg* (1979) **63**:44.

42. Gross D, Cardiac arrhythmia during phenol face peeling, *Plast Reconstr Surg* (1984) **73**:590–4.

43. McCullough EG, Langsdon PR, *Dermabrasion and chemical peel: a guide for facial plastic surgeons* (Thieme Medical Publishers: New York 1988) 43–54.

44. Stagnone GJ, Orgel MG, Stagnon JJ, Cardiovascular effects of topical 50% trichloroacetic acid and Baker's phenol solution, *J Dermatol Surg Oncol* (1987) **13**:999–1002.

45. Klein DR, Little JH, Laryngeal edema as a complication of chemical peel, *Plast Reconstr Surg* (1983) **71**:419–20.

46. Dmytryshyn JR, Chemical face peel complicated by toxic shock syndrome, *Arch Otolaryngol* (1983) **109**:170.

47. LoVerme WE et al, Toxic shock syndrome after chemical face peel, *Plast Reconstr Surg* (1987) **80**:115–18.

Chapter 49

DERMABRASION: REJUVENATION AND SCAR REVISION

Henry H. Roenigk Jr

Dermabrasion is a method of correcting many cutaneous problems from acne scars to removal of tattoos or tumors to the revision of scars.[1] The method has been modified over the past 30 years, from the sandpaper-type equipment to the fast and convenient motor-driven hand engines used today.[2-4] The skill of the operator, judgment in selecting patients, and understanding of the cutaneous lesions are necessary to get good cosmetic results and to avoid serious complications that can result from dermabrasion.

LASERBRASIONS

The CO_2 laser has been used to perform dermabrasion. The CO_2 laser vaporizes tissue without bleeding and possibly with less pain than the standard dermabrasion. The healing time and postoperative care are similar. There is more delineation between normal and laser abrasioned skin (Figures 49.1 and 49.2) because it is more difficult to feather the edges as can be done with standard dermabrasion. These procedures can be combined.

The CO_2 laser has been suggested as ideal treatment of multiple trichoepitheliomas, rhinophyma, epidermal nevi, syringoma, neurofibromas and tattoos. These problems have all been treated satisfactorily with standard dermabrasion. The CO_2 laser is probably the treatment of choice for rhinophyma, and actinic cheilitis.

POSTOPERATIVE CARE AND DRESSING

The new synthetic wound healing dressings have greatly improved the postoperative healing following dermabrasion.[5] The healing time is reduced to 5–7 days with virtually no pain and infrequent infections.

Op-site and Biobrane are new surgical dressings that provide some special benefits. The biggest benefit is that the postoperative burning pain is reduced or completely eliminated. Op-site is a polyurethane material with an adhesive that will stick to stratum corneum but not to wet wounds. When using this, it is necessary to have a nonabraded section of skin around the hairline and in the preauricular area so that the Op-site can stick. On the other hand, Biobrane will stick to moist wounds and can be placed over the completely dermabraded face.

Vigilon is another synthetic dressing that absorbs moisture and reduces the

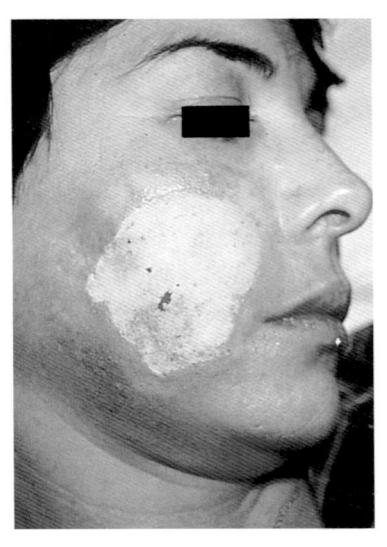

Figure 49.1
Acne scars with white crust immediately after CO_2 laserabrasion.

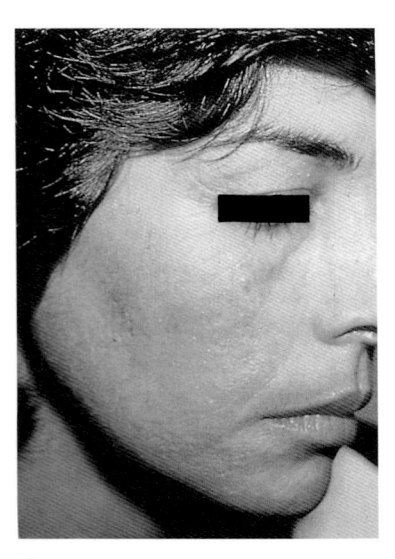

Figure 49.2
Three months later there is still delineation of the laserabrasion area.

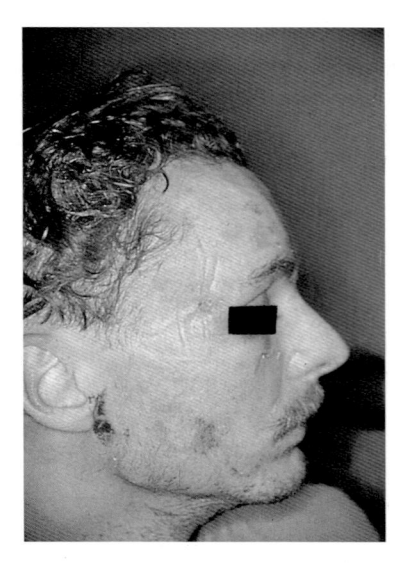

Figure 49.3
Dermabrasion 1 week postoperatively with Vigilon dressing.

postoperative pain. We find that the continuous use of Vigilon allows the skin to re-epithelialize in about 7 days without going through the crusting phase and it is the author's preferred dressing today (Figure 49.3). Prior to application, a polyethylene film is removed from one side of the dressing that will cover the wound. The dressings are changed daily by the patient. Vigilon, unlike other occlusive dressings, permits a moist environment while allowing for absorption of wound exudate. It is also nonadherent.

CURRENT USES OF DERMABRASION

Dermabrasion was developed as a method of treating acne scars. It has been used to treat a variety of problems, including hypertrophic scars, traumatic scars,

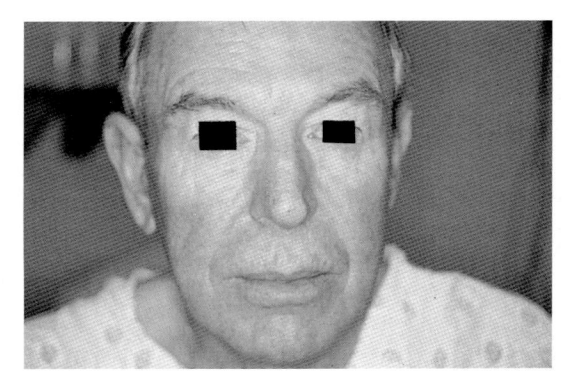

Figure 49.4
Severe actinic damage with multiple actinic keratoses.

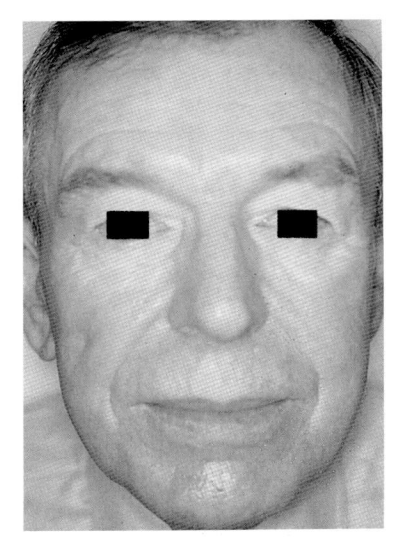

Figure 49.5
Six months after dermabrasion.

actinically damaged and wrinkled skin, and correction of pigmentary abnormalities. Among the cosmetic indications for dermabrasion are: acne scars, fine wrinkling, scar revision, melasma, perioral pseudorhagades, and tattoo removal.[6,7]

There are many other therapeutic reasons for selecting dermabrasion: epidermal nevus, epithelioma adenoides cysticum, rhinophyma, nevus angiomatosus, syrinoma, adenoma sebaceum, keloids, discoid lupus erythematosus, actinic keratosis and solar elastosis (Figure 49.4 and 49.5), seborrheic keratosis, basal cell carcinoma, and Darier's disease. Hanke provided a list of 50 conditions that have been treated with dermabrasion (Table 49.1).

The correction of old and new scars by dermabrasion is very effective. Superficial sharply demarcated scars can often be completely removed while soft saucer-like depressions can be improved but not eliminated. Emphasize to the patient that improvement is expected, but do not promise to eliminate all scars. Dermabrasion will soften sharp edges and improve the crater-like appearance of these scars caused by shadows in the depression. Deep icepick-type scars will require scar revision excision, punch elevation, or punch graft-

ing prior to dermabrasion. Dermabrasion can also be used for cysts or to marsupialize epithelialized sinuses when chronically infected. Scars from excisional surgery or trauma can be dermabraded 6–8 weeks after sutures are removed, to camouflage these wounds by forming a more natural epidermal surface. Older wounds do not respond so well unless they are re-excised, followed by dermabrasion.

SCAR REVISION

The traditional approach for the revision of scars with dermabrasion has been to perform abrasion 6 months or longer after the original surgery or injury with the best aesthetic results being obtained when the scar was older.[8] It was only 12 years ago that earlier intervention was first suggested. In his book, Burks stated that 'pox scars, like other scars, may be dermabraded 6–8 weeks after their appearance.'[3]

Table 49.1
Various entities treated with dermabrasion

Postacne scars	Adenoma sebaceum
Traumatic scars	Neurotic excoriations
Smallpox or chicken pox scars	Multiple trichoepitheliomas
Rhinophyma	Darier's disease
Professionally applied tattoos	Fox–Fordyce
Amateur-type tattoos (India Ink)	Lichenified dermatoses
Blast tattoos (gunpowder)	Porokeratosis of Mibelli
Multiple seborrheic keratoses	Favre–Racouchot syndrome
Multiple pigmented nevi	Lichen amyloidosis
Actinically damaged skin	Verrucous nevus
Age- and sun-related wrinkle lines	Molluscum contagiosum
Active acne	Keratoacanthoma
Freckles	Xanthalasma
Pseudofolliculitis barbae	Hemangioma
Telangiectasia	Leg ulcer
Acne rosacea	Scleromyxedema
Chloasma	Striae distensae
Vitiligo	Early operative scars
Congenital pigmented nevi	Hair transplantation (elevated recipient sites)
Syringocystadenoma papilliferum	Linear epidermal nevus
Nevus flammeus	Syringoma
Keloids	Angiofribromas of tuberous sclerosis
Dermatitis papilaris capilliti	Chronic radiation dermatitis
Lupus erythematosus	Xeroderma pigmentosum
Basal-cell carcinoma (superficial type)	Lentigines

Collins and Farber[9] reported that, in selective cases, diamond fraise dermabrasion effectively enhanced the cosmetic outcome of nasal scars when treated 2–6 weeks after suture removal.

Yarborough[10] found that facial scars, when planed with a wire brush 4–8 weeks after injury, healed without evidence of residual scarring. These were compared to mature scars that were abraded 3 months to 13 years after injury, which were not eradicated.

The correction of scars by dermabrasion is very effective for both old and new scars. The more superficial icepick type of scars can often be completely removed, whereas deeper, more saucer-like scars can be improved but not eliminated. Dermabrasion will remove sharp edges of acne scars and reduce the crater-like appearance of these scars. Occasionally, other procedures should be done to remove deep scars prior to dermabrasion. Fresh scars from excision surgery or traumatic accident repairs can be dermabraded about 6–8 weeks after sutures are removed and greatly enhance the cosmetic appearance of these wounds by forming a more natural epithelial surface over the healing wounds. Older wounds that have a white line are not usually improved much unless there is re-excision with scar revision followed by dermabrasion.

Larger, deep scars that do not respond well to dermabrasion alone should be treated by either:

1. Punch excision of the wound usually with a circular punch and then suture closing of the wound.
2. Punch excision of the depressed scar and elevation of the plug to the flush surface of the surrounding skin. It can be held in place by a Steri-strip dressing.
3. Punch excision with full-thickness graft replacement usually taken from the postauricular area.

Dermabrasion is usually then done about 6 weeks after these procedures have corrected the deeper scars so there is a more uniform smoothing of all the skin surface.

Examples of the results obtained with this technique are as follows:

1. Chicken pox scars—before, during and after punch elevation and dermabrasion (Figures 49.6, 49.7 and 49.8).
2. Dermabrasion of traumatic wounds (Figures 49.9 and 49.10).
3. Dermabrasion of surgical scars (Figures 49.11, 49.12 and 49.13).

Katz[11] has done a controlled study using a split-scar paradigm. Linear scars that were produced by full-thickness surgical excisions on the face, trunk and extremities were chosen randomly for abrasion 4, 6 or 8 weeks postsurgery. The results of spot dermabrasion of the left half of each scar were compared to the untreated right half of each scar. Ratings were performed by physicians, lay persons and the patients themselves after viewing color photographs of the scars taken at various time intervals. One operator performed all of the abrasions. The summary of findings was as follows: (1) dermabrasion significantly improved the appearance of surgical scars; (2) the appearance of the scars was not worsened by dermabrasion; (3) scars improved with dermabrasion at all time intervals, but were significantly improved ($p<0.05$) at 8 weeks postsurgery (50% of the scars disappeared); and (4) the face,

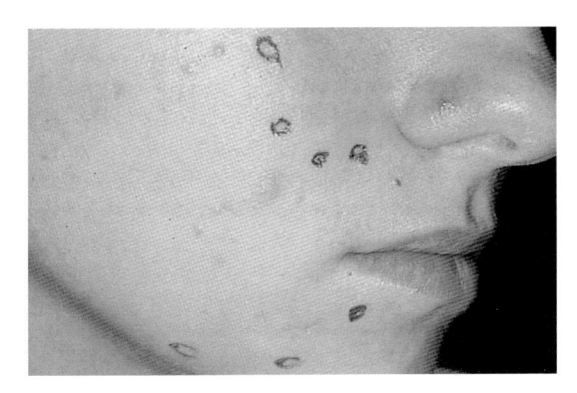

Figure 49.6
Chicken pox scars on face outline with gentian violet.

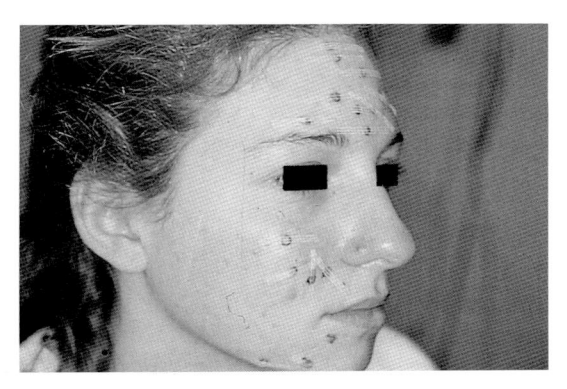

Figure 49.7
Immediately after a combination of punch excision and suturing, punch elevation and punch grafting. Full-face dermabrasion was done 6 weeks later.

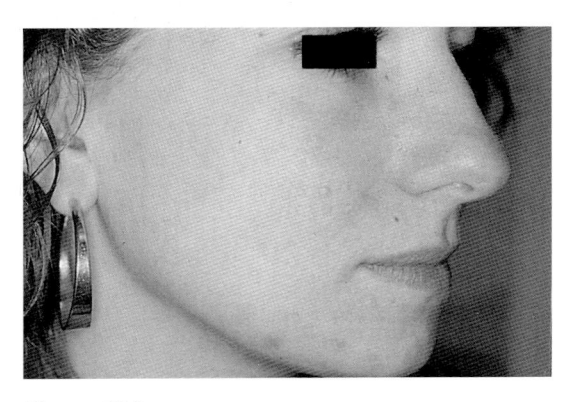

Figure 49.8
Postoperative results at 4 weeks post-dermabrasion for chicken pox scars.

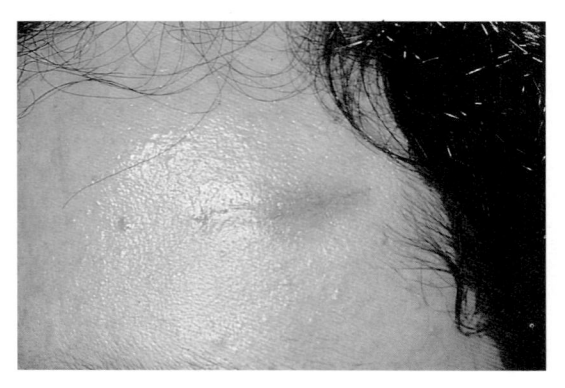

Figure 49.9
Traumatic scar that was sutured and developed a hypertrophic scar.

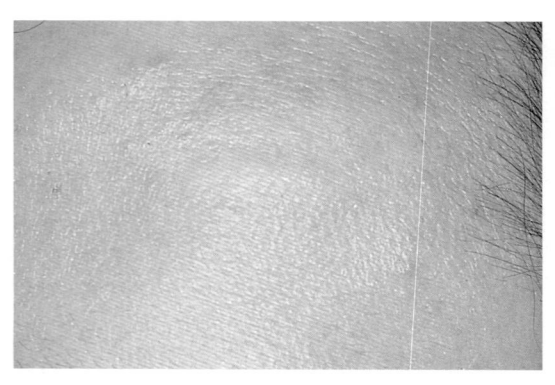

Figure 49.10
Postoperative at 6 weeks, the scar is almost imperceptible.

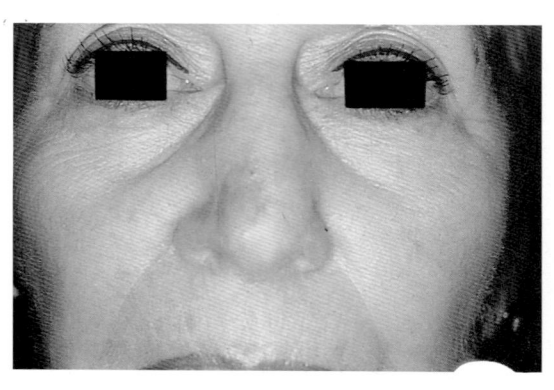

Figure 49.11
Patient with basal cell carcinoma of tip of nose treated by Mohs surgery and full-thickness skin graft 2 months previously.

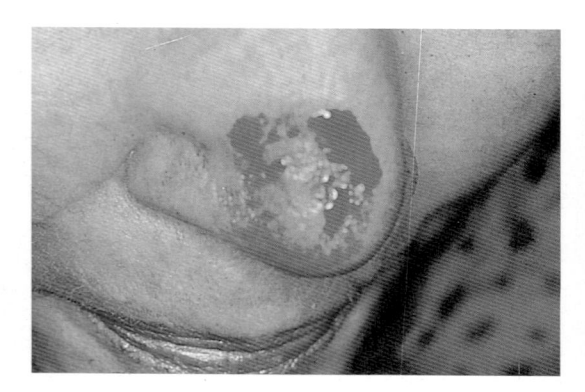

Figure 49.12
Dermabrasion of the graft.

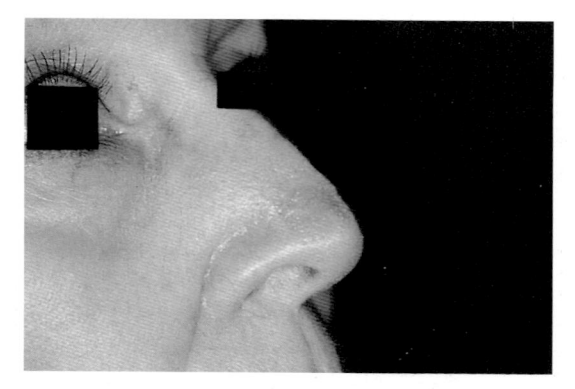

Figure 49.13
Five weeks postdermabrasion with satisfactory cosmetic improvement of the graft.

trunk and extremities showed comparable improvement with dermabrasion. The authors coined the term 'scarabrasion' for this procedure.

PHOTOAGING SKIN

There has been increasing attention paid to methods that can improve skin damaged by prolonged exposure to ultraviolet light. Many topical agents such as Retin-A and alpha-hydroxy acids will cause slow but gradual improvement in actinically damaged skin. Topical 5-fluorouracil has been advocated for patients with extensive

DERMABRASION: REJUVENATION AND SCAR REVISION

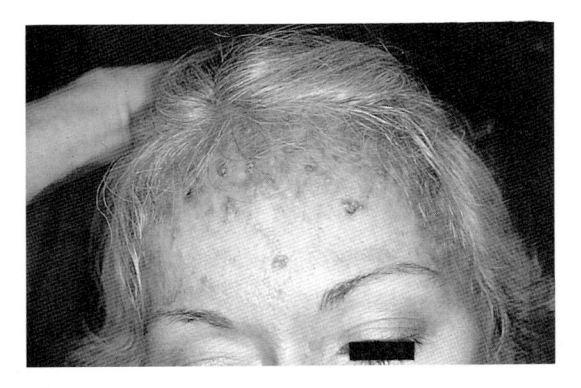

Figure 49.14
Severe actinic damage and multiple actinic keratoses of the forehead.

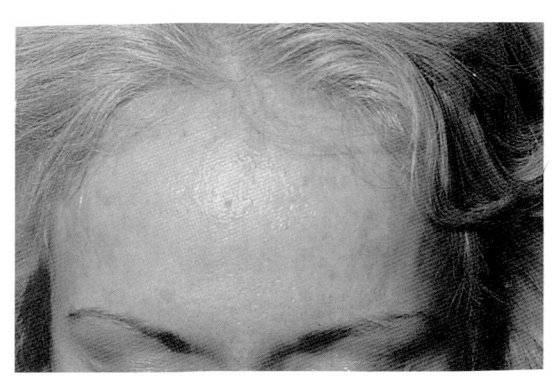

Figure 49.15
Postoperative cosmetic improvement.

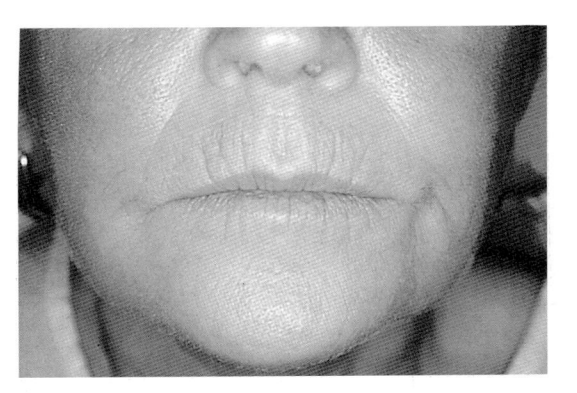

Figure 49.16
Preoperative, deep wrinkles of lips.

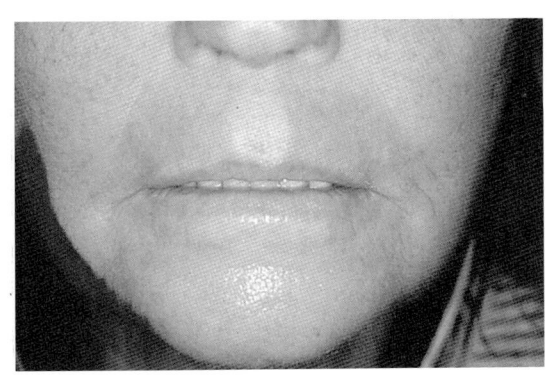

Figure 49.17
Postdermabrasion results at 5 weeks.

actinic keratosis. These agents take a long time to show the improvement and sometimes are very irritating to the skin.

An alternative approach to improving photoaged skin has been the use of chemical peels and dermabrasion. Burks, in his original book on dermabrasion,[3] showed the significant improvement that could be obtained by dermabrasion of one half of the face of actinically damaged skin and observing the changes at 1 year with the nondermabraded skin serving as a control. Dermabrasion done superficially with a diamond fraise is an effective and rapid method of rejuvenating the skin of the face or scalp. The major problem that can occur is that aged skin heals more slowly than young skin and postoperative care may be more difficult and prolonged.

The following are examples of cosmetic improvement of photoaging skin following dermabrasion:

1. Photoaging skin before and after dermabrasion (Figures 49.4 and 49.5).
2. Actinic keratosis of forehead before, during and after dermabrasion (Figures 49.14 and 49.15).
3. Perioral deep wrinkles before and after dermabrasion (Figures 49.16 and 49.17).

515

Problems

Hypertrophic scars or keloids may occur in a small number of patients. A personal or family history of keloid formation is a relative contraindication. Black patients tend to form keloids more frequently. The use of refrigerants, especially on the mandible, may be partially responsible. Atypical keloids develop in locations such as the buccal skin after dermabrasion of patients still on or having recently taken isotretinoin (Accutane). Keloids have also been seen in patients undergoing chemical peel and laser surgery after recent exposure to isotretinoin. Patients now wait 1 year after taking Accutane before the procedure. This has resulted in no atypical keloids in a follow-up study performed by the author. Treatment of these scars with intralesional triamcinolone is helpful. Topical steroids may be used early for suspicious area of hypertrophic scars.

Patients with a history of recurrent cold sores, possibly herpes simplex, should be approached with caution. The surgeon should avoid dermabrasion in the trigger areas of previous herpes simplex. Oral acyclovir (Zovirax), 200 mg five times a day for 3 days before and until the skin has re-epithelialized, can be given prophylactically. If disseminated herpes simplex develops, hospitalization and intravenous acyclovir are indicated.

Hypopigmentation and hyperpigmentation are common but usually temporary. Pigmentary problems are more common in dark-skinned patients (skin types IV–VI). They are most noticeable at the edges of the dermabrasion or in spot dermabrasion. Postinflammatory hyperpigmentation usually fades in several months, and no treatment is necessary. Topical hydroquinone 4% and Retin-A cream 0.05% may cause fading.

Dermabrasion is usually contraindicated in patients with chronic radiodermatitis, pyoderma, herpes simplex, psychosis, severe psychoneurosis, alcoholism, xeroderma pigmentosum, verrucae planae, or burn scars.

References

1. Roenigk HH Jr, Dermabrasion. In: Roenigk RK, Roenigk HH Jr, eds, *Dermatologic surgery principle and practice* (Marcel Dekker: New York 1989) 959–78.
2. Burks JW, *Wire brush surgery* (Charles C Thomas: Springfield, IL 1956).
3. Burks J, *Dermabrasion and chemical peeling in the treatment of certain cosmetic defects and diseases of the skin* (Charles C Thomas: Springfield, IL 1979).
4. Hanke CW, O'Brian JJ, Solow EB, Laboratory evaluation of skin refrigerants used in dermabrasion, *J Dermatol Surg Oncol* (1985) **11**:45–9.
5. Pinski JB, Dressing for dermabrasion: occlusive dressings and wound healing, *Cutis* (1986) **37**:471–6.
6. Roenigk HH Jr, Dermabrasion for miscellaneous cutaneous lesions (exclusive of scarring from acne), *J Dermatol Surg Oncol* (1977) **3**:322–8.
7. Roenigk HH Jr, Dermabrasion: state of the art, *J Dermatol Surg Oncol* (1985) **11**:306–14.
8. Roenigk HH Jr, Scar camouflage using dermabrasion, *Facial Plast Surg* (1984) **1**:249–57.
9. Collins PS, Farber GA, Postsurgical dermabrasion of the nose, *J Dermatol Surg Oncol* (1984) **10**:476–7.
10. Yarborough JM, Ablation of facial scars by programmed dermabrasion, *J Dermatol Surg Oncol* (1988) **14**:292–4.
11. Katz BE, Oca AG, A controlled study of the effectiveness of spot dermabrasion ('scarabrasion') on the appearance of surgical scars, *J Am Acad Dermatol* (1991) **24**:462–6.

Chapter 50

MINIGRAFTS IN HAIR REPLACEMENT

Jean Arouete

Orentreich's technique of hair transplantation was founded on the use of circular punch grafts, but after several years of practice, two drawbacks became obvious. First, the quality of instrumentation available at that time was inadequate. Second, manually obtaining grafts was not a reliable procedure. The grafts were often poor quality, and those that were smaller (2.5 mm) yielded very few viable hairs. For this reason, in the beginning, 4–4.5 mm grafts were performed which provided 10–15 hairs each, centrally in the graft. Consequently, the concept of minigrafting progressed rapidly in an attempt to improve and naturalize the anterior hairline. Presently, minigrafts are also used at the beginning of a procedure for better distribution even in cases of extensive baldness.

DEFINITION OF THE GRAFT

The number of hairs per graft can define the graft. A micrograft contains one to two hairs. A minigraft contains three to eight hairs. However, it should be noted that eight hairs in close proximity provide the undesirable tufted effect. When considering the entire surface of the bald scalp, hairs placed more sparsely will give a less tufted effect that appears more natural.

Another definition of grafts is based on size. Normal grafts are 3–3.5 mm, maxigrafts (not routinely used terminology) are 4–4.5 mm, and minigrafts are those less than 3 mm in diameter. Harvesting grafts less than 2 mm in diameter is difficult, but when one is successful in obtaining one to two hairs, this would be considered a micrograft.

TECHNIQUE OF HARVESTING MINIGRAFTS

'Maxigrafts' cut into four quarters

Minigrafts can be obtained by quartering a 4–4.5 mm graft. The graft is held with curved jeweler's forceps, and is bisected with a scalpel, carefully following the direction of the hair follicles. Both halves are then cut into two other grafts. This is generally performed with a magnification lens (4×). Some authors recommend removing the epidermis from these grafts but, in so doing, the hairs from the graft are cut. Therefore, it is usually best to leave the epidermis intact to facilitate the angling of the hair shaft into the desired direction when it is placed in the recipient site.

Square minigrafts

Minigrafts can also be obtained from narrow strips of occipital hair-bearing scalp. The first step is excising a vertical strip 2–2.5 mm wide from the occipital region. The donor area is immediately sutured. The strip is then fixed at one end with a pin on a block of wood or plastic. The other end is grasped with the forceps and cut at 1.5-, 2.0- or 2.5-mm intervals, depending on the density of the hair on the strip and the number of hairs desired in each minigraft. The cuts must be accurate and parallel to the oblique direction of the hair.

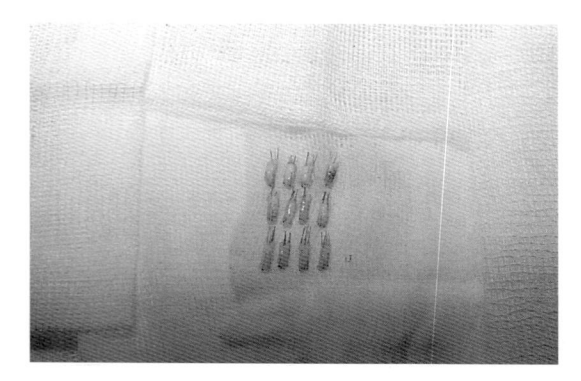

Figure 50.1
Minigrafts harvested with a 2.25-mm punch.

Minigrafts harvested with a punch

The punch graft remains a simple means to harvest minigrafts. As compared to other methods, harvesting with a punch in a simple single motion is easy to perform with some practice. Nevertheless, grafts of less than 2.5 mm in size become more difficult to harvest than larger grafts (3.5–4.0 mm). The procedure, as described by Pinski, to obtain the perfect plug is of utmost importance in harvesting minigrafts.

The punch should be of the best quality with a double bevel, exquisitely sharp, and perfectly polished inside. These are the characteristics of the Australian punch but are also available in other brands. Harvesting should be performed with a power-driven punch and never with a hand-driven punch. The donor site should be infiltrated with a sufficient amount of saline to obtain maximum tissue turgor. Just before cutting, the power punch is positioned close to the skin parallel to the hair shaft. The switch is turned on and the power punch is slowly driven in a linear motion. When cutting small grafts, the risk of transecting hair follicles is great so it is important to have good visibility with as little bleeding as possible. It is important to continually monitor the plugs to see that they are properly angled after each is removed. After the circular cut is made, the grafts are gently grasped with a fine-tooth jeweler's forceps, and the subcutaneous base is cut 1–2 mm deep to the hair follicle. The minigrafts are then placed on moistened gauze in a Petri dish (Figure 50.1).

Micrografts

Micrografts are normally obtained by harvesting conventional grafts and then cutting a portion of the graft longitudinally with a scalpel and fine scissors. Micrografts can also be obtained by teasing hair from the periphery of a good plug which has not had the bulb transected.

Recipient sites for micrografts are made with a needle by making a stab wound. Then dilators (Marritt) are placed in the wound to dilate the hole, making insertion of the micrografts easier. Micrografts are used to refine the anterior hairline.

Preparing the recipient site for minigrafts

There are two ways to prepare the recipient sites from minigrafts based on whether or not tissue is removed from the recipient area. If tissue is not removed from the recipient site, the incisional slit grafting technique is performed. In this technique, all the minigrafts are put into simple incisions made in the scalp. These incisions are made with either a 10 or 15 blade cut to the bone. No recipient tissue is removed. The slit should be perpendicular to the planned hairline. When the slit is made at an acute angle, the 'shingling' effect is obtained with oblique emergence of hair as it grows. The slits are usually separated by 2–4 mm. If the slits are made too close together, it becomes increasingly difficult to place the grafts, as the pressure from the insertion of one graft causes the expulsion of adjacent grafts.

Minigrafts are inserted in the stab wound by grasping its base with a fine pair of nontoothed reverse jeweler's forceps and pushing the graft to the bottom of the slit. It is possible to use the Marritt dilators as well. When the epidermis is not removed from the minigraft, the hair shafts help orient the graft in the proper direction. However, it is not quite as important that all the hair is oriented in the same direction as it is with larger grafts.

Some authors claim that the key principle behind incisional slit grafting is that no tissue is removed from the recipient site prior to transplantation and, although it is difficult to quantify, some authors claim that the yield of growing hairs from grafts placed in incisional slits is greater than that from traditional round grafts. Some authors believe that the difference in yield may be related to a difference in the vascular insult to the subcutaneous tissue.[2]

The recipient site for minigrafts can also be prepared by the removal of a small amount of tissue using a small punch (1.5–2.0 mm). The recipient area can be infiltrated with saline to prevent inadvertent incision of larger vessels. For up to 48 h after grafting, the tissue is nourished by osmotic exchange and the degree of vascularity may play a role in the success of minigrafts. When a 2.5 mm round plug is inserted in a recipient site created with a 2.0 mm punch, the fit is perfect and easier to perform than placing a quarter-graft into a slit. I feel that the fit of the skin to the plug is particularly important. However, when we are dealing with the same number of hairs per graft, whether it be small, round or large and cut into four pieces, the yield should be approximately the same when the procedure is performed by an experienced surgeon. The most important reason for making the recipient hole with the power punch is that the angle of the recipient hole is much more accurate and the graft holds and remains stable with the precise angle of emergence desired by the surgeon.

THE ANGLE OF IMPLANTATION OF MINIGRAFTS

When constructing the anterior hairline, one has two choices: whether the graft provides a transplanted hair hiding its emergence from the skin when styled; or whether it does not. When the emergence is visible (hair at right angles), the result often looks unnatural. To obtain a better result, the hair should hide its emergence from the skin. This can be obtained by grafting the hair at a very acute angle, for example, when repairing a temporal recess (Figure 50.2) or constructing the anterior hairline, the last graft at both ends of the line should be nearly parallel to the neighboring hair. Therefore, from one end to the other, there is not simply one angle for the grafted hairs, but a progressive variation of the angle of emergence from the skin (Figures 50.3 and 50.4).

To understand the variation of the angles of the hair, it is important to think of the scalp three-dimensionally first by looking at the horizontal and then at the sagittal plane. In the horizontal plane, the orientation of the grafts is likened to a divergent fan-shaped configuration. If we look at the horizontal plane of the scalp, the central plug will be directed straight forward. This graft is used as a reference (0°). The graft neighboring the temporal hairline should be placed roughly at 30° so that the entire fan making up the anterior hairline spans a 60° angle. From one graft to the next, the angle of the hair will vary progressively by degree (Figure 50.5).

When looking at the sagittal view, one appreciates the acute angle of the recipient hole. Figure 50.6 helps visualize the different possible angles in which one can direct the hair, either perpendicular, anterior or posterior. Implanting the hair at an acute

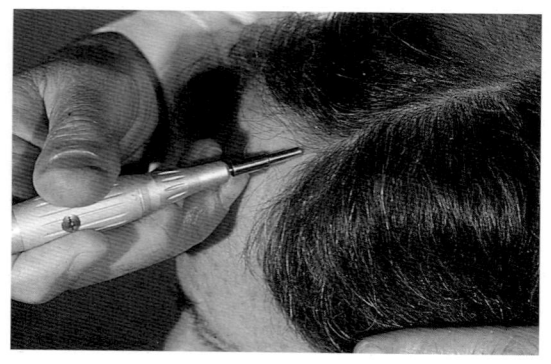

Figure 50.2
The power punch ready for engagement at the junction of the anterior and temporal hairline. Notice the acute angle and that it is parallel to the temporal hairs.

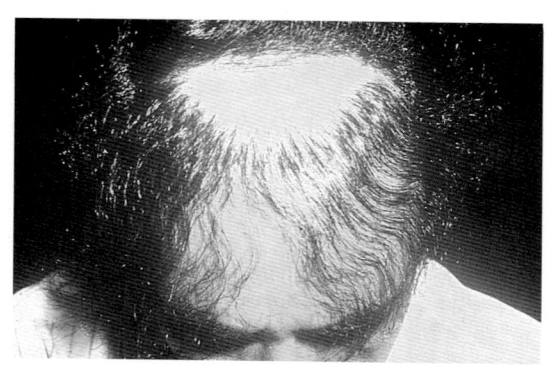

Figure 50.3
A frontal area with minigrafts placed in a 'fan-shaped' configuration. The posterior area will be operated on later.

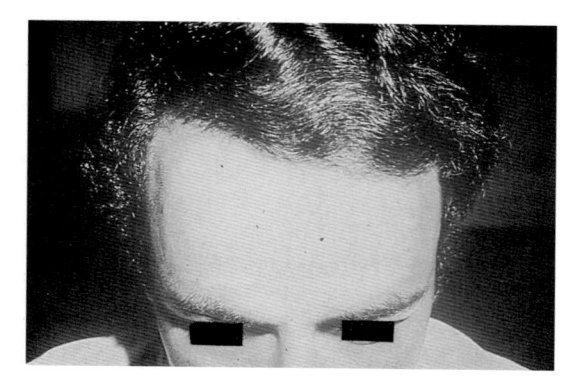

Figure 50.4
Same patient as in Figure 51.3 with the hair styled.

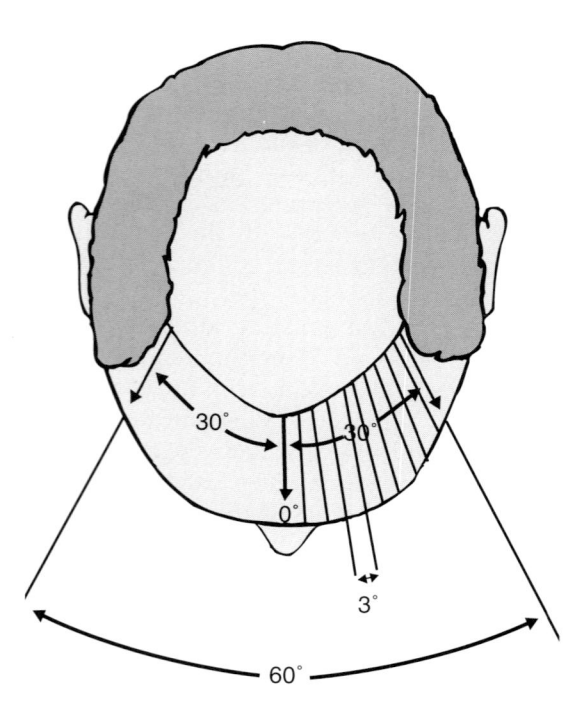

Figure 50.5
Projection in a horizontal plane. Fan-shaped configuration. From one extremity to the opposite, the angle of approach of the power punch should vary degree by degree.

anterior angle can be done in many ways. Often, the recipient hole is tunneled towards the occiput, forcing the hair in an anterior growth direction. This can be done with scissors after the recipient plug has been removed. This is similar to tunneling the stab wound using the incisional technique.[3] Another method is to use the hand-driven punch with a long handle which allows for a change in direction after initial penetration of the punch (Figure 50.7).[4] As soon as the cutting edge has completely penetrated the skin, the axis of the instrument is changed, with point A being fixed and point B brought to point C rotating the punch around point A. The direction of the hand was therefore brought from an initial angle (x) to the shaper angle (y), with the difference denoted by arrow D. After this rotation, the punch is driven to its desired depth.

When the power punch is used, cutting occurs too rapidly to allow for precise change of angle.

When the power punch is used, cutting occurs too rapidly to allow for a precise change of angle. Therefore the power punch should be advanced only in the desired (acute) angle of implantation without changing the angle. The following motion should be performed for each recipient hole to obtain the correct oval-shaped area of cut skin. The power punch is brought to the skin at the desired angle and switched on at low speed. As soon as contact is made between the cutting edge of the power punch and the skin such that a complete circle is cut in the epidermis, slight pressure is applied in the direction of the arrow (Figure 50.8A). This produces an oval-shaped recipient hole by crushing the skin. As soon as the power punch is through the epidermis, the pressure is released and the punch is taken to the desired depth, without changing the axis of linear motion (Figure 50.8B).

We feel that the best way to make the recipient holes is to use the power punch, which allows the angles of the hole to be very accurate. The most acute angle is required at the sideburn area and lateral alopecia after face-lifting. The acute anterior angle technique should be continued back behind the hairline even if this hair is routinely styled posteriorly.

Bleeding

For most well-trained hair transplant surgeons, bleeding is not a problem. Indeed, the scalp is very well vascularized and as soon as the initial incisions are made, the operative field can be flooded with blood. This is reduced by the use of epinephrine with the anesthetic and cold saline for

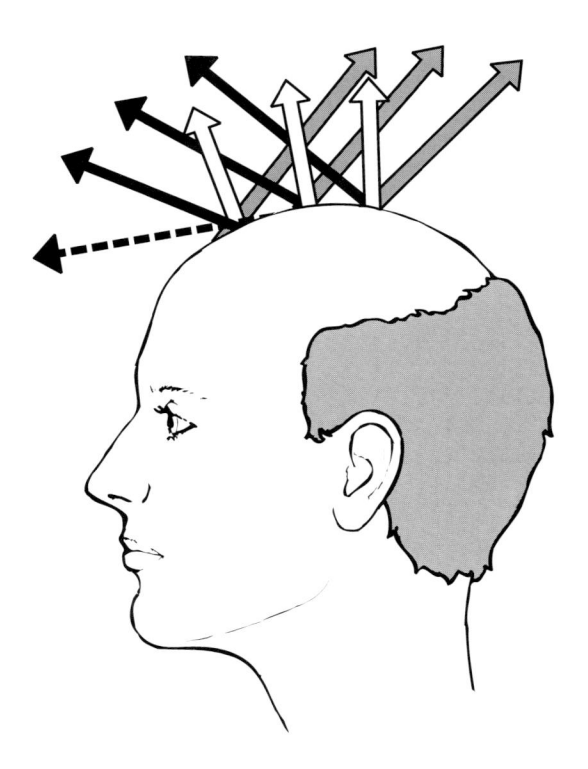

Figure 50.6
Projection in a sagittal plane. ⟹, *backward implantation.* ⇒, *implantation at right angle.* ➡ *forward implantation.* ┄┄▶, *implantation at a very acute angle.*

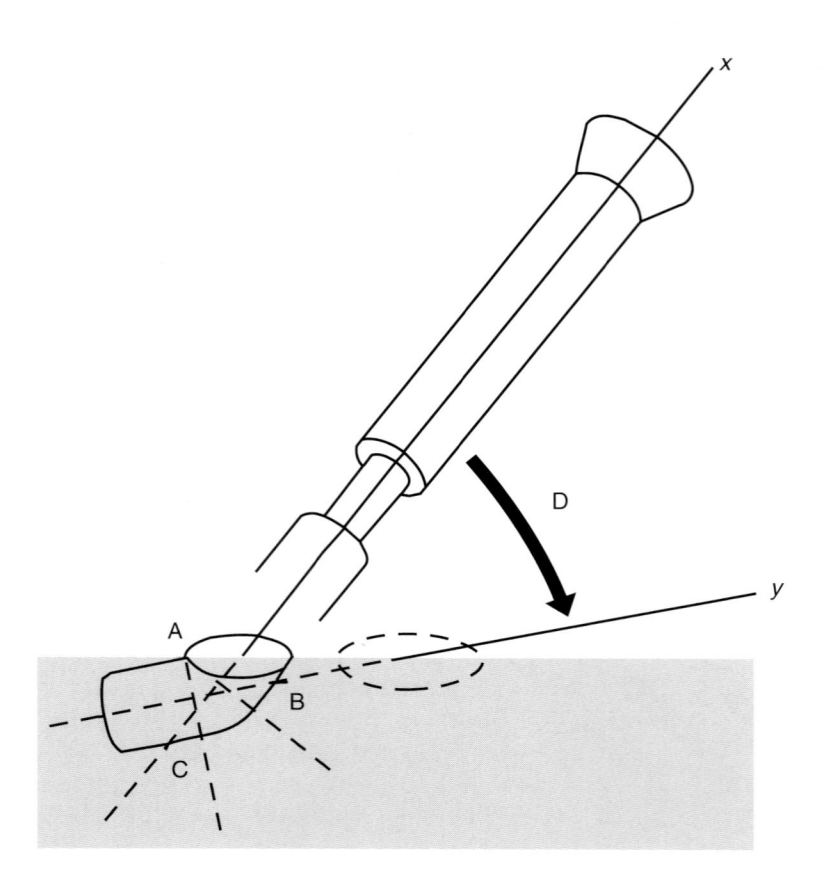

Figure 50.7
How to realize a recipient hole at a very acute angle with a hand-driven punch.

buffer infiltration. It can also be reduced with the use of an Arouete hemostat.[4]

Occipital hemostat

The occipital hemostat (Figure 50.9) is composed of a long rectangular metal frame with a double curvature which, together with the elasticity and flexibility of the metal used, allows it to fit closely onto the scalp. A rectangular opening in the back allows space for the incisions to be made. Its concave side is equipped with an inflatable pneumatic cavity. It is tightly fixed to the head with a strap across the forehead and is screwed in place at two ends of the frame using two articulated ball-and-socket joints. These joints make it possible to obtain homogeneous distribution of pressure. A manometer bulb controls the hemostat inflation. The device is inflated to a level somewhat above arterial pressure. By circumscribing the donor operative field with controlled pneumatic pressure, the occipital hemostat allows the incisions to remain in a bloodless field.

Frontal hemostat

The frontal hemostat (Figure 50.10) is a long flexible metallic band fitted with a pneumatic cavity similar to the occipital

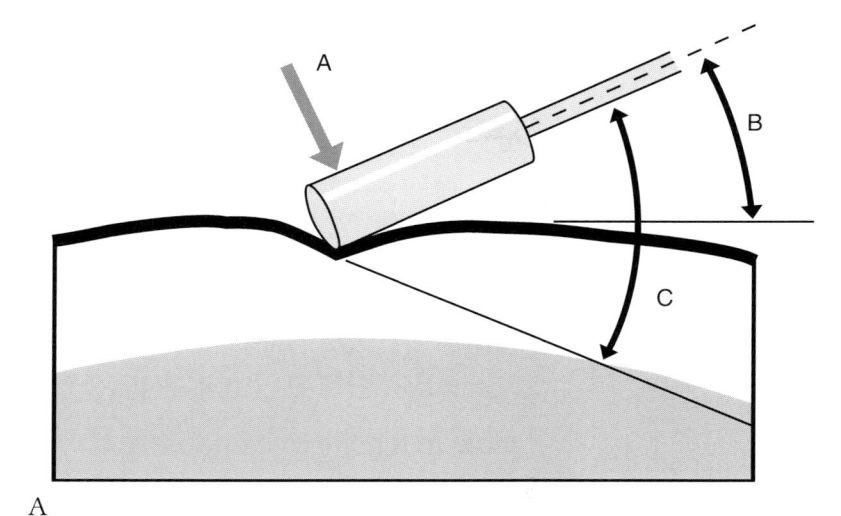

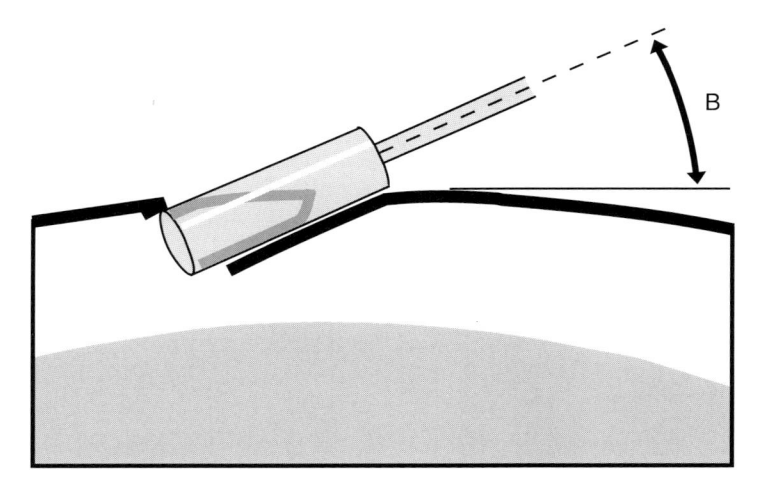

MINIGRAFTS IN HAIR REPLACEMENT

Figure 50.8
(A) The power punch is positioned at the desired acute angle B close to the skin. At the very first touch, the hand holding the power punch and driving it slowly exerts simultaneously a pressure following the arrow A. The pressure is maintained until the cutting edge has penetrated the skin. This pressure modifies the angle of the portion of skin involved with the fixed linear motion of the power punch C. This results in the cutting of a smaller oval shape of skin. (B) As soon as the cutting edge has disappeared into the skin, the pressure is released and the power punch continues its progression following angle B.

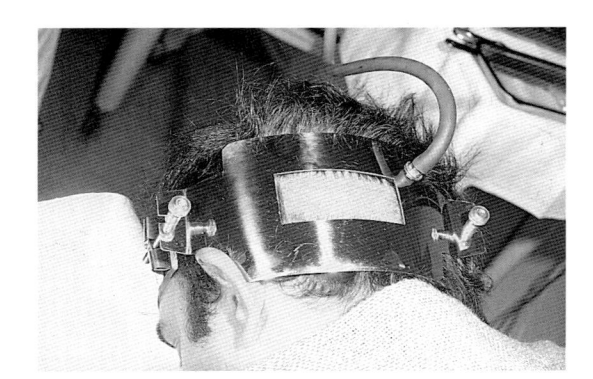

Figure 50.9
Occipital hemostat in position.

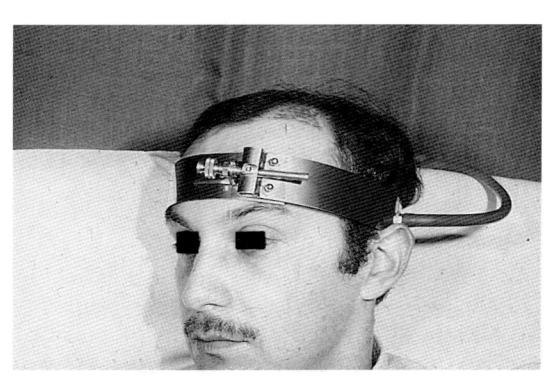

Figure 50.10
Frontal hemostat in position.

523

hemostat. It can be closely fitted to the head and positioned in such a way that it is stable when inflated.

When harvesting the grafts, the patient is positioned on his stomach and the donor field prepared. The hair is cut in a rectangular fashion corresponding to the opening in the occipital hemostat. The assistant holds the frame in a stable position, and the forehead strap is fitted at the end of the frame. After the strap is tightened, the manometer bulb is adjusted and the pressure is set at 20–25 cmHg. With the use of the occipital hemostat, intraoperative problems associated with bleeding are minimized. When the subcutaneous infiltration of saline is performed, the circular block of the occipital hemostat prevents resorption of the saline and therefore this infiltration requires a single step rather than repeated injections. Harvesting of grafts is performed through the window of the occipital hemostat. Depending on the size of the punch used for minigrafts, five to seven rows of plugs can be harvested with 15–20 plugs per row.

When the grafts have been removed, the assistant is asked to reduce the pressure gradually while the donor sites are being carefully observed. It is then possible to determine if there is arterial bleeding which needs suture ligature. By increasing or decreasing the pressure on the tourniquet, it is possible to identify and control arterial bleeding.

Closure of the donor area is controversial. Second intention healing of these wounds has worked well; however, others prefer primary closure to minimize scarring. In 30 years, the author has never closed the donor sites. He harvests the plugs quite close together and never goes back to the same area to harvest a second time.

After the donor site is completed, the patient is turned and the frontal hemostat positioned at the center of the forehead but not onto the arches of the eyebrows. Again, air pressure is applied and saline infiltrated as with the donor area to provide a cushion and avoid transection of deeper structures. When the holes or slits have been created in the recipient area, the frontal hemostat is released and hemostasis obtained with simple manual pressure. Usually, it is not necessary to reinflate the frontal tourniquet but it may be left in place for occasional usage.

STRATEGY OF HAIR REPLACEMENT BY MINIGRAFTS

Slow inconspicuous approach

For many people, surgical correction of baldness is a problem because they want to hide the fact that they have had surgery. To maximally hide the procedure, it is helpful to have the patient's hair styled prior to surgery in such a way that the operated area will be covered. Therefore, when dealing with extensive baldness, the frontal region should be the last area corrected. The first area transplanted should be the apical region in the vertex of the scalp. Hair can be easily combed to cover this site. The patient may be instructed to part his hair a little lower than usual and let it grow long to provide coverage. This is quite common in people who try to cover their baldness and is not unnatural. After the first session, hair that was previously grafted is used to cover the subsequent session of grafts, especially if the hairs have been implanted at an acute anterior angle. These steps are repeated with each subsequent session of transplants. This strategy normally takes at least 2 years to complete. The change in appearance is progressive but less dramatic. The frontal region is finally treated, and the grafts can be completely hidden by lateral and posterior hair (Figures 50.11–50.15).

Rapid strategy

When the patient is in a hurry to have hair replacement achieved and is indiffer-

MINIGRAFTS IN HAIR REPLACEMENT

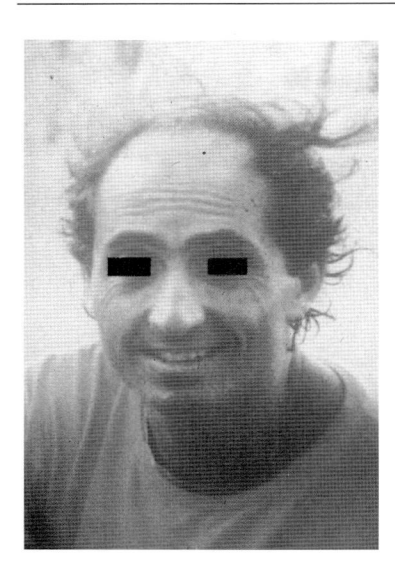

Figure 50.11
A case of extensive baldness.

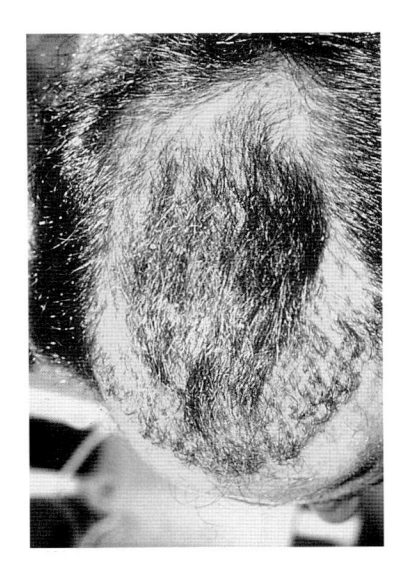

Figure 50.12
Vertex area transplanted first. Notice the angle of implantation. The hair is almost parallel to the skin. The frontal area is operated on after the posterior area.

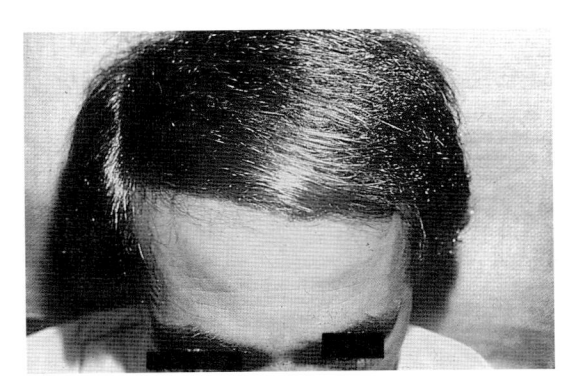

Figure 50.13
The hair is parted lower to hide the procedure.

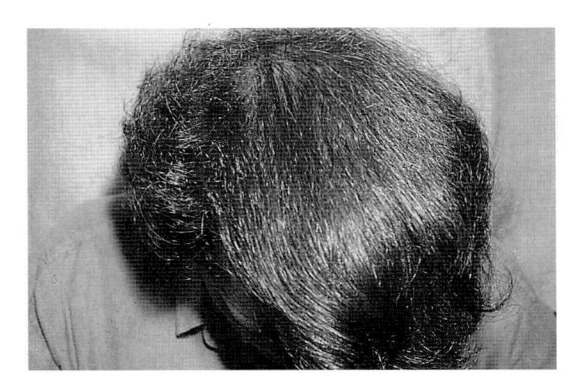

Figure 50.14
Final result with hair combed forward for critical evaluation.

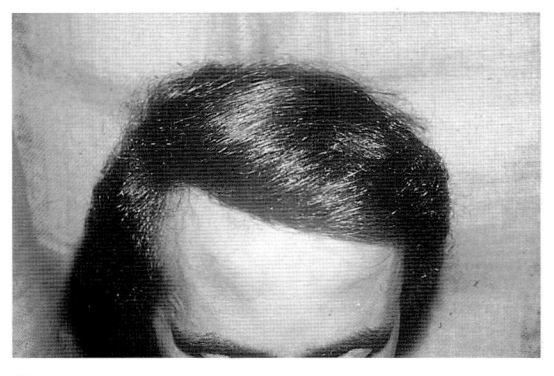

Figure 50.15
Final result with hair styled. Hair grafts are well hidden.

ent to the procedure being conspicuous, or when the patient may wear a wig or toupee, the anterior frontal region can be transplanted first. There are various approaches described in the literature. The first included four steps in a checkerboard pattern filling in the spaces between grafts to get very dense correction. This strategy was initially described for normal grafts but can be used for minigrafts and refined for micrografts as well.

Other approaches have been described. In the three-step approach (Brandy), at each operation normal 4-mm grafts, minigrafts cut from 4.5-mm grafts, and micrografts with one or two hairs are used. This is performed in such a way that the final result is a gradation from one-haired grafts anteriorly to two-haired grafts, minigrafts and then conventional grafts posteriorly. In this way the denser grafts are well hidden and the hair can by styled directly backwards, if desired.

REFERENCES

1. Pinski J, How to obtain the perfect plug, *J Dermatol Surg Oncol* (1984) **10**:953.
2. Nelson BR, Stough DB, Johnson T, Hair transplantation in advanced male pattern alopecia, *J Dermatol Surg Oncol* (1989) **17**:517–73.
3. Norwood OT, Transplanting temporal points, side burns and feminine hair lines, *J Dermatol Surg Oncol* (1984) **12**:959.
4. Arouete J, Special instruments. In: Unger WP, Nordstrom REA, *Hair transplantation,* 2nd edn (Marcel Dekker: New York 1988) 59.

Chapter 51

NEWER TECHNIQUES IN HAIR REPLACEMENT

Pierre Bouhanna

INTRODUCTION

At this present time numerous techniques are available for hair replacement and, together with a better assessment of their reliability and cosmetic effects, it is possible to arrive at clear indications for the correction of male or female baldness.[1] However, a checklist of the pros and cons will always be necessary. Short and long term plans must be individualized to include detailed information from the patient on the possible continuation of his or her alopecia. In this review, for practical reasons, this matter will be considered under four headings: (1) techniques performed in office surgery under local anesthesia; (2) surgery under general anesthesia; (3) marginal techniques; and (4) selection of the most suitable technique.

HAIR SURGERY PERFORMED IN THE OFFICE UNDER LOCAL ANESTHESIA

Local anesthesia combines nerve block anesthesia by injection into the frontal and occipital nerves and infiltration anesthesia using 1% lidocaine with 1% epinephrine of the areas of the scalp on which the operation is to be performed. Frontal and occipital nerve block anesthesia is combined with a 'bracketing' infiltration of the area of the operation.

Long-haired grafts

The technique of long-haired grafts developed by the author[2] makes it possible to transplant grafts of varying shapes and sizes from which the hairs have not been shaved. The advantage of this process is that the area of the operation can be masked immediately. The long hair on the graft will develop in one of two possible ways: either it will fall out during the third week and regrowth will appear three months after the operation; or, all or part if the hair will continue to grow if 2% minoxidil is used during the pre- and postoperative periods. The patient can look presentable enough to resume domestic and professional pursuits 24–48 h later (Figure 51.1).

Three types of long-haired grafts are used: fusiform grafts; micro- and minigrafts; and rectangular or square grafts. The indications for these different autografts are almost the same as for those used in standard practice. This procedure

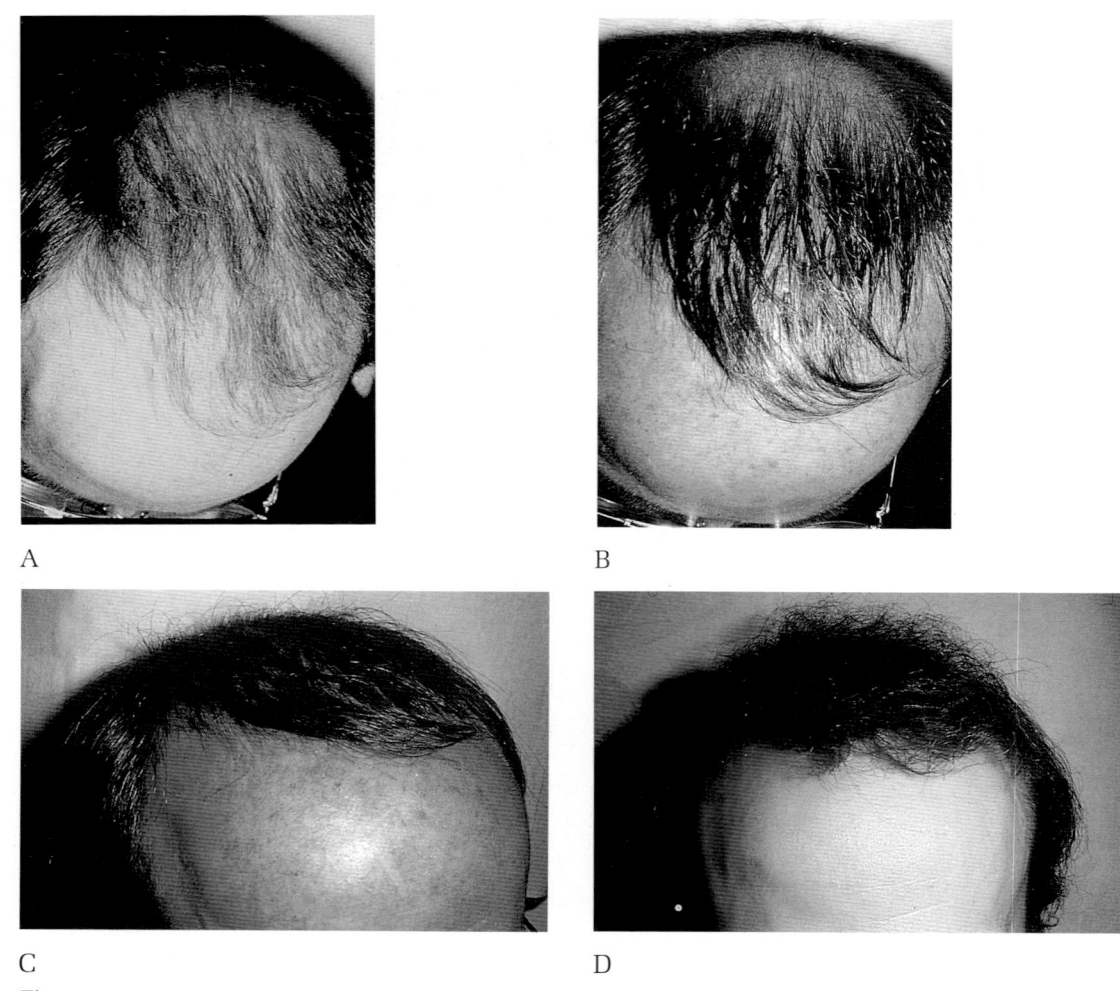

Figure 51.1
Male frontal baldness (A) before; (B) immediately after the first long hair grafting session; (C) immediately after the second session; and (D) 4 months later.

is particularly useful for covering completely hairless areas. In order to make the hair thicker in areas where it is thinning, a shaft length of only 2–3 mm is left.

Removal from the occipital area[2]

Either one or two 10 cm long × 3.5 mm wide strips for fusiform grafts, or, one strip 10–15 cm long and 1–2 cm wide cut into mini- or micrografts are taken according to the shape and size of the grafts required, the density, laxity of the scalp and diameter of the hairs (Figure 51.2A). The grafts are taken horizontally from the lateral occipital areas in males and the median occipital areas in females.[3] The strip is removed using a No. 11 blade, taking care

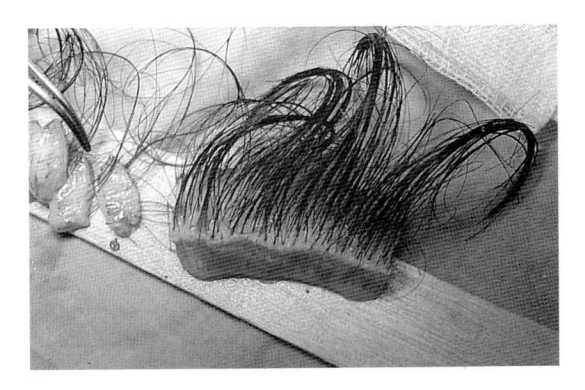

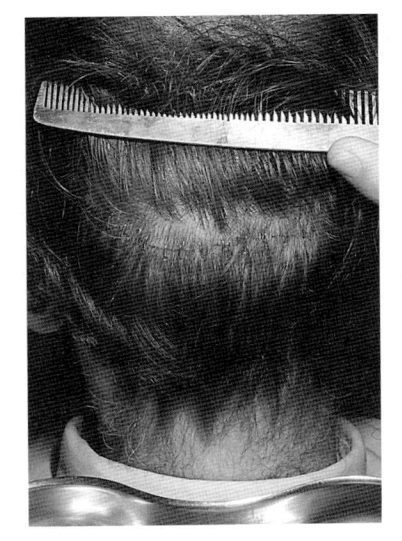

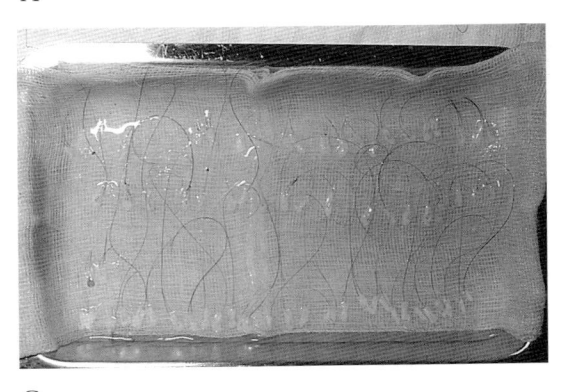

Figure 51.2
(A) Segmentation of a strip into mini or micrografts with long hair. (B) Suture of the strip donor site. (C) Micrografts with long hair placed in saline.

to cut parallel to the bulbs of the hairs. Double or triple bladed knives help provide perfectly parallel incisions. This strip of scalp, excised with scissors down to the subcutaneous layer, is placed in a Petri dish in physiological saline. The excision is closed with staples or sutures (Figure 51.2B).

Cutting the strip of scalp

A distinction is made between: the fusiform strips, which are on average 10 cm long × 3.5 mm wide and may be comprised of 250–300 long hairs; 3 mm square grafts with 7–12 hairs, which are similar in appearance to cylindrical grafts; rectangular grafts, which are 3 mm long × 1.5 mm wide with 5–6 hairs; 1.5 mm square minigrafts with 3–4 hairs; and 1 mm square micrografts with 1–2 hairs. Using a No. 11 blade and cutting parallel to the bulb, the strip, held by the epidermis with forceps on a tongue depressor, is divided into smaller grafts according to the number, size, and shape of grafts required. On average, 300 grafts are cut in this way and each of them is cleared of all fragments of hair shaft or hypodermal debris before being replaced in the dish of physiological saline (Figure 51.2C).

Preparation of the receiving area

The area which is to receive the grafts is marked out with a dermographic pencil, adopting the same criteria as for transplanting standard grafts. The areas chosen

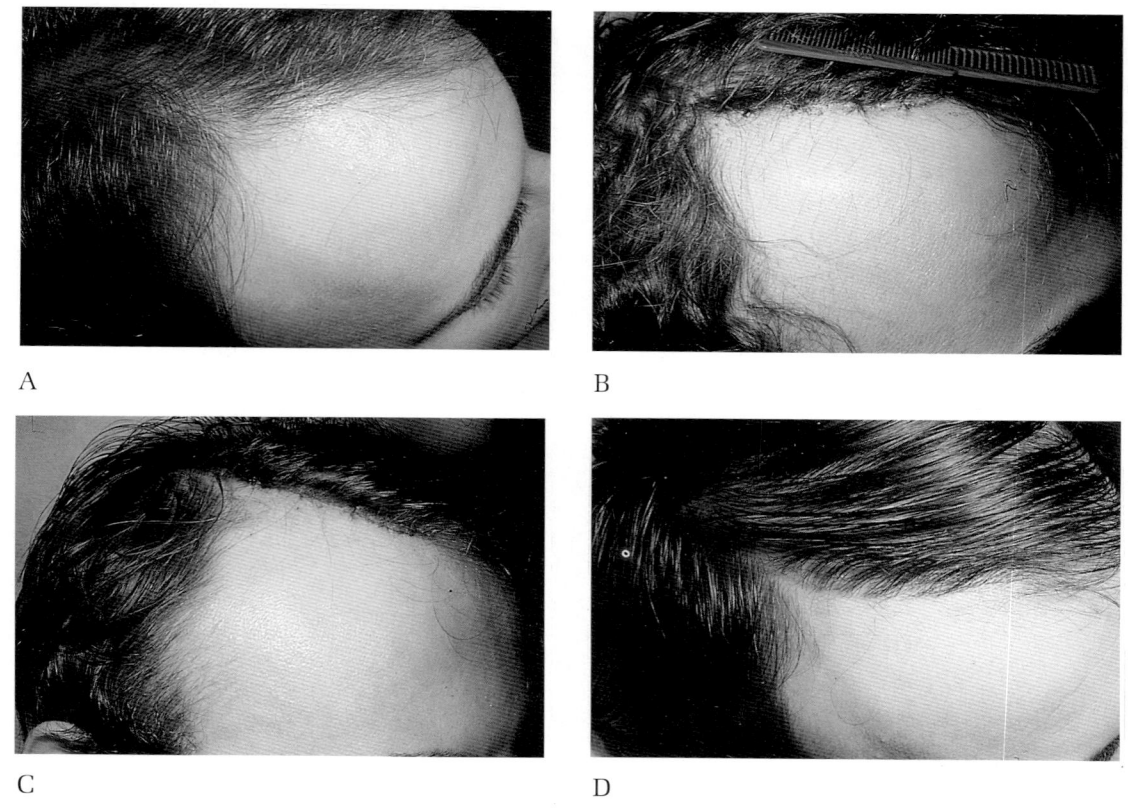

Figure 51.3
Frontal receding hairline (A) before; (B) immediately after the insertion and suture of a fusiform strip with long hairs; (C) 6 days after; and (D) 4 months after.

for each type of graft must be determined and marked accurately. Only fusiform strips must be transplanted separately. Other types of grafts may be combined in one session. Preparation of the grafting site is governed by the size and shape of the grafts.

Fusiform strips with long hairs[2] are inserted between the lips of an incision of the same length. Few, if any, incisions of the glabrous area are needed. Perfect hemostasis of the lips and the bottom of the incision is essential. The graft is held in place by an overcast stitch using a single 5-0 suture going over the graft (Figure 51.3). The long hairs, pointing forwards, enable the frontal hairline to be reconstructed immediately. A strip can be positioned on each fronto–temporal recession during one session.

For all other grafts, preparation of the receiving site is fairly specific (Figure 51.4A,B).[3] First, the surgeon must drill along a 45°–60° axis, using an Orentreich-type hand-operated punch. The diameter depends on the size of the graft to be inserted. The minimum space between holes must be equal to the diameter of the receptor site (ie a 1 mm diameter punch for micrografts; a 1.5 mm diameter punch for minigrafts; a 2 mm diameter punch for rectangular grafts; and a 2.5–3 mm diameter punch for square grafts). Before inserting the grafts into the recipient sites, insert, from front to back, the small, curved point of a Swann Norton stitch cutter. This is a small, cutting hook with which a small incision can be made at the top rear of the hole and the subjacent dermo-hypodermal structures can be notched. This simple step provides each graft with a site suited to its size and prevents it from being extruded when grafts are inserted in the neighboring holes.

Before implantation, a careful check must be made to ensure that no fragments of skin are left in the holes. Each long-haired graft is picked up with jeweler's forceps and inserted into each hole. Micrografts are arranged in two rows along the anterior frontal line (Figure 51.4C,D). Further back, a choice is made between the three other kinds of grafts (minigrafts, rectangular or square grafts) according to the type (fine or coarse), color (light or dark), and shape (straight or curly) of the hair. In one session alone up to 300 grafts can be transplanted. To reconstruct an anterior frontal line, the use of micrografts along the anterior line,[4,5] followed by minigrafts and larger grafts along the rows further back is recommended (Figure 51.4E).

Pre- and postoperative care

The grafted area is compressed manually with gauze soaked in hydrogen peroxide. No dressing is usually necessary. Three hours of observation and rest are required. An antiseptic shampoo is used 1–2 days later.

The fusiform strip technique may require a dressing for 24 h. In order to remove this dressing easily the following day, a paper covering with perforations to release drainage directly on the graft is applied. The donor site is covered with compresses and a pressure bandage. Whichever procedure is chosen, the sutures and staples are removed on the tenth day.

Development

Every graft, regardless of its shape or size, follows the same healing pattern as cylindrical grafts. The scabs which form drop off between the second and third week.

Mini- and micrografts are extremely reliable, a point that must be emphasized. A complication which is less frequently seen with long-haired mini- and micrografts is secondary cysts due to the inadvertent insertion of skin fragments. This complication, which is unusual with cylindrical grafts, has become more common with the use of short-haired mini- and micrografts.[3] The long-haired grafting procedure provides the patient with natural-looking hair immediately after the transplantation session (Figure 51.5).

To enable all or part of the transplanted hair to continue to grow, the patient must apply a lotion based on 2% minoxidil to the receiving area six weeks prior to the treatment. This topical treatment must be continued on the untreated areas for three months after the operation.

Other advantages

For the long-haired graft technique motor-operated punches are not used to take the grafts, thus the difficulties inherent in their maintenance are eliminated. Because of the different shapes and sizes of the grafts, a choice suited to individual cosmetic requirements can be made. The linear scar in the donor area is readily concealed by hair (Figure 51.1B,C, 51.3B and 51.5C). The number of grafts being equal, the operation takes a much shorter time than when a motor-operated punch is used. On the other hand, this type of operation warrants additional help from one or two assistants. If all or part of the long hair

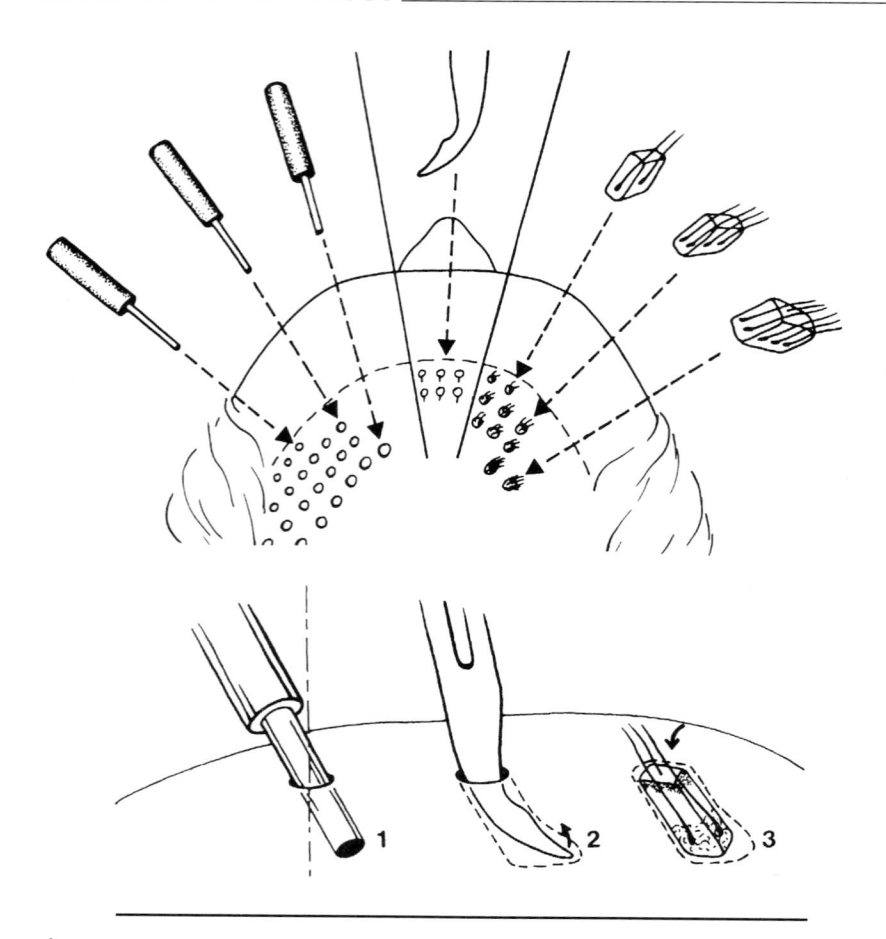

SURGICAL DERMATOLOGY

A

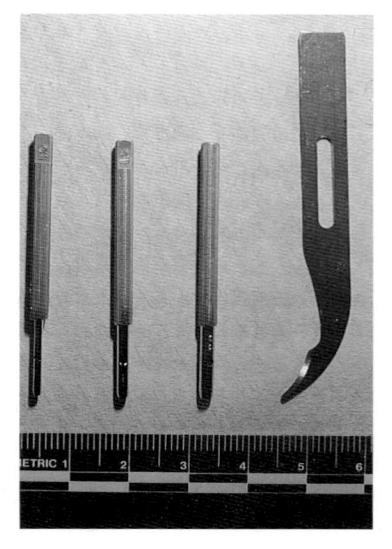

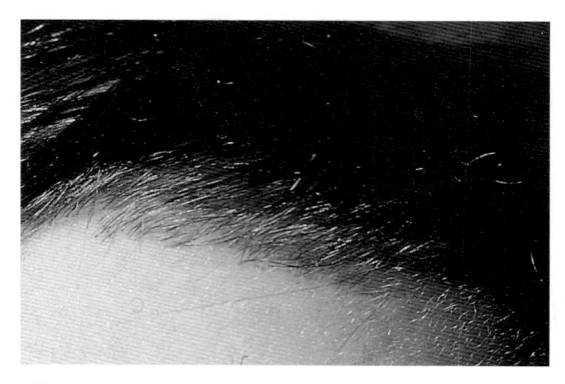

B   C

532

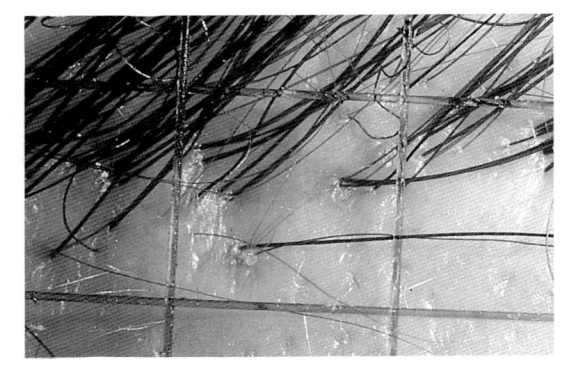

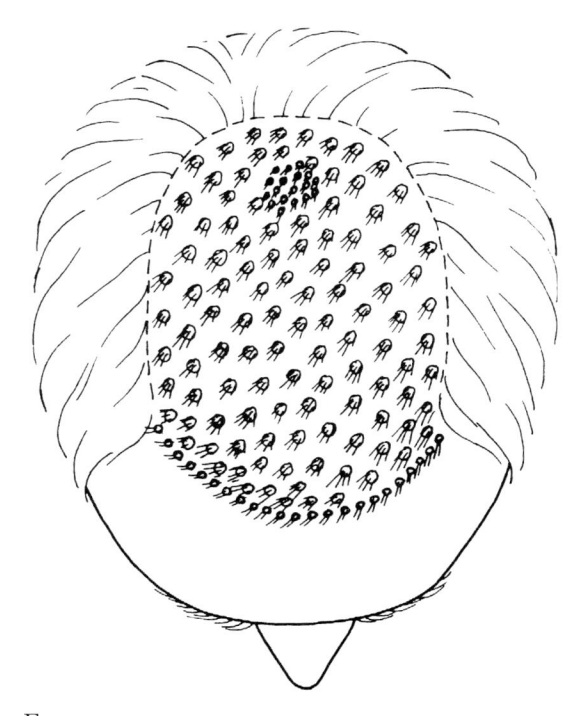

grafts undergo effluvium, the patient would nonetheless have had the benefit of temporary concealment of the operation during that time.

The procedure for preparing the site to take mini- and micrografts has five basic advantages (Figure 51.2D): (1) it is easier to insert the mini- or micrograft; (2) the deep site distends easily and does not cause the transplant to be expelled; (3) the superficial incision allows the initial circle to change shape and thus adjust to the graft's geometrical shape; (4) drilling with a punch has made it possible to excise many small glabrous areas and thus reduce the bald area; (5) it is possible to avoid the use of dilators.

Minoxidil's effect on hair transplants[6]

Ordinarily 2–4 weeks after a hair transplant, the scabs on the grafts fall off taking the bulbs of the transplanted hairs with them. It has been demonstrated that this is a dystrophic anagen process and not telogen in type as stated in the literature. Even though temporary and followed by regrowth three months later, this hair loss is nonetheless cosmetically embarrassing.

It has also been proved that application of a lotion based on 2% minoxidil before and after transplanting autografts enabled part or all of the hair to continue growth in more than two-thirds of grafts, and resulted in a loss of less than half the transplanted hairs from less than one-third of the grafts. It seems, therefore, that pre- and postoperative application of minoxidil allows the anagen phase of a large number of transplanted hairs to continue. This effect of minoxidil led to the development of the long-haired graft procedure.

Vertical flaps

Since the early part of the century (Tilman's flaps), many kinds of flaps have been suggested for the treatment of male baldness.[7–9]

Figure 51.4
(A) The 3 steps on the recipient area: (1) holes made with small hand punch (1 or 2 mm); (2) incision in the hole with a stitch cutter blade; (3) insertion of the grafts with long hairs. (B) The instruments used are small hand punch and a stitch cutter. (C,D) Frontal hairline with micro and minigrafts. (E) Micro- and minigrafts arranged on a wide male baldness.

A   B   C

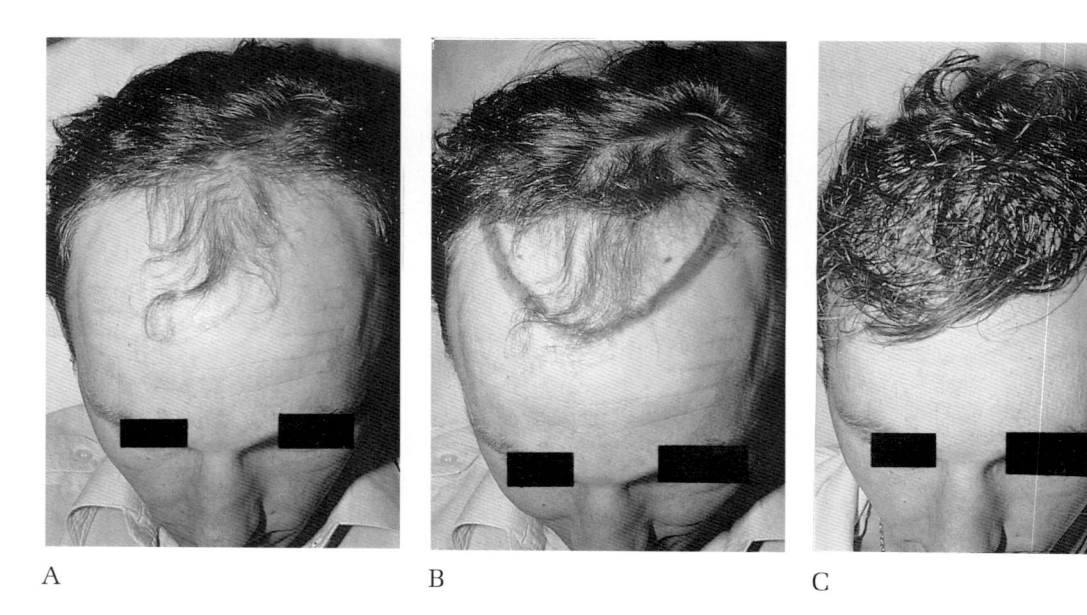

Figure 51.5
(A) Frontal baldness before transplantation. (B) The area is marked out. (C) Immediately after 180 minigrafts with long hairs.

The impractical design of some flaps (Juri-type flaps taken horizontally from the crown),[10,11] and the unfortunate results and injudicious indications of other flaps which are nonetheless regarded as being entirely practical (flaps taken vertically from the crown) long caused this procedure to be rejected. Since the vertical flap was described,[11,12] its design and applications have been diversified and its reliability and cosmetic utility analyzed statistically. It use has now been fully mastered and its indications are more clearly defined.[13] Indeed, more often than not, this technique has come to be used as a first-line treatment. It may usefully be combined with scalp reductions and minigrafts transplants.

Operating technique common to all flaps

The transposition technique itself must be very precise, though simple and unconstricting. Performing a vertical flap is fairly specific, regardless of its size and design.[13] All of these operations have been performed under local anesthesia with 1% lidocaine with 1% epinephrine diluted 50:50 with physiological saline after standard premedication.[11]

The outlines of the flap on the donor area and the receiving area (Figure 51.6) are incised with a No. 11 blade down to the epicranial aponeurosis, taking care to remain in the axis of the bulbs. The flap is lifted after detachment in the subaponeurotic space. After an undermining of the fronto–temporo–parieto–occipital areas under the epicranial aponeurosis, the edges of the donor area are closed together without strain or depth, using skin staples. If there is strain, incisions into the epicranial aponeurosis are used, but cautiously.

After excision of the recipient area, which should be slightly smaller than the flap, the latter is transposed and sutured with staples on its posterior edge and an

NEWER TECHNIQUES IN HAIR REPLACEMENT

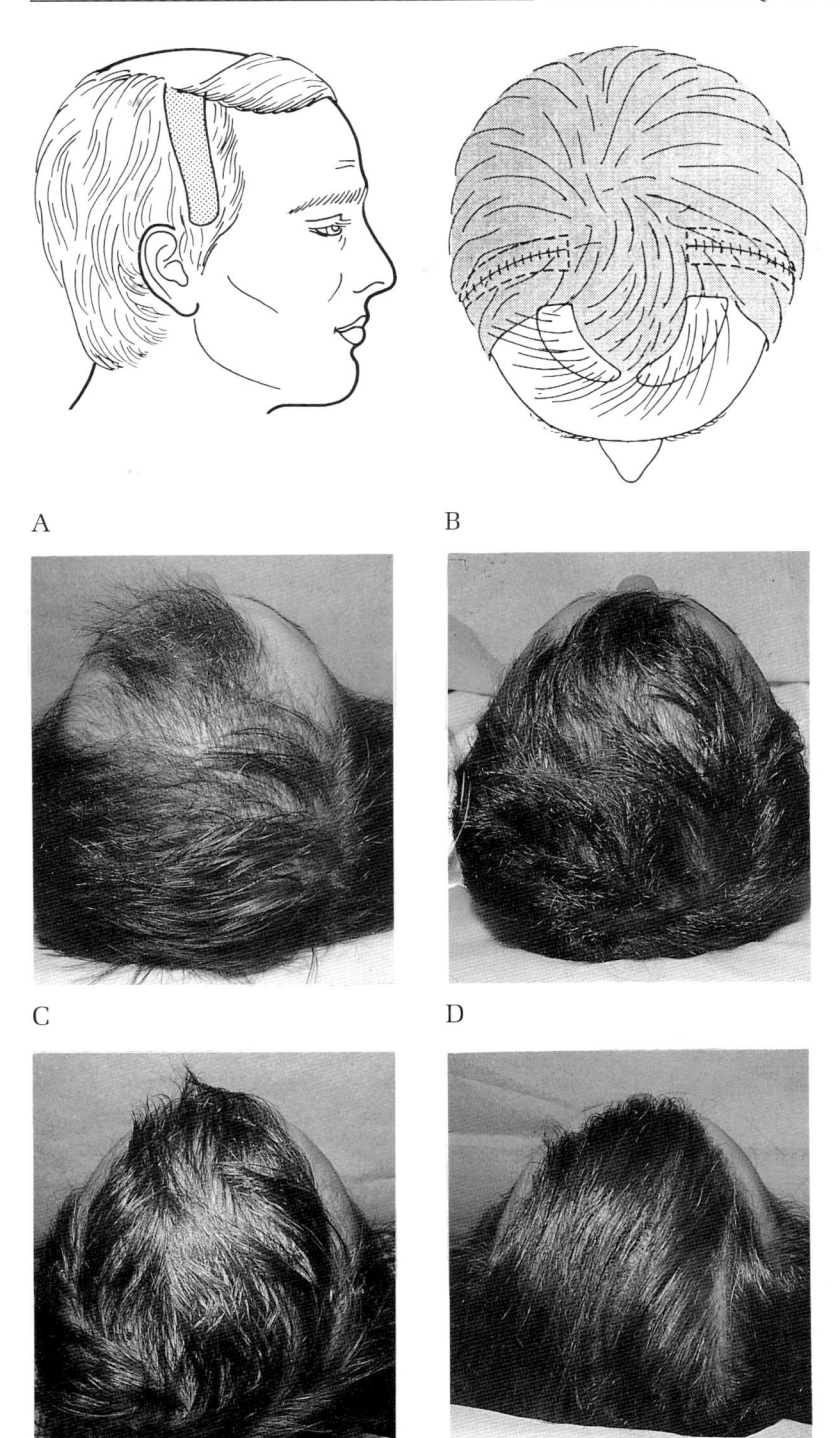

Figure 51.6
(A) Outline of a temporo-frontal vertical flap and (B) of temporo-frontal vertical flaps transposed in one session. (C) Frontal baldness before and (D) immediately after transposition of two flaps in one session. (E) Six days after and (F) 10 months after.

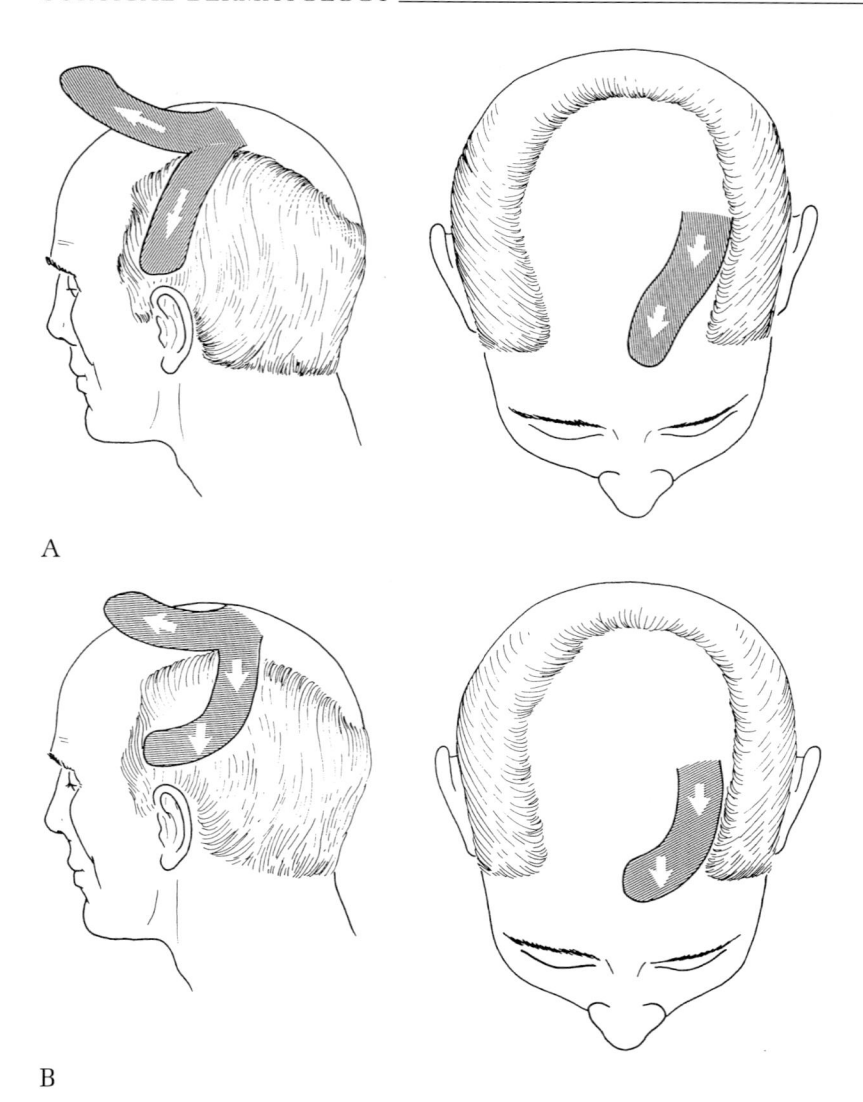

Figure 51.7 A,B
Different designs of the vertical flaps with superior pedicle: (A) Small temporo-frontal vertical flap convex at the front (Nataf), (B) concave at the front (Dardour)

intradermal overcast stitch using a single, non-resorbable 5-0 suture. A drain inserted through the 'dog-ear' space, formed when the flap is turned, is left in position for 24–48 h. An antiseptic shampoo is applied two days later. Sutures and staples are removed from the flap on the seventh day and from the donor area on the 15th day. Prior separation of the flap is unusual but may be necessary in patients whose vascularization is precarious or when the flap is more than 15–16 cm long.

Different designs of vertical flaps with superior pedicle

1. Small, temporo–frontal vertical flap
   Shape: Convex at the front (Nataf[13]) (Figure 51.7A)

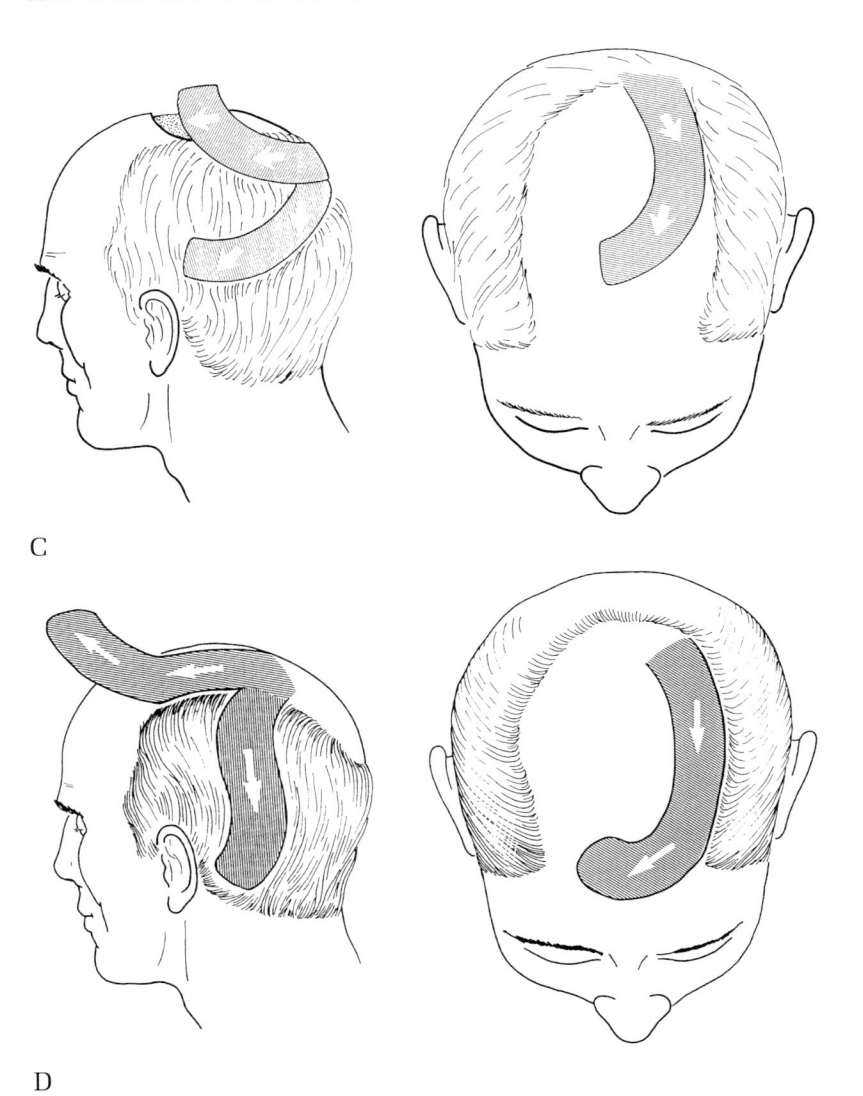

Figure 51.7 C,D
(C) small occipital flap (Bouhanna); (D) large retro-auricular flap (Nataf).

Rectilinear (Bouhanna[14]) (Figure 51.6A)
Concave at the front (Dardour[15]) (Figure 51.7B)
Size: 10–15 cm long × 3 cm wide.

2. Small, occipital vertical flap
   Shape: Concave at the front (Bouhanna[14]) (Figure 51.7C)
   Concave at the rear (Nataf[11])
   Size: 10–15 cm long × 3 cm wide.

3. Large, retro-auricular vertical flap[16,17] (Figure 51.7D)
   Sigmoid, taken vertically from the crown in the retro-auricular area (Nataf).
   Size: 18–22 cm long × 3.5–4 cm wide
   Special features: because of its size, this flap is delayed 1–3 months before transposition.

Complications

It is essential to monitor the flap (at 6 h, 24 h and even 48 h) to remove the drain and to evacuate any subjacent hematoma. The reliability of these flaps has improved in recent years.[14] Necrosis of the tip of the flap occurs in less than 3% of cases. Unfavorable factors such as thin, poorly vascularized skin, poor circulation, and smoking contribute to the risk of necrosis.

It must be reiterated that pre- and postoperative minoxidil[18] is useful in improving flap viability. It has, on rare occasions, been necessary to perform prior delay of flaps less than 15 cm long. It is relatively easy to correct necrosis of the tip of a flap by transplanting minigrafts (Figure 51.8).

The scar along the anterior frontal hairline[14] is invisible in almost all cases when four basic rules are observed (Figure 51.9A): (1) the epidermis is removed and the flap 'buried';[19] (2) fine intraepidermal superficial sutures are used; (3) there is no tension on the wound edges; and (4) there is no exposure to sunlight for three months. In 2% of cases, some noticeable scarring is hidden using micrografts (Figure 51.9).

An unsatisfactory scar due to tension in the donor area[14] is present in less than 10% of cases. This percentage is reduced by further slackening the donor area by making incisions in the epicranial aponeurosis or by sliding in an adjacent rotation flap. At worst, simple transplantation of 10–12 grafts can cover any residual scar.

Temporary hair loss[14] may occur 2–6 weeks after the operation in the donor area, or the area around the tip of the flap in 5% of cases. This alopecia is due to a dystrophic change in the hairs in anagen, similar to grafts. This loss seems to be related to tension on the incision. Spontaneous regrowth appears three months later; earlier if 2% minoxidil lotion has been applied. 'Dog-earing'[14] is present in 50% of cases, but disappears spontaneously in 2–4 weeks. Excision is necessary in less than 1% of cases.

Advantages of the vertical flap[13,14]

The anterior frontal line is of good quality, with a natural outline and normal growth of the emergent hair. The quick cosmetic result allows work to be resumed in 1–2 days (Figure 51.6C,D,E). Remaining bald patches are masked and can be covered later by transplanting minigrafts.

The simple reduction technique

Reduction consists of excising a hairless area of varying size and bringing the hairy areas of the crown as close together as possible.[20] This procedure has the advantage of being simple, quick and safe.

Theoretically, it is sensible to try to reduce the glabrous areas but, in practice, this procedure displaces hairy areas destined to become hairless in the future. Closure of the edges under tension causes redistension of the hairless area (the stretching effect).

It is evident that reduction performed at the limits of the hairless and hairy areas reduces this stretching effect by

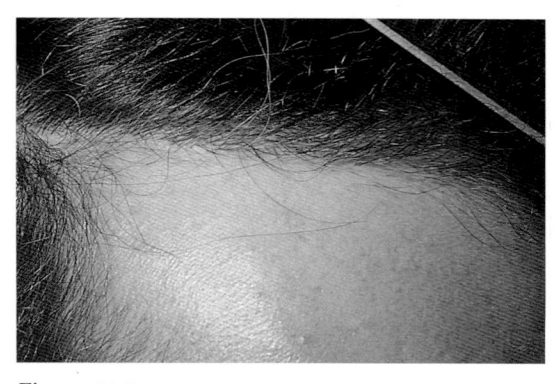

Figure 51.8
Correction of the tip necrosis of a vertical flap by transplantation of minigrafts.

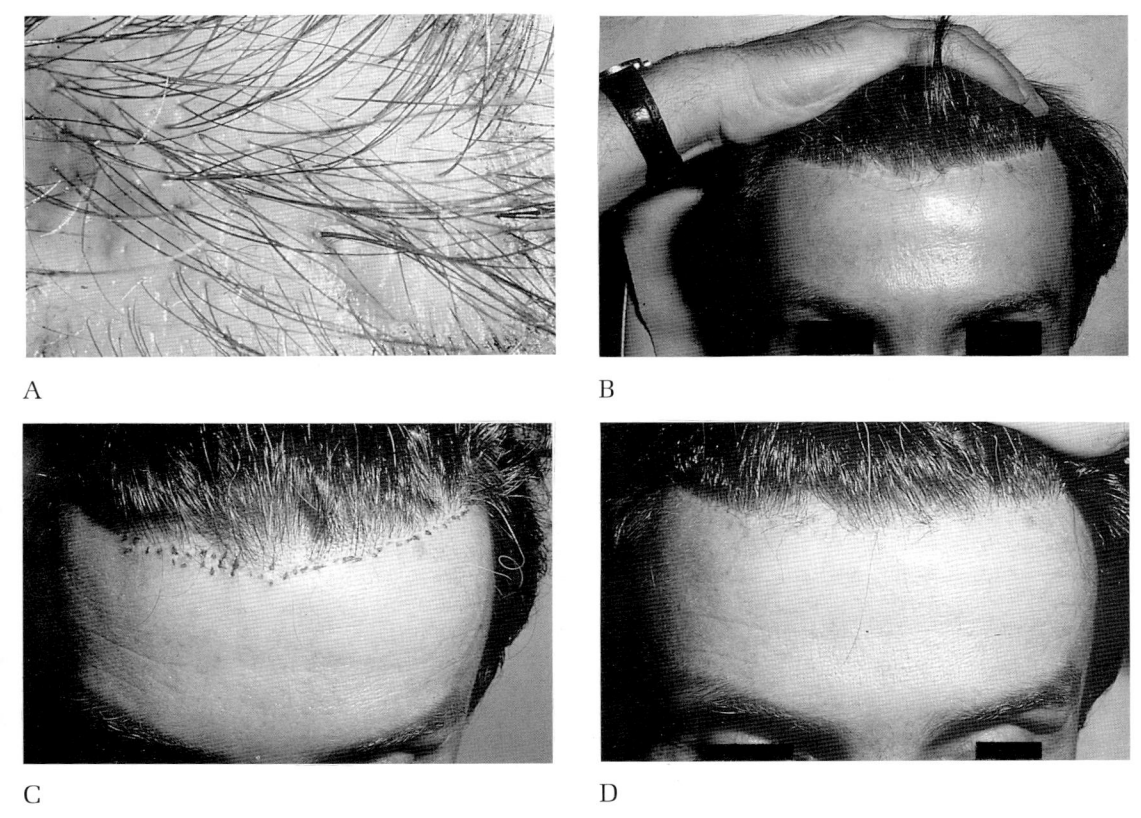

Figure 51.9
(A) Hair growing through the vertical flap frontal scar. (B) A too visible frontal scar of two flaps before correction by micrografts. (C) Immediately after and (D) 1 month after the micro transplantation.

half. To achieve a better quality scar, the tension on the closed edges must be minimal and no releasing incisions should be made in the epicranial aponeurosis. The scar must be positioned in a hairy area (paramedian according to Alt[21]) in order to camouflage it. Three to five reductions may be performed every three months on average.

The amount of skin resected at each session depends on the flexibility of the scalp and particularly the slackness of the epicranial aponeurosis. According to Nordstrom, one-third of the reduction's effect, on average, is lost in the ensuing two months.[22]

Common operating technique

The incision must be parallel to the bulbs. The scalp is undermined in the excisable sub-aponeurotic space using large, curved, blunt-pointed scissors. This bloodless undermining is performed in all directions except the occipital muscle insertions. The area to be resected can be assessed by bringing together one incised edge and the planned opposite edge using towel forceps. Staples are preferable for flat closure. Deep sutures are only used in special cases. Shampooing is done the day after. The staples are removed on the 12th to 15th day.

Different kinds of reduction[21–23]

1. *Midsagittal reduction*
   a) The median scar may be visible until the reductions are completed.
   b) There is maximum secondary skin distension.
   c) The scar at the occiput may look unsightly.
   d) This can be avoided either by slanting this portion of the scar by 45° or making a Z-plasty to change the direction of the hairs.
2. *Paramedian reduction*[22]
   This technique allows maximum elevation of the hairy crown. In order to avoid the stretching effect as much as possible, the remaining hairless area is not undermined. Therefore, the time between two reductions is six weeks, alternating between the left and right sides. The crescent shape of the excised area makes it possible to avoid the unsightly distortion of the occiput.
3. *Transversal reduction*[23]
   This technique has two significant problems:
   a) it is inefficient because maximum elasticity is rarely anteroposterior;
   b) it is not safe because the undermining of the occipital area does not occur as easily as on other areas of the scalp. There is no cleavable subaponeurotic space.
4. *Mixed V–Y reduction*
   This technique takes advantage of the scalp's elasticity along three axes, combining the results of midsagittal and transversal reduction. The reliability of the occipital flap is emphasized; provided two basic factors are observed: (1) the angle of its apex must always exceed 90°; (2) a check must be made to ensure that there are no occipital scars which could hinder its vascularization.

In summary, scalp reduction is a simple procedure which complements the correction of some hairless areas where there is adequate laxity (Figure 51.10). It is

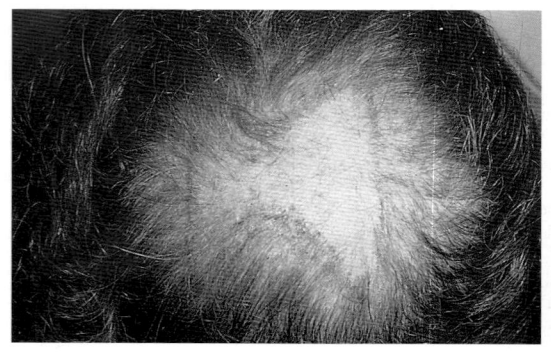

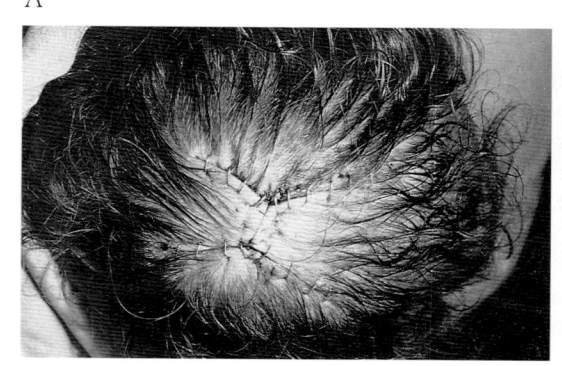

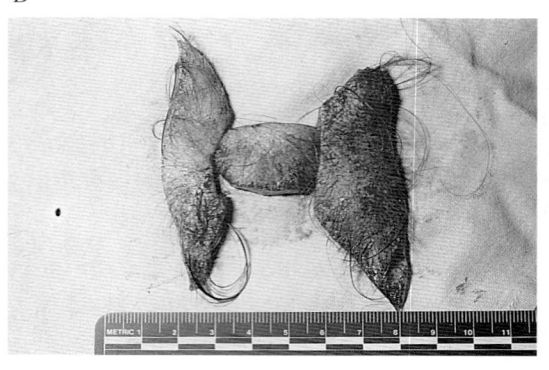

Figure 51.10
(A) Outline of a reduction. (B) Immediately after reduction. (C) The amount of bald scalp excised.

essential that scalp reduction be properly programmed into a long-term plan. It must be performed after flap transposition and before transplanting minigrafts.[24]

HAIR SURGERY UNDER GENERAL ANESTHESIA

Giant reduction

The principle of this procedure is twofold: (1) complete detachment of the whole of the scalp; (2) occipital detachment extended to the bottom of the hairy area at the nape of the neck. The occipital vessels must be sacrificed and the temporal vessels are preserved. This reduction is similar to the modified Fleming flap described by Blanchard.

A U-shaped incision is made from one anterior temporal edge to the other through the hairy part of the crown. The supra-auricular, retro-auricular, and occipital areas in the sup-aponeurotic plane are then detached. This is particularly difficult at the external occipital protuberance, and deep subcutaneous attachment of the cervical area. The occipital arteriovenous pedicles and Arnold's nerve are sectioned.

This vast undermining of the occipital cervical area makes it possible, on average, to raise the parieto–occipital hair border by 4 cm and to advance the anterior temporal hairy area by 2 cm. Suction drains and dressings are left in position for 2–3 days. Different technical variants have been described by Brandy[25] (Figure 51.11A), Marzola[26] and Dardour.[27]

Complications

Possible complications include:

1. Secondary necrosis due to ischemia[28] (closure under tension, pre-existing scars, undermining that is too superficial, absence of temporal arteries, compressive hematoma).

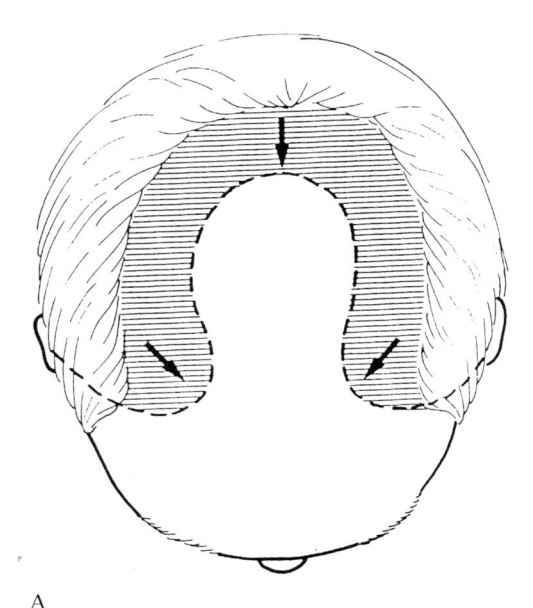

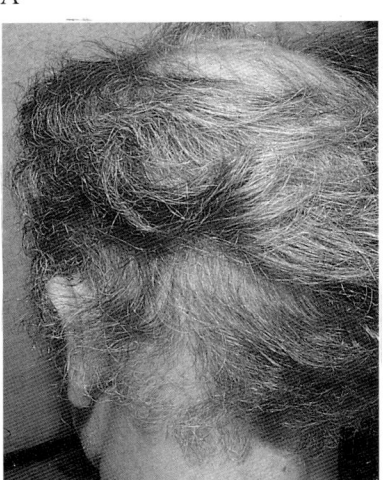

Figure 51.11
(A) Diagram of the scalp lift procedure. (B) Alopecia of the lower occipital area after a wide scalp reduction (scalp lift procedure).

2. Permanent alopecia due to ischemia, without complete skin necrosis.
3. Alopecia of the lower occipital area because of excessive advancement of the hairy crown (Figure 51.11B).

4. Persistent pain and dysesthesia in the occipital area due to cutting Arnold's occipital nerve. This effect could be avoided by gradually stretching the vasculo-nervous pedicle without cutting it.

Scalp expanders

The principle of this procedure, described by Radovan and Manders,[29] consists of progressively distending all or part of the donor area of the scalp in order to distribute it better. A silicone balloon fitted with a check valve is positioned under the scalp. This expander is distended by the injection of physiological saline.

Technical principles

There are many styles of implants available and the choice is made according to size and shape (rectangular, cylindrical, crescent-shaped). The filling valve may be remote, with a connecting tube, or it may be incorporated in the prosthesis (Figure 51.12).

The expander is positioned in a pocket made in the sub-aponeurotic space through an incision, under local or general anesthesia. This pocket must be equal to the area of the implant base. A tunnel is created in order to place the filling valve away from the prosthesis.

Two to three weeks after insertion of this implant, it is inflated progressively with physiological saline twice per week for an average of two months. When the desired degree of filling is achieved, the implant is removed, and the expanded flap is placed over the area to be covered. There are two types of expanded flaps: advancement or transpositional with closure of the donor area (Figure 51.13).

This procedure makes it possible (1) to double the size of the bald area that may be treated; (2) to increase the width of a transposition flap, at the same time making closure of the donor area easier; (3) to

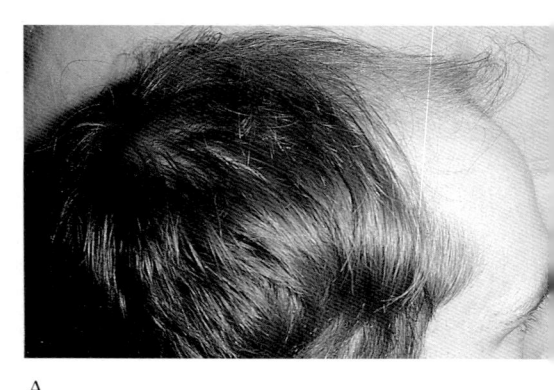

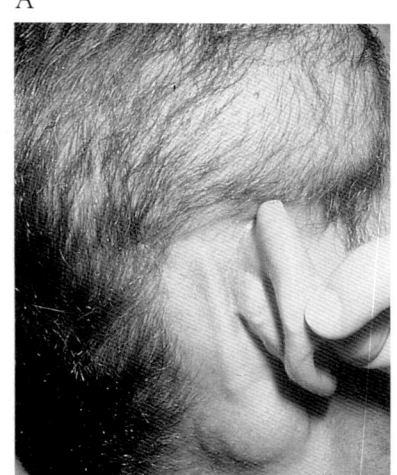

Figure 51.12
(A) Patient before insertion of the expander. (B) Two months after progressive inflation of the prosthesis by injection of physiological saline through the valve. (C) Macrophotographic evaluation of the diminution of the hair density on the expanded scalp (phototrichogram).

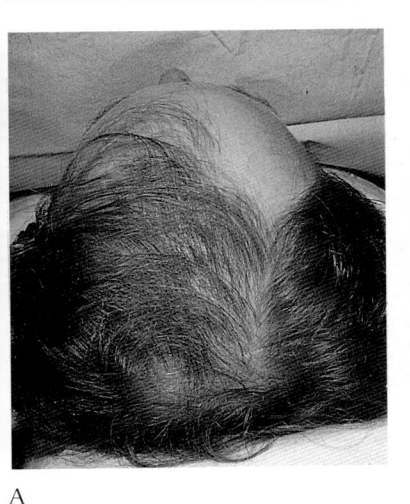

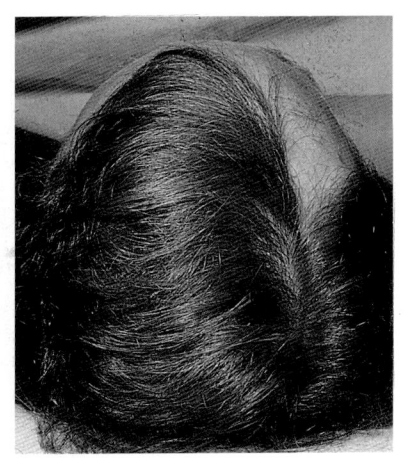

Figure 51.13
Male baldness (A) before and (B) 4 months after transposition of a large vertical expanded flap. (C) A diagram of the procedure.

ensure better vascularization of the expanded scalp; and (4) to ensure homogeneous distribution of capillary densities.

Drawbacks
1. At least two operations are necessary and, more often than not, under general anesthesia.
2. Twice-weekly filling of the implant for at least two months.
3. Unsightly distension, sometimes with painful tension which may warrant 1–2 months away from work.

Complications
The complications are the same as for flap surgery in general:[21] hematoma; skin pain; infection; and, in particular, deflation of the prosthesis or exposure of the prosthesis or the valve.

SURGICAL DERMATOLOGY

Special techniques

Special techniques for scalp expanding include: Manders' technique,[29] in which he uses 2 × 600 cc sigmoid prostheses to obtain two large advancement flaps; Anderson's technique to expand Juri's flaps (this procedure combines drawbacks of expansion with the irrationality of Juri's flaps; Ozun's technique in which two large, 800–1000 cc quadrangular expanders make it possible, in two months, to expand a very wide (10–12 cm) verticle flap with a top pedicle whose transposition is followed by raising of the contralateral crown (Figure 51.13C).

The major use for these techniques, which allow considerable distension of remaining hairy areas, would seem to be the possibility of correcting extreme cases of hair loss. On the other hand, these procedures have a major drawback in that they lead to substantial deformation, warranting the patient's complete withdrawal from social life. It is therefore understandable that these patients' motivation lies more in the context of repair by reconstructive surgery than of correction by cosmetic surgery.

MARGINAL TECHNIQUES

Implants of synthetic or natural hair

For many years, various procedures have been put forward for implantation of Japanese, American and Italian synthetic hair, or natural hair shafts. Whatever the implant, it is inexorably rejected after a few months or years (Figure 51.14). Many papers (Lepaw,[30] Bouhanna[31]) have assessed the speed of rejection of these implants and determined the percentage of complications such as folliculitis, follicular seborrheic deposits, scar pitting and foreign body granuloma (Figure 51.15). The progress made by conventional hair surgery and, in particular, mini- and micrografts has

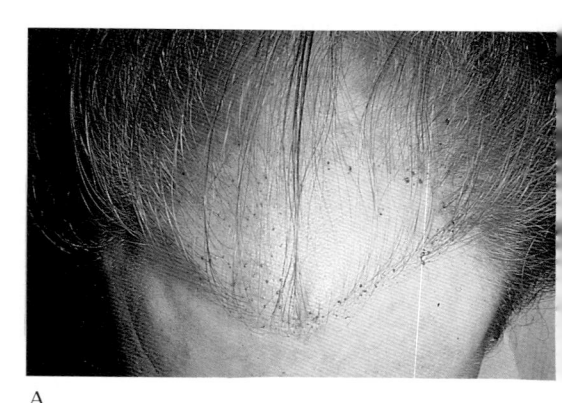

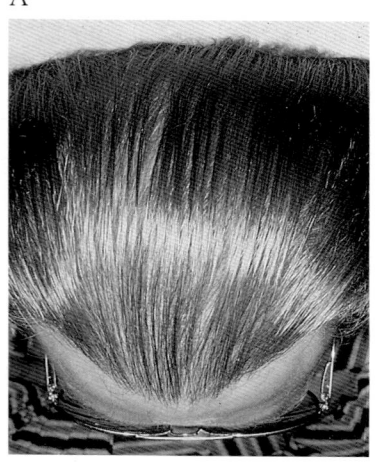

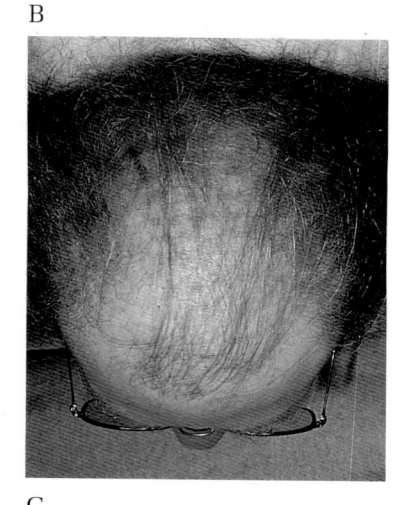

Figure 51.14
Male baldness immediately after implantation of (A) 500 synthetic hairs (B) 2000 synthetic hairs and (C) the same patient 1 year after the implantation.

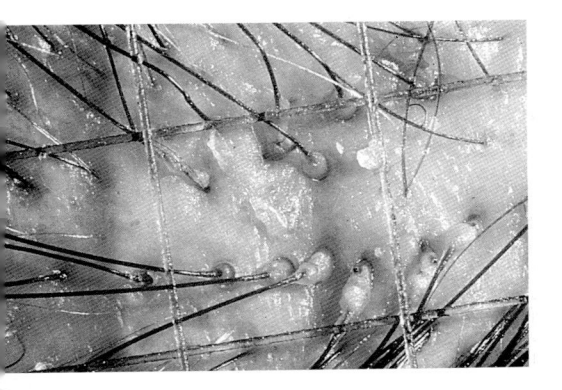

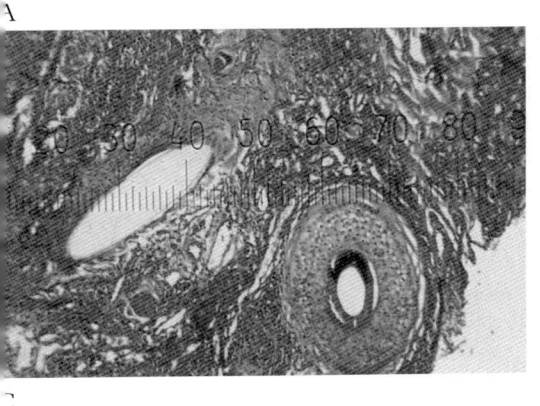

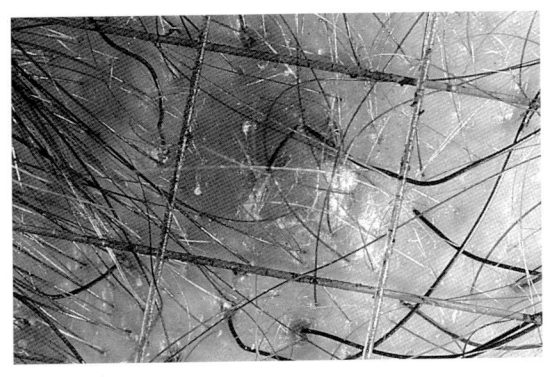

Figure 51.15
Synthetic hair implants rejected with (A) follicular seborrheic deposits or (B) a foreign body granuloma. (C) Histological aspect of the inflammatory granuloma around a synthetic hair and a normal hair.

considerably restricted the indications for synthetic or natural hair implants. The procedure is not approved for use in many countries and should be avoided.

Skin pigmentation[32]

Skin pigmentation or tattooing is only used on the scalp in areas where the hair is permanently diffuse and not on completely glabrous areas (Figure 51.16). The equipment used is a motor whose regular vibrations allow the needle to penetrate. This needle, supplied in a sterile pack, may have either a single point when the intention is to imitate the hair's appearance, or a line of points for coloring a whole area (eg, a scalp whose skin is too pale). This needle is inserted into the dermatograph handle, which is itself connected to the motor. The pigments used are medical grade, approved by the FDA. The colors most often used are black and tobacco brown or opossum.

The indications for skin pigmentation are many and varied. It can be used to complement minigrafts and to make temporal lifting scars[3] or flap donor areas.

SELECTION OF THE MOST SUITABLE TECHNIQUES FOR EACH PATIENT

Females

More often than not, androgenic alopecia causes midsagittal hair loss from the

SURGICAL DERMATOLOGY

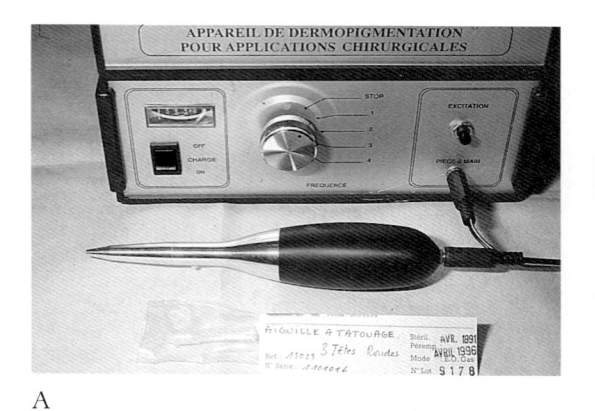

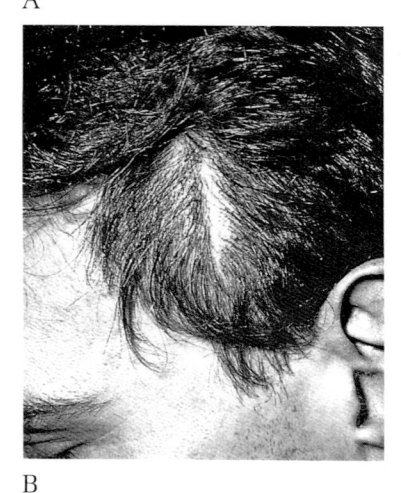

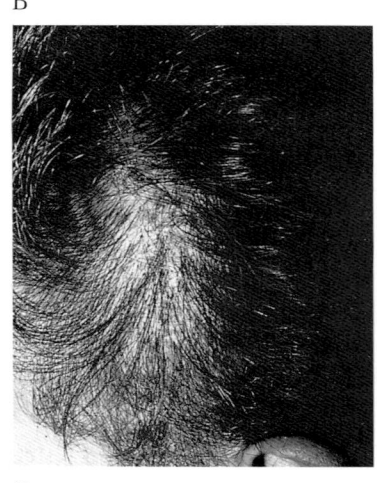

Figure 51.16
(A) The skin pigmentation equipment. A visible scalp scar (B) before and (C) after one tattooing session.

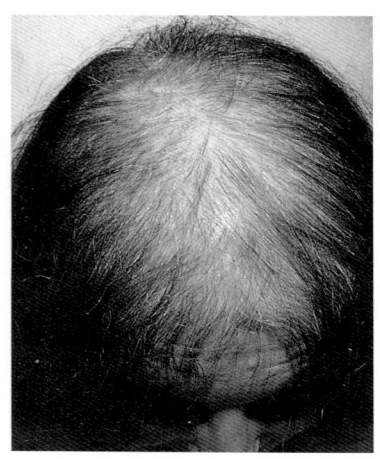

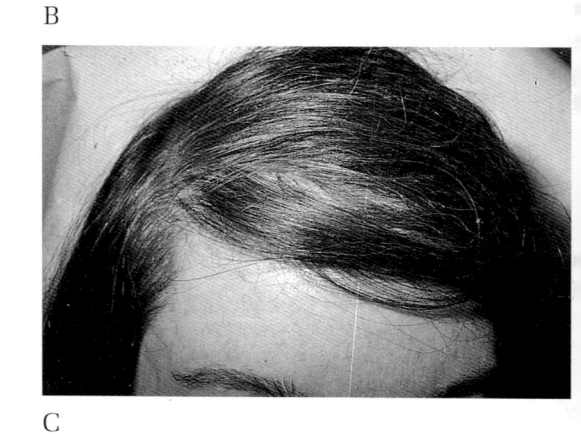

Figure 51.17
Female midsagittal hair loss (A) before and (B,C) one year after 3 sessions of minigraft transplantation.

forehead to the vertex[33] with a persisting frontal hairline and occasional diffuse tempo–occipital thinning. Only the lower median occipital area escapes.[34] Consequently, the minigraft transplant technique is the only one recommended.[35] According to the location of the hair loss, one to three 100–150 minigraft sessions are distributed over the frontal area, the occipital area or possibly the paramedian area if there is lateral coverage (Figure 51.17).[3] Occasionally, skin pigmentation is recommended either to attenuate the paleness of the scalp skin under thin hair or to simulate hair among what hair remains.[3]

Males

The indications in males are more complex and are determined by many objective and subjective factors. The essential points to consider are: (1) the degree of baldness in accordance with one of the three stages in Bouhanna's and Nataf's 1976 classification[12] (Figure 51.18); (2) the diameter, shape and color of the hair; (3) the flexibility, thickness and degree of circulation of the scalp; (4) a harmonious balance between the patient's cosmetic ambitions, age and state of mind on the one hand, and the possibilities offered by present day surgical techniques on the other.

Stage I

Stage I is defined as a receding hairline over the two fronto-temporal recessions (Figure 51.19). This can be treated by:

1. Transposition of two flaps in one session (Figure 51.6).
2. Transplantation of 100–300 minigrafts in 1–2 sessions (Figure 51.1).
3. Transplantation of two fusiform grafts and 100 minigrafts in two sessions (Figure 51.3).

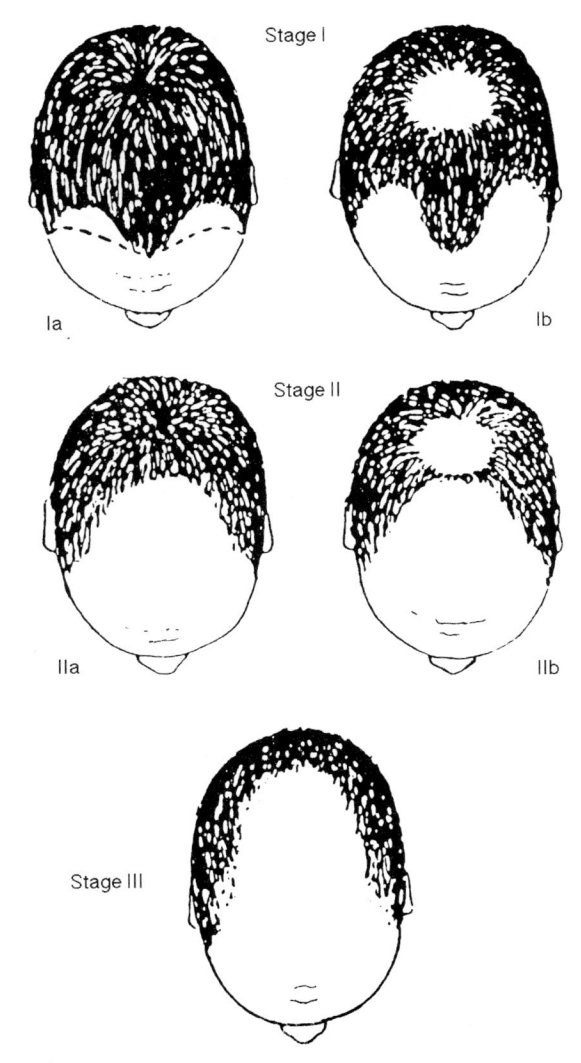

Figure 51.18
The three stages of a male baldness according to Bouhanna's and Nataf's 1976 classification.

Stage II

Stage II is defined as complete frontal baldness, which is treated by:

1. Successive transposition of two vertical flaps, complemented by a scalp reduction or transplantation of 200–300 minigrafts in 1–2 sessions (Figure 51.20 and Figure 51.21).

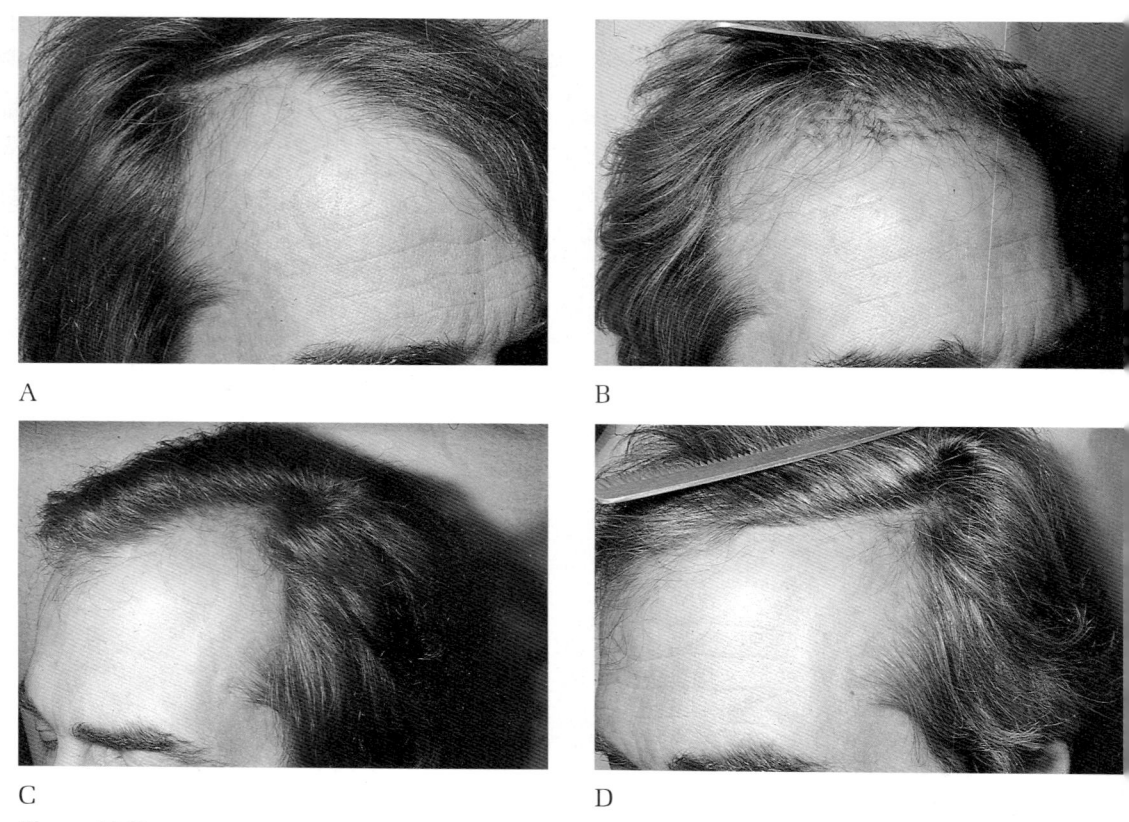

Figure 51.19
The same patient aspect before and 3 months after treatment of the frontal receding hairline. (A,B) On the right after one session of a minigraft transplantation. (C,D) On the left after one transposition of a flap.

2. Transplantation of 300 minigrafts in two successive sessions, finishing off the anterior frontal line with micrografts (Figure 51.1).

   Vertex alopecia
   This may be corrected by:

   1. Transplanting 200–300 minigrafts in 1–2 successive sessions.
   2. One or several reductions complemented by transplanting 100–200 minigrafts.

3. By transposing 1–2 vertical flaps complemented by reduction and/or a 1 × 100 minigraft transplant session (Figure 51.22).

   Stage III
   At Stage III the indications for surgery should be easier to define. In these cases only the crown remains, compared with the preceding stages where one anticipates the continuation of hair loss. Apart from the factors already mentioned, great importance should be attached to the precise

NEWER TECHNIQUES IN HAIR REPLACEMENT

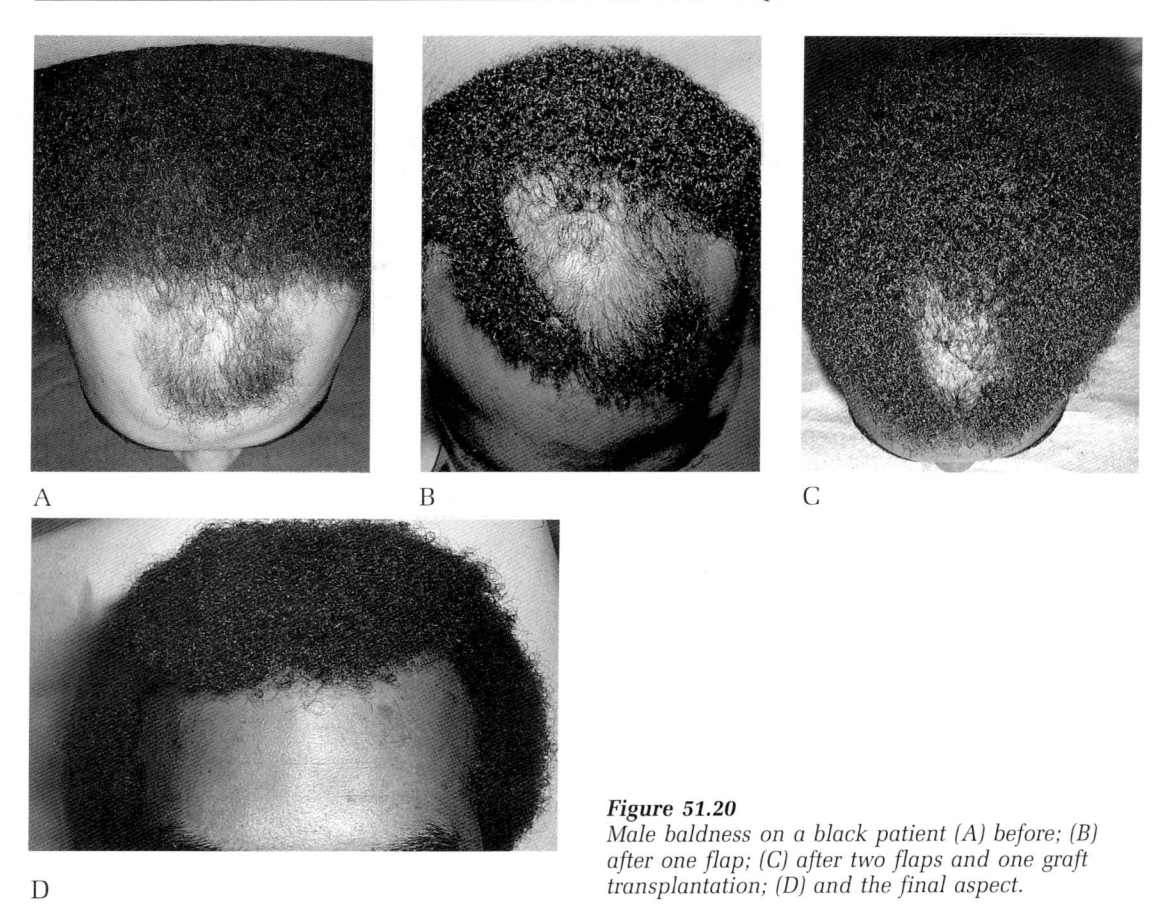

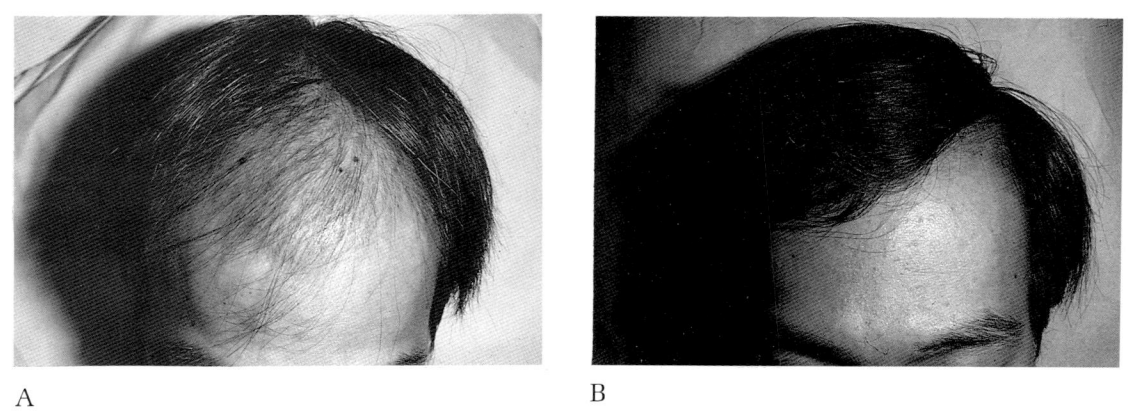

Figure 51.20
Male baldness on a black patient (A) before; (B) after one flap; (C) after two flaps and one graft transplantation; (D) and the final aspect.

Figure 51.21
Male baldness on an Asiatic patient (A) before and (B) after two flaps and one session of minigrafts.

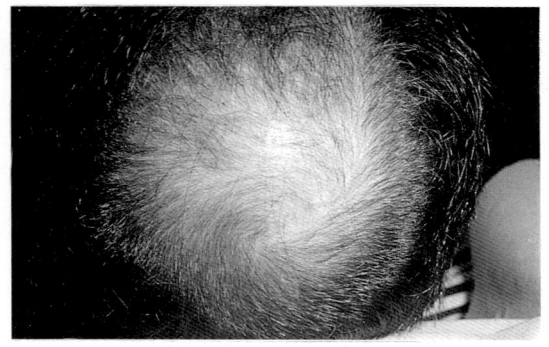

Figure 51.22
(A) Vertex alopecia corrected by (B) two vertical flaps and (C) complemented by a reduction and (D) a minigraft transplant session.

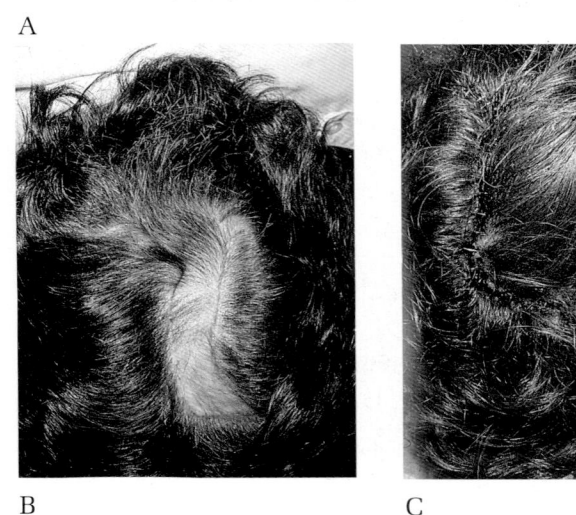

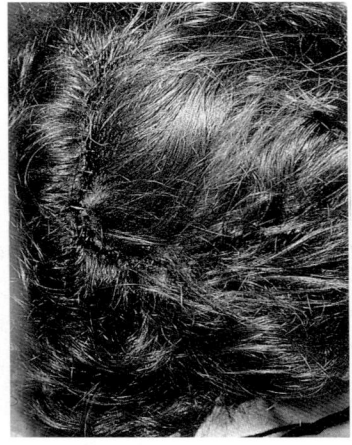

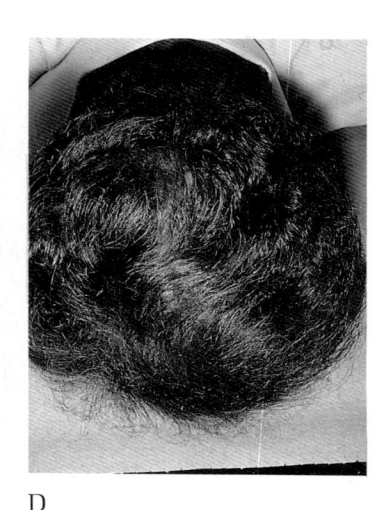

nature of the patient's cosmetic ambitions and his psychological profile.

Progressive transplantation of 3–4 hair minigrafts (4–5 hairs for Blacks, 2–3 hairs for Asians) in 200–300 fragment sessions will correct this type of baldness in 3–4 sessions.

Transposition of vertical flaps is preferable for patients whose temporal crown is more than 10 cm high, whose scalp is flexible and who have no circulation problems. Thus, either two large flaps or 3 small flaps with on reduction and one minigraft session are combined (Figure 51.23).

Scalp reduction is a complementary procedure which is recommended before transplanting minigrafts or after transposing flaps.

A big reduction or expanders have limited indications. They are performed to complement transposition of a large flap.

Skin pigmentation is useful to lessen the contrast between pale or cicatricial skin and hair grafted on to it.

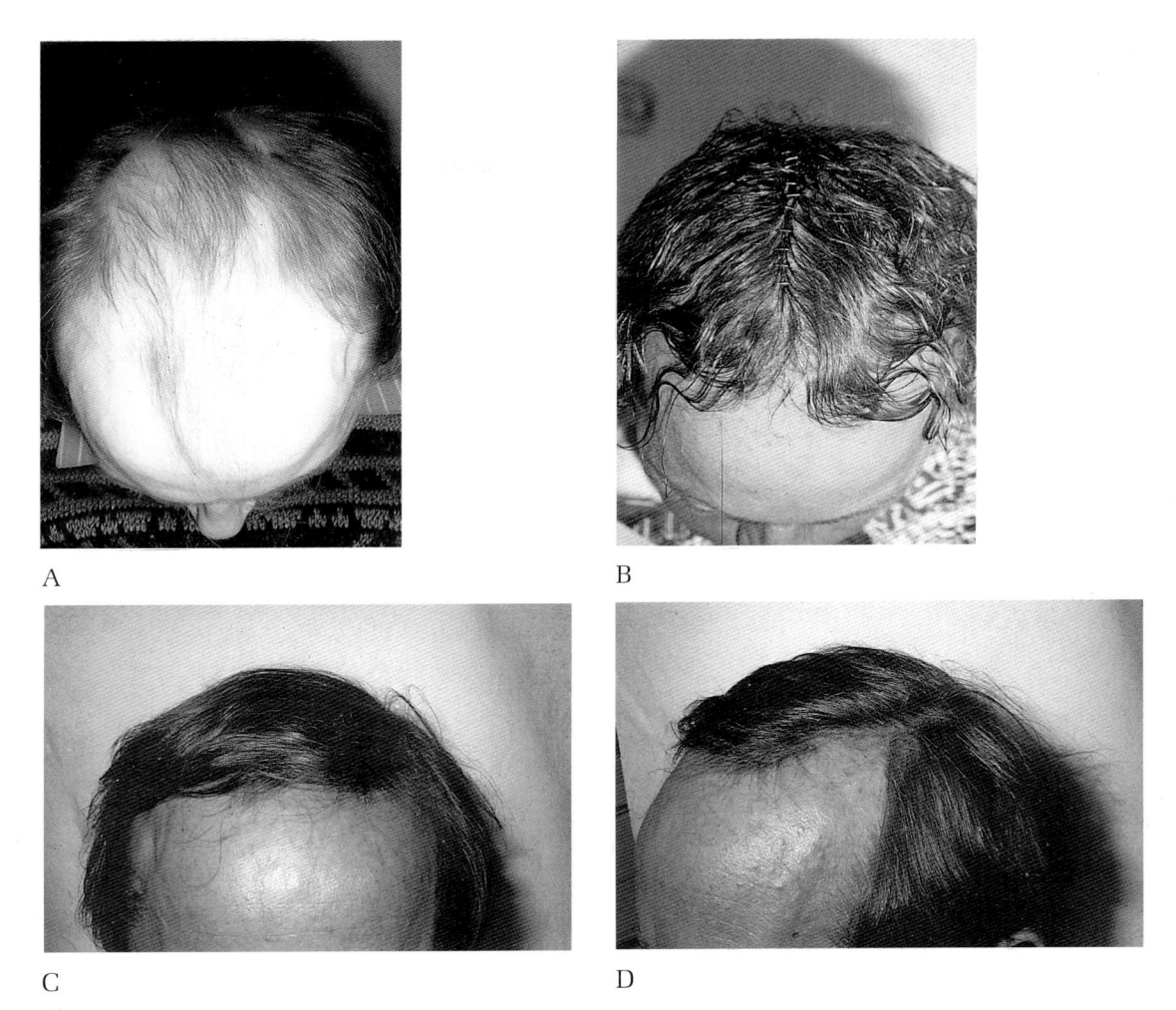

Figure 51.23
(A) Male baldness (B) after transposition of two large vertical flaps, (C,D) complemented by reduction and a minigraft transplant session.

Synthetic hair implants have very limited indications, such as some kinds of alopecia disseminata or cicatricial alopecia.

Cylindrical grafts Many surgeons have permanently abandoned the use of these because, with the exception of black patients,[36] it is difficult to regularly obtain sightly, homogeneous hair.[12]

Juri's flap Many surgeons have also abandoned this kind of transposition of horizontal flaps with a bottom pedicle, of the Juri[10] or Elliot[8] type, because of the rectilinear, unsightly appearance of the anterior frontal line, with hair pointing backwards[12] leaving scars visible, and hair loss from a large part of the flap due to normal continuation of androgenic alopecia.

Conclusion

Hair surgery has been totally transformed by many new techniques. By way of conclusion seven basic points are emphasized:

1. Make an accurate evaluation of the patient's psychological profile.
2. Draw up a schedule of indications, explaining the advantages and drawbacks of each procedure.
3. Make an immediate and prospective evaluation of the cosmetic result, bearing in mind the possible continuation of the alopecia process.
4. Reject irrational or unreliable techniques.
5. As best as possible, select the procedure which has the fewest postoperative risks.
6. Be well aware of complications in order to better avoid or correct them.
7. See the patient every year in order to observe developments and determine whether further surgery or finishing is necessary.

Finally, always bear in mind that learning a technique is simply a matter of seeing it and repeating it many times. The difficult decision is determining indications accurately.

References

1. Bouhanna P, The phototrichogram: an objective technique used in hair replacement surgery evaluation. In: Unger WP and Nordström REA, *Hair transplantation*, 2nd edn. (Marcel Dekker: New York 1988).
2. Bouhanna P, Greffes à cheveux longs immédiats, *Nouv Dermatol* (1989) **8**(4):418–20.
3. Bouhanna P, Technique personnelle de minigreffes pour le traitement de l'alopécie de la femme ménopausée. In: Mole B, ed. *Actualités de Chirurgie Esthétique SOFCEP* (Editions Masson: Paris 1992) 46–59.
4. Marritt E, Single hair transplantation for hairline refinement: a practical solution, *J Dermatol Surg Oncol* (1984) **10**:962–6.
5. Norwood OT, Micrografts and minigrafts for refining grafted hairlines, *Dermatol Clin* (1987) **5**(3):545–52.
6. Bouhanna P, Topical minoxidil used before and after hair transplantation surgery, *J Dermatol Surg Oncol* (1989) **15**:50–3.
7. Bouhanna P, Le cuir chevelu. Les alopécies définitives et leurs traitements, *Thèse de médecine* (Université de Paris – Créteil 1976) 63–73.
8. Elliott RA, Lateral scalp flaps for instant results in pattern baldness, *Plast Reconstr Surg* (1977) **60**:699–703.
9. Flemming RW, Mayer TG, Short and long scalp flaps in the treatment of male pattern baldness, *Arch Oto Laryngol* (1981) **107**(7):403–8.
10. Juri J, Use of parieto-occipital flaps in the surgical treatment of baldness, *Plast Reconstr Surg* (1975) **55**:456–60.
11. Nataf J, Elbaz J-S, Pollet J, Etude critique des transplantations de cuir chevelu et proposition d'une optique, *Ann Chir Plast* (1976) **21**:199–206.
12. Bouhanna P, Nataf J, A propos des transplantations de cuir chevelu. Critiques et propositions, *Rev Chir Esth* (1976) **7**:17–23.
13. Nataf J, Lambeaux de cuir chevelu et étude comparative avec les autres techniques de transplantation, *Ann Chir Plast* (1978) **23**:176–82.
14. Bouhanna P, Les lambeaux de cuir

chevelu à charnière haute, *Ann Chir Plast Esth* (1990) **35**(5):397–404.

15. Dardour J-C, Treatment of male baldness with a one-stage flap, *Aesthetic Plast Surg* (1985) **9**:109.

16. Nataf J, Surgical treatment for frontal baldness: the long temporal vertical flap, *Plast Reconstr Surg* (1984) **74**:628.

17. Bouhanna P, The post auricular vertical hair-bearing transposition flap, *J Dermatol Surg Oncol* (1984) **10**:551–4.

18. Bouhanna P, New aspects of minoxidil, *Nouv Dermatol* (1991) **10**(1):24–34.

19. Nataf J, Réflexions sur 7 années d'utilisation du lambeau 'enfoui', *Ann Chir Plast* (1984) **29**(1):53–7.

20. Blanchard G, Blanchard B, Obliteration of alopecia by hair lifting. A new concept and technique, *J Nat Med Assoc* (1977) **69**:639–41.

21. Alt T, Scalp reduction as an adjunct to hair transplantation, *J Dermatol Surg Oncol* (1980) **6**(2):1011–188.

22. Unger WP, Nordström REA, *Hair transplantation*, 2nd edn. (Marcel Dekker: New York 1988).

23. Norwood OT, Shiell RC, *Hair transplant surgery*, 2nd edn. (Charles C Thomas: Springfield Illinois 1984).

24. Bouhanna P, Considérations sur le traitement chirurgical des alopécies masculines, *J Med Esth Chir Dermatol* (1981) **29**:182–4.

25. Brandy D, The bilateral occipitoparietal flap. *J Dermatol Surg Oncol* (1986) **12**(10):1062–6.

26. Marzola M, An alternative hair replacement method, In: Norwood OT, Shiell RC, eds. *Hair transplant surgery*, 2nd edn. (Charles C Thomas: Springfield Illinois 1984) 315–24.

27. Dardour J-C, Les réductions de tonsure. Principes et innovations: le lifting du scalp, *Ann Chir Plast Esth* (1989) **34**(3):234–42.

28. Unger MG, Post operative necrosis following bilateral scalp reduction, *J Dermatol Surg Oncol* (1988) **14**(5):541–3.

29. Manders EK, Graham WP, Alopecia reconstruction by scalp expansion, *J Dermatol Surg Oncol* (1984) **10**:967.

30. Lepaw MI, Complications of implantation of synthetic fibers into scalps for 'hair' replacement, *J Dermatol Surg Oncol* (1979) **5**:201–4.

31. Bouhanna P, Clinical and macrophotographic study of the percutaneous implantation of synthetic hair (NIDO SHI). In: Van Neste D, Lachapelle J-M, Antoine J-L, eds. *Trends in human hair growth and alopecia research* (Kluwer Acad Publishers: Boston 1989) 257–65.

32. Tiziano J-P, Semeria E, Levy J-L, *La dermographie, technique du tatouage* (Solal Editions: Marseille 1990).

33. Ludwig E, Classifications of the types of androgenetic alopecia (common baldness) occurring in the female sex, *Br J Dermatol* (1977) **97**:249–57.

34. Bouhanna P, Les alopécies de la femme mémopausée, *Reproduction humaine et hormones* (1988) **1**(1):33–41.

35. Villodres RE, Microinjerto de cabello en mujeres con alopecia comun de patron femenico, *Piel* (1989) **4**:407–9.

36. Earles MR, Hair transplantation, scalp reduction and flap rotation in black men, *J Dermatol Surg Oncol* (1986) **12**(1):87–96.

INDEX

Note: Page numbers in **bold** refer to tables; those in *italics* refer to figures

abscesses, soft tissue 32
acantholytic solar keratoses 78
Accutane 516
acetaminophen (paracetamol) 166, 169, 171
acitretin 81
acne, body image in 343
    see also acne scarring
acne keloidalis nuchae, carbon dioxide laser treatment of 295–6
acne rosacea, isotretinoin in treatment of 375
acne scarring
    carbon dioxide laser treatment of 293, 295–6
    cryo peeling 87
    dermabrasion 385, 511
    isotretinoin in treatment of 375, 376, 378, 379
    microlipoinjection of 455, *456, 458*
    phenol chemical peel in 484
acquired immunodeficiency syndrome (AIDS) 41
    cryosurgery and 61
    giant basal cell carcinoma in 96
    metastatic basal cell carcinoma and 109, 117
    treatment of Kaposi's sarcoma in 63–4, 174
    warts in 311
acquired periungual fibrokeratoma 223
acrolentiginous melanoma 232
actinic cheilitis
    carbon dioxide laser treatment of 285, *286*, 293
    laserbrasions 509
actinic keratoses (solar keratoses) 73–82
    Bowenoid keratosis 78
    carbon dioxide laser treatment of *286*, 287
    causes other than solar exposure 79
    chemotherapy 80–2
    clinical features 74–6
    cryosurgery 90, 91
    cutaneous horn 74, *75*
    Darier-like keratosis 78, *79*
    dermabrasion 511, 515
    epidemiology 73–4
    of the eyelid 212
    histologic variants 77–9
    interferon in treatment of 173
    lichenoid keratosis 77–8
    lupus erythematosus-like keratosis (lupoid AK) 75
    mucosal lesions 75–6
    multiple 160
    natural history and immunological aspects 79–80
    pathology and pathophysiology 76–7
    phenol chemical peeling 482
    pigmented actinic keratosis (spreading pigmented AK) 75
    treatment 80–2
actinomycin D 118
acyclovir 502
adenoma sebaceum
    carbon dioxide laser treatment of 287
    dermabrasion 511
adnexal tumors, carbon dioxide laser treatment of 293
adrenal insufficiency as contraindication to sedation 14
Adriamycin 51
AIDS *see* acquired immunodeficiency syndrome
AIDS-related complex (ARC) and metastatic basal cell carcinoma 109, 117
Alzheimer's disease 94
amelanotic melanoma 224
aminophylline 16
amyloidosis 109, 301
analgesia, definition 13
anesthetic creams 7
angiofibromas, carbon dioxide laser treatment of 298

INDEX

angioma 91
  cavernous 224
  cherry, Nd:YAG laser in treatment of 370
  spider 330
angiomatoid malignant fibrohistiocytoma 206
antibiotics 31–8
  in endocarditis prophylaxis 31–4
  new antimicrobials 37–8
  to prevent wound infection 34–7
antihistamines, sedating 24–5
antimicrobials 37–8
apocrine hidrocystoma, carbon dioxide laser treatment of 293
arotinoids 81
arsenical toxication 79
atrophic keratosis 76
atypical fibroxanthoma 201, 202–4
atypical mole syndrome 178, 244, 247
autocrine motility factors 182
Autolase 336
autologous collagen implants 441, 448
axillary hyperhidrosis, tumescent local anesthesia in 10
azalides 38
azithromycin 38

bacitracin 271
bacteriochlorophyll a 349
Baker–Gordon phenol peel 480, *481*, *483*, *485*, *487*, 488, 492, 493, *496*, 498, 501
balanitis xerotica obliterans, carbon dioxide laser treatment of 301, 303
barbiturates 15
basal cell carcinoma
  carbon dioxide laser treatment 287
  cryosurgery and 90, 91
  dermabrasion 511
  giant *see* giant basal cell carcinoma
  interferon in treatment of 165–72
  metastatic *see* metastatic basal cell carcinoma
  metastatic potential 181
  of the nail 222
  Nd:YAG laser in treatment of 371
  photodynamic therapy in 350
  recurring following radiotherapy 101–6
    current data 102–3
    historical background 101–2
    hypotheses and explanations 103–5
    treatment recommendations 105–6
  risk of developing another 178
  surgical margins 139–40, 142
  treatment and prevention with oral isotretinoin 155–62
    chemoprophylaxis 156–7
    chemotherapy 156
    multicenter trial 159–60
    pilot study 156–7
    toxicities 157
  and UV light 56, 57

  vs connective tissue cells, immunohistochemical diagnosis 134–6
  vs hair follicles, immunohistochemical diagnosis 134
  vs sweat glands, immunohistochemical diagnosis 134
  wound healing 85
basal cell nevus syndrome 109
  Nd:YAG laser in treatment of 371
basaloma 93
basaloma terebrans 93
Bednar tumors 192
benzodiazepines 15–18
benzophenoxonines 349
Biobrane 509
blastomycosis, carbon dioxide laser treatment of 296
Blenderm tape 63
bleomycin
  in treatment of keratoacanthoma 220
  in treatment of multiple basal cell carcinoma 118–19
  in treatment of warts 67, 312
bleomycin sulfate in treatment of warts 313
blepharoconjunctivitis 211
blood pressure measurement 26
botryomycoma 224
botryomycosis 296
Bourneville–Pringle disease 223
Bowen's disease 78, 160, 212
  Mohs surgery in 195–8
  of the nail 221–2
  Nd:YAG laser in treatment of 371
  papillomavirus and 310, 311, 312
  photodynamic therapy in 351
Bowenoid keratosis 78
Bowenoid papulosis 309, 310
  carbon dioxide laser treatment of 287
  Nd:YAG laser in treatment of 371
Breslow technique 263
Brodie–Trendelenburg test *429*
bromochlorofluorocarbons 56
bupivacaine 488
burn scars as contraindication to dermabrasion 516

cancerophobia 94
cannula 463–4
  basket–style *463*
  cobra–style 463, *464*
cantharidin 219, 312
cantharone 219
carbolic acid 34
carbon dioxide laser therapy
  acne scarring 293, 295–6
  disorders of keratinization 298–9
  genodermatoses 299–301
  infectious processes 296–7
  inflammatory diseases 301–2
  laserbrasion using 509

carbon dioxide laser therapy (*contd*)
   metabolic diseases 301
   newer uses 293–303
   of papillomavirus 312, 319
   pigmentation disorders 293, 297–8
   tumors 293–4
   vascular tumors 298
   of verrucae 67
carboxyquinolone 37, 38
carcinoembryonic antigen (CEA) 134
carcinoma
   cervical, papillomavirus and 311–12
   cutaneous, embrologic structural development in 145–51
   Merkel cell 106
   review 146–8
   sebaceous, of the eyelid 211–16
   tumor spread and fusions 148–51
   verrucous, papillomavirus and 311
carcinoma segregans 78
cataracts 56
cathepsin B 182
cavernous angioma 224
cefadroxil 36
cephadrine 36
cephalexin 36, 38
cephalosporins 37
Chataigne skin 481
chemical peel
   with phenol 479–505
      application of tape 490–4
      chemical agent application 488–90
      complications 500–4
         cardiac arrhythmia 503–4
         changes in texture 503
         cutaneous atrophy 502–3
         laryngeal edema 504
         persistent erythema 502
         postoperative infection 502
         scarring 501–2
         toxic shock syndrome 504
      histological changes 484–5
      history 479
      indications 479–84
      mask removal 494–8
      postoperative events 499–500
      preoperative preparation 486–8
      relative contraindications 505
      repeat peeling 499
      side-effects 504–5
      technical factors 486
      variations 498–9
   with trichloroacetic acid 469–77
      histological effects 471–6
         advantages **476**
         immediate 472–4
         long–term 474–6
cherry angioma, Nd:YAG laser in treatment of 370
chlorhexidine 35
chlorins 349

chlorofluorocarbons (CFCs) 55–6, 57–8
chlorpromazine 20
chromated glycerin 435–6
chromoblastomycosis 61, 64–5
chromomycosis, carbon dioxide laser treatment of 296
cigarette smoking
   benzodiazepine metabolism inhibition by 16
   and flap survival 404
cimetidine 16
ciprofloxacin 37
cisplatin 119
Cladosporium carrionii 65
collagenase, type IV 182
colony-stimulating factor 47
condylline therapy 67
condyloma acuminata
   anogenital 310
   carbon dioxide laser treatment of 293
   IF-α in treatment of 313
   oral 309, 310
   treatment by cryosurgery 61, 63, 67
condylomas
   genital, local anaesthesia during 3
   Nd:YAG laser in treatment of 371
   use of EMLA as anesthesia in 5
   vaginal and cervical 470
conjunctivitis 211
connective tissue cells vs basal cell carcinoma, immunohistochemical diagnosis 134–6
conscious, definition 13
conscious sedation, definition 13
contact allergy 57
continuous-wave scanners 335–7, 338–9
copper vapor lasers 333–4
corticosteroids 50
coumarin 15
Cowden's disease, carbon dioxide laser treatment of 287
croton oil 486
cryo peeling, full-face 87–8
cryoanesthesia 4, 7
cryoprobes 61
cryosurgery
   AIDS and 61
   cutaneous malignant melanoma (CMM) 88–9
   for cutaneous oncology 85–91
   full-face cryo peeling 87–8
   indications for 61–7
      avoiding cross-contamination 61–2
      disposable devices 62–3
      limiting devices 63
   keloids, shave excision and 85, *86–7*
   with liquid nitrogen treatment of solar lentigines 275–6
   of myxoid pseudocysts of the digits 227
   new equipment 90–1
   other tumors 91
   of papillomavirus 312
   for sebaceous carcinoma of the eyelid 214–15

INDEX

use of ultrasound in 89–90
wound healing after 85–7
cutaneous carcinoma, embryologic structural
    development in 145–51
  review 146–8
  tumor spread and fusions 148–51
cutaneous horn 74, 75
cutaneous malignant melanoma (CMM) 88–9,
    177–8
cutaneous melanoma 56, 57
cutaneous oncology, cryosurgery for 85–91
cutaneous T cell lymphoma 160
cyclophosphamide 118
cylindroma, carbon dioxide laser treatment of 294
cyst
  epidermoid, implantation 220
  myxoid, carbon dioxide laser treatment of 294
cytokeratin 134, 273–4
cytokine 47

Darier's disease 78
  carbon dioxide laser treatment of 299–300, 303
  dermabrasion 511
  isotretinoin in treatment of 375
Darier-like keratosis 78, 79
decorin 51
dermabrasion 52, 509–16
  current uses 510–11
  and isotretinoin 376–80, 381
  laserabrasions 509
  photoaging skin 514–15
  postoperative care and dressing 509–10
  problems 516
  for scar revision 385–93, 511–14
  tumescent local anesthesia in 10
Dermascan shuttered delivery system (ADS) 275
dermatofibroma 90, 201
  of the nail, fibrous 222
  pseudosarcomatous 202
dermatofibrosarcoma protuberans (DFSP) 106,
    191–8, 201
  biological behavior 193–4
  clinical appearance 191
  histology 191–2
  incidence 191
  Mohs surgery 195
  treatment 194–5
  variants 192–3
desmoplakin 134
diabetes
  as contraindication to methoxyflurane use 23
  wounds in 50
diaminobenzidine 274
diazepam 15, 16–17
dichlorotetrafluoroethane 386
dicloxacillin 33
dihematoporphyrin ester/ether (DHE) 349
dinitrochlorobenzene in treatment of warts 313
diphencyprone 219
disseminated superficial actinic porokeratosis 90

disulfiram 16
Doppler ultrasound 429–31
doxorubicin 208
Duplex sonography 431
dyskeratosis, malignant 77
dysplasia 76
dysplastic nevus syndrome 178, 228, 244

eccrine poroma, malignant 160
eczema 220
elastase 182
elastosis, solar, dermabrasion of 511
electrocautery of condyloma acuminata 67
enchondroma of the nail 225
endocarditis prophylaxis 31–4
ephelides, carbon dioxide laser treatment of 287
ephelis 483
epidermal grafts see flaps and grafts
epidermal growth factor (EGF) 47, 50, 51
epidermal nevi
  carbon dioxide laser treatment of 287, 293
  dermabrasion 511
  laserbrasions 509
epidermodysplasia verruciformis (EV) 160, 310–11,
    312
epidermoid cyst, implantation 220
epidermolysis bullosa, epidermal autografts in
    396–7
epilation, use of EMLA as anesthesia in 5
epiloia 223
epinephrine 5, 6, 9, 452, 462
epithelial hyperplasia, focal 309, 310
epithelioma adenoides cysticum, dermabrasion in
    511
epithelioma cuniculatum 222
erythromycin 33, 36
erythroplasia of Queyrat 79, 415
Escherichia coli 38
ethanol 15
ethanolamine oleate 434
etretinate 81
European Society for Micrographic Surgery 127–8
Eutectic Mixture of Local Anesthetics (EMLA) 5–7
exostosis of the nail 225

fentanyl 20–1
fentanyl citrate 488
Fibrel 446–8
  adverse reactions 448
  history and development 446
  indications, contraindications and skin testing
      446–7
  injection technique 447–8
fibrinopeptides A and B 49
fibroblast growth factor (FGF) 48, 50, 51
fibroblastoma, giant cell 192–3
fibrohistiocytic tumors 201
fibrohistiocytoma
  angiomatoid malignant 206
  giant cell malignant 206

fibrohistiocytoma (contd)
  malignant (MFH) 201, 204–8
    inflammatory malignant 206
    storiform–pleomorphic malignant 205
fibrokeratoma, periungual, acquired 223
fibromatosis, infantile (juvenile) digital 223–4
fibromous tumors of the nail 222–4
fibrosarcoma, paradoxical 202
fibrous dermatofibroma of the nail 222
fibroxanthoma, atypical 201, 202–4
flaps and grafts 403–19
  cheek 412
  chin 415
  composite or in vitro reconstituted grafts 397–8
  digits 415–16
  epidermal grafts 395–9
    preparation and transplantation methods 395–6
    structural and functional characterization 398–9
    surgical applications 396–8
  eyelids 406–8
  facilitation of movement 404–5
  fat, longevity of 452–8
  forehead and temple 405–6
  glans penis 415
  harvesting, use of EMLA as anesthesia in 5
  improvement of flap appearance 418
  improvement of survival 404
  keratinocyte allgrafts 397
  keratinocyte autografts 396–7
  lip commissure 414–15
  lower lip 414
  nasal root and glabella 408–9
  new flaps 416
  nose 409–11
  preparation of mesh grafts 419
  reversed dermal graft 418–19
  rotation flap modification to avoid tip and margin necrosis 417
  skin graft survival 418
  technique of movement 405
  upper lip 412–13
  Z-plasties and V-Y advancement 416
  see also hair replacement; hair replacement minigrafts
Flashlamp excited dye laser (FEDL) 327, 333, 337–9
flumazenil 15, 18
5-fluorocytosine (5-FC) 65
5-fluorouracil 469, 470
  in treatment of metastatic basal cell carcinoma 118
  in treatment of keratoacanthoma 220
  in treatment of actinic keratoses 81, 514
  in treatment of warts 310, 312
Fonsecaea pedrosoi 65
formalin in treatment of warts 312
forme bourgeonnate et vegetante 93
freckling 483

Freundenthal funnel 76, *77*
Frigiderm Asepticator 61
full–face cryo peeling 87–8

G-proteins 49
general anesthesia
  definition 13
  stages of 13–14
genital condylomas, local anaesthesia during 3
genodermatoses, carbon dioxide laser treatment of 293
giant basal cell carcinoma 93–7
  associations 93–6
    duration of tumor, age of patient 94
    effects of radiation exposure 95
    effects of wound grafting 95–6
    genetics 96
    histological subtype 94–5
    immunity 96
    neglect 94
    recurrence 94
    tumor location 96
  complications 96–7
  treatment 97
giant basaloma 93
giant cell fibroblastoma 192–3
giant cell malignant fibrohistiocytoma 206
giant cell tumor of the nail 226
giant exophytic basaloma 93
giant pigmented nevi 178
glaucoma as contraindication to use of benzodiazepines 16
glomus tumor of the nail 224
glutaraldehyde in treatment of warts 312
grafts *see* flaps and grafts
granuloma
  pseudopyogenic 224
  pyogenic, of the nail 224
granuloma faciale, carbon dioxide laser treatment of 301
granuloma telangiectaticum 224
growth factors and wound healing 47–52
  acute and chronic wounds 50
  animal studies 50–1
  human wounds 51–2
  mechanism of action 48–9
  nomenclature 47–8
  presence in wounds 49–50
  TGF–beta and scarring 51

Hailey–Hailey disease, carbon dioxide laser treatment of 299–300, 303
hair follicles vs basal cell carcinoma, immunohistochemical diagnosis 134
hair replacement 52, 527–52
  under general anesthesia 541–4
    giant reduction 541–2
    scalp expanders 542–4
      complications 543
      drawbacks 543

special techniques 544
  technical principles 542–3
under local anesthesia 527
  long-haired grafts 527–33
    cutting the strip of scalp 529
    development 531
    minoxidil's effect on 533
    other advantages 531–3
    pre- and postoperative care 531
    preparation of the receiving area 529–31
    removal from the occipital area 528–9
  simple reduction technique 538–41
    common operating technique 539–40
    different kinds of reduction 540–1
  vertical flaps 533–8
    advantages 538
    complications 538
    different designs, with superior pedicle 536–7
    operating technique common to all flaps 534–6
marginal techniques 544–5
  skin pigmentation 545
  synthetic or natural hair implants 544–5
selection of most suitable technique 545–51
  females 545–7
  males 547–51
    big reduction or expanders 550
    cylindical grafts 551
    Juri's flap 551
    progressive transplantation 550
    scalp reduction 550
    skin pigmentation 550
    stages of baldness 547–50
    synthetic hair implants 551
    transposition of vertical flaps 550
tumescent local anesthesia in 10
see also hair replacement minigrafts
hair replacement minigrafts 517–26
  angle of implantation of minigrafts 519–24
    bleeding 521–2
    frontal hemostat 522–4
    occipital hemostat 522, 523
  definition of the graft 517
  strategy of hair replacement by minigrafts 524–6
    rapid strategy 524–6
    slow inconspicuous approach 524
  technique of harvesting 517–19
    maxigrafts cut into four quarters 517
    micrografts 518
    minigrafts harvested with a punch 518
    preparing the recipient site for minigrafts 518–19
    square minigrafts 518
halons 56, 57
hamartomas
  renal 223
  vascular 90
hemangioma 91
  age 342
  body image 341–2

cosmetic changes 342
  in dermatology 343
  factors which may modify 342
  psychological disabilities 341–5
  social norms 342
  strawberry, Nd:YAG laser in treatment of 370
hemangiosarcoma 224
hematoma as risk factor for flap survival 404
hematoporphyrin 347–8
hematoporphyrin derivative 348–9
Hemophilus influenzae 38
heparitinase 182
heparsol 435
hepatic disease as contraindication to sedation 14
hepatitis, cryosurgery and 61
hepatitis B, laser treatment of 319
hepatitis B virus 61
hepatitis C virus 61
herpes simplex 502, 516
  contraindication to dermabrasion 516
Hexascan scanners 337
hidradenitis 466
hidradenitis suppurativa 91, 301
hidrocystoma, apocrine, carbon dioxide laser treatment of 293
histiocytoma, malignant fibrous 192, 204–8
HIV see human immunodeficiency virus
Hodgkin's disease, warts in 311
horrifying basaloma 93
human immunodeficiency virus (HIV) 41–5
  as contraindication to phenol chemical peel 505
  and the laser plume 319
  risk of developing cutaneous malignant melanoma 178
Hutchinson's sign 228, 232
hyaluronic acid 85, 387
hyaluronic acid verum cream 85
hydrochlorofluorocarbons (HCFCs) 57
hydrocystoma 90, 287
hydrofluorocarbons (HFCs) 57
hydroxyzine 24–5, 88
hyperhidrosis 466
  axillary, tumescent local anesthesia in 10
hyperkeratosis 221
hyperpigmentation 516
  following phenol chemical peel 500
  postinflammatory 470
hyperplasia, focal epithelial 309, 310
hyperthyroidism as contraindication to sedation 14
hypertonic saline 434–5
hypertrophic scars 516
hypopigmentation 516
hypothyroidism as contraindication to sedation 14
hypoxia following sedation 26

immunostains **132–3**
infantile digital fibromatosis 223–4
inflammatory malignant fibrohistiocytoma 206
inhalation anesthetics 14
inhalation sedatives 22–3

interferon
  adverse effects **170**, 171
  alpha-interferon 67, 165
  beta-interferon 165
  gamma-interferon 49, 165
  intralesional interferon α2β 82
  for skin cancer 165–75
  in treatment of warts 313
  in treatment of actinic keratoses 173
  interferon α2β, intralesional 82
interleukin 47
interleukin 1 (IL-1) 47
involucrin 274
iontophoresis 6–7
isoniazid 16
isotretinoin 81, 82, 375
  chemical peels and 380–1
  dermabrasion and 376–80, 393
  keloids following 516
  treatment and prevention of basal cell
      carcinoma 155–62
    chemoprophylaxis 156–7
    chemotherapy 156
    multicenter trial 159–60
    pilot study 156–7
    toxicities 157

Jossalind cream 87
juvenile digital fibromatosis 223–4

Kaposi's sarcoma
  AIDS and 63–4
  interferon in treatment of 174–5
  photodynamic therapy in 351
keloid scars
  following dermabrasion 511, 516
  Nd:YAG laser in treatment of 370–1
  retinoids in treatment of 375–6
  shave excision and cryosurgery for 85, *86–7*
  silastic gel sheeting and 391
keratoacanthoma 137, 220
  multiple (Ferguson–Smith) 160
  papillomavirus and 312
  solitary large 160
keratoses
  acantholytic solar 78
  actinic *see* actinic keratoses
  atrophic 76
  flat seborrheic 75
  lichenoid 77–8
  seborrheic 90, 287, 511
  solar *see* actinic keratoses
Ki-67 137
Klebsiella pneumoniae 38
Klein minicannula 464
Klein needle 8, 9, 462
Koebner phenomenon 308
Koenen's tumor 223
KTP-YAG lasers (KTP) 328, 334–5

L-dopa 118
laser abrasions 509
laser plume 319–20
lasers
  carbon dioxide *see* carbon dioxide laser therapy;
      superpulsed carbon dioxide lasers;
      low-fluence carbon dioxide lasers
  continuous-wave 335–7, 338–9
  copper vapor 328, *332*, 333–4
  energy density 329
  general thermal principles 325–6
  iontophoresis and 6
  key principles and terms 325–30
  KTP 328, 334–5
  laser–skin interaction 325
  laser–tissue interaction 281–3
  Nd:YAG *see* Nd:YAG lasers
  pulsed dye *see* pulsed dye lasers
  Q-switched KTP-YAG (Q-KTP) 335
  Q-switched Nd:YAG 277
  Q-switched ruby lasers *see* Q-switched ruby
      lasers
  Q-switched YAG-KDP 329
  quasi-continuous-wave 328
  superficial vascular, selection of 337–9
  superpulsed carbon dioxide *see* superpulsed
      carbon dioxide lasers
  systems comparison 330–7
  terminology 279–81, 325
    duty cycle 281
    energy 280
    fluence 280–1
    power 280
    power density 280
    pulse 281, 328–9
    selectivity, tissue exposure time and energy
        density 328–9
    spot size 280, 329–30
    thermal relaxation time 281
    wavelength and depth 326–7
  tunable-dye (argon-dye) 330–3
  yellow light and 532 NM 323–39
Laugier–Hunziker–Baran's syndrome 229
laurocapram azone 352
leishmaniasis
  carbon dioxide laser treatment of 296–7
  cryosurgery treatment 65, 66
  cutaneous 61
lentigines
  cryosurgery of 275–6
  laser treatment of 271–5, 297, 364
  senile 75
lentigo maligna 75, 90, 484
lentigo maligna melanoma
  interferon in 173, **174**
  Mohs surgery for 257, *259*
lentigo senilis 483
lentigo simplex 470, *472*, 483
lentigos, carbon dioxide laser treatment of 287
leukemia, chronic lymphocytic, warts in 311

INDEX

leukonychia, circumscribed 220
leukoplakia
   genital, Nd:YAG laser in treatment of 371
   oral 160
levodopa 178
lichen planus 77
lichen sclerosis et atrophicus, vaginal, carbon
     dioxide laser treatment of 301, *302*, 303
lichenoid keratosis 77–8
lidocaine 3, 4–5, 461
   30% in acid mantle cream 5
   contact sensitivity to 6
   dosage 7, 8
   for Mohs micrographic surgery 4–5
light reflection rheography 431
linear porokeratosis, carbon dioxide laser
     treatment of 298–9
lipectomy, suction-assisted *see* liposuction
lipomas, removal of, tumescent local anesthesia in
     10
liposuction 461–7
   adjuvant cryoanesthesia for 4
   cannula design 463–4
   controversy in postoperative care 465–6
   hyperhidrosis and hidradenitis 466
   liposculpture 464–5
   local anesthesia in 3, 461–3
   results 467
   tumescent local anesthesia in 8, 9, 10
local anesthesia 3–10
   dry technique 7, 9
   hair replacement under 527–41
   in liposuction 461–3
   tumescent 7–10
   wet technique 7
low-fluence carbon dioxide lasers 271–7
   controlled comparative trials with other lasers
      and nonlasers 275–7
   of lentigines 271–5
     clinical studies 271–2
     histological study 272–3
     immunohistochemical study 273–5
lupus erythematosus, discoid, scarring
   dermabrasion 511
   microlipoinjection of 455
lupus erythematosus-like keratosis (lupoid AK)
   75
lymphangioma, carbon dioxide laser treatment of
     287
lymphangioma circumscripta
   carbon dioxide laser treatment of 298
   cryosurgery of 91
lymphoma, cutaneous T cell 160

macrophages 49
malignant dyskeratosis 77
malignant eccrine poroma 160
malignant fibrohistiocytoma 201, 206
malignant melanoma of the nail 232
masoprocol 82

melanocytic nevi 91
melanoma
   acrolentiginous 232
   amelanotic 224
   cutaneous 56, 57
   cutaneous malignant (CMM) 88–9, 177–8
   excision of 235–8
   excisional biopsy 237
   immunohistochemical diagnosis 136–7
   incisional biopsy 237–8
   interferon in treatment of 173–4
   malignant 160, 173–4, 235–8
   Mohs surgery for 251–61
   of the nail, malignant 232
   nodular 256
   with nonmelanoma skin cancers, risk of
     developing another 178–9
   periorbital, Mohs surgery for 258–61
   review of literature 235–7
   superficial spreading 232, 256–7
   thin *see* thin melanoma
   tumor thickness, surgical approach 237
   ultrasound use in measuring depth 89–90
   wide excision 237
melanonychia, longitudinal, of the nail 228–32
   biopsy methods 229–32
     bands (3–6 mm in width) 230–1
     bands (wider than 6 mm in width) 231–2
     lateral third of the nail plate involved 229
     midportion of the nail plate involved 229
     periungual pigmentation present 229
     thin band (> 3 mm in width) 229–30
melasma, dermabrasion 511
meperidine 19–20, 488, 494
meperidinic acid 20
6-mercaptopurine 118
Merkel cell carcinoma 106
metalloproteinases 182
metastasis
   basic mechanisms and applications in
     dermatology 181–8
   clinical patterns 186–8
   of the nail 227–8
   steps of 182–6
metastatic basal cell carcinoma 109–19
   AIDS and 109, 117
   age of onset of primary tumor 111
   criteria for diagnosis 109
   gender 112–13
   hematologenous versus lymphatic spread 117
   histology 114–16
   history of radiation therapy as a risk factor 117
   immune deficiency states as possible risk factor
     117–18
   incidence 109–11
   interval from onset of primary tumor to
     metastasis 109–12
   location of primary tumor 113
   metastatic potential 119
   multiple primary tumors 113

metastatic basal cell carcinoma (contd)
  skin color 113
  small primary tumors 113–14
  survival 114
  timing of repairs for large Mohs surgery defects 116–17
  treatment 118–19
  work-up for suspected 119
metastatic potential 119, 181
metastatic squamous cell carcinoma 109–19
methadone 118
methotrexate 118
methoxsalen 271
methoxyflurane (MOF) 22–3
8-methoxypsoralen 347
methyl sulfone 81
microlipoinjection 441, 451–9
  cosmetic problems **453**
  donor sites for autologous fat transplantation **453**
  long-term follow-up 452–8
  recipient sites of autologous fat transplants **453**
  technique 451–2
midazolam 15, 17–18, 488
minicannula, Klein 464
minimal sclerosant concentration (MSC) 431–2
minoxidil 533
mithramycin 118
mitral valve prolapse (MVP) 31–3
Mohs micrographic surgery (MMS) 102, 105, 112, 115
  in dermatofibrosarcoma protuberans 195–8
  effect of type of melanoma on width of margins 255–7
  European experience of 125–8
  fixed-tissue technique (MMS-fixed) 252
  fresh-tissue technique (MMS-fresh) 252, 257–8
  in Germany 125
  important technical details 252–4
  lessons learned from some melanoma cases 254–5
  for melanoma 251–61
  naming of the method 251–2
  periorbital melanoma 258–61
  in Portugal 125–6
  results 261
  for sebaceous carcinoma of the eyelid 214
  in Spain 126
  timing of repairs for large defects of metastatic basal cell carcinoma 116–17
  in the UK 126–7
  wound 36, 50, 52, 93, 94, 96, 97
molluscum, use of EMLA as anesthesia in 5
molluscum contagiosum 61, 63
  treatment by cryosurgery 64
monoamine oxidase inhibitor use as contraindication to sedation 14
morphine-like drugs 18–19
Muir–Torre syndrome 211
mycobacteria, atypical, carbon dioxide laser treatment of 297

Mycobacterium marinum 297
mycosis fungoides 160
myxoid cyst, carbon dioxide laser treatment of 294
myxoid malignant fibrohistiocytoma 206
myxoid pseudocysts of the digits 226–7

nail dystrophy 220
naloxone 18, 21–2
naphthalocynanne 349
narcotics 14
Nd:YAG lasers 335, 357, 362–5, 369–71
  capillary and cavernous hemangiomas and AV malformations 370
  condyloma 371
  indications and uses in dermatology 369–70
  keloid scars 370–1
  malignant and premalignant skin tumors 371
  treatment of benign pigmentation 363–5
    mechanism of action 363–4
    results 364–5
    treatment techniques 364
  treatment of tattoos 363
neoplasms in the nail 219–32
neurofibromas, laserbrasions of 509
neurofibromatosis, carbon dioxide laser treatment of 287, 300–1
neutrophils 49
nevi
  epidermal
    carbon dioxide laser treatment of 287, 293
    dermabrasion 511
    laserbrasions 509
  giant pigmented 178
  local anaesthesia during 3
  melanocytic 91
  verrucous epidermal 91
nevoid basal cell carcinoma syndrome 160, 161
nevus angiomatosus, dermabrasion of 511
nitrogen mustard 118
nitrous oxide–oxygen sedation 21, 23–4
nonmelanoma skin cancer 80
  risk of developing another 178
  surgical margins 139–43
nordiazepam 16
norfloxacin 38
normeperidine 20
normeperidinic acid 20

obesity
  as contraindication to methoxyflurane use 23
  as contraindication to sedation 14
ochronosis, carbon dioxide laser treatment of 297–8
ofloxacin 38
onychomycosis 220
Op-site 509
opioids 15, 18–22
oral contraceptives 16
ornipressin 415
osteochondroma of the nail 225

osteoid osteoma of the nail 225–6
otoscope cone 63
oxazepam 16
oxymorphone 21
ozone crisis 55–6

papillomas
　conjunctival 309, 310
　nasal 309, 310
papillomatosis
　laryngeal 309, 310
　oral florid 309
　vulvar 310
papillomavirus 79, 307–13
　cancer and 311–12
　clinical manifestations 309–10
　detection of 311
　epidemiology and natural history of infection 308–9
　in immunosuppressed patients 310–11
　laser treatment of 312, 319
　therapy 312–13
　types and their clinical associations **308**
　virology 307
　see also warts
papulosis, Bowenoid 309, 310
　carbon dioxide laser treatment of 287
　Nd:YAG laser in treatment of 371
paradoxical fibrosarcoma 202
parahormone 118
PDGF-like peptides 49
pearly penile papules, carbon dioxide laser treatment of 294
penicillin 36
peptides 47
perifolliculitis capitis abscedens et suffodiens, carbon dioxide laser treatment of 297
periorbital melanoma, Mohs surgery for 258–61
Perthe's test 429
phenol chemical peeling 479–505
phenothiazines 19
Phialophora verrucosa 65
photochemotherapy 347
photodynamic therapy for skin cancer 347–53
　advantages 352
　clinical applications in cutaneous malignancy 350–2
　disadvantages 352
　future 352
　history 347–8
　light 349–50
　photodynamic effects 348
　photosensitizers 348–9
photofrin 349
photoplethysmography 431
photoradiation therapy 347
photothermolysis, selective 358
physostigmine 17
pigmentation disorders, carbon dioxide laser treatment of 293

pigmented actinic keratosis (spreading pigmented AK) 75
pigmented nevi, giant 178
pitted acne scarring, carbon dioxide laser treatment of 295
pityriasis rubra pilaris, isotretinoin in treatment of 375
plasminogen activator 182
platelet-derived growth factor (PDGF) 48, 49, 51, 52
podophyllin therapy
　in condyloma acuminata 67
　in warts 312, 313
podophyllotoxin
　treatment of condyloma acuminata 67
　treatment of warts 312–13
Podophyllum peltatus 312–13
polidocanol 434
polyiodide iodide 435
polypeptides 47
porokeratosis, linear, carbon dioxide laser treatment of 298–9
porokeratosis of Mibelli 160, 298
portwine stains
　body image 341
　clinical experiences of patients 343–4
　laser treatment 298, 324
　in the newborn, treatment 345
　psychological disability and 344–5
　pulsed dye laser treatment of 7
　use of EMLA as anesthesia in 5
prednisone 118
pregnancy
　accelerated growth of malignant fibrohistiocytoma in 204
　as contraindication to sedation 14
　as contraindication to use of nitrous oxide 24
　detection of early cutaneous melanoma in 246–7
pressure-induced wounds 50
prilocaine, contact sensitivity to 6
Propionibacterium acnes 33
propofol (2,3-diisopropylphenol) 25
proto-oncogenes 49
pseudocysts, myxoids, of the digits 226–7
Pseudomonas aeruginosa 37, 38
pseudopyogenic granuloma 224
pseudorhagades, perioral, dermabrasion of 511
pseudosarcoma of the skin 202
pseudosarcomatous dermatofibroma 202
psoriasis 220
　isotretinoin in treatment of 375
　photodynamic therapy for 347
psychoneurosis as contraindication to dermabrasion 516
psychosis as contraindication to dermabrasion 516
pulse oximeter 26
pulsed dye lasers 277
　use of EMLA as anesthesia in 5
　treatment of port-wine stains 7
purpurins 349

pyoderma as contraindication to dermabrasion 516
pyogenic granuloma of the nail 224

Q-switched ruby lasers 277, 357, 358–62
   treatment of benign pigmented lesions 361–2
      mechanism of action 361
      results 362
      treatment techniques 361
   treatment of tattoos 358–61
      mechanism of action 358
      results 360–1
      treatment techniques 359–60
quinoline antibiotics 37

radiation therapy
   for sebaceous carcinoma of the eyelid 215–16
radiodermatitis 220–1
   as contraindication to dermabrasion 516
reconstruction, tumescent local anesthesia in 10
recurring digital fibrous tumors of childhood 223–4
renal hamartomas 223
Rendu–Osler–Weber disease 33
Retin-A 514
retinoids 81
   dermabrasion, chemical peel and keloids 375–81
   in treatment of warts 313
rhinophyma
   carbon dioxide laser treatment of 287, 293
   dermabrasion 511
   laserbrasions 509
rhodamines 349
Ro14-9706 81

salicylic acid in treatment of warts 312
scalp reduction, tumescent local anesthesia in 10
scar revision, traditional approach to 385–6
scarabrasion
   controlled study 386–7
   full-thickness grafts and flaps 390–1
   and isotretinoin (Accutane) 393
   mechanism of action 387
   punch grafts for icepick scars 388–9
   silastic gel sheeting and scar revision 391–2
   skin necrosis after injection of Zyplast collagen 392–3
   of traumatic scars 388
   varicella scars 389–90
sclerodex 435
sclerotherapy 425–37
   postsclerosis compression 436–7
   presclerotherapy evaluation 426–31
      noninvasive diagnostic technique 429–31
      physical examination 427–9
      sclerosing solutions 431–3
         chemical irritants 435–6
         detergent solutions 433–4
         osmotic solutions 434–5
scopolamine 16

sebaceous carcinoma of the eyelid 211–16
   conclusions and controversies 216
   etiologic considerations 213–14
   histopathology 212–13
   incidence and risks 211–12
   treatment strategies 214–16
seborrheic keratosis 90, 287, 511
sedation 13–27
   definition 13
   intravenous, contraindications 14
   suggestions, standards, precautions and monitoring 25–7
sedative hypnotics 14, 15–18
selective photothermolysis 358
Sezary syndrome 160
shaking chills 4
shave biopsy, iontophoresis in 6
silicone implantation 441, 448–9
skin cancer 36
   immunohistochemical diagnosis 131–7
   interferon for 165–75
   malignant and premalignant, Nd:YAG laser in treatment of 371
   mitotic index of 137
   risk of developing another 177–9
   sun, ozone depletion and 55–8
   ultraviolet radiation and 56–7
   ultrasound use in measuring depth 89–90
   see also carcinoma
skin grafts see flaps and grafts
skin lesions, cautery of, use of EMLA as anesthesia in 5
sodium morrhuate 433–4
sodium stibogluconate (Pentostam) 65
sodium tetradecyl sulfate 434
soft tissue augmentation 441–9
solar cheilitis 75–6
solar keratoses see actinic keratoses
spider angiomas 330
spot dermabrasion 386
spray tips 61, 62
spreading pigmented actinic keratosis 75
squamous cell carcinoma (SCC)
   cryosurgery and 90
   cutaneous horn in 74
   flaps 414, 415
   interferon in treatment of 172–3
   metastatic 109–19
   metastatic potential 181
   Mohs surgery in 195
   in the nail 221–2
   Nd:YAG laser in treatment of 371
   papillomavirus and 311, 312
   photodynamic therapy in 350–1
   relation to actinic keratoses 73
   risk of developing another 178
   surgical margins 139–41, 142
   treatment 160
   UV light and 56, 57
squaric acid dibutyl ester in treatment of warts 313

INDEX

Staphylococcus aureus 33, 38, 158, 296, 504
Staphylococcus epidermidis 33
storiform–pleomorphic malignant
    fibrohistiocytoma 205
Streptococcus pyogenes 38
Streptococcus viridans 33
Styrofoam cup 61
subungual melanocytic lesions of the nail 228–32
sufentanyl 21
superficial basal cell carcinoma, carbon dioxide
    laser treatment of 287
superficial spreading melanoma (SSM) 232, 256–7
superpulsed carbon dioxide lasers 283–9
    clinical applications 285–9
        incision 287–9
        vaporization 285–7
sweat glands vs basal cell carcinoma,
    immunohistochemical diagnosis 134
Synamap 26
synovioma, benign *see* giant cell tumor of the
    nail
syringes, spring-loaded 8, 9
syringoma
    carbon dioxide laser treatment of 287, 294
    dermabrasion 511
    laserbrasions 509

T cell lymphoma, cutaneous 160
tattoo removal
    with carbon dioxide laser 288
    dermabrasion 379, 511
    laserbrasions 509
    Nd:YAG laser 363
    trichloroacetic acid peels 380
tattooing on the scalp 545, *546*
telangiectasia
    cauterization, iontophoresis in 6
    cauterization, local anesthesia during 3
    compression of 436–7
    hereditary hemorrhagic 33
    phenol chemical peel in 484
    sclerotherapy and 436–7
tetracyclines 37
TGF-alpha 50
TGF-beta 49, 51
thin melanoma
    biopsy technique 243–4
    clinical evaluation 244–5
    clinical features 242
    definition 241–2
    follow-up of patients 245–6
    histological evaluation 244
    histological features 242
    initial surgical therapy 245
    management of 241–7
    metastasis and death from 263–8
    methods to maximize early detection 246–7
        advances in diagnostic techniques 247
        early screening 246
        and pregnancy 246–7

surveillance 265–8
    adequate psychosocial support 267–8
    histology 266
    progressive symptoms or rapidly accelerating
        disease 266–7
thiopental 25
tissue lensing 329
TNF-alpha 49
TNKH-1 134, **135**, 137
topical anesthesia
    agents 3–5
    use of 7
Toradol 88
transplantation, organ, cutaneous malignant
    melanoma in 178
tretinoin 81, 88, 376, 470
triamcinolone 85, 516
triamcinolone diacetate 502
trichloroacetic acid 503
    facial chemical peel 469–77
    in treatment of warts 312
trichoepitheliomas
    carbon dioxide laser treatment of 287
    laserbrasions 509
tricyclic antidepressant 14, 18, 20
triphenylmethanes 349
tumescent local anesthesia 3
    advantages 9–10
    formula **8**
    methods of delivery 8–9
    other uses 10
    regional requirements **8**
    technique 8
tumors
    adnexal, carbon dioxide laser treatment of 293
    Bednar 192
    carbon dioxide laser therapy 293–4, 298
    fibrohistiocytic 201
    fibromous, of the nail 222–4
    Koenen's 223

ulcers
    leg, epidermal autografts in 396
    venous 50
    wound healing 52
ulcus terebrans 93
ultrasound, use in dermatology 89–90
ultraviolet radiation and skin cancer 56–7

varicella scars 389–90
varicose veins, sclerotherapy and 436, **437**
vascular hamartoma 90
venous lakes, Nd:YAG laser in treatment of 370
verdins 349
verruca plana (flat warts) 309
    contraindication to dermabrasion 516
    plana, treatment by cryosurgery 66
verruca vulgaris (common warts) 61, 309, 310
    carbon dioxide laser treatment of 287, 293
    treatment by cryosurgery 65, 66

verrucae *see* warts
verrucous carcinoma, papillomavirus and 311
verrucous epidermal nevi 91
Vigilon 509–10
villonodular pigmented synovitis *see* giant cell tumor of the nail
vulvodynia 310

warts
  in AIDS 311
  anogenital 309, 310
  Butcher's 309
  cervical 309
  common 61, 65, 66, 309, 310
  filiform 65, 66, 309
  flat 65, 66, 309, 516
  keratotic palmar 65, 66
  myrmecia 310
  periungual 65, 66
  plantar 65, 66, 309, 310
  subungual 219–20
  treatment by cryosurgery 63, 65–7
  tumorigenesis in 181
  viral, in transplant patients 80
  see also papillomavirus
wounds
  acute and chronic 50
  and growth factors 47–52
    acute and chronic wounds 50
    animal studies 50–1
    human wounds 51–2
    mechanism of action 48–9
    nomenclature 47–8

presence in wounds 49–50
TGF-beta and scarring 51
healing after cryosurgery 85–7
pressure-induced 50
ulcers 52
wrinkling 52

xanthelasma, carbon dioxide laser treatment of 287
xanthoma, atypical fibrous 202–4
xanthomatous giant cell tumors *see* giant cell tumor of the nail
xeroderma pigmentosum 74
  contraindication to dermabrasion 516
  isotretinoin treatment in 81
  risk of developing cutaneous malignant melanoma 178
  treatment and prevention with oral isotretinoin 155, 157–9, 160, 161
  UV light and 57

zidovudine 175
Zyderm 441–6
  adverse reactions 445–6
  history and development 441–2
  indications, contraindications and skin testing 442–3
  injection technique and results 443–4
Zyplast 441–6
  adverse reactions 445–6
  history and development 441–2
  indications, contraindications and skin testing 442–3
  injection technique and results 443–4
  skin necrosis after injection of 392–3